PN Adult Medical Surgical Nursing
REVIEW MODULE EDITION 10.0

P9-DFM-896

Consultants

Tracey Bousquet, BSN, RN

Candy L. Madera, MSN, RN

Christi Blair, MSN, RN

Deb Johnson-Schuh, RN, MSN, CNE

LaKeisha Wheless, MSN, RN

Lisa Bass, MSN, RN, CRNI, CNE

Margaret Hendrix, MSN, RN, CNOR

Maureen D. Abraham, RNC, MSN, CNE

Pam DeMoss, MSN, RN

Margaret Hendrix, MSN, RN, CNOR

Maureen D. Abraham, RNC, MSN, CNE

Pam DeMoss, MSN, RN

Ronda Points, RN, MSN/Ed

Virginia Tufano, EdD, MSN, RN

Contributors

Norma Jean E. Henry, MSN/Ed, RN

Honey C. Holman, MSN, RN

Brenda S. Ball, MEd, BSN, RN

Debborah Williams, MSN, RN

Kellie Wilford, MSN, RN

Marsha S. Barlow, MSN, RN

Mary Jane Janowski, RN, MA

Peggy L. Leehy, MSN, RN

Robin A. Hertel, EdS, MSN, RN, CMSRN

Terri Lemon, DNP, MSN, RN

Director of content review: Kristen Lawler

Director of development: Derek Prater

Project management: Nicole Burke

Coordination of content review: Norma Jean E. Henry, Honey C. Holman

Copy editing: Kelly Von Lunen, Bethany Phillips

Layout: Spring Lenox, Randi Hardy, Charves Hervey, Rachel Cohen

Illustrations: Randi Hardy

Online media: Morgan Smith, Ron Hanson, Nicole Lobdell, Brant Stacy

Cover design: Jason Buck

Interior book design: Spring Lenox

IMPORTANT NOTICE TO THE READER

User's Guide

Welcome to the Assessment Technologies Institute® PN Adult Medical Surgical Nursing Review Module Edition 10.0. The mission of ATI's Content Mastery Series® Review Modules is to provide user-friendly compendiums of nursing knowledge that will:

- Help you locate important information quickly.
- Assist in your learning efforts.
- Provide exercises for applying your nursing knowledge.
- Facilitate your entry into the nursing profession as a newly licensed nurse.

This newest edition of the Review Modules has been redesigned to optimize your learning experience. We've fit more content into less space and have done so in a way that will make it even easier for you to find and understand the information you need.

ORGANIZATION

This Review Module is organized into units covering the foundations of nursing care (Unit 1), body systems and physiological processes (Units 2 to 13), and perioperative nursing care (Unit 14). Chapters within these units conform to one of three organizing principles for presenting the content.

- Nursing concepts
- Procedures
- System disorders

Nursing concepts chapters begin with an overview describing the central concept and its relevance to nursing. Subordinate themes are covered in outline form to demonstrate relationships and present the information in a clear, succinct manner.

Procedures chapters include an overview describing the procedure(s) covered in the chapter. These chapters provide nursing knowledge relevant to each procedure, including indications, nursing considerations, interpretation of findings, and complications.

System disorders chapters include an overview describing the disorder(s) and/or disease process. These chapters address assessments, including risk factors, expected findings, laboratory tests, and diagnostic procedures. Next, you will focus on patient-centered care, including nursing care, medications, therapeutic procedures, interprofessional care, and client education. Finally, you will find complications related to the disorder, along with nursing actions in response to those complications.

ACTIVE LEARNING SCENARIOS AND APPLICATION EXERCISES

Each chapter includes opportunities for you to test your knowledge and to practice applying that knowledge. Active Learning Scenario exercises pose a nursing scenario and then direct you to use an ATI Active Learning Template (included at the back of this book) to record the important knowledge a nurse should apply to the scenario. An example is then provided to which you can compare your completed Active Learning Template. The Application Exercises include NCLEX-style questions, such as multiple-choice and multiple-select items, providing you with opportunities to practice answering the kinds of questions you might expect to see on ATI assessments or the NCLEX. After the Application Exercises, an answer key is provided, along with rationales.

NCLEX® CONNECTIONS

To prepare for the NCLEX-PN, it is important to understand how the content in this Review Module is connected to the NCLEX-PN test plan. You can find information on the detailed test plan at the National Council of State Boards of Nursing's website, www.ncsbn.org. When reviewing content in this Review Module, regularly ask yourself, "How does this content fit into the test plan, and what types of questions related to this content should I expect?"

To help you in this process, we've included NCLEX Connections at the beginning of each unit and with each question in the Application Exercises Answer Keys. The NCLEX Connections at the beginning of each unit point out areas of the detailed test plan that relate to the content within that unit. The NCLEX Connections attached to the Application Exercises Answer Keys demonstrate how each exercise fits within the detailed content outline. These NCLEX Connections will help you understand how the detailed content outline is organized, starting with major client needs categories and subcategories and followed by related content areas and tasks. The major client needs categories are:

- Safe and Effective Care Environment
  - Management of Care
  - Safety and Infection Control
- Health Promotion and Maintenance
- Psychosocial Integrity
- Physiological Integrity
  - Basic Care and Comfort
  - Pharmacological and Parenteral Therapies
  - Reduction of Risk Potential
  - Physiological Adaptation

An NCLEX Connection might, for example, alert you that content within a unit is related to:

- Reduction of Risk Potential
  - Diagnostic Tests
    - Monitor the results of diagnostic testing and intervene as needed.

QSEN COMPETENCIES

As you use the Review Modules, you will note the integration of the Quality and Safety Education for Nurses (QSEN) competencies throughout the chapters. These competencies are integral components of the curriculum of many nursing programs in the United States and prepare you to provide safe, high-quality care as a newly licensed nurse. Icons appear to draw your attention to the six QSEN competencies.

Safety: The minimization of risk factors that could cause injury or harm while promoting quality care and maintaining a secure environment for clients, self, and others.

Patient-Centered Care: The provision of caring and compassionate, culturally sensitive care that addresses clients' physiological, psychological, sociological, spiritual, and cultural needs, preferences, and values.

Evidence-Based Practice: The use of current knowledge from research and other credible sources, on which to base clinical judgment and client care.

Informatics: The use of information technology as a communication and information-gathering tool that supports clinical decision-making and scientifically based nursing practice.

Quality Improvement: Care related and organizational processes that involve the development and implementation of a plan to improve health care services and better meet clients' needs.

Teamwork and Collaboration: The delivery of client care in partnership with multidisciplinary members of the health care team to achieve continuity of care and positive client outcomes.

ICONS

Icons are used throughout the Review Module to draw your attention to particular areas. Keep an eye out for these icons.

(N) This icon is used for NCLEX Connections.

(G) This icon indicates gerontological considerations, or knowledge specific to the care of older adult clients.

Qs This icon is used for content related to safety and is a QSEN competency. When you see this icon, take note of safety concerns or steps that nurses can take to ensure client safety and a safe environment.

QPCC This icon is a QSEN competency that indicates the importance of a holistic approach to providing care.

QEBP This icon, a QSEN competency, points out the integration of research into clinical practice.

QI This icon is a QSEN competency and highlights the use of information technology to support nursing practice.

QQI This icon is used to focus on the QSEN competency of integrating planning processes to meet clients' needs.

QTC This icon highlights the QSEN competency of care delivery using an interprofessional approach.

 This icon appears at the top-right of pages and indicates availability of an online media supplement, such as a graphic, animation, or video. If you have an electronic copy of the Review Module, this icon will appear alongside clickable links to media supplements. If you have a hard copy version of the Review Module, visit www.atitesting.com for details on how to access these features.

FEEDBACK

ATI welcomes feedback regarding this Review Module. Please provide comments to comments@atitesting.com.

Table of Contents

UNIT 5   Nursing Care of Clients Who Have Hematologic Disorders

UNIT 6   Nursing Care of Clients Who Have Fluid/Electrolyte/Acid-Base Imbalances

When reviewing the following chapters, keep in mind the relevant topics and tasks of the NCLEX outline, in particular:

Health Promotion and Maintenance

HEALTH PROMOTION/DISEASE PREVENTION
Monitor the client's actions to maintain health and prevent disease (smoking cessation, exercise, diet, stress management).

Monitor incorporation of healthy behaviors into lifestyle by the client (screening examinations, immunizations, limiting risk-taking behaviors).

Physiological Adaptation

ALTERATIONS IN BODY SYSTEMS: Reinforce education to the client regarding care and condition.

FLUID AND ELECTROLYTE IMBALANCES: Provide interventions to restore the client's fluid and/or electrolyte balance.

MEDICAL EMERGENCIES: Review and document the client's response to emergency interventions (restoration of breathing, pulse).

CHAPTER 1

CHAPTER 1 *Health, Wellness, and Illness*

Health and wellness combine to form a state of optimal physical functioning and a feeling of emotional and social contentment. Wellness involves the ability to adapt emotionally and physically to a changing state of health and environment.

Illness is an altered level of functioning in response to a disease process. Disease is a condition that results in the physiological alteration in the composition of the body.

Nurses must understand the variables affecting health, wellness, and illness, and how they relate to clients' individual perceptions of health needs.

Health and wellness

The level of health and wellness is unique to each individual and relative to the individual's usual state of functioning. For example, a person who has rheumatoid arthritis, a strong support system, and positive outlook might consider himself healthy while functioning at an optimal level with minimal pain.

VARIABLES Qpcc
- **Modifiable:** Can be changed (smoking, nutrition, access to health education, sexual practices, exercise)
- **Nonmodifiable:** Cannot be changed (sex, age, developmental level, genetic traits)

ASPECTS OF HEALTH AND WELLNESS

- **Physical:** Performs activities of daily living
- **Emotional:** Adapts to stress; expresses and identifies emotions
- **Social:** Interacts successfully with others
- **Intellectual:** Effectively learns and disseminates information
- **Spiritual:** Adopts a belief that provides meaning to life
- **Occupational:** Balances occupational activities with leisure time
- **Environmental:** Creates measures to improve standards of living and quality of life

ENVIRONMENT

- A client's state of health and wellness is constantly changing and adapting to a continually fluctuating external and internal environment.
- THE EXTERNAL ENVIRONMENT
  - **Social:** Crime vs. safety, poverty vs. prosperity, peace vs. social unrest, and presence vs. absence of support from social networks
  - **Physical:** Access to health care, sanitation, availability of clean water, and geographic location
- THE INTERNAL ENVIRONMENT includes cumulative life experiences, cultural and spiritual beliefs, age, developmental stage, gender, emotional factors, and perception of physical functioning.

DESIRED OUTCOMES

- Desired outcomes are to obtain and maintain optimal state of wellness and function through access to and use of health promotion, wellness, and illness-prevention strategies.
- Health education and positive action (stress management, smoking cessation, weight loss, immunizations, seeking health care) promote health and wellness.

ILLNESS-WELLNESS CONTINUUM

The Illness-Wellness Continuum is a tool used to measure the level of wellness to premature death.
- Use the Illness-Wellness Continuum as a guide or tool to set goals and find ways to improve a client's state of health or to have the client return to a previous state of health. The health care professional can assist the client to see where he is on the continuum and seek ways to move toward optimal wellness.
- At the center of the continuum is the client's normal state of health.
- The range of wellness to illness runs from optimal wellness to severe illness.
- The degree of wellness is relative to the usual state of wellness for a client and is achieved through awareness, education, and personal growth.

Illness

- Illness is the impairment of a client's physical, social, emotional, spiritual, developmental, or intellectual functioning.
- Illness encompasses the effects of a disease on a client. However, illness and disease are not synonymous.

Response to illness can be influenced by
- Degree of physical changes as a result of a disease process.
- Perceptions by self and others of the illness, which can be influenced by various reliable and unreliable sources of information (friends, magazines, TV, the Internet).
- Cultural values and beliefs.
- Denial or fear of illness.
- Social demands, time constraints, economic resources, and health care access.

HEALTH PROMOTION AND DISEASE PREVENTION

Use health education and awareness to reduce risk factors and promote health care.

HEALTH/WELLNESS DATA COLLECTION Qᴘᴄᴄ

- Physical data collection
- Evaluating health perceptions
- Identifying risks to health/wellness
- Identifying access to health care

Identifying obstacles to compliance and adherence
- Perceptions of illness: awareness of the severity of the illness
- Confidence in the provider
- Belief in the prescribed therapy
  - A client who has had a negative experience with the health care system might not trust the provider, follow the advice, or comply with the treatment prescribed.
  - Cultural or religious beliefs might not align with prescribed treatment.
- Availability of support systems
- Family role and function: One family member might be the family caregiver but neglect caring for herself.
- Financial restrictions that can lead to prioritized health care
  - Prescription medication costs
  - A parent might seek medical care for children but not for herself

NURSING CARE

Evaluate the health needs of a client, and create strategies to meet those needs. Qᴘᴄᴄ

INTERVENTIONS

- Provide resources to strengthen coping abilities. Qᴘᴄᴄ
- Identify and encourage use of support systems during times of illness and stress.
- Identify obstacles to health and wellness, and create strategies to reduce these obstacles.
- Identify ways to reduce health risks and improve compliance.
- Review health education materials to improve health awareness and reduce health risks.

Application Exercises

1. A nurse is caring for an older adult client who has a new diagnosis of type 2 diabetes mellitus and reports difficulty following the diet and remembering to take the prescribed medication. Which of the following actions should the nurse take to promote client adherence to the treatment plan? (Select all that apply.)

   A. Ask the dietitian to assist with meal planning.

   B. Contact the client's support system.

   C. Tell the client he should follow the provider's instructions.

   D. Encourage the use of a daily medication dispenser.

   E. Provide educational materials for home use.

2. A nurse in a health care clinic is evaluating the level of wellness for clients using the Illness-Wellness Continuum tool. The nurse should identify which of the following clients as being at the center of the continuum?

   A. A college student who has influenza

   B. An older adult who has a new diagnosis of type 2 diabetes mellitus

   C. A new mother who has a urinary tract infection

   D. A young male client who has a long history of well-controlled rheumatoid arthritis

3. A nurse is evaluating clients at a health fair for modifiable variables affecting health and wellness. The nurse should identify which of the following variables as modifiable? (Select all that apply.)

   A. Smoking on social occasions

   B. BMI of 28

   C. Alopecia

   D. Trisomy 21

   E. History of reflux

4. A nurse is caring for a client who was just told she has breast cancer. The nurse evaluates the client's response. Which of the following statements by the client reflects a negative response to the illness?

   A. "I have no family history of breast cancer."

   B. "I need a second opinion. There is no lump."

   C. "I am glad we live in the city near several large hospitals."

   D. "I will schedule surgery next week, over the holidays."

PRACTICE Active Learning Scenario

A nurse in a clinic is caring for a client who has a family history of cardiovascular disease and continues to smoke despite numerous attempts to quit. What nursing interventions should the nurse use to meet the health needs of this client? Use the ATI Active Learning Template: Basic Concept to complete this item.

RELATED CONTENT: Include one statement identifying the goal.

UNDERLYING PRINCIPLES: Include one statement regarding health promotion and disease prevention.

NURSING INTERVENTIONS: Include a minimum of four.

1. A. **CORRECT:** The nurse provides resources to strengthen coping abilities by asking the dietitian to assist the client with meal planning. This will improve client adherence.

    B. **CORRECT:** With the client's consent, the nurse can contact members of the client's support system and encourage the client to use this support during times of illness and stress to improve compliance.

    C. Telling the client he should follow the provider's instructions will not likely improve the client's adherence to the treatment plan. The nurse should determine why the client is not following the treatment plan.

    D. **CORRECT:** The nurse encourages the use of a daily medication dispenser to reduce health risks and improve medication adherence by the client.

    E. **CORRECT:** The nurse provides educational materials to the client to improve health awareness and reduce health risks after discharge.

    Ⓝ *NCLEX® Connection: Coordinated Care, Establishing Priorities*

2. A. The client who has influenza has deviated from the normal level of health for the client and would not be in the center of the continuum.

    B. The client who has a new diagnosis of type 2 diabetes has deviated from the normal level of health for the client and would not be in the center of the continuum.

    C. The client who has a urinary tract infection has deviated from the normal level of health for the client and would not be in the center of the continuum.

    D. **CORRECT:** The client who has well-controlled rheumatoid arthritis is measured at the center of the continuum, which is the client's normal state of health.

    Ⓝ *NCLEX® Connection: Health Promotion and Maintenance, Health Promotion/Disease Prevention*

3. A. **CORRECT:** The nurse identifies smoking as a modifiable variable that a client can change. The nurse should provide the client with educational materials and information on smoking cessation.

    B. **CORRECT:** The nurse identifies a BMI of 28 as a modifiable variable that a client can change. The nurse should provide the client with educational materials and information on weight reduction and exercising.

    C. The nurse identifies alopecia as a nonmodifiable variable, because alopecia is a genetic disorder.

    D. The nurse identifies trisomy 21 as a nonmodifiable variable because trisomy 21 is genetic in origin.

    E. **CORRECT:** The nurse identifies reflux as a modifiable variable that a client can change. The nurse should provide the client with step-by-step educational information about treatment.

    Ⓝ *NCLEX® Connection: Health Promotion and Maintenance, Health Promotion/Disease Prevention*

4. A. The client's lack of a family history of cancer can cause the client to wonder about the cause of the cancer, but this statement does not reflect a negative response to the illness.

    B. **CORRECT:** The nurse should identify this statement as an indication of denial, which is a negative response to illness. Other factors that can influence the response to illness include physical changes, self-perception, and cultural beliefs.

    C. The nurse should consider the client's recognition of access to health care resources as an indication the client will seek treatment, which is a positive response to the illness.

    D. The nurse should consider the client's readiness to schedule surgery as an indication the client will seek treatment, which is a positive response to the illness.

    Ⓝ *NCLEX® Connection: Psychosocial Integrity, Coping Mechanisms*

PRACTICE Answer

Using the ATI Active Learning Template: Basic Concept

RELATED CONTENT: Identify obstacles for compliance and adherence.

UNDERLYING PRINCIPLES: Many factors can influence health promotion and disease prevention that a nurse should address for client success.

NURSING INTERVENTIONS
- Provide the client with resources to strengthen coping abilities.
- Encourage use of support systems (family, support group).
- Identify ways to improve compliance.
- Develop health education methods to reduce health risks.
- Identify the client's obstacles to health and wellness.
- Create strategies to reduce the client's obstacles.

Ⓝ *NCLEX® Connection: Health Promotion and Maintenance, High Risk Behaviors*

CHAPTER 2

CHAPTER 2   *Emergency Nursing Principles and Management*

Emergency nursing principles are the guidelines that nurses follow to review and manage emergency situations for one or more clients.

Nurses must be able to identify emergent situations and rapidly check and intervene when life-threatening conditions exist. Emergent conditions are common to all nursing environments.

Emergency nursing principles include triage, primary survey, the ABCDE principle, poisoning, rapid response team, cardiac emergency, and postresuscitation. Q EBP

Emergency departments often implement the five-level system of triage: resuscitation (level one), emergent (level two), urgent (level three), less urgent (level four), and nonurgent (level five). Time and experience are required for the nurse to become an effective member of the triage team. The nurse, provider, and other members of the health care team work together in the triage area to determine the needs of the client.

Resuscitation triage requires immediate treatment to prevent death.

Nonurgent conditions are non-life-threatening conditions that require simple evaluation and care management.

PRIMARY SURVEY

- A primary survey is a rapid assessment of life-threatening conditions.
- The primary survey should be completed systematically so life-threatening conditions are not missed.
- Standard precautions—gloves, gowns, eye protection, face masks, and shoe covers—must be worn to prevent contamination with bodily fluids.
- The ABCDE principle guides the primary survey.

ABCDE PRINCIPLE

AIRWAY/CERVICAL SPINE

- This is the most important step in performing the primary survey. If a patent airway is not established, subsequent steps of the primary survey are futile. As a result of hypoxia, brain injury or death will occur within 3 to 5 min if the airway is not patent. Qs
- If a client is awake and responsive, the airway is open. Check for manifestations of airway occlusion (respiratory distress, stridor, inability to speak). Coarse or muffled speech can indicate a partial airway obstruction.
- If the client is unresponsive without suspicion of trauma, the airway should be opened with a head–tilt/chin–lift maneuver. Qs
  ○ Do NOT perform the head–tilt/chin–lift maneuver on clients who have a potential cervical spine injury.
  ○ To perform the head–tilt/chin–lift maneuver, the nurse should assume a position at the head of the client, place one hand on his forehead, and place the other hand underneath the client's chin. Tilt his head while lifting his chin upward and forward. This maneuver lifts the tongue away from the laryngopharynx and provides for a patent airway. Qs
- If the client is unresponsive with suspicion of trauma, the airway should be opened with a modified jaw thrust maneuver. The nurse should assume a position at the head of the client and place both hands on either side of the client's head. Locate the connection between the maxilla and the mandible. Lift the jaw superiorly while maintaining alignment of the cervical spine.
- After opening the airway, inspect it for blood, broken teeth, vomitus, and secretions. If present, clear any obstructions with suction or the finger–sweep method if the object is clearly visible.
- The open airway can be maintained with airway adjuncts, such as an oropharyngeal or nasopharyngeal airway.
- A bag valve mask with a 100% oxygen source is indicated for clients who need additional support during resuscitation until an advanced airway is established.
- A nonrebreather mask with 100% oxygen source is indicated for clients who are spontaneously breathing.

BREATHING

Once a patent airway is achieved, the nurse should check for the presence and effectiveness of breathing.

BREATHING DATA COLLECTION

- Auscultate breath sounds.
- Observe for chest expansion and respiratory effort.
- Note rate and depth of respirations.
- Look for indications of chest trauma.
- Determine tracheal position.
- Check for jugular vein distention.

If a client is not breathing or is breathing inadequately, provide manual ventilation by using a bag valve mask with supplemental oxygen (or mouth-to-mask ventilation until a bag valve mask can be obtained).

CIRCULATION

- Once adequate ventilation is accomplished, check the client's circulation.
- Check heart rate, blood pressure, peripheral pulses, and capillary refill for adequate perfusion.
- Nurses should consider cardiac arrest, myocardial dysfunction, and hemorrhage as precursors to shock and leading to ineffective circulation.

INTERVENTIONS

- **Restoring effective circulation**
  - CPR Qᴘᴄᴄ
  - Check for external bleeding.
  - Hemorrhage control—Apply direct pressure to visible, significant external bleeding.
  - Ensure IV access is obtained using large-bore IV catheters inserted into the antecubital fossa of both arms, unless there is obvious injury to the extremity.
  - Infuse isotonic IV fluids such as lactated Ringer's and 0.9% sodium chloride, and/or blood products.
- **Alleviating shock:** A compromise in circulation can lead to shock. Shock is the body's response to inadequate tissue perfusion and oxygenation. It manifests with an increased heart rate and hypotension and can cause tissue ischemia and necrosis. Qᴘᴄᴄ
  - Administer oxygen.
  - Apply pressure to obvious bleeding.
  - Elevate lower extremities to shunt blood to vital organs.
  - Administer IV fluids and blood products.
  - Monitor vital signs.
  - Remain with the client, and provide reassurance and support for anxiety.

DISABILITY

Disability involves a quick check to determine the client's level of consciousness.
- The AVPU mnemonic is useful. **(2.1)** Qᴱᴮᴾ
- The Glasgow Coma Scale is a widely used method. **(2.2)** Qᴱᴮᴾ
- Neurologic assessment must be repeated at frequent intervals to ensure immediate response to any change.

EXPOSURE

- The nurse removes the client's clothing for a complete physical assessment. The nurse might need to cut off the client's clothing to accomplish this task.
- Always remove clothing during a resuscitation situation to check for additional injuries or those related to chemical and thermal burns involving the clothing.
- Preserve items that could be considered evidence (clothing, bullets, drugs, weapons).
- Monitor for hypothermia. Hypothermia occurs when core temperature is 35 °C (95 °F) or less.
- Victims of trauma are at risk for hypothermia due to exposure, unwarmed oxygen, and cold IV fluids.
- Hypothermia can lead to eventual coma, hypoxemia, and acidosis.

To prevent hypothermia
- Remove wet clothing from the client.
- Cover the client with warm blankets.
- Increase the temperature of the room.
- Use a heat lamp to provide additional warmth.
- Infuse warmed IV fluids.

POISONING

Poisoning is exposure to a toxic agent.
- Medications, illicit drugs, ingestion of chemicals
- Environmental (pollutants, snake and spider bites, plants)

Poisoning is considered a medical emergency and requires rapid management therapy.
- Obtain a client history to identify the toxic agent.
- Prevent further absorption of the toxin.
- Extract or remove the poison.
- Implement supportive care.
- Administer antidotes when necessary.

2.1 AVPU mnemonic

A **A**lert

V Responsive to **V**oice

P Responsive to **P**ain

U **U**nresponsive

2.2 Glasgow Coma Scale

EYE-OPENING RESPONSE		✚ VERBAL RESPONSE		✚ MOTOR RESPONSE	
Spontaneous	4	Oriented	5	Obeys commands	6
To voice	3	Confused	4	Localizes pain	5
To pain	2	Inappropriate words	3	Withdraws	4
None	1	Incomprehensible sounds	2	Flexion (decorticate)	3
		None	1	Extension (decerebrate)	2
				None	1

A score of 8 or less indicates a comatose state. A low score of 3 indicates a client who is totally unresponsive, and a high score of 15 indicates a client who is within normal limits neurologically.

- A snakebite from a venomous snake is a medical emergency.
  - Children 1 to 9 years old are at highest risk for snakebites.
  - The nurse should be familiar with indigenous snakes in the community.
  - Generally, ice, tourniquets, heparin, and corticosteroids are contraindicated in the first 6 to 8 hr after the bite.
  - Antivenom based on the type and severity of a snakebite is most effective if administered within 4 to 12 hr.

Interventions to manage the clinical status of the client exposed to or who ingested a toxic agent
- Provide measures for respiratory support (oxygen, airway management, mechanical ventilation).
- Monitor compromised circulation (resulting from excess perspiration, vomiting, diarrhea).
- Restore fluids with IV fluid therapy.
- Monitor blood pressure, cardiac monitoring, ECG.
- Monitor for tissue edema every 15 to 30 min for snake or spider bite.
- Administer opioid medications for pain due to snake or spider bite.
- Monitor ABGs, blood glucose levels, coagulation profile.
- For ingested poison, three procedures are available: activated charcoal, gastric lavage (if done within 1 hr of ingestion), and aspiration. Syrup of ipecac is not recommended.
- Administer diazepam if seizures occur.
- Reverse heroin and other opiate toxicity with naloxone.
- Implement dialysis and an exchange blood transfusion as a nonpharmacologic technique to remove toxic agents.

RAPID RESPONSE TEAM

The team is a group of critical care experts (ICU nurse, respiratory therapist, critical care provider, hospitalist). Q**EBP**
- Responds to an emergency call from nurses or family members when a client exhibits indications of a rapid decline.
- Provides early recognition and response before a respiratory or cardiac arrest or stroke occurs.
- Policies and procedures are established in a health care setting.
- Facility staff learn about criteria for calling for assistance when a client's condition changes toward a crisis situation.
- SBAR (Situation, Background, Assessment, Recommendation) communication techniques are used for contacting the team and documentation of event.
- Participate in follow-up, education, and sharing of information (debriefing) for participants after the call.
- Discuss information to identify system failures (not recognizing a crisis, lack of adequate communication, failure in the plan of care).
- Retrieve more information at www.ihi.org.

CARDIAC EMERGENCY

Cardiac arrest: The sudden cessation of cardiac function caused most commonly by ventricular fibrillation or ventricular asystole.

Ventricular fibrillation (VF): A fluttering of the ventricles causing loss of consciousness, pulselessness, and no breathing. This requires collaborative care to defibrillate immediately using ACLS protocol.

Pulseless ventricular tachycardia (VT): An irritable firing of ectopic ventricular beats at a rate of 140 to 180/min. The client over time will become unconscious and deteriorate into VF.

Ventricular asystole: A complete absence of electrical activity and ventricular movement of the heart. The client is in complete cardiac arrest and requires implementation of BLS and ACLS protocol.

Pulseless electrical activity (PEA): A rhythm that appears to have electrical activity but is not sufficient to stimulate effective cardiac contractions and requires implementation of BLS and ACLS protocol.

EMERGENCY NURSE CERTIFICATIONS

- Basic Life Support (BLS), Advanced Cardiac Life Support (ACLS), and Pediatric Advanced Life Support (PALS) are certifications required for nurses practicing in United States emergency departments.
- BLS involves a hands-on approach for management to restore airway, breathing, and circulation.
- ACLS builds on the BLS skills to include advanced concepts.
  - Cardiac monitoring for specific resuscitation rhythms
  - Invasive airway management
  - Electrical therapies (defibrillation or cardioversion)
  - Obtaining IV access
  - Administration of IV antidysrhythmic medications
  - Management of the client postresuscitation
- PALS is built on the BLS protocol for neonatal and pediatric assessment and management skills to include advanced concepts for resuscitation of children.
- Certification courses are based on evidence-based practice management theory, and the basic concepts and techniques for cardiopulmonary resuscitation (CPR). Q**EBP**
- BLS and ACLS guidelines are available from the American Heart Association (AHA) at www.americanheart.org.

AHA ACLS PROTOCOLS

Protocols address management of life-threatening dysrhythmias.
- VF or pulseless VT
- PEA

Nursing actions for clients who have a life-threatening arrhythmia
- Verify the rhythm and check the client.
- Activate help following the facility protocol. Initiate the CPR component of BLS until further help arrives
- Assist with treatment of the underlying cause. **(2.3)**

POSTRESUSCITATION

PHARMACOLOGICAL MANAGEMENT
- Medication therapy following a successful cardiac arrest includes IV medications that cause a catecholamine adrenergic agonist's effect.
- Catecholamine adrenergic agonists cannot be taken orally, do not cross the blood-brain barrier, and have a short duration of action.

- Medications include epinephrine, dopamine, and dobutamine.
- These medications respond to an identifiable receptor and produce specific effects. **(2.4, 2.6)**

CONTRAINDICATIONS/PRECAUTIONS (2.5)
- Pregnancy Risk Category C: epinephrine, dopamine, dobutamine
- These medications are contraindicated in clients who have tachydysrhythmias and ventricular fibrillation.
- Use cautiously in clients who have hyperthyroidism, angina, history of myocardial infarction, hypertension, and diabetes mellitus.

NURSING INTERVENTIONS AND CLIENT EDUCATION
- Use IV pump to control continuous infusions.
- Monitor blood pressure response and heart rate to facilitate titration for therapeutic response. (These medications affect heart rate and blood pressure.)
- Stop the infusion at the first sign of infiltration. Extravasation can be treated with a local injection of an alpha adrenergic blocking agent, such as phentolamine.
- Monitor for chest pain. Notify the provider if the client experiences chest pain.
- Provide continuous ECG monitoring. Notify the provider if the client experiences tachycardia or dysrhythmias.

2.3 Common causes of pulseless electrical activity

5 H's

Hypovolemia

Hypoxia

Hydrogen ion accumulation, resulting in acidosis

Hyperkalemia or hypokalemia

Hypothermia

5 T's

Toxins (accidental or deliberate drug overdose)

Tamponade (cardiac)

Tension pneumothorax

Thrombosis (coronary)

Thrombosis (pulmonary)

2.4 Receptor sites and responses

Alpha₁

Activation of receptors in arterioles of skin, viscera and mucous membranes, and veins lead to vasoconstriction

Beta₁

Heart stimulation leads to increased heart rate, increased myocardial contractility, and increased rate of conduction through the atrioventricular (AV) node.

Activation of receptors in the kidney leads to the release of renin.

Beta₂

Bronchial stimulation leads to bronchodilation.

Activation of receptors in uterine smooth muscle causes relaxation.

Activation of receptors in the liver causes a breakdown of glycogen into glucose.

Skeletal muscle receptor activation leads to muscle contraction, which can lead to tremors.

Dopamine

Activation of receptors in the kidney cause the renal blood vessels to dilate.

2.5 Medication interactions

MAOIs promote the release of norepinephrine from sympathetic nerves and thereby prolong and intensify the effects of epinephrine and can cause hypertensive crisis.

NURSING INTERVENTIONS: Avoid the use of MAOIs in clients who are receiving epinephrine.

Tricyclic antidepressants block the uptake of epinephrine, which will prolong and intensify the effects of epinephrine.

NURSING INTERVENTIONS: Clients taking these medications concurrently can need a lower dose of epinephrine.

General anesthetics can cause the heart to become hypersensitive to the effects of epinephrine, which leads to dysrhythmias.

NURSING INTERVENTIONS

Perform continuous ECG monitoring.

Notify the provider if the client experiences chest pain, dysrhythmias, or an elevated heart rate.

Beta adrenergic blocking agents, such as propranolol, block the action at beta receptors.

NURSING INTERVENTIONS: Propranolol may be used to treat chest pain, hypertension, myocardial infarction, and dysrhythmias.

Diuretics promote the beneficial effect of dopamine.

NURSING INTERVENTIONS: Monitor for therapeutic effects.

2.6 Emergency medications

RECEPTORS	PHARMACOLOGICAL ACTION	THERAPEUTIC USE	ADVERSE EFFECTS	NURSING ACTIONS
Epinephrine				
Alpha$_1$	Vasoconstriction	Slows absorption of local anesthetics Manages superficial bleeding Reduces congestion of nasal mucosa Increases blood pressure	Vasoconstriction from activation of alpha$_1$ receptors in the heart can lead to hypertensive crisis.	Provide continuous cardiac monitoring. Report changes in vital signs to the provider.
Beta$_1$	Increases heart rate Strengthens myocardial contractility Increases rate of conduction through the AV node	Treatment of AV block and cardiac arrest	Beta$_1$ receptor activation in the heart can cause dysrhythmias. Beta$_1$ receptor activation also increases the workload of the heart and oxygen demand, leading to the development of angina.	Provide continuous cardiac monitoring. Monitor closely for dysrhythmias, change in heart rate, and chest pain. Monitor for hyperglycemia in clients who have diabetes mellitus.
Beta$_2$	Bronchodilation	Asthma	The activation of beta$_2$ receptors in the liver and skeletal muscles can cause hyperglycemia from the breakdown of glycogen.	Notify the provider if the client experiences dysrhythmias, an elevated heart rate, or chest pain, and treat per protocol.
Dopamine				
Dopamine	Low dose—dopamine (2 to 5 mcg/kg/min) Renal blood vessel dilation			
Beta$_1$	Moderate dose—dopamine (5 to 10 mcg/kg/min) Renal blood vessel dilation Increases: • Heart rate • Myocardial contractility • Rate of conduction through the AV node • Blood pressure	Shock Heart failure Acute kidney injury	Beta$_1$ receptor activation in the heart can cause dysrhythmias. Beta$_1$ receptor activation also increases the workload of the heart and oxygen demand, leading to the development of angina.	Provide continuous cardiac monitoring. Monitor closely for dysrhythmias, change in heart rate, and chest pain. Notify the provider of signs of dysrhythmias, elevated heart rate, and chest pain, and treat per protocol. Monitor for urinary output less than 30 mL/hr. Do not confuse dopamine with dobutamine.
Beta$_1$ Alpha$_1$	High dose—dopamine (greater than 10 mcg/kg/min) Renal blood vessel vasoconstriction Increases: • Heart rate • Myocardial contractility • Rate of conduction through the AV node • Blood pressure • Vasoconstriction		Necrosis can occur from extravasation due to high doses of dopamine.	Infuse dopamine into the central line. Monitor the IV site carefully. Discontinue the infusion at first sign of irritation.
Dobutamine				
Beta$_1$	Increases: • Heart rate • Myocardial contractility • Rate of conduction through the AV node	Heart failure	Increased heart rate	Provide continuous cardiac monitoring. Report changes in vital signs to the provider. Monitor for urinary output less than 30 mL/hr. Do not confuse dobutamine with dopamine.

Application Exercises

1. A nurse on a medical-surgical unit is caring for a group of clients. The nurse should notify the rapid response team for which of the following clients?

    A. Client who has an ulceration of the right heel whose blood glucose is 300 mg/dL

    B. Client who reports right calf pain and shortness of breath

    C. Client who has blood on a pressure dressing in the femoral area following a cardiac catheterization

    D. Client who has dark red coloration of left toes and absent pedal pulse

2. A nurse is caring for a client who has ingested a toxic agent. Which of the following actions should the nurse plan to take? (Select all that apply.)

    A. Induce vomiting.

    B. Instill activated charcoal.

    C. Perform a gastric lavage with aspiration.

    D. Administer syrup of ipecac.

    E. Ensure the cleint has IV fluids infused.

3. A nurse at a rural community clinic is caring for a client who fell through the ice on a pond, is unresponsive, and is breathing slowly. Which of the following actions should the nurse take? (Select all that apply.)

    A. Remove wet clothing.

    B. Maintain normal room temperature.

    C. Apply warm blankets.

    D. Apply a heat lamp.

    E. Ensure the cleint has warmed IV fluids infused.

4. A nurse encounters an unresponsive client during a walk. The client's partner states, "He was pulling weeds in the yard and slumped to the ground." Which of the following techniques should the nurse use to open the client's airway?

    A. Head-tilt/chin-lift

    B. Modified jaw thrust

    C. Hyperextension of the head

    D. Flexion of the head

5. A nurse discovers an assistive personnel was splashed with a large amount of chemicals and is lying on the floor and calls for assistance. After checking to make sure the AP has an adequate airway and is breathing, which of the following actions should the nurse take next?

    A. Remove the AP's clothing.

    B. Rate the AP using the Glasgow Coma Scale.

    C. Check for adequate tissue perfusion.

    D. Measure the AP's temperature.

PRACTICE Active Learning Scenario

A nurse orienting to an emergency department (ED) is reviewing the five-level triage system. Use the ATI Active Learning Template: Basic Concept to complete this item.

RELATED CONTENT: Identify the five levels of the ED triage system.

UNDERLYING PRINCIPLES: Define each of the five triage levels.

NURSING INTERVENTIONS: Describe a client who meets the criteria for each of the five triage levels.

Application Exercises Key

1. A. The situation does not indicate the beginning of a rapid decline in the client's condition. The nurse should notify the provider of the glucose level to obtain a prescription for treatment.

   B. **CORRECT:** The nurse should identify that the client is at risk for respiratory arrest due to a possible embolism. The nurse should call the rapid response team because this can cause a rapid decline in the client's condition.

   C. This situation does not indicate the beginning of a rapid decline in the client's condition at this time. The nurse should monitor the dressing and notify the provider if the bleeding increases.

   D. The situation does not indicate the beginning of a rapid decline in the client's condition. The nurse should notify the provider if this is a change in the client's condition.

   Ⓝ *NCLEX® Connection: Physiological Adaptation, Medical Emergencies*

2. A. Vomiting places the client at risk for aspiration.

   B. **CORRECT:** Activated charcoal adsorbs toxic substances, and the charcoal does not pass into the bloodstream.

   C. **CORRECT:** Gastric lavage with aspiration removes the toxic substance when the instilled fluid is suctioned from the gastrointestinal tract.

   D. The nurse should avoid administering syrup of ipecac because it induces vomiting, which increases the client's risk for aspiration.

   E. **CORRECT:** Intravenous fluids help dilute the toxic substances in the bloodstream and promote elimination from the body through the kidneys.

   Ⓝ *NCLEX® Connection: Physiological Adaptation, Alterations in Body Systems*

3. A. **CORRECT:** Removing wet clothing will help increase the body temperature.

   B. The nurse should increase the temperature of the room to help return the client to a body temperature within the expected range.

   C. **CORRECT:** Applying warm blankets will help increase the client's body temperature.

   D. **CORRECT:** Using a heat lamp will help increase the client's body temperature.

   E. **CORRECT:** Infusing warmed IV fluids will help increase the client's body temperature.

   Ⓝ *NCLEX® Connection: Physiological Adaptation, Alterations in Body Systems*

4. A. **CORRECT:** The nurse should open the client's airway by the head-tilt/chin-lift method, because the client is unresponsive without suspicion of trauma.

   B. The nurse should use the modified jaw thrust for a client who is unresponsive with suspected traumatic neck injury.

   C. The nurse should not hyperextend a client's head, because it can close off the airway and cause injury.

   D. The nurse should recognize that flexion of the head will close the airway further.

   Ⓝ *NCLEX® Connection: Physiological Adaptation, Medical Emergencies*

5. A. The nurse should remove the AP's clothing to check the skin and remove contaminants. However, there is another action the nurse should take first.

   B. The nurse should use the Glasgow Coma Scale or other tool to determine the AP's level of consciousness. However, there is another action the nurse should take first.

   C. **CORRECT:** The next action the nurse should take when using the ABCDE principle is to check for adequate tissue perfusion. The nurse should measure blood pressure, heart rate, and peripheral pulses to determine problems with circulation.

   D. The nurse should measure the AP's temperature to see if the chemical exposure caused temperature abnormalities. However, there is another action the nurse should take first.

   Ⓝ *NCLEX® Connection: Physiological Adaptation, Medical Emergencies*

PRACTICE Answer

Using the ATI Active Learning Template: Basic Concept

RELATED CONTENT
- Resuscitation
- Emergent
- Urgent
- Less urgent
- Nonurgent

UNDERLYING PRINCIPLES
- Resuscitation: The client needs immediate treatment to prevent death.
- Emergent: The client requires time sensitive treatment for a problem that has the potential to become a life or limb-threatening situation.
- Urgent: The client requires treatment but the situation is not life-threatening.
- Less Urgent: The client is able to wait for a period of time without immediate treatment.
- Nonurgent: The client requires simple evaluation and minor management of care.

NURSING INTERVENTIONS
- Resuscitation: A client who is experiencing cardiac arrest, stroke, pulmonary emboli, or drug overdose.
- Emergent: A client who has sustained a traumatic amputation, head or neck injury, snake or spider bite.
- Urgent: A client who has a kidney stone, gallbladder colic, or fracture.
- Less Urgent: A client who has a bladder infection, laceration, or infected toe.
- Nonurgent: A client who has a rash, minor cut, or backache.

Ⓝ *NCLEX® Connection: Coordinated Care, Establishing Priorities*

When reviewing the following chapters, keep in mind the relevant topics and tasks of the NCLEX outline, in particular:

Safety and Infection Control

HOME SAFETY: Provide the client with information on home safety.

Basic Care and Comfort

MOBILITY/IMMOBILITY: Check the client for mobility, gait, strength, and motor skills.

NONPHARMACOLOGICAL COMFORT INTERVENTIONS: Provide nonpharmacological measures for pain relief (imagery, massage or repositioning).

NUTRITION AND ORAL HYDRATION: Monitor the client's ability to eat (chew, swallow).

Pharmacological Therapies

ADVERSE EFFECTS/CONTRAINDICATIONS/SIDE EFFECTS/ INTERACTIONS: Reinforce client teaching on possible effects of medications (common side effects or adverse effects, when to notify the primary health care provider).

EXPECTED ACTIONS/OUTCOMES: Monitor the client's use of medications over time (prescription, over-the-counter, home remedies).

PHARMACOLOGICAL PAIN MANAGEMENT: Identify the client's need for pain medication.

Reduction of Risk Potential

DIAGNOSTIC TESTS: Perform diagnostic testing (blood glucose, oxygen saturation, testing for occult blood).

POTENTIAL FOR ALTERATIONS IN BODY SYSTEMS: Perform neurological checks.

POTENTIAL FOR COMPLICATIONS OF DIAGNOSTIC TESTS/TREATMENTS/PROCEDURES: Identify the client's risk and implement interventions.

THERAPEUTIC PROCEDURES: Reinforce client teaching on treatments and procedures.

CHAPTER 3 Neurologic Diagnostic Procedures

Neurologic assessment and diagnostic procedures are tools to evaluate neurologic function by testing indicators such as mental status, motor function, electrical activity, and intracranial pressure.

Neurologic assessment and diagnostic procedures that nurses should be knowledgeable about include cerebral angiography, cerebral computed tomography (CT) scan, electroencephalography (EEG), Glasgow Coma Scale (GCS), intracranial pressure (ICP) monitoring, lumbar puncture (spinal tap), magnetic resonance imaging (MRI), positron emission tomography (PET), single-photon emission computed tomography (SPECT), and radiography (x-ray).

Cerebral angiography

Cerebral angiography provides visualization of the cerebral blood vessels.
- Digital subtraction angiography hides the bones and tissues from the images, providing x-rays with only the vessels apparent.
- The procedure detects defects, narrowing, or obstruction of arteries or blood vessels in the brain.
- The procedure is performed within the radiology department, because iodine-based contrast dye is injected into an artery during the procedure.

INDICATIONS

Cerebral angiography is used to assess the blood flow to and within the brain, identify aneurysms, and define the vascularity of tumors (useful for surgical planning). It is also used therapeutically to inject medications that treat blood clots or to administer chemotherapy.

CONSIDERATIONS

PREPROCEDURE

If the client is pregnant, a determination of the risks to the fetus versus the benefits of the information obtained by this procedure should be made.

NURSING ACTIONS
- Instruct the client to refrain from consuming food or fluids for 8 to 12 hr prior to the procedure.
- Check for allergy to shellfish or iodine, which would require the use of a different contrast media.
- Any history of bleeding or anticoagulant medication requires additional considerations and monitoring to ensure clotting after the procedure. Qs
- Review BUN and serum creatinine to determine kidney's ability to excrete the dye.
- Ensure that the client is not wearing any jewelry.
- The client may take a mild sedative for relaxation prior to or during the procedure and will require continuous vital sign monitoring.

CLIENT EDUCATION
- The importance of not moving during the procedure and the need to keep the head immobilized.
- Void immediately before the test.
- There can be a metallic taste in the mouth and a warm sensation over the face, jaw, tongue, lips, and behind the eyes from the dye injected during procedure

INTRAPROCEDURE
- The client is placed on a radiography table, where the head is secured.
- A catheter is placed into an artery (usually in the groin or the neck), dye is injected, and x-ray images are taken.
- Once all images are taken, the catheter is removed and an arterial closure device is used or pressure is held over the artery to control bleeding by thrombus formation sealing the artery.

POSTPROCEDURE

NURSING ACTIONS
- Closely monitor the catheter site to ensure that clotting occurs.
- Restrict movements, depending on the type of procedure used to seal the artery, to prevent rebleeding at the catheter site.
- Monitor vital signs.
- Perform neurologic checks.
- Check for dysphagia and respiratory distress, which could indicate internal bleeding in the neck.

COMPLICATIONS

There is a risk for bleeding or hematoma formation at the entry site.

NURSING ACTIONS
- Check the insertion site frequently.
- Check the affected extremity distal to the puncture site for adequate circulation (color, temperature, pulses, capillary refill).
- If bleeding occurs, apply pressure over the artery and notify the provider. Q̃EBP

Cerebral computed tomography scan

A CT scan provides cross-sectional images of the cranial cavity. Contrast media can be used to enhance the images.

INDICATIONS

CT scanning can be used to identify tumors and infarctions, detect abnormalities, monitor response to treatment, and guide needles used for biopsies.

CONSIDERATIONS

PREPROCEDURE

If the client is pregnant, the provider will help the client weigh risks to the fetus versus the benefits of the procedure.

NURSING ACTIONS
- If contrast media or sedation is expected:
  - Instruct the client to refrain from consuming food or fluids for at least 3 hr prior to the procedure.
  - Check for allergy to shellfish or iodine, which would require the use of a different contrast media.
  - Determine renal function (BUN and creatinine), because contrast media is excreted by the kidneys. Q̃s
- Because this procedure is performed with the client in a supine position, placing pillows in the small of the client's back can assist in preventing back pain. The head must be secured to prevent unnecessary movement during the procedure.
- Ensure that the client's jewelry is removed prior to this procedure. In general, clients wear a hospital gown to prevent any metals from interfering with the x-rays.
- Premedicate as prescribed to prevent claustrophobia.

INTRAPROCEDURE
- The client must lie supine with the head stabilized during the procedure.
- Instruct client regarding warm flush feeling or metallic taste in mouth associated with contrast dye.
- Advise and reassure client of expected noises from the CT scanner.

POSTPROCEDURE

NURSING ACTIONS
- If contrast media is injected, monitor for allergic reaction and changes in kidney function.
- If sedation is administered, monitor the client until stable.
- If a lumbar puncture is needed for an intrathecal contrast-enhanced CT (also called cisternography), follow the same postprocedural care as for lumbar puncture.

Electroencephalography

This noninvasive procedure assesses the electrical activity of the brain and is used to determine if there are abnormalities in brain wave patterns. An EEG provides information about the ability of the brain to function and highlights areas of abnormality.

INDICATIONS

EEGs are most commonly performed to identify and determine seizure activity, but they are also useful for detecting sleep disorders and behavioral changes. The provider can also prescribe evoked potential studies in conjunction with EEG.

CONSIDERATIONS

PREPROCEDURE

NURSING ACTIONS: Withhold or discontinue medications prior to this procedure as indicated by the provider.

CLIENT EDUCATION
- Wash hair prior to the procedure and eliminate all oils, gels, and sprays.
- If indicated, the client should be sleep-deprived, because this provides cranial stress, increasing the possibility of abnormal electrical activity (such as seizure potentials) occurring during the procedure.
- Increased electrical activity can be stimulated with exposure to bright flashing lights, or by requesting the client to hyperventilate for 3 to 4 min.
- Avoid taking any sedative medication the night prior to the procedure and withhold stimulants for 24 to 48 hr prior to the procedure.

INTRAPROCEDURE

- The procedure generally takes 45 min to 2 hr.
- There are no risks associated with this procedure.
- With the client resting in a chair or lying in bed, small electrodes are placed on the scalp and connected to a brain wave machine or computer.
- Electrical signals produced by the brain are recorded by the machine or computer in the form of wavy lines. This documents brain activity.
- Notations are made when stimuli are presented or when sleep occurs. (Flashes of light or pictures can be used during the procedure to assess the client's response to stimuli.)

POSTPROCEDURE

CLIENT EDUCATION
- Resume normal activities.
- Shampoo hair to remove electrode paste.

Glasgow Coma Scale

This assessment concentrates on neurologic function. It is useful to determine the level of consciousness and monitor response to treatment. The GCS is reported as a number that allows providers to immediately determine if neurologic changes have occurred.

INDICATIONS

GCS scores are helpful in determining changes in the level of consciousness for clients who have head injuries, space-occupying lesions or cerebral infarctions, and encephalitis. This is important because complications related to neurologic injuries can occur rapidly and require immediate treatment.

CONSIDERATIONS

GCS scores are calculated by using appropriate stimuli (a painful stimulus can be necessary) and then measuring the client's response in three areas. Q̲ᴇʙᴘ
- **Eye opening (E):** The best eye response, with responses ranging from 4 to 1
  - 4 = Eye opening occurs spontaneously.
  - 3 = Eye opening occurs secondary to sound.
  - 2 = Eye opening occurs secondary to pain.
  - 1 = Eye opening does not occur.
- **Verbal (V):** The best verbal response, with responses ranging from 5 to 1
  - 5 = Conversation is coherent and oriented.
  - 4 = Conversation is incoherent and disoriented.
  - 3 = Words are spoken, but inappropriately.
  - 2 = Sounds are made, but no words.
  - 1 = Vocalization does not occur.
- **Motor (M):** The best motor response, with responses ranging from 6 to 1
  - 6 = Commands are followed.
  - 5 = Local reaction to pain occurs.
  - 4 = There is a general withdrawal to pain.
  - 3 = Decorticate posture (adduction of arms, flexion of elbows and wrists) is present.
  - 2 = Decerebrate posture (abduction of arms, extension of elbows and wrists) is present.
  - 1 = Motor response does not occur.

Responses within each subscale are added, with the total score quantitatively describing level of consciousness.

E + V + M = Total GCS

- In critical situations, where head injury is present and close monitoring is required, subscale results may also be documented. Thus, a GCS may be reported as either a single number indicating the sum of the subscales (3 to 15), or as three numbers, one from each subscale result, and the total (E3 V3 M4 = GCS 13). This allows providers to determine specific neurologic function.
- Intubation limits the ability to use GCS summed scores. If intubation is present, the GCS may be reported as two scores, with modification noted. This is generally reported as "GCS 5t" (with the t representing the intubation tube).

INTERPRETATION OF FINDINGS

The best possible GCS score is 15. In general, total scores of the GCS correlate with the degree or level of coma.
- A score less than 8 is associated with severe head injury and coma.
- A score of 9 to 12 indicates a moderate head injury.
- A score greater than 13 is associated with minor head trauma.

Intracranial pressure monitoring

An ICP monitor is a device inserted into the cranial cavity that records pressure and is connected to a monitor that shows a picture of the pressure waveforms. Q̲s
- Monitoring ICP facilitates continual assessment and is more precise than vague manifestations.
- ICP monitoring is useful for early identification and treatment of increased intracranial pressure. Clients who are comatose or have GCS scores of 8 are candidates for ICP monitoring.
- Clients are kept in a critical care unit for ICP monitoring.

Lumbar puncture (spinal tap)

A lumbar puncture is a procedure during which a small amount of CSF is withdrawn from the spinal canal and then analyzed to determine its constituents.

INDICATIONS

This procedure is used to detect the presence of some diseases (multiple sclerosis, syphilis, meningitis), infections, and malignancies. A lumbar puncture may also be used to reduce CSF pressure, instill a contrast medium or air for diagnostic tests, or administer medication or chemotherapy directly to spinal fluid.

CONSIDERATIONS

PREPROCEDURE

The risks versus benefits of a lumbar puncture should be discussed with the client prior to this procedure.

- A lumbar puncture can be associated with rare but serious complications, such as brain herniation, especially when performed in the presence of increased ICP.
- Lumbar punctures for clients who have bleeding disorders or who are taking anticoagulants can result in bleeding that compresses the spinal cord.

NURSING ACTIONS

- Ensure that all of the client's jewelry is removed and the client is wearing only a hospital gown.
- Instruct the client to void prior to the procedure.
- Clients should be positioned to stretch the spinal canal. This can be done by having the client assume a "cannonball" position while on one side or by having the client stretch over an overbed table, if sitting is preferred. (3.1)

INTRAPROCEDURE

- Obtain a sterile lumbar tray and anesthetic.
- Medical and nursing personnel should don a mask during the procedure.
- The provider will cleanse the area of the needle insertion and inject a local anesthesia.
- The provider will insert the needle and withdraw the CSF, then remove the needle.
- A manometer can be used to determine the opening pressure of the spinal cord, which is useful if increased pressure is a consideration.

POSTPROCEDURE

- CSF is sent to the pathology department for analysis.
- NURSING ACTIONS: Monitor the puncture site. The client should remain lying for several hours to ensure that the site clots and to decrease the risk of a post-lumbar puncture headache, caused by CSF leakage. Qᴇʙᴘ
- CLIENT EDUCATION: Once stable, advise the client that normal activities may be resumed.

COMPLICATIONS

If clotting does not occur to seal the dura puncture site, CSF can leak, resulting in a headache and increasing the potential for infection.

NURSING ACTIONS

- Encourage the client to lie flat in bed. Provide fluids for hydration, and administer pain medication.
- Prepare the client for an epidural blood patch to seal the hole in the dura if the headache persists.

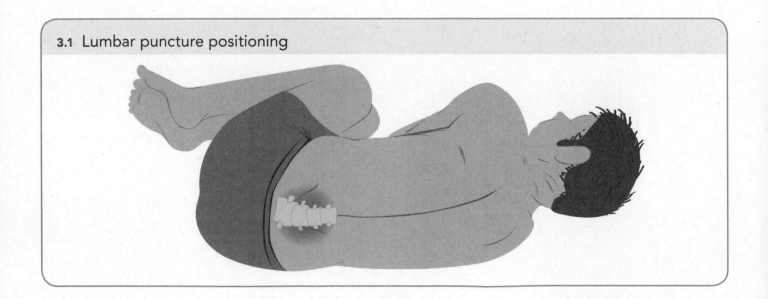

3.1 Lumbar puncture positioning

Magnetic resonance imaging scan

An MRI scan provides cross-sectional images of the cranial cavity. A contrast media may be used to enhance the images.

- Unlike CT scans, MRI images are obtained using magnets. Thus, the consequences associated with radiation are avoided. This makes this procedure safer for women who are pregnant.
- The use of magnets precludes the ability to scan a client who has an artificial device (pacemaker, surgical clip, intravenous access port) Qs
- Use MRI-approved equipment to monitor vital signs, and provide ventilator/oxygen assistance to clients undergoing MRI scans.

INDICATIONS

- MRI scans are used to detect abnormalities, monitor response to treatment, and guide needles used for biopsies.
- MRIs are capable of discriminating soft tissue from tumor or bone. This makes the MRI scan effective in determining tumor size and blood vessel location.

CONSIDERATIONS

PREPROCEDURE

NURSING ACTIONS
- Remove any transdermal patches with a foil backing, as these can cause burn injuries. Qs
- Ensure that the client's jewelry is removed prior to this procedure. The client should wear a hospital gown to prevent any metals from interfering with the magnet.
- If sedation is expected, the client should refrain from food or fluids for 4 to 8 hr prior to the procedure.
- Determine if the client has a history of claustrophobia, and explain the tight space and noise.
- Ask the client about any implants containing metal (pacemaker, orthopedic joints, artificial heart valves, intrauterine devices, aneurysm clips).
- All people in the scanning area while the magnet is on must remove all jewelry, electronics, and phones to prevent damage to themselves or the magnet.
- Because this procedure is performed with the client in a supine position, placing pillows in the small of the client's back can assist in preventing back pain. The head must be secured to prevent unnecessary movement during the procedure.

INTRAPROCEDURE

- The client must lie supine with the head stabilized.
- MRI scanning is noisy, and earplugs or sedation may be provided.

POSTPROCEDURE

NURSING ACTIONS
- If contrast media is injected, monitor the site to ensure that clotting has occurred, and monitor for any indications of an allergic reaction.
- If sedation is administered, monitor the client until stable.

PET and SPECT scans

Positron emission tomography and single-photon emission computed tomography scans are nuclear medicine procedures that produce three-dimensional images of the head. These images can be static (depicting vessels) or functional (depicting brain activity).

PET/SPECT scans use radioactive tracers, which are injected into the bloodstream. This initiates metabolic activity (areas of increased blood flow will collect more of the isotope), which is then documented by the scanner.

INDICATIONS

A PET/SPECT scan capture of regional metabolic processes is most useful in determining tumor activity and response to treatment. PET/SPECT scans are also able to determine the presence of dementia, indicated by the inability of the brain to respond to the tracer.

CONSIDERATIONS

PREPROCEDURE

PET/SPECT scans use radiation. Thus, the risks and benefits to a client who might be pregnant must be discussed.

NURSING ACTIONS: Check for a history of diabetes mellitus. While this condition does not preclude a PET/SPECT scan, alterations in medications can be necessary to avoid hyperglycemia or hypoglycemia before and after this procedure. Qs
- Instruct clients to avoid sedatives or tranquilizers prior to the diagnostic test.
- Advise clients to empty bladder prior to the diagnostic test.

INTRAPROCEDURE

- While the pictures are being obtained, the client must lie flat with the head restrained.
- This procedure is not painful, and sedation is rarely necessary.

POSTPROCEDURE

NURSING ACTIONS
- If radioisotopes are used, monitor for allergic reaction.
- There is no follow-up care after a PET/SPECT scans.

Radiography (x-ray)

An x-ray uses electromagnetic radiation to capture images of the internal structures of an individual.

- A structure's image is light or dark relative to the amount of radiation the tissue absorbs. The image is recorded on a radiograph, which is a black-and-white image that is held up to light for visualization. Some are recorded digitally and available immediately.
- X-rays are interpreted by a radiologist, who documents the findings.

INDICATIONS

X-ray examinations of the skull and spine can reveal fractures, curvatures, bone erosion and dislocation, and possible soft tissue calcification, all of which can damage the nervous system.

CONSIDERATIONS

PREPROCEDURE

NURSING ACTIONS
- There is no specific preprocedure protocol for x-rays that do not use contrast. X-rays are often the first diagnostic tool used after an injury (to rule out cervical fracture in head trauma), and they can be done without any preparation.
- Determine if the client is pregnant.
- Ensure that the client's jewelry is removed and that no clothes cover the area.

CLIENT EDUCATION: The amount of radiation used in contemporary x-ray machines is very small.

INTRAPROCEDURE

CLIENT EDUCATION: Remain still during the procedure.

POSTPROCEDURE

NURSING ACTIONS: Inform the client when results will be available.

Application Exercises

1. A nurse is caring for a client who is postprocedure following lumbar puncture and reports a throbbing headache when sitting upright. Which of the following actions should the nurse take? (Select all that apply.)

   A. Use the Glasgow Coma Scale to evaluate the client.

   B. Assist the client to a supine position.

   C. Administer an opioid medication.

   D. Encourage the client to increase fluid intake.

   E. Remove the bandage on the client's puncture site.

2. A nurse is reinforcing teaching with a client who is scheduled for a cerebral computed tomography (CT) scan with contrast. Which of the following statements by the client indicates understanding of the teaching?

   A. "I should not have caffeine 48 hr before the procedure."

   B. "I will have my kidney function checked before the test."

   C. "I should tape my wedding band in place before the procedure."

   D. "I will have my brain activity monitored during the test."

3. A nurse is using the Glasgow Coma Scale (GCS) to check a client for changes in the level of consciousness. The client opens his eyes when spoken to, speaks incoherently, and moves his extremities when pain is applied. Which of the following GCS scores should the nurse document?

   A. E2 + V3 + M5 = 10

   B. E3 + V4 + M4 = 11

   C. E4 + V5 + M6 = 15

   D. E2 + V2 + M4 = 8

4. A nurse is reviewing the plan of care for a client who is scheduled for cerebral angiography with contrast dye. Which of the following statements by the client should the nurse report to the provider? (Select all that apply.)

   A. "I think I might be pregnant."

   B. "I take warfarin."

   C. "I take antihypertensive medication."

   D. "I am allergic to shrimp."

   E. "I ate a light breakfast this morning."

5. A nurse is reinforcing teaching with a client who is to undergo an electroencephalogram (EEG) the next day. Which of the following information should the nurse include in the teaching?

   A. "Do not wash your hair the morning of the procedure."

   B. "Try to stay awake most of the night prior to the procedure."

   C. "The procedure will take approximately 15 minutes."

   D. "You will need to lie flat for 4 hours after the procedure."

PRACTICE Active Learning Scenario

A nurse is reviewing the plan of care for a client who is scheduled for a magnetic resonance imaging (MRI) scan with contrast dye. What should the nurse include in the plan of care? Use the ATI Active Learning Template: Diagnostic Procedure to complete this item.

PROCEDURE NAME: Define this diagnostic test.

NURSING INTERVENTIONS (PRE, INTRA, POST): Identify three preprocedure actions, one intraprocedure action, and one postprocedure action.

Application Exercises Key

1. A. The Glasgow Coma Scale is used to assess a client's level of consciousness and is not necessary following a lumbar puncture.

   B. **CORRECT:** The nurse should assist the client to a supine position, which can relieve a headache following a lumbar puncture.

   C. **CORRECT:** The nurse should administer an opioid medication for a client's report of headache pain.

   D. **CORRECT:** The nurse should encourage an increased fluid intake to maintain a positive fluid balance, which can relieve a headache following a lumbar puncture.

   E. Leaking CSF can cause a headache following lumbar puncture. The client can require a patch to seal the puncture site if the headache doesn't resolve.

   (N) NCLEX® Connection: Physiological Adaptation, Unexpected Response to Therapies

2. A. The nurse should recognize that a client should withhold stimulants, such as caffeine, 24 to 48 prior to electroencephalography. The client should be NPO 3 to 4 hr prior to a CT scan.

   B. **CORRECT:** Contrast media used for the CT is excreted by the kidneys. The nurse should check kidney function prior to the CT to prevent harm to the client.

   C. The nurse should remind the client to remove jewelry and all forms of metal prior to the procedure to promote accurate results.

   D. The nurse should recognize that a client will undergo monitoring of brain activity during electroencephalography.

   (N) NCLEX® Connection: Reduction of Risk Potential, Diagnostic Tests

3. A. The calculation is incorrect. E2 represents eyes opening secondary to pain, V3 represents verbal response with words spoken inappropriately, and M5 represents motor response to pain with a local reaction.

   B. **CORRECT:** The score is calculated correctly, indicating moderate head injury. E3 represents opening eyes secondary to voice stimulation, V4 represents verbal conversation that is incoherent and disoriented, and M4 represents motor response as a general withdrawal to pain.

   C. The score is calculated incorrectly. E4 represents eyes opening spontaneously, V5 represents verbal conversation as coherent and oriented, and M6 indicates a client is able to follow commands.

   D. The score is calculated incorrectly. E2 represents eyes opening secondary to pain, V2 represents verbal response by the client making sounds but speaking no words, and M4 is a motor response with a general withdrawal to pain.

   (N) NCLEX® Connection: Reduction of Risk Potential, Diagnostic Tests

4. A. **CORRECT:** The nurse should report the client's statement of possible pregnancy to the provider because the contrast dye can place the fetus at risk.

   B. **CORRECT:** The nurse should report that the client is taking warfarin to the provider due to the potential for bleeding following angiography.

   C. There is no contraindication related to contrast dye for a client who is taking antihypertensive medication.

   D. **CORRECT:** The nurse should report a client's report of allergy to shrimp, which is a shellfish, to the provider because of a potential allergic reaction to the contrast dye.

   E. **CORRECT:** The nurse should report a client's intake of food to the provider since the client should remain NPO for 8 to 12 hr prior to the procedure.

   (N) NCLEX® Connection: Reduction of Risk Potential, Potential for Complications of Diagnostic Tests/Treatments/Procedures

5. A. The nurse should instruct the client to wash her hair on the morning of the procedure to remove oils, gels, and sprays, which can affect the EEG readings.

   B. **CORRECT:** The nurse should tell the client to remain awake most of the night to provide cranial stress and increase the possibility of abnormal electrical activity.

   C. The nurse should inform the client that the procedure will take approximately 45 min to 2 hr.

   D. The nurse should include that the client can resume normal activity immediately following the procedure.

   (N) NCLEX® Connection: Reduction of Risk Potential, Diagnostic Tests

---

PRACTICE Answer

Using the ATI Active Learning Template: Diagnostic Procedure

PROCEDURE NAME: Magnetic resonance imaging (MRI) scan relies on magnetic field to take multiple images of the body.

NURSING INTERVENTIONS (PRE, INTRA, POST)
- Preprocedure
  - Remove all client jewelry.
  - Determine if the client has claustrophobia.
  - Question the client concerning implants containing metal.
  - Question the client regarding allergies.
- Intraprocedure: Stabilize the client's head.
- Postprocedure: Monitor for allergic reaction to the contrast dye used during the MRI.

(N) NCLEX® Connection: Reduction of Risk Potential, Potential for Complications of Diagnostic Tests/Treatments/Procedures

CHAPTER 4   *Pain Management*

Effective pain management includes the use of pharmacological and nonpharmacological pain management therapies.

Clients have a right to adequate assessment and management of pain. Nurses are accountable for the assessment of pain. Professional organizations and The Joint Commission have mandates requiring pain assessment and management. The nurse's role is that of an advocate, member of the health care team, and educator for effective pain management.

Nurses have a priority responsibility for the continual assessment of the client's pain level and to provide individualized interventions. They should evaluate the effectiveness of the interventions 30 to 60 min after implementation. Qᴘᴄᴄ

Assessment challenges can occur with clients who are cognitively impaired, critically ill, or on a ventilator.

PHYSIOLOGY

- Transduction is the conversion of painful stimuli to an electrical impulse through peripheral nerve fibers (nociceptors) to the spinal cord.
- Transmission occurs as the electrical impulse travels along the nerve fibers, to the spinal cord, where the impulse moves up into the cerebral cortex and thymus.
- Perception or awareness and interpretation of pain occurs in various areas of the brain, with influences from thought and emotional processes

- Modulation occurs in the spinal cord, causing the body to decrease the perception of pain by releasing natural endorphins.
- The pain threshold is the point at which a person feels pain.
- Pain tolerance is the amount of pain a person is willing to bear before discussing it or seeking treatment.

Substances that increase pain transmission and cause an inflammatory response include substance P, prostaglandins, bradykinin, and histamine.

Substances that decrease pain transmission and produce analgesia include serotonin and endorphins.

DATA COLLECTION

Pain is whatever the person experiencing it says it is, and it exists whenever the person says it does. The client's report of pain is the most reliable diagnostic measure of pain. Self-report using standardized pain scales is useful for clients older than 7 years old.

- Specialized pain scales are available for use with younger children. Qᴘᴄᴄ
- Monitor for and document pain (the fifth vital sign) according to the client's condition and agency guidelines. Pain is categorized by duration (acute or chronic) or by origin (nociceptive or neuropathic). (4.1)
- Use a focused assessment to obtain subjective data. (4.2)

4.1 Pain categories

Acute pain

Acute pain is protective, temporary, usually self-limiting, and resolves with tissue healing.

Physiological responses (sympathetic nervous system) are fight-or-flight responses (tachycardia, pale skin, shallow breathing and tachypnea, hypertension, anxiety, diaphoresis, muscle tension).

Behavioral responses include grimacing, moaning, flinching, and guarding. The nurse should be aware that a client not exhibiting physiological or behavioral responses does not mean that pain is absent.

Interventions include treatment of the underlying problem.

Chronic pain

Chronic pain is not protective. It is ongoing or recurs frequently, lasting longer than 3 months and persisting beyond tissue healing of the original condition.

Physiological responses do not usually increase vital signs. The client's vital signs can actually be lower than normal in response to chronic pain. Clients can have depression, fatigue, decreased level of functioning, irritability, or disability.

Chronic pain might not have a known cause, and the client might not respond to interventions.

Management aims at pain relief and improving client quality of life and coping.

Chronic pain can be classified as chronic cancer pain or chronic noncancer pain.

Nociceptive pain

Nociceptive pain arises from damage to or inflammation of tissue other than that of the peripheral and central nervous systems.

Nociceptive pain is the activation of normal processing of painful stimuli.

It is usually throbbing, aching, and localized.

This pain typically responds to opioids and nonopioid medications.

TYPES OF NOCICEPTIVE PAIN

Somatic: in bones, joints, muscles, skin, blood vessels, or connective tissues.

Visceral: in internal organs such as the stomach or intestines. It can cause referred pain in other body locations separate from the stimulus.

Neuropathic pain

Neuropathic pain arises from abnormal or damaged pain nerves.

It differs from nociceptive pain as it is the abnormal processing of painful stimuli by the central or peripheral nerve system.

It includes phantom limb pain, pain below the level of a spinal cord injury, and diabetic neuropathy.

Neuropathic pain is usually intense, shooting, burning, or described as "pins and needles."

This pain typically responds to adjuvant medications (antidepressants, antispasmodic agents, skeletal muscle relaxants).

4.2 Focused pain assessment

Location

USE ANATOMICAL TERMINOLOGY AND LANDMARKS TO DESCRIBE LOCATION.

Ask: *"Where is your pain?"*

Ask: *"Does it radiate anywhere else?"*

Ask: *"Is the pain superficial or deep?"*

Ask clients to point to the location.

Quality

QUALITY REFERS TO HOW THE PAIN FEELS: sharp, dull, aching, burning, stabbing, pounding, throbbing, shooting, gnawing, tender, heavy, tight, tiring, exhausting, sickening, terrifying, torturing, nagging, annoying, intense, or unbearable.

Ask: *"What does the pain feel like?"* Give more than two choices (*"Is the pain throbbing, burning, or stabbing?"*).

Measures

INTENSITY, STRENGTH, AND SEVERITY ARE "MEASURES" OF PAIN. Use visual analog scales (description scale, number rating scale) to measure pain, monitor pain, and evaluate the effectiveness of interventions.

Ask: *"How much pain do you have now?"*

Ask: *"What is the worst/best the pain has been?"*

Ask: *"Rate your pain on a scale of 0 to 10."*

Timing

ONSET, DURATION, FREQUENCY

Ask: *"When did it start?"*

Ask: *"How long does it last?"*

Ask: *"How often does it occur?"*

Ask: *"Is it constant or intermittent?"*

Setting

HOW THE PAIN AFFECTS DAILY LIFE OR HOW ACTIVITIES OF DAILY LIVING (ADLs) AFFECT THE PAIN

Ask: *"Where are you when the symptoms occur?"*

Ask: *"What are you doing when the symptoms occur?"*

Ask: *"How does the pain affect your sleep?"*

Ask: *"How does the pain affect your home life, work, and social interactions?"*

Associated manifestations

DOCUMENT ASSOCIATED MANIFESTATIONS: fatigue, depression, nausea, anxiety, anorexia, insomnia.

Ask: *"What other symptoms do you have when you are feeling pain?"*

Aggravating/relieving factors

Ask: *"What makes the pain better?"*

Ask: *"What makes the pain worse?"*

Ask: *"What seems to trigger the pain?"*

Ask: *"Are you currently taking any prescription, herbal, or over-the-counter medications?"*

RISK FACTORS

Risk factors for undertreatment of pain

- Cultural and societal attitudes
- Lack of knowledge
- Fear, anxiety
- Exaggerated fear of respiratory depression
- Populations at risk for undertreatment of pain
- Infants
- Children
- Older adults
- Clients who have substance use disorder
- Causes of acute and chronic pain
- Trauma
- Surgery
- Inflammation
- Cancer (tumor invasion, nerve compression, bone metastases, associated infections, immobility)
- Arthritis
- Fibromyalgia
- Neuropathy
- Diagnostic or treatment procedures (injection, intubation, radiation)

Factors that affect the pain experience

- Age
  - Infants cannot verbalize or understand their pain.
  - Older adult clients can have multiple pathologies that cause pain and limit function. ©
- Fatigue can increase sensitivity to pain.
- The meaning associated with the pain can influence pain tolerance.
- Genetic sensitivity can increase or decrease pain tolerance.
- Cognitive function: Clients who are cognitively impaired might not be able to report pain or report it accurately.
- Prior experiences can increase or decrease sensitivity depending on whether clients obtained adequate relief.
- Anxiety and fear can increase sensitivity to pain.
- Support systems can decrease sensitivity to pain.
- The use of relaxation or distraction techniques can decrease sensitivity to pain.
- Culture can influence how clients express pain or the meaning they give to pain.

EXPECTED FINDINGS

- Behaviors complement self-report and assist in pain assessment of nonverbal clients.
  - Facial expressions (grimacing, wrinkled forehead), body movements (restlessness, pacing, guarding)
  - Moaning, crying
  - Decreased attention span
- Blood pressure, pulse, and respiratory rate can temporarily increase with acute pain. Eventually, increases in vital signs will stabilize despite the persistence of pain. Therefore, physiologic indicators might not be an accurate measure of pain over time.

PATIENT-CENTERED CARE

NONPHARMACOLOGICAL PAIN MANAGEMENT

- Cutaneous (skin) stimulation: transcutaneous electrical nerve stimulation (TENS), heat, cold, therapeutic massage **Qᴘᴄᴄ**
  - Interruption of pain pathways
  - Cold for inflammation
  - Heat to increase blood flow and to reduce stiffness
- Distraction: includes ambulation, deep breathing, visitors, television, and music
- Hypnotism
- Massage
- Relaxation: includes meditation, yoga, and progressive muscle relaxation
- Imagery
  - Focusing on a pleasant thought to divert focus
  - Requires an ability to concentrate
- Acupuncture: vibration or electrical stimulation via tiny needles inserted into the skin and subcutaneous tissues at specific points
- Reduction of pain stimuli in the environment
- Elevation of edematous extremities to promote venous return and decrease swelling

PHARMACOLOGICAL INTERVENTIONS

Analgesics are the mainstay for relieving pain. The three classes of analgesics are nonopioids, opioids, and adjuvants.

Nonopioid analgesics

Nonopioid analgesics (acetaminophen, nonsteroidal anti-inflammatory drugs [NSAIDs], including salicylates) are appropriate for treating mild to moderate pain. Nonopioid analgesics can have antipyretic and anti-inflammatory properties.

- Be aware of the hepatotoxic effects of acetaminophen. Clients who have a healthy liver should take no more than 4 g/day. Make sure clients are aware of opioids that contain acetaminophen, such as hydrocodone bitartrate 5 mg/acetaminophen 500 mg. **Qs**
- Monitor for salicylism (tinnitus, vertigo, decreased hearing acuity).
- Prevent gastric upset by administering NSAIDs with food or antacids.
- Monitor for bleeding with long-term NSAID use. NSAIDs can increase the effects of warfarin.

Opioid analgesics

Opioid analgesics (morphine, fentanyl, oxycodone) are appropriate for treating moderate to severe pain. The term "narcotic" is not synonymous with opioid analgesics. Narcotics can also refer to illegal substances, such as cocaine.

- Managing acute severe pain with short-term (24 to 48 hr) around-the-clock administration of opioids is preferable to following a PRN schedule.
- The IV route works best for immediate, short-term relief of acute pain. When parenteral administration is necessary, the subcutaneous route is preferred over the intramuscular. The oral route is better for chronic, nonfluctuating pain. Opioids are available in transdermal, transmucosal, and buccal routes.
- Consistent timing and dosing of opioid administration provides consistent pain control.
- It is essential to monitor and intervene for adverse effects of opioid use.
  - Constipation: Use a preventative approach (monitoring of bowel movements, fluids, fiber intake, exercise, stool softeners, stimulant laxatives, enemas).
  - Orthostatic hypotension: Advise clients to sit or lie down if lightheadedness or dizziness occur. Instruct clients to avoid sudden changes in position by slowly moving from a lying to a sitting or standing position. Provide assistance with ambulation.
  - Urinary retention: Monitor I&O, monitor for distention, administer bethanechol, and catheterize.
  - Nausea/vomiting: Administer antiemetics, advise clients to lie still and move slowly, and eliminate odors.
  - Sedation: Monitor level of consciousness, and take safety precautions. Sedation usually precedes respiratory depression. **Qs**
  - Respiratory depression: Monitor respiratory rate and depth prior to and following administration of opioids. Encourage deep breathing every 15 to 30 min to counteract respiratory depression. Initial treatment of respiratory depression and sedation is generally a reduction in opioid dose. If necessary, administer naloxone to reverse opioid effects.

Adjuvant analgesics

Adjuvant analgesics enhance the effects of nonopioids, help alleviate other manifestations that aggravate pain (depression, seizures, inflammation), and are useful for treating neuropathic pain.

- Anticonvulsants: carbamazepine
- Antianxiety agents: diazepam
- Tricyclic antidepressants: amitriptyline
- Serotonin norepinephrine reuptake inhibitors (SNRIs): duloxetine
- Anesthetics: lidocaine
- Antihistamine: hydroxyzine
- Glucocorticoids: dexamethasone
- Antiemetics: ondansetron

Patient-controlled analgesia (PCA)

PCA is a medication delivery system that allows clients to self-administer safe doses of opioids.

- Small, frequent dosing ensures consistent plasma levels.
- Clients have less lag time between identified need and delivery of medication, which increases their sense of control and can decrease the amount of medication they need.
- Morphine and hydromorphone are typical opioids for PCA delivery.
- Clients should tell the nurse if using the pump does not control the pain.
- To prevent inadvertent overdosing, the client is the only person who should push the PCA button.

Other strategies

- Other strategies for effective pain management include the following.
  - Taking a proactive approach by giving analgesics before pain becomes too severe. It takes less medication to prevent pain than to treat pain.
  - Instructing clients to report developing or recurrent pain and not wait until pain is severe (for PRN pain medication).
  - Explaining misconceptions about pain. Qᴘᴄᴄ
  - Helping clients reduce fear and anxiety.
  - Creating a treatment plan that includes both nonpharmacological and pharmacological pain-relief measures.
- Strategies specific for relieving chronic pain include the above interventions, plus:
  - Administering long-acting or controlled-release opioid analgesics (including the transdermal route).
  - Administering analgesics around the clock rather than PRN.

COMPLICATIONS

- Undertreatment of pain is a serious complication and can lead to increased anxiety with acute pain and depression with chronic pain. Check clients for pain frequently, and intervene as appropriate.
- Sedation, respiratory depression, and coma can occur as a result of overdosing. Sedation always precedes respiratory depression. Qs
  - Identify high-risk clients (such as older adult clients). Ⓖ
  - Carefully titrate doses while closely monitoring respiratory status.
  - Stop the opioid and give the antagonist naloxone if respiratory rate is less than 8/min and shallow, or the client is difficult to arouse.
  - Monitor the client closely following administration of naloxone. The duration of the certain opioids can last longer than the effectiveness of the naloxone, creating a need for additional doses.
  - Identify the cause of sedation.
  - Use a sedation scale in addition to a pain rating scale to monitor pain, especially when administering opioids.

Application Exercises

1. A nurse is evaluating the pain level of a client who reports severe abdominal pain. The nurse asks the client whether he has nausea and has been vomiting. The nurse is determining which of the following components of a pain assessment?

   A. Presence of associated manifestations

   B. Location of the pain

   C. Pain quality

   D. Aggravating and relieving factors

2. A nurse is collecting data from a client who reports continued pain despite analgesia. Which of the following actions should the nurse take to determine the intensity of the client's pain?

   A. Ask the client what precipitates his pain.

   B. Question the client about the location of his pain.

   C. Offer the client a pain scale to measure his pain.

   D. Use open-ended questions to identify the sensation of his pain.

3. A nurse is caring for a client who is receiving morphine via a patient-controlled analgesia (PCA) infusion device after abdominal surgery. Which of the following client statements indicates that the client understands how to use the device?

   A. "I'll wait to use the device until it's absolutely necessary."

   B. "I'll be careful about pushing the button so I don't get an overdose."

   C. "I should tell the nurse if the pain doesn't stop after I use this device."

   D. "I will ask my son to push the dose button when I am sleeping."

4. A nurse is discussing pain assessment with a newly licensed nurse. Which of the following information should the nurse include?

   A. Most clients exaggerate their level of pain.

   B. Pain must have an identifiable source to justify the use of opioids.

   C. Objective data are essential in measuring pain.

   D. Pain is whatever the client says it is.

5. A nurse is monitoring a client who is receiving opioid analgesia. Which of the following findings should the nurse identify as adverse effects of opioid analgesics? (Select all that apply.)

   A. Urinary incontinence

   B. Diarrhea

   C. Bradypnea

   D. Orthostatic hypotension

   E. Nausea

PRACTICE Active Learning Scenario

A nurse at a long-term care facility is reviewing with a group of newly licensed nurses the various types of pain clients can experience. Use the ATI Active Learning Template: Basic Concept to complete this item.

UNDERLYING PRINCIPLES: List the four different types of pain, their definitions, and characteristics.

Application Exercises Key

1. A. **CORRECT:** Nausea and vomiting are common manifestations clients have when they are in pain.

   B. The location of the pain is where the client feels the pain.

   C. Pain quality is what the pain feels like, such as throbbing and dull.

   D. Aggravating and relieving factors are what might make the pain better or worse.

   ⓝ *NCLEX® Connection: Pharmacological Therapies, Medication Administration*

2. A. Assessment of pain triggers will provide valuable information to help select pain-control interventions, but it does not provide information about the intensity of pain.

   B. Identification of the location of the client's pain provides valuable information to help select pain-control interventions, but it does not provide information about the intensity of pain.

   C. **CORRECT:** The nurse should use a pain scale to help the client measure the amount of pain he has and its intensity.

   D. Asking open-ended questions is important in pain assessment, but it does not provide for quantification of pain intensity.

   ⓝ *NCLEX® Connection: Pharmacological Therapies, Pharmacological Pain Management*

3. A. The client may use the device when he begins to feel pain. It will help prevent unnecessary worsening of the pain and more doses of analgesia to provide relief.

   B. A feature of PCA devices is the timing control or lockout mechanism, which enforces a preset minimum interval between medication doses. This safety feature is one means of preventing an overdose, because the client cannot self-administer another dose of medication until that time interval has passed.

   C. **CORRECT:** The nurse should identify that PCA is a method of delivering pain medication through an electronic infusion device that allows the client to self-administer pain medication on an as-needed basis. If the client is not achieving adequate pain control, he should let the nurse know so that she can initiate a reevaluation of the client's pain management plan.

   D. The client is the only one who should operate the PCA pump. In situations where the client is not able to do so, the provider may authorize a nurse or a family member to operate the pump.

   ⓝ *NCLEX® Connection: Pharmacological Therapies, Pharmacological Pain Management*

4. A. A misconception about pain is that clients exaggerate their pain level.

   B. Clients can have pain without being able to identify the source.

   C. Objective data are not always present when clients have pain.

   D. **CORRECT:** The nurse should identify that pain is a subjective experience, and the client is the best source of information about it.

   ⓝ *NCLEX® Connection: Basic Care and Comfort, Nonpharmacological Comfort Interventions*

5. A. Urinary retention, not urinary incontinence, is a common adverse effect of opioid analgesia.

   B. Constipation, not diarrhea, is a common adverse effect of opioid analgesia.

   C. **CORRECT:** Respiratory depression, which causes respiratory rates to drop to dangerously low levels, is a common adverse effect of opioid analgesia.

   D. **CORRECT:** Dizziness or lightheadedness when changing positions is a common adverse effect of opioid analgesia.

   E. **CORRECT:** Nausea and vomiting are common adverse effects of opioid analgesia.

   ⓝ *NCLEX® Connection: Pharmacological Therapies, Expected Actions/Outcomes*

PRACTICE Answer

Using the ATI Active Learning Template: Basic Concept

UNDERLYING PRINCIPLES

Acute pain
- Definition: Protective, temporary, usually self-limiting, resolves with tissue healing
- Physiological responses: Tachycardia, hypertension, anxiety, diaphoresis, muscle tension
- Behavioral responses: Grimacing, moaning, flinching, guarding

Chronic pain
- Definition: Not protective; ongoing or recurs frequently, lasts longer than 3 months, persists beyond tissue healing, can be chronic cancer pain or chronic noncancer pain
- Physiological responses: No change in vital signs, depression, fatigue, decreased level of functioning, disability

Nociceptive pain
- Definition: Arises from damage to or inflammation of tissue other than that of the peripheral and central nervous systems, is usually throbbing, aching, localized; pain typically responds to opioids and nonopioid medications
- Types of nociceptive pain
  - Somatic: In bones, joints, muscles, skin, or connective tissues
  - Visceral: In internal organs such as the stomach or intestines, can cause referred pain

Neuropathic pain
- Definition: Arises from abnormal or damaged pain nerves (phantom limb pain, pain below the level of a spinal cord injury, diabetic neuropathy), usually intense, shooting, burning, or "pins and needles"
- Physiological responses to adjuvant medications (antidepressants, antispasmodic agents, skeletal muscle relaxants)

ⓝ *NCLEX® Connection: Physiological Adaptation, Basic Pathophysiology*

CHAPTER 5

CHAPTER 5 *Meningitis*

Meningitis is an inflammation of the meninges, which are the membranes that protect the brain and spinal cord. Infection is the cause of inflammation.

Viral, or aseptic, meningitis is the most common form of meningitis and commonly resolves without treatment. Fungal meningitis is common in clients who have AIDS. Bacterial (or septic) meningitis is a contagious infection with a high mortality rate. Early treatment and care improves the client's prognosis.

There are three vaccines for different pathogens that cause bacterial meningitis. One is available for high-risk populations, such as residential college students.

HEALTH PROMOTION AND DISEASE PREVENTION

Haemophilus influenzae type b (Hib) vaccine
Ensure infants receive the vaccine for bacterial meningitis on schedule. Provide a series of four doses beginning at 2 months of age, with the final dose at 12 to 15 months.

Pneumococcal polysaccharide vaccine (PPSV)
Though primarily intended to prevent respiratory infection, this immunization also decreases the risk for central nervous system (CNS) infections. Immunize adults who are immunocompromised, have a chronic disease, smoke cigarettes, have cochlear implants, have cerebrospinal fluid leakage, or live in a long-term care facility. Follow CDC guidelines for reimmunization. Give one dose to adults older than 65 who do not have history of disease or prior immunization.

Meningococcal vaccine (MCV4) (*Neisseria meningitidis*)
Ensure that adolescents receive the vaccine on schedule and prior to living in a residential setting in college. Individuals in other communal living conditions (such as military) also should be immunized. Provide an initial dose for healthy children between the ages of 11 to 12, with a booster administered at age 16.

DATA COLLECTION

RISK FACTORS

Viral meningitis
- Viral illnesses (the mumps, measles, herpes, cytomegalovirus, arboviruses [West Nile]).
- There is no vaccine against viral meningitis.

Fungal meningitis: Fulminant fungal-based infection of the sinuses are from the organism *Cryptococcus neoformans.*

Bacterial meningitis: Bacterial-based infections (otitis media, pneumonia, sinusitis) in which the infectious microorganism is *Neisseria meningitidis, Streptococcus pneumoniae,* or *Haemophilus influenzae*

Immunosuppression

Direct contamination of spinal fluid

Invasive procedures, skull fracture, or penetrating wound

Overcrowded living conditions

EXPECTED FINDINGS

SUBJECTIVE DATA
- Excruciating, constant headache that worsens with head movement
- Nuchal rigidity (stiff neck)
- Photophobia (sensitivity to light)

OBJECTIVE DATA: Physical findings
- Fever and chills
- Nausea and vomiting
- Altered level of consciousness (confusion, disorientation, lethargy, difficulty arousing, coma)
- Positive Kernig's sign (resistance and pain with extension of the client's leg from a flexed position)
- Positive Brudzinski's sign (flexion of the knees and hips occurring with deliberate flexion of the client's neck)
- Hyperactive deep tendon reflexes
- Seizures
- Red macular rash (meningococcal meningitis)
- Restlessness, irritability

LABORATORY TESTS

- **Urine, throat, nose, and blood culture and sensitivity**: Perform culture and sensitivity of various body fluids to identify possible infectious bacteria and an appropriate broad-spectrum antibiotic. Not definitive for meningitis, but can guide initial selection of antimicrobial.
- **CBC**: Elevated WBC count

DIAGNOSTIC PROCEDURES

Cerebrospinal fluid (CSF) analysis performed via lumbar puncture (spinal tap)

- CSF analysis is the most definitive diagnostic procedure. CSF is collected during a lumbar puncture performed by the provider.
- Results indicative of meningitis
  - Appearance of CSF: cloudy (bacterial) or clear (viral)
  - Elevated WBC
  - Elevated protein
  - Decreased glucose (bacterial)
  - Elevated CSF pressure
- Counterimmunoelectrophoresis (CIE) of CSF can determine whether the infectious agent is viral or protozoa. Clients who received antibiotics before CSF was collected should have CIE.

CT scan and MRI: A CT scan or an MRI helps identify increased intracranial pressure (ICP) or an abscess.

PATIENT-CENTERED CARE

NURSING CARE

- Isolate any client suspected to have meningitis.
- Maintain isolation precautions per hospital policy.
  - The nurse should initiate droplet precautions, which require a private room. Discontinue droplet precautions once 24 hr of antibiotic therapy is complete and nasal secretions are no longer infectious. Clients who have bacterial meningitis might need to remain on droplet precautions continuously.
  - Implement standard precautions for all clients who have meningitis.
- Implement fever-reduction measures, such as a cooling blanket, if necessary.
- Report meningococcal infections to the public health department.
- Decrease environmental stimuli.
- Provide a quiet environment.
- Minimize exposure to bright light (natural and electric).
- Maintain bed rest with the head of the bed elevated to 30°.
- Monitor for increased ICP.
- Monitor the abdomen for distension and bowel sounds
- Tell the client to avoid coughing and sneezing, which increase ICP.
- Maintain client safety, such as seizure precautions. **Qs**
- Replace fluid and electrolytes as indicated by laboratory values.
- Older adult clients are at an increased risk for secondary complications, such as pneumonia. **©**

MEDICATIONS

The client usually requires a combination of oral and IV antibiotic therapy.

- **Ceftriaxone or cefotaxime in combination with vancomycin**: Antibiotics given until culture and sensitivity results are available. These are effective for treating bacterial infections.
- **Phenytoin**: Anticonvulsants given if ICP increases or client experiences a seizure.
- **Dexamethasone**: Given to decrease inflammation.
- **Mannitol, furosemide**: Administer to reduce cerebral edema.
- **Acetaminophen, ibuprofen**: Analgesics given to treat headache and fever. Use nonopioids to avoid masking changes in the level of consciousness.
- **Ciprofloxacin, rifampin, or ceftriaxone**: Prophylactic antibiotics given to individuals in close contact with the client.

COMPLICATIONS

Increased ICP

Meningitis can cause ICP to increase, possibly to the point of brain herniation.

NURSING ACTIONS

- Monitor for indications of increasing ICP (decreased level of consciousness lethargy, pupillary changes, impaired extraocular movements, hypertension, bradycardia, vomiting).
- Provide interventions to reduce ICP (position the head of the bed elevation at 30° with the head and neck midline, and prevent coughing and straining). **Qs**
- The provider can prescribe mannitol IV.

SIADH

SIADH can be a complication of meningitis due to abnormal stimulation to the hypothalamic area of the brain, causing excess secretion of antidiuretic hormone (vasopressin).

NURSING ACTIONS

- Monitor for manifestations (dilute blood, concentrated urine, polydipsia).
- Provide interventions (administer demeclocycline, and restrict fluids).
- Monitor weight daily, I&O, and electrolyte balance.

Septic emboli

- Septic emboli can form during meningitis and travel to other parts of the body, particularly the hands, but can occur in the feet as well.
- Development of gangrene can necessitate an amputation.
- Septic emboli can lead to disseminated intravascular coagulation or stroke.

NURSING ACTIONS

- Monitor circulatory status of extremities and coagulation studies.
- Report any alterations immediately to the provider.

Application Exercises

1. A nurse is collecting data from a client who reports severe headache and a stiff neck. Data collection reveals positive Kernig's and Brudzinski's signs. Which of the following actions should the nurse perform first?

   A. Administer antibiotics.

   B. Implement droplet precautions.

   C. Obtain an IV access.

   D. Decrease bright lights.

2. A nurse is checking for the presence of Brudzinski's sign in a client who has suspected meningitis. Which of the following actions should the nurse take? (Select all that apply.)

   A. Place client in supine position.

   B. Flex client's hip and knee.

   C. Place hands behind the client's neck.

   D. Bend client's head toward chest.

   E. Straighten the client's flexed leg at the knee.

3. A nurse is contributing to the plan of care for a client who has meningitis and is at risk for increased intracranial pressure (ICP). Which of the following interventions should the nurse recommend? (Select all that apply.)

   A. Implement seizure precautions.

   B. Perform neurological checks four times a day.

   C. Administer morphine for the report of neck and generalized pain.

   D. Turn off room lights and television.

   E. Monitor for impaired extraocular movements.

   F. Encourage the client to cough frequently.

4. A health department nurse is reviewing the use of the meningococcal vaccine (MCV4) for the prevention of meningitis with a newly licensed nurse. Which of the following information should the nurse include?

   A. The vaccine reduces the risk of respiratory infection.

   B. Administer this vaccine in a series of four doses.

   C. Recommend this vaccine for adolescents before starting college.

   D. The vaccine series begins at 2 months of age.

5. A nurse is contributing to the plan of care for a client who has bacterial meningitis. Which of the following interventions should the nurse include? (Select all that apply.)

   A. Monitor for hypotension.

   B. Provide an emesis basin at the bedside.

   C. Administer antipyretic medication.

   D. Perform a skin assessment.

   E. Keep the head of the bed flat.

PRACTICE Active Learning Scenario

A nurse is reviewing the plan of care for a client who has bacterial meningitis. Use the ATI Active Learning Template: System Disorder to complete this item.

ALTERATION IN HEALTH (DIAGNOSIS):
Define bacterial meningitis.

MEDICATIONS: Identify three medications, their actions, and the reason for administration.

COMPLICATIONS: Describe two complications of meningitis.

Application Exercises Key

1. A. The nurse should administer antibiotics to stop the microorganisms from multiplying, but this is not the priority action.

    B. **CORRECT:** The client is exhibiting manifestations of possible meningitis. When using the urgent vs. nonurgent approach to care, the nurse determines the priority action is to initiate droplet precautions to prevent spread of the disease to others.

    C. The nurse should initiate IV access to allow IV medication and fluid administration, but this is not the priority action.

    D. The nurse should decrease bright lights because photophobia is a manifestation of meningitis, but this is not the priority action.

    Ⓝ *NCLEX® Connection: Basic Care and Comfort, Nonpharmacological Comfort Interventions*

2. A. **CORRECT:** The nurse should place the client in supine position when checking for Brudzinski's sign.

    B. The nurse should flex the client's hip and knee when checking for Kernig's sign.

    C. **CORRECT:** The nurse should place her hands behind the client's neck when checking for Brudzinski's sign, in order to flex the client's neck.

    D. **CORRECT:** The nurse should bend the client's head toward the chest when checking for Brudzinski's sign.

    E. The nurse should straighten the client's flexed leg at the knee when checking for Kernig's sign.

    Ⓝ *NCLEX® Connection: Reduction of Risk Potential, Diagnostic Tests*

3. A. **CORRECT:** The client is at risk for seizures due to possible increased ICP. Therefore, the nurse should implement seizure precautions to reduce the client's risk for injury.

    B. The nurse should perform neurological checks more frequently due to the client's risk for increased ICP.

    C. The nurse should avoid administering opioids to a client who is at risk for increased ICP. Opioids can mask changes in the client's level of consciousness.

    D. **CORRECT:** The nurse should turn off room lights and the television, because they can increase neuron stimulation and cause a seizure when a client is at risk for increased ICP.

    E. **CORRECT:** The nurse should monitor for impaired extraocular movements because this finding can indicate increased ICP.

    F. The nurse should instruct the client to avoid coughing because this action can cause increased ICP.

    Ⓝ *NCLEX® Connection: Physiological Adaptation, Alterations in Body Systems*

4. A. The pneumococcal vaccine reduces the risk of respiratory infection. However, it also reduces the risk of CNS infection.

    B. The HIB vaccine is administered to infants in a series of four doses.

    C. **CORRECT:** The nurse should recommend the meningococcal vaccine for adolescents prior to starting college due to the increased risk for infection in communal living facilities.

    D. The HIB vaccine series begins for infants at 2 months of age.

    Ⓝ *NCLEX® Connection: Health Promotion and Maintenance, Health Promotion/Disease Prevention*

5. A. The nurse should plan to monitor for hypertension when a client has meningitis.

    B. **CORRECT:** The nurse should provide an emesis basin at the bedside, because the client who has meningitis can have nausea and vomiting.

    C. **CORRECT:** The nurse should plan to administer antipyretic medication for fever to a client who has meningitis.

    D. **CORRECT:** The nurse should perform a skin assessment to determine whether the client has a red macular rash associated with meningococcal meningitis.

    E. The nurse should elevate the head of the client's bed 30° to promote venous drainage from the head and prevent increased ICP.

    Ⓝ *NCLEX® Connection: Pharmacological Therapies, Dosage Calculations*

PRACTICE Answer

Using the ATI Active Learning Template: System Disorder

ALTERATION IN HEALTH (DIAGNOSIS): Bacterial meningitis is a bacterial infection that causes an inflammation of the meninges, the membranes that protect the brain and spinal cord.

MEDICATIONS
- Ceftriaxone with vancomycin: antibiotics administered to treat the infection.
- Acetaminophen: an antipyretic used to treat a fever.
- Phenytoin: an anticonvulsant given to prevent the client from experiencing a seizure when at risk of ICP.

COMPLICATIONS
- Increased ICP, which can lead to seizures, coma, and death.
- Syndrome of inappropriate antidiuretic hormone (SIADH), which is due to pressure from inflammation abnormally stimulating the hypothalamus, causing increased secretion of antidiuretic hormone (vasopressin).
- Septic emboli can occur as a result of meningitis. This complication can lead to disseminated intravascular coagulation, stroke, or gangrene.

Ⓝ *NCLEX® Connection: Pharmacological Therapies, Dosage Calculations*

UNIT 2   NURSING CARE OF CLIENTS WHO HAVE
NEUROSENSORY DISORDERS
SECTION: CENTRAL NERVOUS SYSTEM DISORDERS

CHAPTER 6 *Seizures and Epilepsy*

Seizures are abrupt, abnormal, excessive, and uncontrolled electrical discharge of neurons within the brain that can cause alterations in the level of consciousness and changes in motor and sensory ability and behavior.

Epilepsy is chronic recurring abnormal brain electrical activity resulting in two or more seizures. Seizures resulting from identifiable causes (substance withdrawal, fever) are not considered epilepsy.

The International Classification of Epileptic Seizures uses three broad categories to describe seizures: generalized, partial, and unclassified.

DATA COLLECTION

RISK FACTORS

- **Genetic predisposition:** Absence seizures are more common in children and tend to occur in families.
- **Acute febrile state:** Particularly among infants and children younger than 2 years old.
- **Head trauma:** Early or late onset (up to 9 months). Incidence increases when the head trauma includes a skull fracture.
- **Cerebral edema:** Seizure activity occurs acutely and tends to disappear when edema is successfully treated.
- **Abrupt cessation of antiepileptic drugs (AEDs):** Seizure activity occurs as a rebound response.
- **Infection:** If intracranial, results from an increase in intracranial pressure; if systemic, results from a persistent febrile state.
- **Metabolic disorder:** A seizure is the result of insufficient or excessive chemicals within the brain, such as occurring from hypoglycemia or hyponatremia.
- **Exposure to toxins:** Especially those associated with pesticides, carbon monoxide, and lead poisoning.
- **Stroke:** Usually occurs within the first 24 hr following a stroke as a result of increased intracranial pressure.
- **Heart disease:** Cerebrovascular disease is a common cause for an increase in seizures in older adults. ⓒ

- **Brain tumor:** If benign, seizures are the result of the increased bulk associated with the tumor; if malignant, are associated with the inability of the brain tissue to function.
- **Hypoxia:** Results from a decreased oxygen level of the brain; necessary for neuronal activity.
- **Acute substance withdrawal:** Dehydration accompanies withdrawal, creating a toxic level of the substance in the body.
- **Fluid and electrolyte imbalances:** Results from abnormal levels of nutrients required for neuronal function.

TRIGGERING FACTORS
- Not taking medication for seizures
- Increased physical activity
- Excessive stress
- Hyperventilation
- Overwhelming fatigue
- Acute alcohol ingestion
- Excessive caffeine intake
- Exposure to flashing lights
- Substances such as cocaine, aerosols, and inhaled glue products

EXPECTED FINDINGS

Generalized seizures involve both cerebral hemispheres. Generalized seizures can begin with an aura (alteration in vision, smell, hearing, or emotional feeling).

Clients can experience different types of generalized seizures.
- **Tonic-clonic or grand mal seizure**
  - The tonic episode begins for only a few seconds with stiffening of muscles and loss of consciousness.
  - Clonic episode lasts 1 to 2 min with rhythmic jerking of the extremities and follows the tonic episode.
  - Breathing can stop during the tonic phase and become irregular during the clonic phase.
  - Cyanosis can accompany breathing irregularities.
  - Biting of the cheek or tongue can occur during clonic phase.
  - Incontinence can also accompany a tonic-clonic seizure.
  - Postictal phase (a period of confusion and sleepiness) follows the seizure and can last for several hours. Unconsciousness can last for 30 min, at which time the client awakens slowly and is usually confused and disoriented. Often the client reports headache, fatigue, and muscle aches. The client can have no memory of what happened just before the seizure.
- **Tonic seizure**
  - Only the tonic phase is experienced.
  - The client suddenly loses consciousness and experiences sudden increased muscle contraction and rigidity, loss of consciousness, and autonomic manifestations (arrhythmia, apnea, vomiting, incontinence, salivation).
  - The seizure usually lasts 30 seconds to several minutes.

- **Clonic seizure**
  - Only the clonic phase is experienced.
  - The seizure lasts several minutes.
  - During this type of seizure, the muscles contract and relax.
- **Absence or petit mal seizure**
  - Most common in children
  - The seizure consists of a change of consciousness lasting a few seconds, blank staring (like daydreaming), blinking or fluttering of eyes, and lip smacking.
  - Motor activity is absent during the seizure.
  - The client resumes baseline neurological function after the seizure, with no apparent sequelae.
  - This type of seizure lasts for seconds.

Partial or focal/local seizure: Seizure activity begins in one cerebral hemisphere. The client can experience two types of partial seizures.
- **Complex partial seizure**
  - Associated automatisms (behaviors that the client is unaware of, such as lip smacking or picking at clothes).
  - The seizure can cause a loss of consciousness or blackout for several minutes.
  - Amnesia can occur immediately prior to and after the seizure.
  - The seizure can have an aura.
- **Simple partial seizure**
  - Consciousness is maintained throughout simple partial seizures.
  - Seizure activity can consist of unusual sensations, tingling, hallucinations, or flashing lights.
  - Lasts for seconds.

Unclassified or idiopathic seizures: These types of seizures do not fit into other categories, account for half of all seizure activity, and occur for no known reason.

LABORATORY TESTS

- Tests should include alcohol and illicit substance levels, HIV testing, and if suspected, screen for the presence of excessive toxins.
- Include a comprehensive metabolic panel (CBC) and blood glucose levels.

DIAGNOSTIC PROCEDURES

- Electroencephalogram (EEG) records electrical activity and can identify the origin of seizure activity.
- Magnetic resonance imaging (MRI), computed tomography (CT) imaging/computed axial tomography (CAT) scan, positron emission tomography (PET) scan, cerebrospinal fluid (CSF) analysis, and skull x-ray can be used to identify or rule out potential causes of seizures.

PATIENT-CENTERED CARE

NURSING CARE

During a seizure
- Protect the client's privacy.
- Protect the client from injury (move furniture away, hold head in lap if on the floor). Qs
- Position the client to provide a patent airway.
- Be prepared to suction oral secretions.
- Turn the client to the side to decrease the risk of aspiration.
- Loosen restrictive clothing.
- Do not attempt to restrain the client.
- Do not attempt to open the jaw or insert airway during seizure activity (can damage teeth, lips, and tongue).
- Do not use padded tongue blades.
- Document onset and duration of seizure and findings (level of consciousness, apnea, cyanosis, motor activity, incontinence) prior to, during, and following the seizure.

After a seizure
- This is the postictal phase of the seizure episode.
- Maintain the client in a side-lying position to prevent aspiration and to facilitate drainage of oral secretions.
- Check vital signs.
- Check for injuries.
- Perform neurological checks.
- Allow the client to rest if necessary.
- Reorient and calm the client, who might be agitated or confused.
- Determine if client experienced an aura, which can indicate the origin of seizure in the brain.
- Try to determine possible trigger (fatigue).

MEDICATIONS

Administer AEDs such as phenytoin, carbamazepine, valproic acid, or gabapentin.
- Initial goal is to control seizure activity using one medication.
- Ineffectiveness of the medication can require an increase in the dose or adding or substituting another antiepileptic medication.
- Scheduled routine blood tests to determine therapeutic levels and ensure compliance and effectiveness of the medication. Qebp
- Administer the medications at the same time every day to enhance effectiveness.
- Allergic reactions to an antiepileptic medication are rare but can occur immediately or late in therapy and will require replacement with another antiepileptic medication.
- Notify the provider of the client's use of over-the-counter medications and reinforce the teaching with the client about medication-medication interactions (decreased effectiveness of oral contraceptives), and medication-food interactions.
- Routine oral hygiene and dental visits can minimize oral gum overgrowth, because an adverse effect of some antiepileptic medications is gingival hyperplasia (phenytoin).

- Avoid oral contraceptives when taking phenytoin, which decreases contraceptive effectiveness.
- Phenytoin when administered with warfarin can cause a decrease in the effectiveness of the oral anticoagulants.

INTERPROFESSIONAL CARE

- Ask social services to refer the client and family to a local support group.
- Provide information about seizures from the Epilepsy Foundation.

THERAPEUTIC PROCEDURES

Vagal nerve stimulation and surgical procedures can help the client whose seizures are not controlled with medication therapy.

Vagal nerve stimulator (VNS) (6.1)

- The VNS is a device implanted into the left chest wall and connected to an electrode placed on the left vagus nerve.
- This procedure is performed under general anesthesia.
- The device is then programmed to administer intermittent stimulation of the brain via stimulation of the vagal nerve, at a rate specific to the client's needs.

CLIENT EDUCATION: The VNS can cause temporary hoarseness, mild cough and dyspnea, and change in voice.

Surgical treatment

Surgical procedures are available for clients who experience partial or generalized seizure.
- **Partial corpus callosotomy** is performed to resect the corpus callosum, preventing neuronal discharges across hemispheres to reduce the severity and frequency of seizures.
- **Partial temporal lobe resection** can help to eliminate temporal lobe seizures.

CLIENT EDUCATION
- Seizure management includes monitoring antiepileptic medication serum levels to maintain a therapeutic medication level.
- Possible medication interactions include decreased effectiveness of oral contraceptives.
- Wear a medical identification tag at all times.
- All antiepileptic medication can cause sedation, drowsiness, and lethargy. Research state driving laws. Some states restrict or limit driving for individuals who have a recent history of seizures. Qs
- Do not to drink alcohol or use central nervous system depressants when taking an antiepileptic medication.
- Never stop taking antiepileptic medication unless prescribed by the provider.
- Have routine dental check-ups.

6.1 Vagal nerve stimulator

electrodes

vagus nerve

electrodes

implanted wire
pulse generator

implanted wire

pulse generator

COMPLICATIONS

Status epilepticus

This condition manifests as repeated seizure activity occurring over 30 min, or a single prolonged seizure that lasts more than 5 min.
- The complications associated with this condition relate to decreased oxygen levels, inability of the brain to return to normal functioning, and continued assault on neuronal tissue.
- Status epilepticus is an acute condition requiring immediate treatment to prevent permanent loss of brain function.
- The usual causes are substance withdrawal, sudden withdrawal from AEDs, head injury, cerebral edema, infection, and metabolic disturbances. Qтc

NURSING ACTIONS
- Maintain an airway, provide oxygen, maintain IV access, perform ECG monitoring, and monitor pulse oximetry and ABG results.
- Observe clients after administration of IV diazepam or lorazepam, and administer phenytoin or fosphenytoin.

Application Exercises

1. A nurse is collecting data from a client who has a seizure disorder. The client reports sensing an aura and is about to have a seizure. Which of the following actions should the nurse implement? (Select all that apply.)

   A. Provide privacy.

   B. Ease the client to the floor if standing.

   C. Move furniture away from the client.

   D. Loosen the client's clothing.

   E. Protect the client's head with padding.

   F. Restrain the client.

2. A nurse is caring for a client who just experienced a generalized seizure. Which of the following actions should the nurse perform first?

   A. Keep the client in a side-lying position.

   B. Document the duration of the seizure.

   C. Reorient the client to the environment.

   D. Provide client hygiene.

3. A nurse is reinforcing discharge instructions with a female client who has a prescription for phenytoin. Which of the following information should the nurse include?

   A. Consider taking oral contraceptives when on this medication.

   B. Watch for receding gums when taking the medication.

   C. Take the medication at the same time every day.

   D. Provide a urine sample to determine therapeutic levels of the medication.

4. A nurse is reinforcing education about trigger factors that can cause seizures with a client who has a new diagnosis of generalized seizures. Which of the following information should the nurse include in this review? (Select all that apply.)

   A. Avoid overwhelming fatigue.

   B. Remove caffeinated products from the diet.

   C. Limit looking at flashing lights.

   D. Perform aerobic exercise.

   E. Limit episodes of hypoventilation.

   F. Use of aerosol hairspray is recommended.

5. A nurse is reinforcing discharge teaching to a client who has seizures and received a vagal nerve stimulator to decrease seizure activity. Which of the following statements should the nurse include?

   A. "I will have a sore throat after placement of the stimulator."

   B. "This stimulator will stop my tonic/clonic seizures."

   C. "I can expect to have a temporary voice change."

   D. "The device is inserted under local anesthesia."

PRACTICE Active Learning Scenario

A nurse is contributing to the plan of care for a client who is experiencing status epilepticus. What concepts should the nurse take into consideration when making recommendations? Use the ATI Active Learning Template: Basic Concept to complete this item.

RELATED CONTENT: Define the condition.

UNDERLYING PRINCIPLES: Describe four possible causes.

NURSING INTERVENTIONS: Describe five actions the nurse should plan to take.

Application Exercises Key

1. A. **CORRECT:** The nurse should implement privacy to minimize the client's embarrassment.

    B. **CORRECT:** The nurse should ease the client to the floor to prevent falling and injury.

    C. **CORRECT:** The nurse should move the furniture away from the client to prevent injury.

    D. **CORRECT:** The nurse should loosen the client's clothing to minimize restriction of movement.

    E. **CORRECT:** The nurse should protect the client's head from injury by placing the client's head in her lap or using a pillow or blanket under the head during a seizure.

    F. The nurse should not restrain the client. Restraint can increase the client's risk for injury or more seizure activity.

    Ⓝ *NCLEX® Connection: Reduction of Risk Potential, Potential for Complications of Diagnostic Tests/Treatments/Procedures*

2. A. **CORRECT:** The greatest risk to the client is aspiration during the postictal phase. Therefore, the priority intervention is to keep the client in a side-lying position so secretions can drain from the mouth keeping the airway patent.

    B. The nurse should document the duration of the seizure in the client's medical record, but there is another action that the nurse should take first.

    C. The nurse should reorient the client to the environment because the client can feel confused, but there is another action that the nurse should take first.

    D. The nurse should provide client hygiene if the client experienced incontinence during the seizure, but there is another action that the nurse should take first.

    Ⓝ *NCLEX® Connection: Physiological Adaptation, Alterations in Body Systems*

3. A. Contraceptive effectiveness is decreased when taking phenytoin.

    B. Phenytoin causes overgrowth of the gums.

    C. **CORRECT:** The client should take phenytoin at the same time every day to enhance effectiveness.

    D. The client should have periodic blood tests to determine the therapeutic level of phenytoin.

    Ⓝ *NCLEX® Connection: Pharmacological Therapies, Medication Administration*

4. A. **CORRECT:** Overwhelming fatigue can trigger a seizure by stimulating abnormal electrical neuron activity.

    B. **CORRECT:** Caffeinated products from the diet can trigger a seizure by stimulating abnormal electrical neuron activity.

    C. **CORRECT:** Flashing lights can trigger a seizure by stimulating abnormal electrical neuron activity.

    D. The client should avoid vigorous physical activity, which can help to avoid triggering a seizure.

    E. The client should limit excess hyperventilation, which can trigger a seizure by stimulating abnormal electrical neuron activity.

    F. The client should avoid using aerosol hairspray, which can trigger a seizure by stimulating abnormal electrical neuron activity.

    Ⓝ *NCLEX® Connection: Reduction of Risk Potential, Potential for Complications from Surgical Procedures and Health Alterations*

5. A. The client should expect to have a hoarse throat following the procedure.

    B. The stimulator will stop partial seizures.

    C. **CORRECT:** The client should expect to have a temporary voice change due to stimulation of the device on the vagal nerve.

    D. The stimulator is inserted under general anesthesia into the left chest wall and electrodes are connected to the vagal nerve that stimulates the brain.

    Ⓝ *NCLEX® Connection: Reduction of Risk Potential, Therapeutic Procedures*

PRACTICE Answer

Using the ATI Active Learning Template: Basic Concept

RELATED CONTENT: Status epilepticus is repeated seizure activity over 30 min or a single prolonged seizure that lasts more than 5 min.

UNDERLYING PRINCIPLES
- Substance withdrawal
- Withdrawal from antiepileptic medication
- Infection
- Head injury
- Cerebral edema
- Metabolic disturbances

NURSING INTERVENTIONS
- Maintain a patent airway.
- Assist with ECG monitoring.
- Review ABG results.
- Ensure the client has IV access.
- Provide oxygen.
- Monitor pulse oximetry.
- Assist with administration of medications including lorazepam, diazepam, phenytoin, or fosphenytoin.

Ⓝ *NCLEX® Connection: Physiological Adaptation, Basic Pathophysiology*

UNIT 2 NURSING CARE OF CLIENTS WHO HAVE NEUROSENSORY DISORDERS
SECTION: CENTRAL NERVOUS SYSTEM DISORDERS

CHAPTER 7 *Parkinson's Disease*

Parkinson's disease (PD) is a progressively debilitating disease that grossly affects motor function. It is characterized by four primary manifestations: tremor, muscle rigidity, bradykinesia (slow movement), and postural instability. These manifestations occur due to overstimulation of the basal ganglia by acetylcholine.

The secretion of dopamine and acetylcholine in the body produce inhibitory and excitatory effects on the muscles respectively. In PD, degenerative changes lead to decreased dopamine production, so that acetylcholine overstimulates the basal ganglia. This excessive stimulation without adequate dopamine to inhibit the response makes smooth, controlled movements difficult.

Treatment of PD focuses on increasing the amount of dopamine or decreasing the amount of acetylcholine in a client's brain.

DATA COLLECTION

RISK FACTORS

- Onset of symptoms between age 40 to 70
- More common in males
- Genetic predisposition
- Exposure to environmental toxins and chemical solvents
- Chronic use of antipsychotic medication

EXPECTED FINDINGS

- Report of fatigue
- Report of decreased manual dexterity over time

PHYSICAL ASSESSMENT FINDINGS

- Stooped posture
- Slow, shuffling, and propulsive gait
- Slow, monotonous speech
- Tremors/pill-rolling tremor of the fingers
- Muscle rigidity (rhythmic interruption, mildly restrictive, total resistance to movement)
- Bradykinesia/akinesia
- Masklike expression
- Autonomic symptoms (orthostatic hypotension, flushing, diaphoresis, drooling)
- Difficulty chewing and swallowing
- Dysarthria
- Progressive difficulty with ADLs
- Mood swings
- Cognitive impairment (dementia)

LABORATORY TESTS

- There are no definitive diagnostic procedures.
- The provider will consider manifestations and their progression, and rule out other disorders to diagnose PD. **(7.1)**

PATIENT-CENTERED CARE

NURSING CARE

- Administer medications at prescribed times. Monitor medication effectiveness, and make recommendations for changes in dosage and time of administration to provide best coverage.
- Monitor swallowing, and maintain adequate nutrition and weight. Consult speech-language pathologist to assess swallowing if the client demonstrates a risk for choking. **Qs**
  - Consult the dietitian for appropriate diet, which often includes semisolid foods and thickened liquids.
  - Document the client's weight at least weekly.
  - Keep a dietary intake log.
  - Encourage fluids and document intake.
  - Provide smaller, more frequent meals.
  - Sit the client upright to eat or drink, and keep upright for 1 hr following meals.
  - Consult with occupational therapist for adaptive eating devices. **Qтc**
  - Evaluate need for high-calorie, high-protein supplements to maintain the client's weight.

7.1 The five stages of Parkinson's disease involvement

As Parkinson's disease is a progressive disease, there are five stages of involvement.

Stage I	Stage II	Stage III	Stage IV	Stage V
Unilateral shaking or tremor of one limb.	Bilateral limb involvement occurs, making walking and balance difficult.	Physical movements slow down significantly, affecting walking more.	Tremors can decrease but akinesia and rigidity make day-to-day tasks difficult.	Client unable to stand or walk, is dependent for all care, and might exhibit dementia.

- Maintain client mobility for as long as possible.
  - Encourage exercise, such as yoga (can also improve mental status).
  - Encourage use of assistive devices as disease progresses.
  - Encourage range-of-motion (ROM) exercises at least twice daily.
  - Remind the client to stop occasionally when walking to slow down speed and reduce risk for injury.
  - Pace activities by providing rest periods.
  - Assist with ADLs as needed (hygiene, dressing).
- Promote client communication for as long as possible.
  - Reinforce teaching about facial muscle strengthening exercises.
  - Encourage the client to speak slowly and to pause frequently.
  - Use alternate forms of communication as appropriate (communication board).
  - Recommend client referral to a speech-language pathologist.
- Monitor mental and cognitive status.
  - Observe for signs of depression and dementia.
  - Provide a safe environment (no throw rugs, encourage the use of an electric razor). Qs
  - Identify personal and family coping with the client's chronic, degenerative disease.
  - Provide a list of community resources (support groups) to the client and family.
  - Recommend client referral to a social worker or case manager as condition advances (financial issues, long-term home care, and respite care). Qtc

MEDICATIONS

- Can take several weeks of use before improvement of symptoms is seen.
- While the client is taking a combination of medications, maintenance of therapeutic medication levels is necessary for adequate control.

Dopaminergics

- When given orally, medications such as levodopa are converted to dopamine in the brain, increasing dopamine levels in the basal ganglia.
- Dopaminergics may be combined with carbidopa to decrease peripheral metabolism of levodopa, requiring a smaller dose to make the same amount available to the brain. Adverse effects are subsequently less.
- Due to medication tolerance and metabolism, the dosage, form of medication, and administration times must be adjusted to avoid periods of poor mobility.

NURSING ACTIONS: Monitor for the "wearing-off" phenomenon and dyskinesias (problems with movement), which can indicate the need to adjust the dosage or time of administration or the need for a medication holiday.

Dopamine agonists

Dopamine agonists (bromocriptine, ropinirole, pramipexole) activate release of dopamine. May be used in conjunction with a dopaminergic for better results.

NURSING ACTIONS: Monitor for orthostatic hypotension, dyskinesias, and hallucinations. Qs

Anticholinergics

Anticholinergics (benztropine, trihexyphenidyl) help control tremors and rigidity.

NURSING ACTIONS: Monitor for anticholinergic effects (dry mouth, constipation, urinary retention, acute confusion).

Catechol O-methyltransferase (COMT) inhibitors

- COMT inhibitors, such as entacapone, decrease the breakdown of levodopa, making more available to the brain as dopamine. COMT inhibitors are used in conjunction with a dopaminergic and dopamine agonist for better results.
- Dark urine is a normal finding.

NURSING ACTIONS:
- Monitor for dyskinesia/hyperkinesia when used with levodopa.
- Monitor for diarrhea.

Monoamine oxidase type B (MAO-B) inhibitors

- MAO-B inhibitors (selegiline, rasagiline) inhibit monoamine oxidase type B activity and increase dopamine levels. MAO-B inhibitors reduce the wearing-off phenomenon when administered concurrently with levodopa.
- Severe reactions can occur when these medications are administered with sympathomimetics, meperidine, and fluoxetine.

CLIENT EDUCATION: Avoid foods high in tyramine, which can cause hypertensive crisis. Qs

Antivirals

- Antivirals, such as amantadine, stimulate release of dopamine and prevent its reuptake.
- Clients might experience anxiety, confusion, and anticholinergic effects.

NURSING ACTIONS: Monitor for discoloration of the skin that subsides when amantadine is discontinued.

THERAPEUTIC PROCEDURES

Stereotactic pallidotomy or thalamotomy

- Strict eligibility criteria generally includes those who have not responded to other therapies.
- Stereotactic pallidotomy and thalamotomy causes the destruction of a small portion of the brain within the globus pallidus or thalamus through the use of brain imaging and electrical stimulation.
- Target area is identified with a CT scan or an MRI.
- Mild electrical stimulation is provided through a burr hole to a target area.
- Client is evaluated for a decrease in tremors and muscle rigidity.
- When a decrease is elicited, a temporary lesion is formed and the client is reassessed.
- If symptomatic relief is demonstrated (alleviation of tremors and rigidity), a permanent lesion is made.

NURSING ACTIONS: Monitor for a neurological impairment and brain hemorrhage postoperatively.

Deep brain stimulation (DBS)

- An electrode is implanted in the thalamus.
- A current is delivered through a small pulse generator implanted under the skin of the upper chest. Electrical stimulation from DBS impulses decreases tremors and involuntary movements, and can decrease medications required to control PD.

NURSING ACTIONS: Monitor for infection, brain hemorrhage, and stroke-like symptoms.

INTERPROFESSIONAL CARE

- Because PD is a degenerative neurological disorder, long-term treatment and care must be accommodated.
- During the later stages of the disorder, the client needs referrals to and support from disciplines such as speech therapists, occupational therapists, physical therapists, and social service/case management.

COMPLICATIONS

Aspiration pneumonia

As PD advances in severity, alterations in chewing and swallowing worsen, increasing the risk for aspiration.

NURSING ACTIONS
- Use swallowing precautions to decrease the risk for aspiration. Qs
- Develop an individual dietary plan based on the speech therapist's recommendations, thickening liquids as needed.
- Have a nurse in attendance when the client is eating.
- Encourage the client to eat slowly and chew thoroughly before swallowing. Qs
- Feed the client in an upright position, and have suction equipment on standby.
- Evaluate need for enteral feedings to maintain weight and prevent aspiration as PD progresses.

Altered cognition (dementia, memory deficits)

Clients in advanced stages of PD can exhibit altered cognition in the form of dementia and memory loss.

NURSING ACTIONS
- Acknowledge the client's feelings.
- Provide for a safe environment.
- Review a comprehensive plan of care with the family, client, and interprofessional team. Qᵀᶜ

Application Exercises

1. A nurse is reviewing the plan of care for a client who has PD. Which of the following interventions should the nurse identify as the priority?

   A. Recommend a community support group.

   B. Integrate a daily exercise routine.

   C. Provide a walker for ambulation.

   D. Schedule a swallowing evaluation.

2. A nurse is contributing to a plan of care for the nutritional needs of a client who has stage IV Parkinson's disease. Which of the following actions should the nurse include in the plan of care? (Select all that apply.)

   A. Provide three large balanced meals daily.

   B. Record diet and fluid intake daily.

   C. Document weight every other week.

   D. Place the client in Fowler's position to eat.

   E. Offer nutritional supplements between meals.

3. A nurse is reinforcing teaching with the family of a client who has Parkinson's disease and a new prescription for bromocriptine. Which of the following statements by a family member should the nurse identify as understanding of the teaching?

   A. "This medication can cause dizziness."

   B. "This medication turns into dopamine once in the brain."

   C. "We should see improved mobility in 2 to 3 days."

   D. "We should avoid dopaminergics while taking this medication."

4. A nurse is collecting data from a client who has Parkinson's disease. Which of the following findings should the nurse expect? (Select all that apply.)

   A. Decreased vision

   B. Pill-rolling tremor of the fingers

   C. Shuffling gait

   D. Drooling

   E. Bilateral ankle edema

   F. Lack of facial expression

5. A nurse is caring for a client who has Parkinson's disease and is starting to display bradykinesia. Which of the actions should the nurse take?

   A. Remind the client to walk more quickly when ambulating.

   B. Complete passive range-of-motion exercises daily.

   C. Place the client on a low-protein, low-calorie diet.

   D. Give the client extra time to perform activities.

PRACTICE Active Learning Scenario

A nurse is contributing to the plan of care for a client who has a new diagnosis of Parkinson's disease. What should the nurse include in the plan of care? Use the ATI Active Learning Template: System Disorder to complete this item.

ALTERATION IN HEALTH (DIAGNOSIS): Define Parkinson's disease.

COMPLICATIONS: Identify four.

NURSING CARE: Describe six nursing actions.

Application Exercises Key

1. A. The nurse should recommend a community support group to facilitate coping with PD progression. However, another intervention is the priority.

    B. The nurse should help the client integrate daily exercise to improve balance and cognition. However, another intervention is the priority.

    C. The nurse should help the client obtain a walker to promote safe ambulation. However, another intervention is the priority.

    D. **CORRECT:** When using the airway, breathing, circulation approach to client care, the nurse determines that the priority intervention is to schedule a swallowing evaluation for the client. Impaired swallowing from loss of muscle control places the client at risk for aspiration when consuming food or beverages.

    Ⓝ *NCLEX® Connection: Basic Care and Comfort, Nutrition and Oral Hydration*

2. A. The nurse should provide small frequent meals during the day to maintain adequate nutrition.

    B. **CORRECT:** The nurse should record the client's diet and fluid intake daily to monitor dietary needs and to maintain adequate nutrition and hydration.

    C. The nurse should document the client's weight weekly to identify weight loss and intervene to maintain the client's weight.

    D. The nurse should ensure that the client is sitting upright for meals rather than in a supported Fowler's position, where the client's head is elevated to 45° to 60°.

    E. **CORRECT:** The nurse should offer nutritional supplements between meals to maintain the client's weight.

    Ⓝ *NCLEX® Connection: Basic Care and Comfort, Nutrition and Oral Hydration*

3. A. **CORRECT:** Orthostatic hypotension is a common adverse effect of bromocriptine, a dopamine receptor agonist. The family members should have the client rise slowly when standing up to decrease the risk for dizziness and lightheadedness.

    B. The nurse should remind the family member that bromocriptine stimulates the body to release dopamine. Dopaminergic medications convert to dopamine in the brain.

    C. The nurse should remind the family that medications to treat PD can take weeks to become effective in improving manifestations of the disease.

    D. The nurse should remind the family that dopamine agonists, such as bromocriptine are given along with a dopaminergic medication to increase effectiveness.

    Ⓝ *NCLEX® Connection: Pharmacological Therapies, Expected Actions/Outcomes*

4. A. Decreased vision is not an expected finding in a client who has PD.

    B. **CORRECT:** The client who has PD can manifest pill-rolling tremors of the fingers due to overstimulation of the basal ganglia by acetylcholine, making controlled movement difficult.

    C. **CORRECT:** The client who has PD can manifest shuffling gait because of overstimulation of the basal ganglia by acetylcholine, making controlled movement difficult.

    D. **CORRECT:** The client who has PD can manifest drooling because of overstimulation of the basal ganglia by acetylcholine, making the controlled movement of swallowing secretions difficult.

    E. Bilateral ankle edema is not an expected finding in a client who has PD, but can be an adverse effect of certain medications used for treatment.

    F. **CORRECT:** The client who has PD can manifest a lack of facial expressions due to overstimulation of the basal ganglia by acetylcholine, making controlled movement difficult.

    Ⓝ *NCLEX® Connection: Physiological Adaptation, Basic Pathophysiology*

5. A. The client who has PD develops a propulsive gait and tends to walk increasingly rapidly. The nurse should remind the client to stop occasionally when walking to prevent a propulsive gait and decrease the risk for falls.

    B. The nurse should encourage active, not passive, range-of-motion exercises to promote mobility in the client who has PD and is displaying bradykinesia.

    C. The client who has PD often requires high-calorie, high-protein supplements between meals in order to maintain adequate weight.

    D. **CORRECT:** Bradykinesia is abnormally slowed movement and is seen in clients who have PD. The nurse should give the client extra time to perform activities and encourage the client to remain active.

    Ⓝ *NCLEX® Connection: Basic Care and Comfort, Mobility/Immobility*

PRACTICE Answer

Using the ATI Active Learning Template: System Disorder

ALTERATION IN HEALTH (DIAGNOSIS):
Parkinson's disease is a debilitating condition that progresses to complete dependent care. The disease involves a decrease in dopamine production and an increase in secretion of acetylcholine, causing resting tremor, slowed movement, and muscular rigidity.

COMPLICATIONS
- Aspiration due to pharyngeal muscle involvement making swallowing difficult
- Orthostatic hypotension, slow movement, and muscle rigidity
- Change in speech pattern: slow, monotonous speech
- Altered emotional changes that can include depression and fear

NURSING CARE
- Add thickener to liquids to prevent aspiration.
- Consult with a dietitian about appropriate diet.
- Encourage periods of rest between activities.
- Allow adequate time to rise slowly from a sitting to standing position.
- Encourage slower speech when expressing thoughts.
- Observe for signs of depression and dementia.

Ⓝ *NCLEX® Connection: Physiological Adaptation, Basic Pathophysiology*

CHAPTER 8 *Alzheimer's Disease*

Alzheimer's disease (AD) is a nonreversible type of dementia that progressively develops over many years. A framework of seven stages categorizes the disease and its manifestations. The framework is based on three general stages: early (mild), mid (moderate), and late (severe).

Dementia is defined as multiple cognitive deficits that impair memory and can affect language, motor skills, and abstract thinking. The percentage of dementia attributable to AD ranges from 60% to 90%.

The mean duration of survival after diagnosis is approximately 10 years, but some people can live with the disease for up to 20 years.

AD is most likely to occur in clients in their 60s and 70s. However, it can be diagnosed as early as 40. Age is the No. 1 known risk factor for AD, which usually occurs after age 65. ©

AD is characterized by memory loss, problems with judgment, and changes in personality. As the disease progresses, severe physical decline occurs along with deteriorating cognitive functions.

HEALTH PROMOTION AND DISEASE PREVENTION

- Consume a diet high in omega-3 polyunsaturated fats, fruits, and vegetables.
- Engage in intellectually stimulating activities on a regular basis (reading, debating, learning a new skill).
- Estrogen therapy for females can prevent AD, but it is not useful in decreasing the effects of existing dementia.

DATA COLLECTION

Mini Mental State Examination (MMSE) is used.

RISK FACTORS

- Advanced age
- Chemical imbalances
- Family history of AD or Down syndrome
- Genetic predisposition, apolipoprotein E
- Environmental agents (herpes virus, metal, toxic waste, dichlorodiphenyltrichloroethane [DDT])
- Previous head injury
- Sex (female)
- Ethnicity (African Americans greater risk; Hispanics develop AD earlier)
- Chronic conditions (hypercholesterolemia, diabetes mellitus, cardiovascular disease)
- Poor diet
- Inactivity

EXPECTED FINDINGS

AD progression and manifestations are categorized into seven stages. (8.1)

KEY MANIFESTATIONS USED FOR DIAGNOSING AD

- **Cognitive:** Memory loss, disoriented to place and time, loss of abstract thought, forgetting words, impaired judgment
- **Functional:** Inability to perform familiar tasks (cooking, playing games), misplacing items in unusual places
- **Psychological:** Mood, personality, and behavior changes; withdrawal; passivity

LABORATORY TESTS

- No specific lab test can definitively diagnose AD.
- Several labs can rule out other causes of dementia.
- Genetic test for the presence of apolipoprotein can determine if there is an increased risk of AD, but it does not specifically diagnose AD. The presence of the protein increases the likelihood that dementia is due to AD.

DIAGNOSTIC PROCEDURES

- There is no definitive diagnostic procedure, except brain tissue examination upon death.
- Magnetic resonance imaging (MRI), computed tomography (CT) imaging/computed axial tomography (CAT) scan, positron emission tomography (PET) scan, and electroencephalogram (EEG) may be performed to rule out other possible causes of findings.
- A lumbar puncture may be performed for laboratory testing of cerebral spinal fluid for soluble beta protein precursor (sBPP). Beta amyloid protein normally assists in growth and protection of nerve cells. The presence of low levels of sBPP supports the diagnosis of AD.

PATIENT-CENTERED CARE

NURSING CARE

- Check for cognitive status, memory, judgment, and personality changes.
- Observe and document patterns of behavior to identify client habits that could cause a safety risk (failure to use assistive devices, tendency to wander, times of increased confusion).
- Maintain bowel and bladder program based on a set schedule.
- Encourage the client and family to participate in an AD support group.
- Provide a safe environment. Qs
  - Frequent monitoring/visual checks.
  - Keep client from stairs, elevators, exits.
  - Remove or secure dangerous items in the client's environment.
- Provide frequent walks to reduce wandering.
- Maintain a sleeping schedule, and monitor for irregular sleeping patterns.
- Provide verbal and nonverbal ways to communicate with the client.
- Offer snacks or finger foods if the client is unable to sit for long periods of time.

- Check skin weekly for breakdown.
- Provide cognitive stimulation.
  - Offer varied environmental stimulations (walks, music, craft activities).
  - Keep a structured environment and introduce change gradually (client's daily routine or a room change).
  - Use a calendar to assist with orientation.
  - Use short directions when explaining an activity or care the client needs, such as a bath.
  - Be consistent and repetitive.
  - Use therapeutic touch.
- Provide memory training.
  - Reminisce with the client about the past.
  - Use memory techniques (making lists, rehearsing).
  - Stimulate memory by repeating the client's last statement.
  - Place tags on frequently used objects to help the client identify their purpose
- Avoid overstimulation. Keep noise and clutter to a minimum, and avoid crowds.
- Promote consistency by placing commonly used objects in the same location and using a routine schedule.
  - Reality orientation (early stages)
  - Easily viewed clock and single-day calendar
  - Pictures of family and pets
  - Frequent reorientation to time, place, and person

8.1 Alzheimer's disease stages and manifestations

Mild Alzheimer's (early stage)

NO IMPAIRMENT
- Normal function
- Manifestation: No memory problems.

VERY MILD COGNITIVE DECLINE
- (Can be normal age-related changes or very early signs of AD)
- Manifestations
  - Forgetfulness, especially of everyday objects (eyeglasses or wallet).
  - No memory problems evident to provider, friends, or coworkers.

MILD COGNITIVE DECLINE
- (Problems with memory or concentration can be measurable in clinical testing or during a detailed medical interview)
- Mild cognitive deficits, including losing or misplacing important objects.
- Manifestations
  - Decreased ability to plan.
  - Short-term memory loss noticeable to close relatives.
  - Decreased attention span.
  - Difficulty remembering words or names.
  - Difficulty in social or work situations.

Moderate Alzheimer's (middle stage)

MODERATE COGNITIVE DECLINE
- Medical interview will detect clear-cut deficiencies.
- Manifestations
  - Personality changes: appearing withdrawn or subdued, especially in social or mentally challenging situations.
  - Obvious memory loss.
  - Limited knowledge and memory of recent occasions, current events, or personal history.
  - Difficulty performing tasks that require planning and organizing (paying bills or managing money).
  - Difficulty with complex mental arithmetic.

MODERATELY SEVERE COGNITIVE DECLINE
- Manifestations
  - Increasing cognitive deficits emerge.
  - Inability to recall important details such as address, telephone number, or schools attended, but memory of information about self and family remains intact.
  - Assistance with ADLs becomes necessary.
  - Disorientation and confusion as to time and place.

Severe Alzheimer's (late stage)

SEVERE COGNITIVE DECLINE
- Manifestations
  - Memory difficulties continue to worsen.
  - Loss of awareness of recent events and surroundings.
  - Can recall own name, but unable to recall personal history.
  - Significant personality changes are evident (delusions, hallucinations, and compulsive behaviors).
  - Wandering behavior.
  - Requires assistance with ADLs such as dressing, toileting, and grooming.
  - Normal sleep/wake cycle is disrupted.
  - Increased episodes of urinary and fecal incontinence.

VERY SEVERE COGNITIVE DECLINE
- Manifestations
  - Ability to respond to environment, speak, and control movement is lost.
  - Unrecognizable speech.
  - General urinary incontinence.
  - Inability to eat without assistance and impaired swallowing.
  - Gradual loss of all ability to move extremities (ataxia).

- Validation therapy (later stages)
  - Acknowledge the client's feelings.
  - Don't argue with the client; this will lead to the client becoming upset.
  - Reinforce and use repetitive actions or ideas cautiously.
- Promote self-care as long as possible. Assist with activities of daily living as appropriate.
- Speak directly to the client in short, concise sentences.
- Reduce agitation. (Use calm, redirecting statements. Provide a diversion.)
- Provide a routine toileting schedule.

MEDICATIONS

- Most medications for clients who have dementia attempt to target behavioral and emotional problems (anxiety, agitation, combativeness, depression).
- These medications include antipsychotics, antidepressants, and anxiolytics. Closely monitor clients receiving these medications for adverse effects.
- AD medications temporarily slow the course of the disease and do not work for all clients.
  - Pharmacotherapeutics is based on the theory that AD is a result of depleted levels of the enzyme acetyltransferase, which is necessary to produce the neurotransmitter acetylcholine.
  - Benefits for clients who do respond to medication include improvements in cognition, behavior, and function.
- If a client fails to improve with one medication, a trial of one of the other medications is warranted.
  - **Cholinesterase** inhibitors, such as donepezil, prevent the breakdown of acetylcholine (ACh), which increases the amount of ACh available and increases nerve impulses at the nerve sites.

NURSING ACTIONS

- Observe for frequent stools or upset stomach.
- Monitor for dizziness or headache. The client can feel lightheaded or have an unsteady gait.
- Use caution when administering cholinesterase inhibitors to clients who have asthma or COPD, as lung problems can worsen.

THERAPEUTIC PROCEDURES

ALTERNATIVE THERAPY: Ginkgo biloba, an herbal product taken to increase memory and blood circulation, can cause a variety of side effects and medication interactions. If a client is using ginkgo biloba or other nutritional supplements, that information should be shared with providers.

INTERPROFESSIONAL CARE

- Encourage the client and family to seek legal counsel regarding advanced directives, guardianship, or durable medical power of attorney.
- Recommend referral to social services and case managers for possible adult day care or long-term care facilities.
- Recommend referral to the Alzheimer's Association and community outreach programs. This can include family support groups, in-home care, or respite care.
- Review the resources available to the family as the client's health declines. Include long term care options. A variety of home care and community resources, such as respite care, is available to the family in many areas of the country. Some respite care allows the client to remain at home rather than in a facility.

CLIENT EDUCATION

- Information about illness, methods of care, medications, and adaptation of the home environment.
- Home safety measures. Qs
  - Removing scatter rugs
  - Installing door locks that cannot be easily opened, and placing alarms on doors
  - Keeping a lock on the water heater and thermostat, and keeping the water temperature at a safe level
  - Providing good lighting, especially on stairs
  - Installing handrails on stairs and marking step edges with colored tape
  - Placing the mattress on the floor
  - Removing clutter and clearing hallways for walking
  - Securing electrical cords to baseboards
  - Keeping cleaning supplies in locked cupboards
  - Installing handrails in the bathroom, at bedside, and in the tub; placing a shower chair in the tub
  - Having the client wear a medical identification bracelet or GPS tracking bracelet if living at home with a caregiver; enrolling in Safe Return Home Program (www.alz.org).
  - Facilitating an exercise program to maintain mobility
  - Intervening for seizures that can happen late in the disease
  - Strategies to reduce caregiver stress

Application Exercises

1. A nurse is reinforcing teaching with the partner of an older adult client who has AD and has a new prescription for donepezil. Which of the following statements by the partner indicates the teaching is effective?

   A. "This medication should increase my partner's appetite."

   B. "This medication should help my partner sleep better."

   C. "This medication should help my partner's daily function."

   D. "This medication should increase my partner's energy level."

2. A nurse working in a long-term care facility is caring for a client who has AD. Which of the following actions should the nurse take?

   A. Allow the client to sleep whenever he chooses.

   B. Avoid using gestures when communicating with the client.

   C. Redirect the client when he talks about the past.

   D. Provide finger foods for the client's snacks and meals.

3. A nurse is making a home visit to a client who has AD. The client's partner states that the client is often disoriented to time and place, is unsteady on his feet, and has a history of wandering. Which of the following safety measures should the nurse review with the partner? (Select all that apply.)

   A. Remove floor rugs.

   B. Have door locks that can be easily opened.

   C. Provide increased lighting in stairwells.

   D. Install handrails in the bathroom.

   E. Place the mattress on the floor.

4. A nurse is caring for a client who has AD and falls frequently. Which of the following actions is the priority for the nurse to take to keep the client safe?

   A. Keep the call light near the client.

   B. Place the client in a room close to the nurses' station.

   C. Encourage the client to ask for assistance.

   D. Remind the client to walk with someone for support.

5. A nurse is caring for a client who has AD. A family member of the client asks the nurse about risk factors for the disease. Which of the following information should the nurse include? (Select all that apply.)

   A. Exposure to metal waste products

   B. Long-term estrogen therapy

   C. Sustained use of vitamin E

   D. Previous head injury

   E. History of herpes infection

PRACTICE Active Learning Scenario

A nurse in a long-term care facility is helping prepare a program for assistive personnel about caring for a client who has Alzheimer's disease. What should be included in this program? Use the ATI Active Learning Template: System Disorder to complete this item.

NURSING CARE: Describe three nursing interventions for each of the following areas.
- Providing cognitive stimulation
- Providing memory training

Application Exercises Key

1. A. Donepezil does not affect appetite.

   B. Donepezil does not affect sleep or sleep patterns.

   C. **CORRECT:** Donepezil helps slow the progression of AD and can help improve behavior and daily functions.

   D. Donepezil does not affect energy levels.

   Ⓝ *NCLEX® Connection: Pharmacological Therapies, Expected Actions/Outcomes*

2. A. The nurse should help establish a sleeping schedule for the client and should watch for irregular sleeping patterns.

   B. The nurse should use both verbal and nonverbal communication techniques when interacting with the client.

   C. The nurse should support the client in reminiscing about the past because it can help the client maintain his memory.

   D. **CORRECT:** The nurse should provide the client with finger foods to provide a simple, quick food source. This can help promote adequate nutrition during times when the client is having difficulty focusing or sitting still for meals.

   Ⓝ *NCLEX® Connection: Physiological Adaptation, Basic Pathophysiology*

3. A. **CORRECT:** Removing floor rugs can decrease the risk of falling.

   B. Easy-to-open door locks increase the risk for a client who wanders to get out of his home and get lost.

   C. **CORRECT:** Good lighting can decrease the risk for falling in dark areas, such as stairways.

   D. **CORRECT:** Installing handrails in the bathroom can be useful for the client to hold on to when his gait is unsteady.

   E. **CORRECT:** By placing the client's mattress on the floor, the risk of falling or tripping is decreased.

   Ⓝ *NCLEX® Connection: Safety and Infection Control, Home Safety*

4. A. Keeping the call light within the client's reach promotes safety. However, another action is the priority, because the client might not remember to use the call light.

   B. **CORRECT:** The greatest risk to this client is injury from fall or delay in treatment from a fall. Therefore, the priority action is to place the client in close proximity to the nurse's station. This allows staff to visualize the client more frequently to better prevent falls and provide quick assistance if the client becomes injured.

   C. Encouraging the client to ask for assistance promotes safety. However, another action is the priority because the client might not remember to ask for assistance.

   D. Reminding the client to walk with someone promotes safety. However, another action is the priority because the client might not remember to call for assistance.

   Ⓝ *NCLEX® Connection: Safety and Infection Control, Home Safety*

5. A. **CORRECT:** Exposure to metal and toxic waste is a risk factor for AD.

   B. Long-term estrogen therapy can prevent AD.

   C. Long-term use of vitamin E is not a risk factor for AD. Presence of apolipoprotein E (genetic) increases the risk of AD.

   D. **CORRECT:** A previous head injury is a risk factor for AD.

   E. **CORRECT:** A history of herpes infection is a risk factor for AD.

   Ⓝ *NCLEX® Connection: Health Promotion and Maintenance, Health Promotion/Disease Prevention*

PRACTICE Answer

Using the ATI Active Learning Template: System Disorder

NURSING CARE
- Providing cognitive stimulation
  - Offer varied environmental stimulations (walks, music, craft activities).
  - Keep a structured environment. Introduce change slowly.
  - Use a calendar to assist with orientation.
  - Use short directions when explaining care to be provided, such as a bath.
  - Be consistent and repetitive.
  - Use therapeutic touch.
- Providing memory training
  - Reminisce about the past.
  - Help the client make lists and rehearse.
  - Repeat the client's last statement to stimulate memory.

Ⓝ *NCLEX® Connection: Physiological Adaptation, Alterations in Body Systems*

CHAPTER 9

CHAPTER 9 *Stroke*

Strokes, also known as cerebrovascular accidents or brain attacks, involve a disruption in the cerebral blood flow secondary to ischemia, or hemorrhage. Classifications of strokes are hemorrhagic and ischemic. Ischemic strokes are further classified as thrombotic or embolic.

Hemorrhagic strokes occur secondary to a ruptured artery or aneurysm. The prognosis for a client who has experienced a hemorrhagic stroke is poor due to the amount of ischemia and increased ICP caused by the expanding collection of blood. The prognosis of a hemorrhagic stroke improves significantly with early detection and evacuation of the clot following cessation of the active bleed. **(9.1)**

Ischemic strokes occur secondary to the development of a blood clot (thrombus) on an atherosclerotic plaque in a cerebral artery. This thrombus gradually shuts off the artery and causes ischemia distal to the occlusion. Manifestations of a thrombotic stroke evolve over several hours to days. **(9.2)**

Another type of ischemic stroke is caused by an embolus traveling from another part of the body to a cerebral artery. Blood to the brain distal to the occlusion is immediately blocked, instantly causing neurologic deficits or a loss of consciousness. **(9.3)**

Ischemic strokes (thrombotic or embolic) can be reversed with fibrinolytic therapy using alteplase, also known as tissue plasminogen activator (tPA), if given within 3 to 4.5 hr of the initial manifestations (unless contraindicated by factors such as presence of active bleeding).

Transient ischemic attack (TIA) is a temporary interruption in blood flow to the cerebral hemisphere. TIA can be caused by certain conditions such as vasospasms, partially occluded cerebral arteries, and any medications or conditions that may cause vasoconstriction (constriction of blood vessels). The client can experience the same manifestations as a full stroke, but the manifestations will subside usually within 1 hour. A TIA can be the first warning sign that the client is at increased risk for a neurological event, such as a stroke.

9.1 Hemorrhagic stroke

blood leaks
into brain tissue

9.2 Thrombotic stroke

thrombus

HEALTH PROMOTION AND DISEASE PREVENTION

- Hypertension, diabetes mellitus, smoking, and other related disorders can increase the risk for a stroke. Q EBP
- Early treatment of hypertension, maintenance of blood glucose within expected range, and refraining from smoking will decrease these risk factors.
- Maintaining a healthy weight and getting regular exercise can also decrease the risk of a stroke.
- Monitor for the warning signs of strokes.
  - New onset of weakness, numbness, or loss of function in face, arm, or leg
  - Sudden onset of slurred speech, confusion, or inability to speak or understand what others are saying
  - Sudden onset of severe headache, visual changes, or loss of balance
  - Loss of consciousness

DATA COLLECTION

RISK FACTORS

MODIFIABLE RISK FACTORS
- Diabetes mellitus
- Obesity
- Hypertension
- Hyperlipidemia
- Hypercoagulability
- Atrial fibrillation
- Use of oral contraceptives
- Smoking
- Cocaine use
- Alcohol consumption
- Sedentary lifestyle
- Sleep apnea

NONMODIFIABLE RISK FACTORS
- Age (65 years and older)
- Race (higher incidence for African American clients)
- Sex (higher incidence in male clients)
- History of stroke (individual or family)

EXPECTED FINDINGS

Some clients report transient manifestations (visual disturbances, dizziness, slurred speech, a weak extremity).
- These manifestations can indicate a TIA, which can be a warning of an impending stroke.
- Antithrombotic medication and/or surgical removal of atherosclerotic plaques in the carotid artery can prevent the subsequent occurrence of a stroke.

PHYSICAL FINDINGS
Manifestations vary based on the area of the brain that is deprived of oxygenated blood.
- **The left cerebral hemisphere** is responsible for language, mathematics skills, and analytic thinking.
  - Expressive and receptive aphasia (inability to speak and understand language)
  - Right extremity hemiplegia (paralysis) or hemiparesis (weakness)
  - Slow, cautious behavior
  - Depression, anger, and quick to become frustrated
  - Visual changes, such as hemianopsia (loss of visual field in one or both eyes)
- **The right cerebral hemisphere** is responsible for visual and spatial awareness and proprioception. Q s
  - Altered perception of deficits (overestimation of abilities)
  - Loss of depth perception
  - Poor impulse control and judgment
  - Inability to solve problems
  - Emotional lability
  - Left hemiplegia or hemiparesis
  - Visual changes, such as hemianopsia
- Other manifestations
  - Agnosia (unable to recognize familiar objects)
  - Alexia (reading difficulty)
  - Agraphia (writing difficulty)
  - Unilateral neglect syndrome (ignore affected side of the body: cannot see, feel, or move affected side, so client unaware of its existence).
  - Apraxia (inability to complete common tasks, such as combing the hair, even when paralysis is not a factor)
  - Incontinence of bowel and bladder

9.3 Embolic stroke

blood clot travels through bloodstream toward brain

source of blood clot

blood clot

blood clot

9.4 Communication board

| YES | MAYBE | DON'T KNOW | NO |

A	B	C	D	E	F	G	H	I
J	K	L	M	N	O	P	Q
R	S	T	U	V	W	X	Y	Z

| 1 | 2 | 3 | 4 | 5 | 6 | 7 | 8 | 9 | 10 |

| FOOD | DRINK | STOP | GO | HURT |
| GOOD | BAD | COLD | HOT | MORE |

DIAGNOSTIC PROCEDURES

Magnetic resonance imaging (MRI), computed tomography (CT) imaging, and/or a computed axial tomography (CAT) scan can be used to identify edema, ischemia, and necrosis.

Magnetic resonance angiography or a cerebral angiography are used to identify the presence of a cerebral hemorrhage, abnormal vessel structures (AV malformation, aneurysms), vessel ruptures, and regional perfusion of blood flow in the carotid arteries and brain.

Lumbar puncture is used to assess for the presence of blood in the cerebrospinal fluid. A positive finding is consistent with a cerebral hemorrhage or ruptured aneurysm.

The Glasgow Coma Scale is used when the client has a decreased level of consciousness or orientation. The risk for increased intracranial pressure (ICP) exists related to the swelling of the brain that can occur secondary to ischemic insult.

Electroencephalogram is used to determine brain or seizure activity.

Doppler studies of the carotid arteries can identify blood flow to the brain.

The NIH stroke scale is used to evaluate the presence and extent of neurological deficit as well as recovery.

PATIENT-CENTERED CARE

NURSING CARE

- Monitor vital signs every 1 to 2 hr. Notify the provider immediately if blood pressure exceeds a systolic greater than 180 mm Hg or a diastolic greater than 110 mm Hg. This can indicate the client is experiencing an ischemic stroke. Qs
- Monitor the client's temperature. A fever can cause an increase in intracranial pressure.
- Provide oxygen therapy to maintain oxygen saturation level greater than 92%, or if the client's level of consciousness is decreased.
- Place the client on a cardiac monitor to detect arrhythmias.
- Monitor IV access to ensure delivery of medications and fluids.
- Monitor for changes in level of consciousness, which can indicate increased intracranial pressure.
- Monitor vital signs and electrocardiogram.
- Elevate the head of the bed approximately 30° to reduce ICP and to promote venous drainage. Avoid extreme flexion or extension of the neck, and maintain the client's head in the midline neutral position. QEBP
- Institute seizure precautions.

- Assist with the client's communication skills if speech is impaired. **(9.4)**
  - Determine the ability to understand speech by asking the client to follow simple commands.
  - Observe for consistently affirmative answers when the client actually does not comprehend what is being said.
  - Determine accuracy of yes/no responses in relation to closed-ended questions.
  - Supply the client with a picture board of commonly requested items/needs.
  - For expressive and receptive aphasia, speak slowly and clearly, and use one-step commands.
- Assist with safe feeding. Qs
  - Consult speech-language pathologist (SLP) to assess swallowing and gag reflexes before feeding. The SLP can request a swallowing study that can involve swallowing a barium substrate and radiography of the peristaltic activity of the esophagus. QTC
  - Four liquid consistencies have been identified by a collaborative group of specialists for clients who have dysphagia: thin (water, juice), nectar-like (cream soups, nectars), honey-like (honey, yogurt), and spoon-thick (pudding, cooked cereals). Food levels for dysphagia include pureed, mechanically altered, advanced/mechanically soft, and regular. Use the appropriate consistency and food type as recommended by the SLP to minimize choking.
  - Have the client eat in an upright position and swallow with the head and neck flexed slightly forward.
  - Place food in the back of the mouth on the unaffected side.
  - Have suction on standby.
  - Maintain a distraction-free environment during meals.
  - Collaborate with a dietitian to ensure appropriate caloric intake, because weight loss is common following stroke. QTC
- Prevent complications of immobility, such as atelectasis, pneumonia, pressure sores, and deep-vein thrombosis (DVT). Clients who have experienced strokes are ambulated as soon as possible to prevent complications. However, during periods of inactivity, preventive measures related to complications of immobility should be implemented.
  - Collaborate with physical therapy to assist client with transfers and ambulation. QTC
- Maintain skin integrity.
  - Reposition the client every 2 hr and use pillows to maintain proper body alignment.
  - Monitor bony prominences, paying particular attention to the affected extremities.
  - Instruct the client who has one-sided neglect, to protect and care for the affected extremity by pulling the affected extremity to midline and out of danger from the wheel of the wheelchair or hitting/smashing it against a doorway.

- Encourage passive range of motion every 4 hr to the affected extremities and active range of motion every 4 hr to the unaffected extremities. Reinforce teaching with the client on how to use the unaffected side to exercise the affected side of the body.
- Maintain a safe environment to reduce the risk of falls. Assistive devices (transfer belts, sliding boards) should be used during transfers. Sit-to-stand lifts can also facilitate transfers and reduce strain on the care provider's body. Qs
- Instruct the client who has homonymous hemianopsia (loss of the same visual field in both eyes) to use a scanning technique (turning head from the direction of the unaffected side to the affected side) when eating and ambulating.
- To prevent DVT, provide preventive measures (sequential compression stockings, frequent position changes, mobilization).
- Provide assistance with ADLs as needed. Instruct the client to dress the affected side first and sit in a supportive chair that aids in balance. Have occupational therapy assess the client for adaptive aids (plate guard, utensils with built-up handles, reaching tool to pick things up, shirts and shoes that have hook and loop fasteners or tape instead of buttons and ties). Qtc
- Clients who have experienced strokes have decreased endurance and impaired balance due to paralysis on one side of the body. Provide frequent rest periods from sitting in the wheelchair by returning the client to bed after therapies and meals. When sitting the client up in bed or in a wheelchair, leaning to the affected side typically occurs and should be countered with some manner of support.
- Shoulder subluxation can occur if the affected arm is not supported. The weight of the arm is such that it can cause a painful dislocation of the shoulder from its socket. Support the arm while in bed, the wheelchair, or during ambulation with an arm sling or strategically placed pillows.
- Support the client during periods of emotional lability and depression. Qpcc

MEDICATIONS

Anticoagulants (heparin, enoxaparin, warfarin): Use of anticoagulants is controversial and not recommended due to the high risk of intracerebral bleeding (not given with a hemorrhagic stroke due to increased risk for bleeding).

Antiplatelets (aspirin): Not given with a hemorrhagic stroke due to increased risk for bleeding. Low-dose aspirin is given following a stroke to prevent further clot formation.

Thrombolytic medication alteplase or systemic tissue plasminogen activator (t-PA) are given no later than 4.5 hr after initial onset of manifestations.

Antiepileptic medications (phenytoin, gabapentin) are not commonly given following a stroke unless the client develops seizures.

Antihypertensives (nifedipine) are given if the systolic blood pressure is greater than 220 mm Hg.

THERAPEUTIC PROCEDURES

Systemic or catheter-directed thrombolytic therapy restores cerebral blood flow. It is contraindicated for treatment of a hemorrhagic stroke and for clients who have an increased risk of bleeding due to anticoagulant therapy or other bleeding disorders. Possibility of hemorrhagic stroke is ruled out with an MRI prior to the initiation of thrombolytic therapy, as well as a complete client history.
- Carotid artery angioplasty with stenting (CAS) involves inserting a catheter in the femoral artery and placing a distal/embolic protection device to catch clot debris during the procedure while a stent is being placed in the carotid artery to open a blockage. CAS is less invasive, blood loss is decreased, and length of hospitalization is shorter. Postoperative care is the same as carotid endarterectomy.
- Carotid endarterectomy is performed to open the artery by removing atherosclerotic plaque. This procedure is performed when the carotid artery is blocked or when the client is experiencing TIAs.
- Check for increased headache, neck swelling, and hoarseness of the throat.
- Craniotomy with repair of aneurysm is performed for clients experiencing this type of hemorrhagic stroke. The aneurysm is either removed or wrapped to prevent further rupture.

INTERPROFESSIONAL CARE

- Speech and language therapists can be consulted for language therapy and swallowing exercises.
- Physical therapy can be consulted for assistance with reestablishment of ambulation with or without assistive devices (single or quad cane, walker) or wheelchair support. Wheelchair adaptations, such as an extended brake handle on the client's affected side of the wheelchair, can be necessary. Safety features, such as placing the brakes on when preparing to transfer and the use of a cushion on the seat, may also be initiated by physical therapy.
- Occupational therapy can be consulted for assistance with reestablishment of partial or full function of the affected hand and arm. If function does not return to the extremity, measures such as massage and elastic gloves will be prescribed by occupational therapy to prevent swelling of the extremity. Occupational therapy will also help with activities of daily living (ADLs) (brushing hair, brushing teeth, shaving).
- Social services can be consulted to make arrangements for rehabilitation services and temporary placement on a skilled rehabilitation unit or extended-care facility during provision of these services. Prior to discharge, the social worker may make a home visit with selected therapists and nurses to evaluate the need for environmental alterations in the home and adaptive equipment needed for ADLs.

COMPLICATIONS

Dysphagia and aspiration

- Dysphagia can result from neurological involvement of the cranial nerves that innervate the face, tongue, soft palate, and throat. As a result, the client's risk of aspiration is great. Qs
- Not all clients who have experienced a stroke have dysphagia, but all should be evaluated prior to reestablishing oral nutrition and hydration.

NURSING ACTIONS

- Collaborate with a speech-language pathologist to complete a dysphagia screening prior to initiating oral intake. Qtc
- Keep the client completely NPO until evaluated by the SLP.
- Begin the client with the prescribed liquid-consistency regimen from the National Dysphagia Diet and observe closely for choking. Have suction equipment available, but feed with care because nasotracheal suctioning increases ICP. Qebp
- Some clients require an eating environment without distractions to prevent choking.
- Position the client in an upright (high-Fowler's) position prior to food, fluid, or medication administration.
- Reinforce swallowing techniques recommended by speech language pathologist. Qtc
- Reinforce teaching with the client's family about strategies for eating, and give instructions regarding prescribed consistency of liquids and solid foods.

CLIENT EDUCATION

- Sit upright and to flex his head forward when swallowing to decrease the risk of choking. Qs
- Sit upright for 45 to 60 minutes following a meal.

Unilateral neglect

Unilateral neglect is the loss of awareness of the side affected by the stroke. The client cannot see, feel, or move the affected side of his body; therefore, he forgets that it exists. This lack of awareness poses a great risk for injury to the neglected extremities and creates a self-care deficit.

NURSING ACTIONS

- Check affected extremities for injury (bruises and abrasions of the affected hand and arm, hyperflexion of the foot from it falling off of the wheelchair during transport).
- Apply an arm sling if the client is having difficulty remembering care for the affected extremity.
- Ensure that the foot rest is on the wheelchair and that an ankle brace is on the affected foot.
- Reinforce teaching with the client on how to care for the affected side.

CLIENT EDUCATION

- Dress the affected side first. Qpcc
- Use the unaffected hand to pull the affected extremity to midline and out of danger from the wheel of the wheelchair or from hitting or smashing it against a doorway.
- Look over the affected side periodically.

Application Exercises

1. A nurse is caring for a client who has experienced a right-hemispheric stroke. Which of the following findings should the nurse expect? (Select all that apply.)

   A. Impulse control difficulty

   B. Left hemiplegia

   C. Loss of depth perception

   D. Aphasia

   E. Lack of situational awareness

2. A nurse is caring for a client who has left homonymous hemianopsia. Which of the following interventions should the nurse implement?

   A. Instruct the client to scan to the right to see objects on the right side of her body.

   B. Place the bedside table on the right side of the bed.

   C. Orient the client to the food on her plate using the clock method.

   D. Place the wheelchair on the client's left side.

3. A nurse is contributing to the plan care for a client who has dysphagia and a new dietary prescription. Which of the following interventions should the nurse include in the plan? (Select all that apply.)

   A. Have suction equipment available for use.

   B. Feed the client thickened liquids.

   C. Place food on the unaffected side of the client's mouth.

   D. Assign an assistive personnel to feed the client slowly.

   E. Instruct the client to swallow with her neck flexed.

4. A nurse is contributing to the plan of care for a client who has global aphasia (both receptive and expressive). Which of the following interventions should the nurse include in the client's plan? (Select all that apply.)

   A. Speak to the client at a slower rate.

   B. Assist the client to use flash cards with pictures.

   C. Speak to the client in a loud voice.

   D. Complete sentences that the client cannot finish.

   E. Give instructions one step at a time.

5. A nurse is collecting data on a client who has experienced a left-hemispheric stroke. Which of the following manifestations should the nurse expect?

   A. Impulse control difficulty

   B. Poor judgment

   C. Frustrated about deficits

   D. Loss of depth perception

PRACTICE Active Learning Scenario

A nurse is caring for a client who has dysphagia. Use the ATI Active Learning Template: Nursing Skill to complete this item.

NURSING INTERVENTIONS: List three nursing actions the nurse should include while caring for this client.

Application Exercises Key

1. A. **CORRECT:** A client who has experienced a right-hemispheric stroke can exhibit impulse control difficulty, such as the urgency to use the restroom.

   B. **CORRECT:** A client who has experienced a right-hemispheric stroke can exhibit left-sided hemiplegia.

   C. **CORRECT:** A client who has experienced a right-hemispheric stroke can experience a loss in depth perception.

   D. A client who has experienced a left-hemispheric stroke can experience aphasia.

   E. **CORRECT:** A client who has experienced a right-hemispheric stroke can demonstrate a lack of awareness of surroundings.

   Ⓝ *NCLEX® Connection: Physiological Adaptation, Basic Pathophysiology*

2. A. A client who has left homonymous hemianopsia has lost the left visual field of both eyes. The nurse should instruct the client to turn his head to the left to visualize the entire field of vision.

   B. **CORRECT:** The client is unable to visualize to the left midline of her body. Placing the bedside table on the right side of the client's bed will permit visualization of items on the table.

   C. Using the clock method of food placement is ineffective because the client can only see half of the plate.

   D. The nurse should place the wheelchair to the client's right or unaffected side.

   Ⓝ *NCLEX® Connection: Physiological Adaptation, Alterations in Body Systems*

3. A. **CORRECT:** Suction equipment should be available in case of choking and aspiration.

   B. **CORRECT:** The client should be given liquids that are thicker than water to prevent aspiration.

   C. **CORRECT:** Placing food on the unaffected side of the client's mouth will allow her to have better control of the food and reduce the risk of aspiration.

   D. Due to the risk of aspiration, assistive personnel should not be assigned to feed the client because the client's swallowing ability should be checked, and suctioning can be needed if choking occurs.

   E. **CORRECT:** The client should be taught to flex her neck, tucking the chin down and under to close the epiglottis during swallowing.

   Ⓝ *NCLEX® Connection: Basic Care and Comfort, Nutrition and Oral Hydration*

4. A. **CORRECT:** Clients who have global aphasia have difficulty with speaking and understanding speech. One strategy that can enhance client understanding is speaking to the client at a slower rate.

   B. **CORRECT:** One strategy that can enhance understanding is the use of alternative forms of communication, such as flash cards with pictures or a computer.

   C. For the client who has aphasia, speaking in a loud voice is unnecessary and can be interpreted as patronizing.

   D. The nurse should allow the client adequate time to finish sentences and not complete the sentences for him.

   E. **CORRECT:** One strategy that can enhance understanding is giving instructions one step at a time.

   Ⓝ *NCLEX® Connection: Psychosocial Integrity, Sensory/ Perceptual Alterations*

5. A. A client who has experienced a right-hemispheric stroke can experience difficulty with impulse control.

   B. A client who has experienced a right-hemispheric stroke can experience poor judgment.

   C. **CORRECT:** A client who experienced a left-hemispheric stroke can demonstrate depression and frustration regarding physical limitations due to the stroke.

   D. A client who experienced a right-hemispheric stroke can experience a loss of depth perception.

   Ⓝ *NCLEX® Connection: Physiological Adaptation, Basic Pathophysiology*

PRACTICE Answer

Using the ATI Active Learning Template: Nursing Skill

NURSING INTERVENTIONS

- If the client exhibits difficulty managing food or fluids, a speech therapist should do a swallowing evaluation.
- Position the client in an upright (high-Fowler's) position prior to food, fluid, or medication administration.
- Reinforce swallowing techniques recommended by speech language pathologist.
- Begin the client with a prescribed diet and observe closely for choking. Have suction equipment available.
- Thicker liquids are usually tolerated better than thin liquids. Collaborate with the speech-language pathologist and dietitian to find the proper consistency and type of diet.

Ⓝ *NCLEX® Connection: Basic Care and Comfort, Nutrition and Oral Hydration*

CHAPTER 10 *Multiple Sclerosis*

Multiple sclerosis (MS) is a neurological disease that typically results in impaired and worsening function of voluntary muscles.

MS is an autoimmune disorder that affects nerve cells in the brain and spinal cord. It is characterized by development of plaque in the white matter of the central nervous system (CNS). This plaque damages the myelin sheath and interferes with impulse transmission between the CNS and the body.

MS follows several possible courses. The most common is relapsing and remitting. The disease is marked by relapses and remissions that might not return the client to her previous baseline level of function.

MS is a chronic disease with no known cure that progresses in severity over time, sometimes to quadriplegia. Initial findings can be so vague that diagnosis is not made for several years.

Some forms of MS are aggressive and can shorten the lifespan. In most cases, life expectancy is not adversely affected by this disease.

DATA COLLECTION

RISK FACTORS

- The onset of MS is typically between 20 and 40 years of age. MS occurs two to three times as often in females. The etiology of MS is unknown. There is a family history (first-degree relative) of MS in many cases.
- Because MS is an autoimmune disease, there are factors that trigger relapses.
  - Viruses and infectious agents
  - Living in a cold climate
  - Physical injury
  - Emotional stress
  - Pregnancy
  - Fatigue
  - Overexertion
  - Temperature extremes
  - Hot shower/bath

EXPECTED FINDINGS

- Fatigue, especially of the lower extremities
- Pain or paresthesia
- Diplopia, changes in peripheral vision, decreased visual acuity
- Uhthoff's sign: a temporary worsening of vision and other neurological functions commonly seen in clients who have or are predisposed to MS, just after exertion or in situations where they are exposed to heat
- Tinnitus, vertigo, decreased hearing acuity
- Dysphagia
- Dysarthria (slurred and nasal speech)
- Muscle spasticity
- Ataxia or muscle weakness
- Nystagmus
- Bowel dysfunction (constipation, fecal incontinence)
- Bladder dysfunction (areflexia, urgency, nocturia)
- Cognitive changes (memory loss, impaired judgment)
- Sexual dysfunction

LABORATORY TESTS

Cerebrospinal fluid analysis reveals elevated protein level and a slight increase in WBCs.

DIAGNOSTIC PROCEDURES

Magnetic resonance imaging (MRI) reveals plaques of the brain and spine, which is most diagnostic.

PATIENT-CENTERED CARE

NURSING CARE

- Monitoring of
  - Visual acuity
  - Speech patterns: fatigue with talking
  - Swallowing
  - Activity tolerance
  - Skin integrity
- MS is a potentially debilitating condition. Discuss coping mechanisms and sources of support (family, friends, spiritual figures, support groups).
- Encourage fluid intake and other measures to decrease the risk of developing a urinary tract infection. Assist the client with bladder elimination: intermittent self-catheterization, bladder pacemaker, Credé's maneuver (placing manual pressure on abdomen over the bladder to expel urine).
- Monitor cognitive changes and assist with planning interventions to promote cognitive function. (Reorient the client. Place objects used daily in routine places.)
- Facilitate effective communication for dysarthria using a communication board.
- Apply eye patches to treat diplopia. Alternate eyes every few hours. Reinforce teaching about scanning techniques. Instruct the client to visually scan his environment by moving his head from side to side.
- Exercise and stretch involved muscles. (Avoid fatigue and overheating.)
- Promote energy conservation by grouping care and planning rest periods.
- Promote and maintain safe home and hospital environment to reduce the risk of injury (walking with wide base of support, assistive devices, skin precautions). Qs

MEDICATIONS

Azathioprine and cyclosporine

Immunosuppressive agents reduce the frequency of relapses.

NURSING ACTIONS
- Monitor for long-term effects.
- Be alert for manifestations of infection.
- Monitor for hypertension.
- Check for kidney dysfunction.

Prednisone

Corticosteroids reduce inflammation in acute exacerbations.

NURSING ACTIONS: Monitor for increased risk of infection, hypervolemia, hypernatremia, hypokalemia, hyperglycemia, gastrointestinal bleeding, and personality changes.

Dantrolene, tizanidine, baclofen, and diazepam

- Antispasmodics are used to treat muscle spasticity.
- Intrathecal baclofen can treat severe cases of MS.

NURSING ACTIONS
- Observe for increased weakness.
- Monitor for liver damage with tizanidine or dantrolene.

CLIENT EDUCATION
- Report increased weakness and jaundice to the provider.
- Avoid stopping baclofen abruptly.

Interferon beta

Immunomodulators are used to prevent or treat relapses.

Carbamazepine

Anticonvulsants are used for paresthesia.

Docusate sodium

Stool softeners are used for constipation.

Propantheline

Anticholinergics are used for bladder dysfunction.

Primidone and clonazepam

Beta blockers are used for tremors.

TEAMWORK AND COLLABORATION

- Assist in planning for disease progression. Provide community resources and respite services for the client and family.
- Consider referral to occupational and physical therapy for home environment assessment to determine safety and ease of mobility. Use adaptive devices to assist with activities of daily living.
- Refer to speech-language therapist for dysarthria and dysphagia.
- Emphasize the need to avoid overexertion, stress, extremes of temperatures, humidity, and people who have infections.

Application Exercises

1. A nurse is caring for a client who has multiple sclerosis. Which of the following findings should the nurse expect?

   A. Fluctuations in blood pressure

   B. Loss of cognitive function

   C. Ineffective cough

   D. Drooping eye lids

2. A nurse is collecting data from a client who has a new diagnosis of multiple sclerosis. Which of the following findings should the nurse expect? (Select all that apply.)

   A. Areas of paresthesia

   B. Involuntary eye movements

   C. Alopecia

   D. Increased salivation

   E. Ataxia

3. A nurse is reinforcing teaching with a client who has multiple sclerosis and a new prescription for baclofen. Which of the following statements should the nurse include in the teaching?

   A. "This medication will help you with your tremors."

   B. "This medication will help you with your bladder function."

   C. "This medication may cause your skin to bruise easily."

   D. "This medication may cause your skin to appear yellow in color."

PRACTICE Active Learning Scenario

A nurse is reinforcing teaching with the family members of a client who has a new diagnosis of multiple sclerosis. What should the nurse include in the teaching? Use the ATI Active Learning Template: System Disorder to complete this item.

ALTERATION IN HEALTH (DIAGNOSIS)

LABORATORY TESTS

DIAGNOSTIC PROCEDURES

MEDICATIONS: Describe four medications and one teaching point for each.

Application Exercises Key

1. A. Fluctuations in blood pressure is a manifestation associated with amyotrophic lateral sclerosis. The nurse should expect a client who has MS to exhibit a fluctuation in disease manifestations that worsens with heat exposure or exertion.

   B. **CORRECT:** Loss of cognitive function is a manifestation associated with MS.

   C. Ineffective cough is a manifestation associated with amyotrophic lateral sclerosis. The nurse should expect a client who has MS to exhibit ineffective bowel and bladder function.

   D. Drooping eyelids is a manifestation associated with myasthenia gravis. The nurse should expect a client who has MS to exhibit changes in visual acuity.

   Ⓝ NCLEX® Connection: Physiological Adaptation, Basic Pathophysiology

2. A. **CORRECT:** Areas of loss of skin sensation are a finding in a client who has MS.

   B. **CORRECT:** Nystagmus is a finding in a client who has MS.

   C. Hair loss is not a finding in a client who has MS.

   D. Dysphagia (swallowing difficulty) is a finding in a client who has MS.

   E. **CORRECT:** Ataxia occurs in the client who has MS as muscle weakness develops and there is loss of coordination.

   Ⓝ NCLEX® Connection: Physiological Adaptation, Basic Pathophysiology

3. A. Primidone and clonazepam are beta blockers given to clients who have MS to treat tremors.

   B. Propantheline is an anticholinergic medication that is given to clients who have MS to treat bladder dysfunction.

   C. Prednisone is a corticosteroid medication that is given to clients who have MS to treat inflammation. An adverse effect of this medication is bruising of the skin.

   D. **CORRECT:** Dantrolene and tizanidine are antispasmodic medications that are given to clients who have MS to treat muscle spasms. An adverse effect of this medication is a yellow appearance of the skin, also known as jaundice. The nurse should instruct the client to monitor for this finding, as this can indicate impaired liver function.

   Ⓝ NCLEX® Connection: Pharmacological Therapies, Expected Actions/Outcomes

PRACTICE Answer

Using the ATI Active Learning Template: System Disorder

ALTERATION IN HEALTH (DIAGNOSIS): MS is an autoimmune disorder characterized by the development of plaque in the white matter of the central nervous system. Plaque damages the myelin sheath and interferes with impulse transmission between the CNS and the body.

LABORATORY TESTS:
Cerebrospinal fluid analysis

DIAGNOSTIC PROCEDURES:
MRI of the brain and spine

MEDICATIONS
- Immunosuppressive agents such as azathioprine and cyclosporine: Long-term effects include increased risk for infection, hypertension, and kidney dysfunction.
- Corticosteroids such as prednisone: Increased risk for infection, hypervolemia, hypernatremia, hypokalemia, GI bleeding, and personality changes.
- Antispasmodics such as dantrolene, tizanidine, baclofen, and diazepam are used to treat muscle spasticity. Report increased weakness and jaundice to provider. Avoid stopping baclofen abruptly.
- Immunomodulators such as interferon beta are used to prevent and treat relapses.
- Anticonvulsants such as carbamazepine are used for paresthesia.
- Stool softeners such as docusate sodium are used for constipation.
- Anticholinergics such as propantheline are used for bladder dysfunction.
- Beta blockers such as primidone and clonazepam are used for tremors.

Ⓝ NCLEX® Connection: Physiological Adaptation, Alterations in Body Systems

CHAPTER 11 *Headaches*

Headaches are often classified as acute or chronic, temporary, or life-threatening. Headaches are a common occurrence and affect individuals of all ages. Headaches are associated with conditions such as colds, allergies, and stress or muscle tension.

Primary headaches have no identifiable organic cause. They include migraine, tension-like, and cluster headaches. Management of headaches can occur in the primary care setting.

Secondary headaches are associated with an organic cause (brain tumor, aneurysm) and warrant further investigation and medical management.

This chapter includes migraine headaches and cluster headaches.

HEALTH PROMOTION AND DISEASE PREVENTION

- Promote stress management strategies and recognition of triggers of the onset of a headache.
- Recommend use of a headache diary to help identify type of headache and response to interventions.
- Promote hand hygiene to prevent the spread of viruses that produce cold-like symptoms.
- Review pain management to include over-the-counter medications and herbal remedies.
- Review risk factors (triggers) for both migraine and cluster headaches.
  - Alcohol or environmental allergies
  - Intense odors, bright lights, overuse of some medications
  - Fatigue, sleep deprivation, depression, emotional or physical stress, anxiety
  - Menstrual cycles and oral contraceptive use
  - Foods containing tyramine, monosodium glutamate (MSG), nitrites, or milk products

Migraine headaches

DATA COLLECTION

EXPECTED FINDINGS

- Photophobia and phonophobia (sensitivity to sounds)
- Nausea and vomiting
- Stress and anxiety
- Unilateral pain, often behind one eye or ear
- Health history and family history for headache patterns
- Alterations in ADLs for 4 to 72 hr with some debilitation
- Common in females
- Pain is aggravated by physical activity
- Pallor, unilateral weakness, diaphoresis

Classified by categories

With aura

- Aura precedes onset of headache symptoms and includes visual disturbances (light flashes, bright spots).
- Migraine symptoms appear and include severe, incapacitating, throbbing headache that intensifies over several hours and is accompanied by nausea, vomiting, photophobia, and phonophobia.

Without aura

- Unilateral, pulsating pain
- One or more manifestations: photophobia, phonophobia, nausea, vomiting
- Persists for 4 to 72 hr

DIAGNOSTIC PROCEDURES

- Neuroimaging, electroencephalography, and lumbar puncture if neurologic findings are present to identify potential organic causes
- Allergy testing and serum metabolic profiles

PATIENT-CENTERED CARE

Nursing care focus during headache is pain management.
- Maintain a cool, dark, quiet, and odor-free environment.
- Administer medications as prescribed.
- Cold compresses
- Determine the level of pain
- Offer back massage
- Employ distraction techniques: progressive relaxation, deep breathing

MEDICATIONS

Available in a variety of forms to alleviate discomfort (nasal, rectal, injections)

- **Preventive therapy** is taken consistently to reduce frequency, duration, and intensity of headaches.
  - Beta-adrenergic blocker (propranolol), antiepileptic medications (divalproex, topiramate), tricyclic antidepressants (amitriptyline), or estrogens (for menstrual migraines)
  - Onabotulinum toxin A is approved for adults for chronic migraines. It is injected into specific areas of the head and neck for up to five treatment cycles. It blocks the pain signals from being transmitted to the brain.
- **Abortive therapy** alleviates pain during aura or soon after start of headache.
  - For mild migraines: NSAIDs (ibuprofen, naproxen), acetaminophen/aspirin/caffeine, or acetaminophen/isometheptene/dichloralphenazone formulations
  - Antiemetics (metoclopramide, droperidol) to relieve nausea and vomiting
  - Severe migraines
    - Triptan preparations (zolmitriptan sumatriptan, eletriptan) to produce a vasoconstrictive effect
    - Ergot alkaloids (ergotamine, dihydroergotamine) to narrow blood vessels and reduce inflammation
    - Opioids (butorphanol, meperidine)

COMPLEMENTARY AND ALTERNATIVE THERAPIES

- Pyridoxine (vitamin B_6) for estrogen-related migraines
- Riboflavin (vitamin B_2)
- Herbal products (bay, feverfew, ginger, lemon balm)

CLIENT EDUCATION

- Keep a diary to record headache patterns and triggers.
- Report changes in headache intensity, or new visual or neurological disturbances.
- Remain in a cool, dark, quiet environment.
- Check pulse when taking beta adrenergic blockers.
- Trigger avoidance and management
  - Limit foods with tyramine (pickles, caffeine, beer, wine, aged cheese, artificial sweeteners), MSG, or preservatives.
  - Maintain adequate regular sleep patterns.
  - Avoid light glare or flickering lights.
  - Review menstrual cycle pattern and hormone fluctuations.
  - Avoid intense environmental odors, perfumes, and tobacco smoke.
- Complementary and alternative therapies
  - Join community centers offering yoga, meditation, tai chi, exercise, biofeedback, and massage for relaxation and to alleviate muscle tension.
  - Practice deep-breathing exercises.
  - Use acupuncture and acupressure therapy, which can be helpful for pain management.
  - Review herbal remedies and nutrition supplements with the provider to prevent interactions with prescribed medications.

Cluster headaches

DATA COLLECTION

EXPECTED FINDINGS

- Brief episode of intense, unilateral, nonthrobbing periorbital pain lasting 30 min to 2 hr that can radiate to forehead, temple, or cheek
  - Occurring daily at about the same time for 4 to 12 weeks, often during sleep
  - Followed by period of remission for up to 12 months
- No warning signs; alcohol is a common trigger
- Less common than migraines
- Men between 20 to 40 years of age
- Tearing of the eye with pupillary constriction and ptosis
- Runny nose and nasal congestion
- Facial swelling

DIAGNOSTIC PROCEDURES

Neuroimaging (MRI, MRA, CT) to rule out infectious or other causes

PATIENT-CENTERED CARE

MEDICATIONS

PREVENTATIVE THERAPY

- Glucocorticoids (prednisone)
- Calcium channel blocker (verapamil)
- Neurostabilizers (lithium)

ABORTIVE THERAPY

- Triptans
- Ergot alkaloids
- Lidocaine (intranasal)
- Capsaicin (intranasal)
- 100% oxygen (inhalation)

> ! Opiates are not administered due to the possibility of rebound headaches.

THERAPEUTIC PROCEDURES

Home oxygen therapy at 12 L/min for 15 to 20 min at onset of headache can provide relief within 15 min.

CLIENT EDUCATION

- Maintain safety precautions when using oxygen in the home.
- Prevention strategies Qpcc
  - Avoid triggers such as alcohol.
  - Obtain adequate rest, sleep, exercise, and relaxation.
- Use complementary and alternative therapies to promote relaxation. Qpcc

Application Exercises

1. A nurse in a clinic is caring for a client who has frequent migraine headaches. The client asks about foods that can cause headaches. The nurse should recommend that the client avoid which of the following foods?

   A. Baked salmon
   B. Salted cashews
   C. Frozen strawberries
   D. Fresh asparagus

2. A nurse in a clinic is reinforcing teaching with a client who has a history of migraine headaches about a new prescription for zolmitriptan. Which of the following statements by the client indicates understanding of the teaching?

   A. "This medication will relieve my symptoms by causing my blood vessels to dilate."
   B. "I should take this medication daily to prevent the headache from occurring."
   C. "I should expect facial flushing when I take this medication."
   D. "This medication will lower my sensitivity to food triggers."

3. A nurse in a provider's office is collecting data from a client who has cluster headaches. Which of the following findings should the nurse expect? (Select all that apply.)

   A. Pain is bilateral across the posterior occipital area.
   B. Client experiences altered sleep-wake cycle.
   C. Headache occurs at approximately the same time of the day.
   D. Client describes headache pain as dull and throbbing.
   E. Nasal congestion and drainage occur.

4. A nurse is reinforcing discharge instructions with a client who has a new diagnosis of migraine headaches. Which of the following instructions should the nurse include?

   A. Increase environmental lighting when an aura occurs.
   B. Increase high-impact physical activity when a headache is present.
   C. Drink beverages that contain artificial sweeteners to prevent headaches.
   D. Apply a cool cloth to the face during a headache.

5. A nurse is obtaining a health history from a client who is being evaluated for the cause of frequent headaches. Which of the following questions should the nurse ask to identify the findings of migraine headaches?

   A. "Do the headaches occur at the same time each day?"
   B. "Is your headache accompanied by profuse tearing of the eyes?"
   C. "Does your headache awaken you from sleep?"
   D. "Is there a pattern of headaches among family members?"

PRACTICE Active Learning Scenario

A nurse in a clinic is caring for a client who has migraine headaches and a new prescription for sumatriptan nasal spray 5 mg. Use the ATI Active Learning Template: Medication and the ATI Pharmacology Review Module to complete this item.

EXPECTED PHARMACOLOGICAL ACTION

THERAPEUTIC USES

COMPLICATIONS

NURSING INTERVENTIONS

INTERACTIONS

CLIENT EDUCATION

MEDICATION ADMINISTRATION

EVALUATION OF MEDICATION EFFECTIVENESS

1. A. The client should avoid fish that is smoked because it contains tyramine. Baked salmon does not contain tyramine and is not a trigger for migraine headaches.

   B. **CORRECT:** Nuts contain tyramine, which can trigger migraine headaches.

   C. Fruits are not a source of tyramine.

   D. Vegetables are not a source of tyramine.

   Ⓝ *NCLEX® Connection: Basic Care and Comfort, Nutrition and Oral Hydration*

2. A. Zolmitriptan causes cranial arteries, basilar arteries, and blood vessels in the dura mater to constrict.

   B. Zolmitriptan is used for abortive therapy in treating migraine headaches. It is not used for headache prevention.

   C. **CORRECT:** Zolmitriptan can cause facial flushing, tingling, and warmth.

   D. Zolmitriptan is used as a component of abortive therapy for treatment of migraine headaches and does not affect a client's sensitivity to food triggers.

   Ⓝ *NCLEX® Connection: Pharmacological Therapies, Expected Actions/Outcomes*

3. A. Cluster headaches typically cause pain on one side of the head and radiate to the forehead, temple, or cheek.

   B. **CORRECT:** Cluster headaches can be due to a lack of continuity in the sleep-wake cycle.

   C. **CORRECT:** Cluster headaches occur at about the same time of day for 4 to 12 weeks.

   D. Cluster headaches are described as unilateral, intense, and nonthrobbing.

   E. **CORRECT:** A client can have a runny nose and nasal congestion with a cluster headache.

   Ⓝ *NCLEX® Connection: Physiological Adaptation, Basic Pathophysiology*

4. A. A quiet, dark environment can provide comfort during a migraine headache.

   B. Increasing physical activity during a migraine headache can worsen the pain.

   C. Artificial sweeteners contain tyramine, which can trigger a migraine headache.

   D. **CORRECT:** A cool cloth placed over the client's eyes provides comfort and can relieve pain.

   Ⓝ *NCLEX® Connection: Basic Care and Comfort, Nonpharmacological Comfort Interventions*

5. A. Cluster headaches typically occur at the same time each day.

   B. Facial tearing is typical in the presence of cluster headaches.

   C. Interrupted sleep patterns are associated with cluster headaches.

   D. **CORRECT:** A familial pattern of headaches is a common finding with migraines.

   Ⓝ *NCLEX® Connection: Health Promotion and Maintenance, Data Collection Techniques*

PRACTICE Answer

Using the ATI Active Learning Template: Medication

EXPECTED PHARMACOLOGICAL ACTION: Vasoconstriction of cranial carotid arteries

THERAPEUTIC USES: Abortive treatment of acute migraine attacks with or without aura and cluster headaches

COMPLICATIONS: Chest pressure and tightness; mild vertigo, malaise, fatigue and tingling sensations; coronary vasospasm (rare)

NURSING INTERVENTIONS: Report chest pressure and tightness to provider if does not resolve quickly. Monitor blood pressure.

INTERACTIONS: Do not use concurrent with ergot alkaloids, monoamine oxidase inhibitors, selective serotonin reuptake inhibitors, or serotonin/norepinephrine reuptake inhibitors.

CLIENT EDUCATION: Avoid use of St. John's wort when taking this medication. Limit use to three to four times each month. Do not take medication during pregnancy or if trying to become pregnant, as medication can have teratogenic effects.

MEDICATION ADMINISTRATION: Administer one unit-dose nasal spray in one nostril. Can repeat in 2 hr if headache remains but not to exceed 40 mg in 24 hr.

EVALUATION OF MEDICATION EFFECTIVENESS: The client should note relief of headache pain within 10 min after administration, with complete relief anticipated within 2 hr. Relief of photophobia, phonophobia, nausea and vomiting associated with migraine attack.

Ⓝ *NCLEX® Connection: Pharmacological Therapies, Expected Actions/Outcomes*

CHAPTER 12 *Increased Intracranial Pressure Disorders*

Increased intracranial pressure occurs from lesions, brain tumors, or fluid accumulation from a brain injury in the cranium. The cranium is a closed bony structure that does not expand in an adult. The lesion or fluid takes up space in the cranium resulting in increased intracranial pressure. Pressure increase beyond the expected levels increases edema and decreases brain tissue perfusion, leading to impaired neurological function, and possible death.

Brain tumors

- Brain tumors occur in any part of the brain and are classified according to the cell or tissue of origin. Cerebral tumors are the most common.
- Types of brain tumors include benign and malignant. Examples include malignant gliomas (neuroglial cells), benign meningiomas (meninges), pituitary adenomas, and acoustic neuromas (acoustic cranial nerve).
- A secondary classification, supratentorial tumors occur in the cerebral hemispheres above the tentorium cerebelli. Those below the tentorium cerebelli, such as tumors of the brain stem and cerebellum, are classified as infratentorial tumors.
- Brain tumors apply pressure to surrounding brain tissue, resulting in decreased outflow of cerebrospinal fluid (CSF), increased intracranial pressure (ICP), cerebral edema, and neurological deficits. Tumors that involve the pituitary gland can cause endocrine dysfunction.
- Malignant brain tumors are associated with a high overall mortality rate. Primary malignant brain tumors originate from neuroglial tissue and rarely metastasize outside of the brain. Secondary malignant brain tumors are lesions that are metastases from a primary cancer located elsewhere in the body. Cranial metastatic lesions are most common from breast, kidney, lung, and gastrointestinal tract cancers.
- Benign brain tumors develop from the meninges or cranial nerves and do not metastasize. These tumors have distinct boundaries and cause damage either by the pressure they exert within the cranial cavity and/or by impairing the function of the cranial nerve.

M◇ *Online Videos: Nystagmus, Romberg Sign, Babinski Reflex*

HEALTH PROMOTION/ DISEASE PREVENTION

There are no routine screening procedures to detect brain tumors.

DATA COLLECTION

RISK FACTORS

The cause is unknown, but several risk factors have been identified.
- Genetics
- Environmental agents
- Exposure to ionizing radiation
- Exposure to electromagnetic fields
- Previous head injury

EXPECTED FINDINGS

PHYSICAL FINDINGS
- Dysarthria
- Dysphagia
- Positive Romberg sign
- Positive Babinski sign
- Vertigo
- Hemiparesis
- Cranial nerve dysfunction (inability to discriminate sounds, loss of gag reflex, loss of blink response)
- Papilledema

MANIFESTATIONS SPECIFIC TO
SUPRATENTORIAL BRAIN TUMORS
- Severe headache (worse upon awakening but improving over time)
- Visual changes (blurring, visual field deficit)
- Seizures
- Loss of voluntary movement or the inability to control movement
- Change in cognitive function (memory loss, language impairment)
- Change in personality, inability to control emotions
- Nausea with or without vomiting
- Paralysis

MANIFESTATIONS SPECIFIC TO
INFRATENTORIAL BRAIN TUMORS
- Hearing loss or ringing in the ear
- Visual changes
- Facial drooping
- Difficulty swallowing
- Nystagmus, crossed eyes, or decreased vision
- Autonomic nervous system dysfunction
- Ataxia or clumsy movements
- Hemiparesis
- Cranial nerve dysfunction (inability to discriminate sounds, loss of gag reflex, loss of blink response)

LABORATORY TESTS

- CBC and differential to rule out anemia or malnutrition
- Blood alcohol and toxicology screen to rule out these as possible causes of altered physical findings

DIAGNOSTIC PROCEDURES

- X-ray, computed tomography (CT) imaging scan, magnetic resonance imaging (MRI), brain scan, position emission tomography (PET) scan, and cerebral angiography are used to determine the size, location, and extent of the tumor.
- Lumbar puncture (LP) and electroencephalography (EEG) can provide additional information about the tumor.
- To prevent brain herniation, the client who has or shows manifestations of increasing ICP should not have a lumbar puncture.
- Laboratory tests evaluate endocrine function, renal status, and electrolyte balance.
- Cerebral biopsy identifies cellular pathology.
  - The client will have this procedure in the surgical suite or in a radiology specialty suite.
  - Diagnostic procedures aid the biopsy process, such as a CT or MRI scan. The surgical suite has image guiding systems, which use CT or MRI scan information.
  - The biopsy involves taking a sample of a piece of abnormal cerebral tissue indicated on the CT/MRI scan. Diagnostic testing identifies the pathology of the tissue sample.
  - Benefit: Biopsy is minimally disruptive to the rest of the brain, provides a decreased recovery time, and is not associated with the risks of an open craniotomy.
  - Negative: Biopsy does not remove or debulk the tumor, the diagnostic determination by pathology can be inconclusive (related to insufficient tissue), and a misdiagnosis can occur if the tumor contains many types of tissue or the specimen is taken from one site.

CLIENT EDUCATION

- Continue antiepileptic medications as prescribed to prevent seizure activity. Qs
- Discontinue aspirin products at least 72 hr prior to the procedure to minimize the risk of intracerebral bleeding.
- Resume preprocedure activities after the client recovers from the general anesthetic. Care of the incision should include keeping the area clean and dry. Plan to remove sutures in 1 to 7 days. The client should avoid driving or other dangerous activities until follow-up appointment occurs and diagnosis is known.

PATIENT-CENTERED CARE

NURSING CARE

- Maintain airway (monitor oxygen levels, administer oxygen as needed, monitor lung sounds).
- Monitor neurological status—in particular, for changes in level of consciousness (LOC), neurological deficits, and occurrence of seizures.
- Maintain client safety. (Assist with transfers and ambulation. Provide assistive devices as needed.) Qs
- Implement seizure precautions.
- Administer medications as prescribed.

MEDICATIONS

Nonopioid analgesics are used to treat headaches. Opioid medications are avoided because they tend to decrease LOC.

Corticosteroids are used to reduce cerebral edema.
- Corticosteroid medications quickly reduce cerebral edema.
- Chronic administration is used to control cerebral edema associated with the presence or treatment of benign or malignant brain tumors.

Anticonvulsant medications are used to control or prevent seizure activity.
- Anticonvulsant medications suppress the neuronal activity within the brain, which prevents seizure activity.
- There are several classifications of antiepileptic medications, each specifically designed to treat specific seizure behavior.

H_2-antagonists are used to decrease the acid content of the stomach, reducing the risk of stress ulcers.
- H_2-antagonists are administered during acute or stressful periods (after surgery, at the initiation of chemotherapy, during the first several radiation therapy treatments).
- The effect of these treatments, together with the necessity of corticosteroids, places the client at risk for stress ulcers. This is primarily preventative treatment.

Antiemetics are used if nausea (with or without vomiting) is present.
- Nausea and vomiting is often a result of the increased ICP, the site of the tumor, or the treatment required.
- These medications are administered as prescribed, and are often provided as a preventative intervention, especially when the treatment is associated with nausea or vomiting.

INTERPROFESSIONAL CARE

- Recommend appropriate referrals (social services, support groups, medical equipment, and physical, speech, and occupational therapy).
- Treatments include steroids, surgery, chemotherapy, conventional radiation therapy, stereotactic radiosurgery, and clinical trials. Chemotherapy and conventional radiation therapy are often administered prior to surgery to reduce the bulk of the tumor, or after surgery to prevent tumor recurrence.
- In most cases when the tumor is benign, surgery is a curative treatment. However, these tumors can regrow. Radiation and chemotherapy are often provided to prevent recurrence.
- Some tumors are malignant by location, meaning that while the pathology is benign, the location makes the mortality rate associated with them high.
- In cases where the tumor is a metastatic lesion from a primary lesion elsewhere in the body, treatments are palliative. These treatments can consist of surgery, radiation, and chemotherapy, in any combination, and are aimed at controlling intracerebral lesions.

THERAPEUTIC PROCEDURES

Craniotomy

Complete or partial resection of brain tumor through surgical opening in the skull

PREOPERATIVE NURSING ACTIONS

- Explain the procedure to the client, answering all appropriate questions and providing emotional support.
- Provide written information to address the client's questions regarding the surgery and its outcomes, in an effort to ensure all questions are answered.
- Encourage the presence of the client's partner to hear the responses and avoid miscommunication.
- The client should stop taking aspirin, if prescribed, at least 72 hr prior to the procedure.
- No alcohol, tobacco, anticoagulants, or NSAIDs for 5 days prior to surgery.
- If the client uses alternative/complementary medications or treatments, make these known to the provider.
- The client should complete a living will and durable power for health care decisions.
- Administer medications as prescribed. The client may require an antianxiety or muscle relaxant medication before the procedure.

POSTOPERATIVE NURSING ACTIONS

- Closely monitor vital signs and neurological status, including using the Glasgow Scale.
- Treat pain adequately.
- Elevate the head of the client 30° for clients who had supratentorial surgery and in a neutral position to prevent increased ICP. Turn the client to the side or supine to decrease risk of pressure ulcers and pneumonia. Qs
- Infratentorial craniotomy clients lie flat and side-lying. Turn side to side every 2 hr for 24 to 48 hr.
- Avoid straining activities (moving up in bed and attempting to have a bowel movement) to prevent increased ICP. Postoperative bleeding and seizure activity are the greatest risks.
- Periorbital edema and ecchymosis is not unusual. Treat with cold compresses.
- Monitor head dressing every 1 to 2 hr for drainage.

COMPLICATIONS

Syndrome of inappropriate antidiuretic hormone

Syndrome of inappropriate antidiuretic hormone (SIADH) is a condition where fluid is retained as a result of an overproduction of vasopressin or antidiuretic hormone (ADH) from the posterior pituitary gland.

- SIADH occurs when the hypothalamus has been damaged and can no longer regulate the release of ADH.
- Treatment consists of fluid restriction, administration of tolvaptan, and treatment of hyponatremia.
- If SIADH is present, the client can have disorientation, headache, vomiting, muscle weakness, decreased LOC, irritability, loss of thirst, and weight gain.
- If severe or untreated, this condition can cause seizures and coma.

Diabetes insipidus

Diabetes insipidus (DI) is seen most often after supratentorial surgery, especially when involving the pituitary gland or hypothalamus.

- This is a condition where large amounts of dilute urine are excreted as a result of a deficiency of ADH from the posterior pituitary gland.
- The condition occurs when the hypothalamus has been damaged and can no longer regulate the release of ADH.
- Treatment of DI consists of massive fluid replacement, careful attention to laboratory values, and replacement of essential nutrients as indicated.

Head injury

Head injuries are classified as open or closed. In an open head injury, the integrity of the skull is compromised by either a penetrating object or blunt force trauma. A closed head injury occurs from blunt trauma that causes acceleration of the head and then deceleration. Head injuries are also classified as mild, moderate, or severe, depending upon Glasgow Coma Scale ratings and the length of time the client was unconscious.

TYPES OF BRAIN INJURY

- Types of brain injury include concussion, contusion, diffuse axonal injury, and intracranial hemorrhage.
  - **A concussion, or mild traumatic brain injury**, occurs after head trauma that result in a change in neurological function but no identified brain damage and usually resolves within 72 hr. Post-concussion syndrome includes persistence of cognitive and physical manifestations for an unknown period of time.
  - **A contusion** occurs when the brain is bruised and the client has a period of unconsciousness associated with stupor and confusion.
  - **Diffuse axonal injury** is a widespread injury to the brain that results in coma and is seen in severe head trauma.
  - **Intracranial hemorrhage** can occur in the epidural, subdural, or intracerebral space. It is a collection of blood following head trauma. There can be a delay of weeks to months in presenting manifestations for a subacute or chronic subdural hematoma.
  - **A coup-contrecoup injury** (acceleration-deceleration injury) can occur when the head is moving rapidly and hits a stationary object.
- Open-head injuries pose a high risk for infection. Scalp injuries often result in profuse bleeding due to the poor vasoconstriction of the blood vessels of the scalp.
- Skull fractures can occur following forceful head injury and might result in brain damage. The client can have localized pain at the site of the fracture, and swelling can occur. The nurse should observe for drainage from the ears or eyes (CSF).
- A cervical spine injury should always be suspected when a head injury occurs. A cervical spine injury must be ruled out prior to removing any devices used to stabilize the cervical spine. Qs

HEALTH PROMOTION AND DISEASE PREVENTION

- Wear helmets when skateboarding, riding a bike or motorcycle, skiing, and playing football or any other sport that could cause a head injury.
- Wear seat belts when driving or riding in a car.
- Avoid dangerous activities (speeding, driving under the influence of alcohol or drugs).
- Lock up all firearms.
- Avoid riding in open sections of motor vehicles.
- Promote programs directed at older adults to prevent falls, which are a major cause of neurological injury in adults ages 65 to 75. Older adults who sustain head injuries are at greater risk for complications, such as hematomas due to increased adherence of dura mater to skull and because of higher rates of anticoagulants prescribed to the older population. Ⓖ

DATA COLLECTION

RISK FACTORS

- Motor vehicle or motorcycle crashes
- Drug and alcohol use
- Sports injuries
- Assault
- Gunshot wounds
- Falls

EXPECTED FINDINGS

- Possible presence of alcohol or illicit drugs at time of injury
- Amnesia (loss of memory) before or after the injury
- Loss of consciousness: Length of time the client is unconscious is significant.
- CSF leakage from the nose and ears can indicate a basilar skull fracture ("halo" sign: yellow stain surrounded by blood on a paper towel; fluid tests positive for glucose).

MANIFESTATIONS OF INCREASED ICP
- Severe headache, nausea, vomiting
- Deteriorating LOC, restlessness, irritability
- Dilated or pinpoint nonreactive pupils
- Cranial nerve dysfunction
- Alteration in breathing pattern (Cheyne-Stokes respirations, central neurogenic hyperventilation, apnea)
- Deterioration in motor function, abnormal posturing (decerebrate, decorticate, flaccidity)
- Cushing's triad is a late finding characterized by severe hypertension with a widening pulse pressure (systolic-diastolic) and bradycardia.
- Seizures

LABORATORY TESTS

- ABGs
- CBC with differential
- Blood glucose level
- Electrolyte levels
- Serum and urine osmolarity
- Toxicology screen and electrocardiogram (ECG)
- Monitor antiseizure medication blood levels

DIAGNOSTIC PROCEDURES

- Cervical spine films to diagnose a cervical spine injury
- CT or MRI of the head and neck (with and without contrast if indicated)
- Calculation of cerebral perfusion using the ICP monitor, if it is in place

12.1 Extension posturing (decerebrate)

12.2 Flexion posturing (decorticate)

PATIENT-CENTERED CARE

NURSING CARE

- Support of the family following head injury is of great importance. Effective coping can be very difficult to achieve without support from providers and community members. The Brain Injury Association of America provides families and clients with information needed to cope with this potentially devastating injury. Qpcc
- The family can face difficult decisions following head injury. If brain death has occurred, the family needs support when deciding whether to donate organs.
  - Maintain cervical spine stability until cleared by an x-ray.
  - Implement measures to prevent complications of immobility (turn every 2 hr, footboard, splints). Specialty beds can be used.
  - Monitor fluid and electrolyte values and osmolality to detect changes in sodium regulation, onset of diabetes insipidus, or severe hypovolemia.
  - Monitor IV fluid infusions to maintain cerebral perfusion and minimize cerebral edema, which could increase ICP.
  - Maintain safety and seizure precautions (side rails up, padded side rails, call light within the client's reach). Qs
  - Even if the LOC is decreased, explain to the client the actions being taken and why. (Hearing is the last sense affected by a head injury.)
  - Monitor I&O closely and follow provider's orders regarding encouraging or restricting fluids.

Monitor at regularly scheduled intervals

Respiratory status (the priority assessment): The brain is dependent upon oxygen to maintain function and has little reserve available if oxygen is deprived. Untreated hypoxia leads to brain injury or death if the brain has been denied adequate oxygenation for 3 to 5 min. Changes in LOC, using the Glasgow Coma Scale (GCS), provide the earliest indication of neurological deterioration.

Cranial nerve function: Monitor eye blink response, gag reflex, tongue and shoulder movement

Check pupils for size, equality, and reaction to light: Pupils that are equal, round, and react to light and accommodation (PERRLA) are a normal finding.

Bilateral sensory and motor responses

Increased ICP: Monitored by placing a screw, catheter or sensor through a burr hole into the ventricle, subarachnoid, epidural, or subdural space. Expected reference range is 10 to 15 mm Hg.
- ICP can be increased by
  - Hypercarbia, which leads to cerebral vasodilation
  - Endotracheal or oral tracheal suctioning
  - Coughing or blowing the nose
  - Extreme neck or hip flexion/extension
  - Maintaining the head of the bed at an angle less than 30°
  - Increasing intra-abdominal pressure (restrictive clothing, Valsalva maneuver)

- Implement actions that decrease ICP.
  - Elevate head 20° to 30° to reduce ICP and promote venous drainage.
  - Avoid extreme flexion, extension, or rotation of the head, and maintain the body in a midline neutral position.
  - Maintain a patent airway. Brief periods of hyperventilation for the intubated client can be used after the first 24 hr following injury to help lower ICP. During the first 24 hr, hyperventilation can cause cerebral vasoconstriction, which can cause ischemia.
  - Administer oxygen as indicated to maintain $PaCO_2$ 35 to 45 mm Hg and PaO_2 levels greater than 95%.
  - Administer stool softeners and tell the client to avoid the Valsalva maneuver.
  - Report presence of CSF from nose or ears to the provider.
  - Provide a calm, restful environment. (Limit visitors. Minimize noise.)
  - Use measures to maintain normal body temperature

MEDICATIONS

Mannitol

- Mannitol is an osmotic diuretic that treats cerebral edema. When used for increased ICP, the medication draws fluid from the brain into the blood.
- Administered IV to treat acute cerebral edema.

NURSING ACTIONS

- Insert indwelling urinary catheter to monitor fluid and renal status. Monitor urine osmolality.
- Monitor serum electrolytes and osmolality closely.

Barbiturates

The provider may place the client in a coma (barbiturate coma) to decrease cellular metabolic demand until ICP decreases.
- Pentobarbital and thiopental are the most common medications.
- When barbiturate coma is used, monitoring neurological function is more difficult.
- Medication dosage is adjusted to keep the client completely unresponsive.
- Mechanical ventilation, cardiac and hemodynamic monitoring, and ICP monitoring are required.

Phenytoin

- Phenytoin can prevent or treat seizures. It was the first medication used to suppress seizures that did not depress the entire CNS.
- Dosing for this medication is client-specific and based on therapeutic blood levels.

NURSING ACTIONS: Check for medication interactions.

Histamine$_2$ receptor blockers or proton pump inhibitors

Helps to protect the gastric mucosa

THERAPEUTIC PROCEDURES

Craniotomy

A craniotomy is the removal of nonviable brain tissue that allows for expansion or removal of epidural or subdural hematomas. It is also used to decrease ICP and remove brain tumors. It involves drilling a burr hole or creating a bone flap to permit access to the affected area.
- Treatment of intracranial hemorrhages requires surgical evacuation. There are three surgical approaches: supratentorial (above the tentorial), infratentorial (below the tentorial, brain stem), and transsphenoidal (through the mouth and nasal sinuses).
- Burr holes are circular openings through the skull. The burr hole is used to assess cerebral swelling, injury, size, and position of the ventricles.
- This is a life-saving procedure and is associated with many potential complications (severe neurological impairment, infection, persistent seizures, neurological deficiencies, death).

NURSING ACTIONS

- The goal is to decrease cerebral edema. Administer medications such as mannitol and dexamethasone every 6 hr for 24 to 72 hr postoperatively.
- Phenytoin or diazepam is administered to prevent seizure activity.
- Monitor ICP and follow written protocols to detect for changes in ICP.
- Follow postoperative prescription for positioning to protect the incision and to prevent increased ICP.

INTERPROFESSIONAL CARE

- Care should include professionals from other disciplines as indicated. This can include physical, occupational, recreational, and speech therapists due to neurological deficits that can occur secondary to the area of the brain damaged.
- Contact a case manager to provide links to social service agencies and schools.
- Discuss possible transfer to a rehabilitation facility to compress the time required to recover from a head injury and support re-emergence into society.

COMPLICATIONS

Brain herniation

A brain herniation is the downward shift of brain tissue due to cerebral edema.

- The brain consists of brain tissue, cerebrospinal fluid, and blood. Due to the limited space within the skull, an alteration of any one of the components of the brain results in a compromise in the other components. When trauma creates a shift in these components, and the other components are unable to accommodate, the brain shifts from the cranial vault, or herniates. This can result in brain tissue moving downward, through the foramen magnum.
- Findings include fixed dilated pupils, deteriorating LOC, Cheyne–Stokes respirations, hemodynamic instability, and abnormal posturing.
- Recovery after this occurrence is rare, and urgent medical treatment (mannitol) or surgical (debulking) treatment is indicated.
- With treatment, severe neurological impairment usually persists.

NURSING ACTIONS
- Prevent this situation before treatment is needed.
- Closely monitoring vital signs and neurological status to allow early reporting of changes in the GCS score, an increase in the blood pressure, and an alteration in respiratory pattern and effort. **Qs**

CLIENT EDUCATION
- Frequently update family members on the health status of the client. Frequent updates and repeating medical information is often necessary to ensure comprehension among family members.
- The decision to surgically treat brain herniation is made in the presence of a critical situation. **Qᴛᴄ**
- Social service workers and pastoral personnel provide support for the family while reinforcing the medical situation.

Hematoma and intracranial hemorrhage

- Surgery is required to remove subdural and epidural hematoma.
- Intracranial hemorrhage is treated with osmotic diuretics.

NURSING ACTIONS: Monitor for severe headache, rapid decline in LOC, worsening neurological function and herniation, and changes in ICP.

Pulmonary edema

- Findings mimic acute pulmonary edema without cardiac involvement.
- This is a life–threatening emergency. Immediate, aggressive treatment is used. Survival is rare.

Diabetes insipidus or SIADH

Diabetes insipidus or syndrome of inappropriate antidiuretic hormone (SIADH) is a possible complication.

Cerebral salt wasting (CSW)

- CSW causes decreased serum osmolality and hyponatremia. CSW is the primary cause of hyponatremia following neurosurgery.
- CSW causes hypovolemia, compared with increased extracellular fluid in clients who have SIADH.

NURSING ACTIONS
- Monitor serum electrolytes and osmolality daily.
- Document strict intake and output.
- Weigh client daily.
- Treat electrolyte and fluid imbalance, as prescribed.
- Monitor for dehydration or fluid overload during treatment.

Hydrocephalus

- Excessive accumulation of CSF
- Can cause motor, cranial nerve deficits and decrease cognitive abilities.

NURSING ACTIONS: Facilitate return to the client's previous level of physical and cognitive function.

Application Exercises

1. A nurse is collecting data from a client who has increased intracranial pressure (ICP). Which of the following findings should the nurse expect? (Select all that apply.)

   A. Disoriented to time and place

   B. Restlessness and irritability

   C. Unequal pupils

   D. ICP 15 mm Hg

   E. Headache

2. A nurse is reviewing a prescription for dexamethasone with a client who has an expanding brain tumor. Which of the following are appropriate statements by the nurse? (Select all that apply.)

   A. "It is given to reduce swelling of the brain."

   B. "You will need to monitor for low blood sugar."

   C. "You may notice weight gain."

   D. "Tumor growth will be delayed."

   E. "It can cause you to retain fluids."

3. A nurse is caring for a client who has a benign brain tumor. The client asks the nurse if he can expect this same type of tumor to occur in other areas of his body. Which of the following is an appropriate response by the nurse?

   A. "It can spread to breasts and kidneys."

   B. "It can develop in your gastrointestinal tract."

   C. "It is limited to brain tissue."

   D. "It probably started in another area of your body and spread to your brain."

4. A nurse is reviewing the health record of a client who has a malignant brain tumor and notes the client has a positive Romberg sign. Which of the following actions should the nurse take to check for this manifestation?

   A. Stroke the lateral aspect of the sole of the foot.

   B. Ask the client to blink his eyes.

   C. Observe for facial drooping.

   D. Have the client stand erect with eyes closed.

5. A nurse is assisting with the care of a client following surgical evacuation of a subdural hematoma. Which of the following data is the priority to monitor?

   A. Glasgow Coma Scale

   B. Cranial nerve function

   C. Oxygen saturation

   D. Pupillary response

6. A nursing is caring for a client who is at risk for increased intracranial pressure (ICP). Which of the following actions should the nurse take to decrease the potential for raising the client's ICP? (Select all that apply.)

   A. Suction the client frequently.

   B. Decrease the noise level in the client's room.

   C. Elevate the client's head on two pillows.

   D. Administer a stool softener.

   E. Keep the client well hydrated.

PRACTICE Active Learning Scenario

A nurse is reviewing preoperative teaching with a client who has a brain tumor and will undergo a craniotomy. What should the nurse include in the teaching? Use the ATI Active Learning Template: Therapeutic Procedure to complete this item.

DESCRIPTION OF PROCEDURE

NURSING INTERVENTIONS: Describe three preoperative and three postoperative interventions.

Application Exercises Key

1. A. **CORRECT:** Changes in level of consciousness are an early indicator of increased ICP.

   B. **CORRECT:** Increased ICP can cause behavior changes, such as restlessness and irritability.

   C. **CORRECT:** Unequal pupils indicates pressure on the oculomotor nerve secondary to increased ICP.

   D. An ICP of 15 mm Hg is within the expected reference range.

   E. **CORRECT:** A headache is a manifestation of increased ICP.

   Ⓝ *NCLEX® Connection: Physiological Adaptation, Basic Pathophysiology*

2. A. **CORRECT:** Dexamethasone is a common steroid prescribed to reduce cerebral edema.

   B. The client can experience hyperglycemia as an adverse effect of dexamethasone.

   C. **CORRECT:** Weight gain is an adverse effect of dexamethasone.

   D. Dexamethasone does not affect tumor growth. It is given to prevent cerebral edema.

   E. **CORRECT:** Fluid retention is an adverse effect of dexamethasone.

   Ⓝ *NCLEX® Connection: Pharmacological Therapies, Expected Actions/Outcomes*

3. A. Metastases of a benign brain tumor do not occur.

   B. Metastases of a benign brain tumor do not occur.

   C. **CORRECT:** Benign brain tumors develop from the meninges or cranial nerves and do not metastasize.

   D. Benign brain tumors develop from the meninges or cranial nerves and are not secondary to other types of tumors.

   Ⓝ *NCLEX® Connection: Physiological Adaptation, Alterations in Body Systems*

4. A. A Babinski sign is elicited by stroking the lateral aspect of the sole of the foot.

   B. Asking the client to blink his eyes assesses cranial nerve function and is not part of the Romberg test.

   C. Observing for facial drooping assesses cranial nerve function and is not part of the Romberg test.

   D. **CORRECT:** A positive Romberg sign is indicated when a client loses his balance while attempting to stand erect with his eyes closed.

   Ⓝ *NCLEX® Connection: Reduction of Risk Potential, Diagnostic Tests*

5. A. The Glasgow Coma Scale is important to detect a decline in neurological function. However, the nurse should identify other data as the priority.

   B. Monitoring cranial nerve function is important to detect a decline in neurological function. However, the nurse should identify other data as the priority.

   C. **CORRECT:** When using the airway, breathing, and circulation approach to client care, the priority data to monitor is oxygen saturation. Brain tissue can only survive for 3 min before permanent damage occurs.

   D. Monitoring pupillary response is important to detect a decline in neurological function. However, the nurse should identify other data as the priority.

   Ⓝ *NCLEX® Connection: Reduction of Risk Potential, Potential for Complications of Diagnostic Tests/Treatments/Procedures*

6. A. The nurse should limit suctioning to only when necessary because it can increase ICP.

   B. **CORRECT:** Decreasing the noise level and restricting the number of people in the client's room can help prevent increases in ICP.

   C. The nurse should avoid hyperflexion of the client's neck with pillows because it can increase ICP. The nurse should elevate the head of the bed to at least 30° and maintain the client's head in an upright neutral position.

   D. **CORRECT:** The nurse should administer a stool softener to decrease the need to bear down (Valsalva maneuver) during bowel movements, which can increase ICP.

   E. The nurse should avoid overhydration because it can increase ICP. The nurse should monitor fluid and electrolyte levels closely for the client who has increased ICP.

   Ⓝ *NCLEX® Connection: Physiological Adaptation, Alterations in Body Systems*

PRACTICE Answer

Using the ATI Active Learning Template: Therapeutic Procedure

DESCRIPTION OF PROCEDURE: A craniotomy is a surgical opening in the skull to expose brain tissue. It involves a complete or partial resection of the brain tumor.

NURSING INTERVENTIONS

- Preoperative
  - Explain the procedure, answer appropriate questions, and provide emotional support.
  - Provide written explanations.
  - Include the client's partner in teaching.
  - Remind client to stop taking aspirin at least 72 hr prior to the procedure, if appropriate.
  - Review use of alternative/complementary therapies, and report their use to the provider.
  - Review the need for a living will and durable power for health care decisions.
  - Administer medications (anxiolytics, muscle relaxants) as prescribed.

- Postoperative
  - Monitor vital signs and neurological status to include use of Glasgow Scale.
  - Maintain client's head elevated to 30° and in a neutral position to prevent increased ICP.
  - Monitor for postoperative bleeding and seizures.
  - Prevent client performing any straining activities (moving up in bed, attempting to have a bowel movement).

Ⓝ *NCLEX® Connection: Reduction of Risk Potential, Potential for Complications from Surgical Procedures and Health Alterations*

UNIT 2   NURSING CARE OF CLIENTS WHO HAVE
          NEUROSENSORY DISORDERS
          SECTION: SENSORY DISORDERS

CHAPTER 13 *Disorders of the Eye*

Disorders of the eye are often caused by injury, disease processes, and the aging process. Disorders of the eye include macular degeneration, cataracts, and glaucoma.

Macular degeneration

Macular degeneration, often called age-related macular degeneration (AMD), is the central loss of vision that affects the macula of the eye.
- There is no cure for macular degeneration.
- AMD is a common cause of vision loss in older adults. Ⓖ

TYPES OF MACULAR DEGENERATION

Dry macular degeneration is the most common and is caused by a gradual blockage in retinal capillary arteries, which results in the macula becoming ischemic and necrotic due to the lack of retinal cells.

Wet macular degeneration is a less common form and is caused by the new growth of blood vessels that have thin walls that leak blood and fluid into the macular region of the eye.

DATA COLLECTION

RISK FACTORS

Dry macular degeneration
- Smoking
- Diabetes mellitus
- Hypertension
- Female
- Short body stature
- Family history
- Diet lacking carotene and vitamin E

Wet macular degeneration can occur at any age.

EXPECTED FINDINGS
- Lack of depth perception
- Objects appear distorted
- Dark spot in the center of vision
- Blurred vision
- Loss of central vision
- Blindness

DIAGNOSTIC PROCEDURES

Ophthalmoscopy: An ophthalmoscope is used to examine the back part of the eyeball (fundus), including the retina, optic disc, macula, and blood vessels.

Visual acuity tests: Snellen and Rosenbaum eye charts

Amsler Grid: Detects the progression of the disease

Fluorescein angiography or optical tomography: Determines specific areas of retinal involvement

PATIENT-CENTERED CARE

Wet macular degeneration
- Laser therapy to seal leaking blood vessels
- Ocular injections to inhibit blood vessel growth
- Photodynamic therapy destroys abnormal cells

Dry macular degeneration: No available treatment to restore vision.

CLIENT EDUCATION
- Encourage clients to consume foods high in antioxidants, carotene, and vitamins E and B_{12}. The provider might prescribe a daily supplement high in carotene and vitamin E. Ⓠpcc
- As loss of vision progresses, clients will be challenged with the ability to eat, drive, write, and read, as well as other activities of daily living.
- Refer clients to community organizations that can assist with transportation, reading devices, and large-print books.

Cataracts

A cataract is an opacity in the lens of an eye that impairs vision. **(13.1)**

Common causes of cataracts

Age-related: Drying of lens due to water loss; increase in lens density due to lens fiber compaction

Traumatic: Blunt or penetrating injury or foreign body in the eye, exposure to radiation or ultraviolet light

Toxic: Long-term use of corticosteroids, phenothiazine derivatives, beta blockers, or miotic medications

Congenital: Often caused by the transfer of a maternal infection

Associated: Diabetes mellitus, hypoparathyroidism, Down syndrome, chronic sunlight exposure

Complicated: Intraocular disease such as retinitis pigmentosa, glaucoma, or retinal detachment

13.1 Normal and cataract-clouded lenses

normal lenses	cataract-clouded lenses

HEALTH PROMOTION AND DISEASE PREVENTION

- Reinforce teaching with clients to wear sunglasses while outside.
- Advise clients to wear protective eyewear while playing sports and performing hazardous activities such as welding and yard work. Qs
- Encourage annual eye examinations and good eye health, especially in adults over the age of 40. ⓒ

DATA COLLECTION

RISK FACTORS

- Advanced age
- Diabetes
- Heredity
- Smoking
- Eye trauma
- Alcohol consumption greater than four drinks/day for males and three drinks/day for females
- Excessive exposure to the sun
- Chronic corticosteroid use

EXPECTED FINDINGS

- Decreased visual acuity (prescription changes, reduced night vision, decreased color perception)
- Blurred vision
- Diplopia (double vision)
- Photophobia
- Progressive and painless loss of vision
- Visible opacity
- Absent red reflex
- Increased nearsightedness

DIAGNOSTIC PROCEDURES

- Cataracts are diagnosed upon examination of the lens using an ophthalmoscope.
- Slit lamp visualizes opacities.

PATIENT-CENTERED CARE

NURSING CARE

- Check visual acuity using the Snellen chart.
- Examine external and internal eye structures using an ophthalmoscope.
- Determine the client's functional capacity due to decreased vision.
- Increase the amount of light in a room.
- Provide adaptive devices that accommodate for reduced vision.
  - Magnifying lens and large-print reading materials
  - Talking devices, such as clocks

MEDICATIONS

Anticholinergic agents (atropine 1% ophthalmic solution)

- This medication prevents pupil constriction for prolonged periods of time (mydriasis) and relaxes muscles in the eye (cycloplegia). It is used to dilate the eye preoperatively and for visualization of the eye's internal structures.
- The medication has a long duration, but a fast onset.

CLIENT EDUCATION
- The effects of the medication can last 7 to 12 days.
- The medication can cause photosensitivity, so wear sunglasses to protect the eyes. Qpcc
- Adverse effects can include dry mouth, tachycardia, constipation, fever, and confusion.

INTERPROFESSIONAL CARE

Consult with an ophthalmologist (eye surgeon) for cataract surgery.

THERAPEUTIC PROCEDURES

Surgical removal of the lens

Extracapsular (common): A small incision is made, and the lens is removed in one piece, or in several pieces after being broken up using sound waves (phacoemulsification). The posterior capsule is retained. A replacement or intraocular lens is inserted. Replacement lenses can correct refractive errors, resulting in improved vision.

Intracapsular: The lens and the capsule are removed. Cryosurgery (freezing of the lens before removal) is often performed.

NURSING ACTIONS

- Prior to surgery
  - Reinforce teaching about postoperative restrictions
  - Administer perioperative eye drops as prescribed
- Postoperative care should focus on
  - Preventing an increase in intraocular pressure (IOP)
  - Preventing infection
  - Administering ophthalmic medications
  - Providing pain relief
  - Reinforcing teaching with the client about self-care at home and fall prevention Ⓖ

CLIENT EDUCATION

- Wear sunglasses while outside or in brightly lit areas.
- Report manifestations of infection, such as yellow or green drainage.
- Avoid getting water in the eye.
- Cover the eye with a protective shield at night.
- Avoid activities that increase IOP.
  - Bending over at the waist
  - Sneezing
  - Coughing
  - Straining at bowel movements
  - Head hyperflexion
  - Restrictive clothing, such as tight shirt collars
  - Sexual intercourse
  - Lifting heavy objects greater than 5 lb
- Limit activities.
  - Tilting the head back to wash hair
  - Cooking and housekeeping
  - Rapid, jerky movements, such as vacuuming
  - Driving and operating machinery
  - Playing sports
- Report pain with nausea/vomiting (indications of increased IOP or hemorrhage).
- Best vision is not expected until 4 to 6 weeks following surgery.
- Report if any changes occur (lid swelling, decreased vision, bleeding or discharge, sharp sudden eye pain, flashes of light, floating shapes).
- Administer eye drops as prescribed.
- Keep follow-up appointments.

COMPLICATIONS

Infection

Infection can occur after surgery.

CLIENT EDUCATION: Report yellow or green drainage, increased redness or pain, reduction in visual acuity, increased tear production, and photophobia. Ⓠᴘᴄᴄ

Bleeding

Bleeding is a risk several days following surgery.

CLIENT EDUCATION: Immediately report any sudden change in visual acuity or an increase in pain. Ⓠᴘᴄᴄ

Glaucoma

Glaucoma is a disturbance of the functional or structural integrity of the optic nerve. Decreased fluid drainage or increased fluid secretion increases intraocular pressure (IOP) and can cause atrophic changes of the optic nerve and visual defects. The expected reference range for IOP is 10 to 21 mm/Hg.

- There are two primary types of glaucoma.
  - **Primary open-angle glaucoma (POAG):** This is the more common form. Open-angle refers to the angle between the iris and sclera. The aqueous humor outflow is decreased due to blockages in the eye's drainage system (canal of Schlemm and trabecular meshwork), causing a gradual rise in IOP.
  - **Primary angle-closure glaucoma:** IOP rises suddenly. The angle between the iris and the sclera suddenly closes, causing a corresponding increase in IOP. The onset is sudden and requires immediate treatment.
- Glaucoma is a frequent cause of blindness. Early diagnosis and treatment is essential in preventing vision loss from glaucoma.

HEALTH PROMOTION AND DISEASE PREVENTION

- Encourage annual eye examinations and good eye health, especially for adults over the age of 40. Ⓖ
- Reinforce teaching with clients about the disease process and early indications of glaucoma (reduced vision, mild eye pain).

DATA COLLECTION

RISK FACTORS

- Age
- Infection
- Tumors
- Diabetes mellitus
- Genetic predisposition
- Hypertension
- Eye trauma
- African American ethnicity

EXPECTED FINDINGS

Primary open-angle glaucoma
- Painless
- Gradual reduction of peripheral vision
- Decreased accommodation
- Halos seen around lights
- Elevated IOP (greater than 21 mm Hg: usually 22 to 32)

Primary angle-closure glaucoma
- Rapid onset of elevated IOP (30 mm Hg or greater)
- Severe eye pain and headache
- Decreased or blurred vision
- Colored halos seen around lights
- Pupil nonreactive to light
- Nausea
- Photophobia

DIAGNOSTIC PROCEDURES

Visual data collection: Measures decrease in visual acuity and peripheral vision

Tonometry: Measures IOP (expected reference range is 10 to 21 mm Hg). IOP is elevated with glaucoma, especially angle-closure.

Gonioscopy: Used to determine the depth of the anterior chamber of the eyes

Fundoscopy: Identifies optic disc cupping

PATIENT-CENTERED CARE

NURSING CARE

- Monitor for increased IOP (greater than 21 mm Hg).
- Monitor for decreased vision and light sensitivity.
- Monitor for aching or discomfort around the eye.
- Reinforce information about the disease process and allow clients to express their feelings.
- Treat severe pain and nausea that accompanies angle-closure glaucoma with analgesics and antiemetics.

MEDICATIONS

The priority intervention for treating glaucoma is medication therapy.

CLIENT EDUCATION
- Prescribed eye medication is beneficial if used every 12 hr.
- Instill one drop in each eye once or twice daily.
- Wait 5 to 10 min between eye drops if more than one is prescribed to prevent one medication from diluting another.
- Avoid touching the tip of the application bottle to the eye.
- Always wash hands before and after use.
- Once eye drop is instilled, apply pressure using the punctal occlusion technique (placing pressure on the inner corner of the eye).

Miotics

Pilocarpine ophthalmic solution
Pilocarpine is a miotic medication, which constricts the pupil and allows for improved circulation and outflow of the aqueous humor. Miotics can cause blurred vision. Pilocarpine is considered a second-line drug for POAG.

Beta blockers (timolol)
- Beta blockers are first-line medication therapy for glaucoma. They decrease IOP by reducing aqueous humor production.
- Can be absorbed systemically and cause bronchoconstriction and hypoglycemia. Use with caution in clients who have asthma, COPD, and diabetes mellitus. Can potentiate systemic effects of oral beta-blockers and cause bradycardia and hypotension.

Prostaglandin analogs (latanoprost)
- Increases the outflow of the aqueous humor
- CLIENT EDUCATION: Vision is often blurred following instillation. Instill drops at bedtime. These medications can cause permanent darkening of iris and skin around the eyelid.

Carbonic anhydrase inhibitors

Acetazolamide, dorzolamide, brinzolamide decrease IOP by reducing aqueous humor production.

NURSING ACTIONS: Ask clients whether they are allergic to sulfa. Carbonic anhydrase inhibitors are sulfa-based. Can cause ocular stinging, bitter taste in mouth, conjunctivitis, and eyelid reactions.

IV mannitol

IV mannitol is an osmotic diuretic used in the emergency treatment for primary angle-closure glaucoma to quickly decrease IOP. Adverse effects include headache, nausea, and vomiting.

THERAPEUTIC PROCEDURES

Glaucoma surgery

Cyclocryotherapy freezes the ciliary body and prevents aqueous humor production.

Laser trabeculectomy, iridotomy, or the placement of a shunt are procedures used to improve the flow of the aqueous humor by opening a channel out of the anterior chamber of the eye.

NURSING ACTIONS: Reinforce teaching with clients about the disease and importance of adhering to the medication schedule to treat IOP.

CLIENT EDUCATION

- Wear sunglasses while outside or in brightly lit areas.
- Report manifestations of infection, such as yellow or green drainage.
- Avoid activities that increase IOP.
  - Bending over at the waist
  - Sneezing
  - Coughing
  - Straining
  - Head hyperflexion
  - Restrictive clothing, such as tight shirt collars
  - Sexual intercourse
- Clients should not lie on the operative side and should report severe pain or nausea (possible hemorrhage).
- Clients should report if any changes occur (lid swelling; decreased vision; bleeding; discharge; sharp, sudden pain in the eye; flashes of light; floating shapes).
- Limit activities.
  - Tilting head back to wash hair
  - Cooking and housekeeping
  - Rapid, jerky movements, such as vacuuming
  - Driving and operating machinery
  - Playing sports
  - Report pain with nausea/vomiting (indications of increased IOP or hemorrhage).
- Final best vision is not expected until 4 to 6 weeks after surgery.

INTERPROFESSIONAL CARE

Refer to an ophthalmologist if surgery is necessary.

CLIENT EDUCATION

Set up services (community outreach programs, meals on wheels, services for the blind). Q℠

Complementary therapies

Advise clients that kava can cause pupil dilation, which can increase IOP.

COMPLICATIONS

Blindness

Blindness is a potential consequence of untreated glaucoma.

CLIENT EDUCATION: Encourage adults 40 or older to have an annual examination, including a measurement of IOP. Ⓖ

PRACTICE Active Learning Scenario

A nurse is reinforcing discharge instructions with a client who has a primary open-angle glaucoma and a new prescription for timolol 0.25% eye drops. Use the ATI Active Learning Template: Medication and the ATI Pharmacology Review Module to complete this item.

COMPLICATIONS: List at least three adverse effects to included in the teaching.

Application Exercises

1. A nurse is caring for an older adult client who has diabetes mellitus and reports a gradual loss of peripheral vision. The nurse should recognize this as a manifestation of which of the following diseases?
   - A. Cataracts
   - B. Open-angle glaucoma
   - C. Macular degeneration
   - D. Angle-closure glaucoma

2. A nurse is reinforcing postoperative teaching with a client following cataract surgery. Which of the following statements should the nurse include in the teaching?
   - A. "You can resume playing golf in 2 days."
   - B. "You need to tilt your head back when washing your hair."
   - C. "You can get water in your eyes in 1 day."
   - D. "You need to limit your housekeeping activities."

3. A nurse is collecting data on a male older adult client who has a new diagnosis of glaucoma. Which of the following findings should the nurse recognize as risk factors associated with this disease? (Select all that apply.)
   - A. Gender
   - B. Genetic predisposition
   - C. Eye trauma
   - D. Age
   - E. Diabetes mellitus

4. A nurse is collecting data on a client who has a new diagnosis of cataracts. Which of the following manifestations should the nurse expect? (Select all that apply.)
   - A. Eye pain
   - B. Floating spots
   - C. Blurred vision
   - D. White pupils
   - E. Bilateral red reflexes

5. A nurse is reinforcing teaching with a client who has a new diagnosis of dry macular degeneration. Which of the following instructions should the nurse include in the teaching?
   - A. Increase intake of deep yellow and orange vegetables.
   - B. Administer eye drops twice daily.
   - C. Avoid bending at the waist.
   - D. Wear an eye patch at night.

Application Exercises Key

1. A. A client who has cataracts experiences a decrease in peripheral and central vision due to opacity of the lens.

   B. **CORRECT:** A gradual loss of peripheral vision is a manifestation associated with open angle glaucoma.

   C. A client who has macular degeneration experiences a loss of central vision.

   D. A client who has angle-closure glaucoma experiences sudden nausea, severe pain, and halos around lights.

   Ⓝ *NCLEX® Connection: Reduction of Risk Potential, Potential for Complications from Surgical Procedures and Health Alterations*

2. A. The nurse should not instruct the client to resume playing golf for several weeks. This could cause a rise in intraocular pressure (IOP) or possible injury to the eye.

   B. The nurse should not instruct the client to tilt his head back when washing his hair. This could cause a rise in IOP or possible injury to the eye.

   C. The client should not get water in his eyes for 3 to 7 days following cataract surgery to reduce the risk for infection and promote healing.

   D. **CORRECT:** The nurse should instruct the client to limit housekeeping activities following cataract surgery. This activity could cause a rise in IOP or injury to the eye.

   Ⓝ *NCLEX® Connection: Reduction of Risk Potential, Potential for Complications from Surgical Procedures and Health Alterations*

3. A. Gender is not a risk factor associated with glaucoma.

   B. **CORRECT:** Genetic predisposition is a risk factor associated with glaucoma.

   C. **CORRECT:** Eye trauma is a risk factor associated with glaucoma.

   D. **CORRECT:** Age is a risk factor associated with glaucoma.

   E. **CORRECT:** Diabetes mellitus is a risk factor associated with glaucoma.

   Ⓝ *NCLEX® Connection: Health Promotion and Maintenance, Health Promotion/Disease Prevention*

4. A. Eye pain is manifestation associated with primary angle-closure glaucoma.

   B. Floating spots are a manifestation associated with retinal detachment.

   C. **CORRECT:** Blurred vision is a manifestation associated with cataracts.

   D. **CORRECT:** White pupils are a manifestation associated with cataracts.

   E. Bilateral red reflexes are absent in a client who has cataracts.

   Ⓝ *NCLEX® Connection: Physiological Adaptation, Basic Pathophysiology*

5. A. **CORRECT:** The nurse should instruct the client to increase dietary intake of carotenoids and antioxidants to slow the progression of the macular degeneration.

   B. A client who has primary open-angle glaucoma should administer eye drops once or twice daily.

   C. A client who is at risk for increased intraocular pressure, such as following cataract surgery, should avoid bending at the waist.

   D. A client who has had eye surgery, such as cataract surgery, should wear an eye patch at night to protect the eye from injury.

   Ⓝ *NCLEX® Connection: Basic Care and Comfort, Nutrition and Oral Hydration*

PRACTICE Answer

Using ATI Active Learning Template: Medication

COMPLICATIONS
- Central nervous system: Lethargy, fatigue, anxiety, headache, somnolence, depression
- Cardiovascular: Bradycardia, palpitations, syncope, hypotension, AV conduction disturbances, congestive heart failure
- Specific senses: Eye stinging, tearing, photophobia, eye irritation
- Gastrointestinal: Nausea, dry mouth
- Respiratory: Difficulty breathing, bronchospasm
- Metabolic: Hypoglycemia

Ⓝ *NCLEX® Connection: Pharmacological Therapies, Adverse Effects/Contraindications/Side Effects/Interactions*

UNIT 2 **NURSING CARE OF CLIENTS WHO HAVE NEUROSENSORY DISORDERS**
SECTION: SENSORY DISORDERS

CHAPTER 14 # Middle and Inner Ear Disorders

The ear is a sensory organ with two functions: hearing and balance.

The middle ear consists of the tympanic membrane (eardrum) and the three smallest bones (ossicles) of the body (malleus, incus, and stapes), and connects to the nasopharynx via the Eustachian tube, which equalizes pressure.

The inner ear is located deep within the temporal bone, separated from the middle ear by the oval window. It consists of the cochlea (hearing organ) and semicircular canals (responsible for balance). Cranial nerves VII (facial nerve) and VIII (vestibulocochlear nerve) are part of the inner ear anatomy.

Visual, vestibular, and proprioceptive systems provide the brain with input regarding balance. Problems within any of these systems pose a risk for loss of balance. Qs

Nurses who are knowledgeable can identify the types of middle- and inner ear disorders, including infection, tumors, and issues with balance and coordination.

TYPES OF EAR DISORDERS

Hearing loss

- Environmental or workplace exposure to noise can lead to hearing loss.
- Conductive hearing loss is caused by factors such as otitis media, otosclerosis, and presence of a foreign body (such as impacted cerumen).
- Color of cerumen and external ear canal varies depending on client's race and skin tone. During data collection the nurse should expect these variations. Qpcc

- Sensorineural hearing loss is caused by damage to cranial nerve VIII and is common with noise exposure. Other causes include presbycusis, ototoxic medications, exposure to rubella in utero, and severe infections.
- Combined hearing loss is caused by a combination of conductive and sensorineural problems.
- Changes in the middle and inner ear related to aging include thickening of the tympanic membrane (loss of elasticity), loss of sensory hair cells in the organ of Corti, and limitations to movement of the ossicles. Ⓒ

Conditions of the middle ear

- Conditions of the middle ear are often caused by injury, disease, and the aging process.
- Acute otitis media, which is common in children, is a viral or bacterial infection of the middle ear.
- Manifestations include ear pain, pressure, fever, headache, conductive hearing loss, and purulent or bloody drainage if perforation of the eardrum occurs.
- Otoscopic exam can show redness, bulging tympanic membrane, and inability to visualize usual landmarks.
- Medical management includes general observation to allow resolution on its own, systemic antibiotic therapy, analgesics and application of heat for pain, and decongestants.
- Surgical management includes myringotomy and placement of a grommet to equalize pressure.
- Refer to **PN NURSING CARE OF CHILDREN REVIEW MODULE: CHAPTER 36: ACUTE OTITIS MEDIA**.

Conditions of the inner ear

- Vertigo occurs when the client has the sensation that he or his surroundings are in motion.
- Benign paroxysmal positional vertigo occurs in response to a change in position. It is thought to be caused by the disruption of the debris located within the semicircular canal (small crystals of calcium carbonate). Onset is sudden and can last for a few weeks or years. Bed rest is prescribed along with a short course of meclizine.
- Ménière's disease is caused by excess fluid and pressure in the labyrinth and is characterized by episodic vertigo, tinnitus (ringing in the ears), and fluctuating sensorineural hearing loss.
- Labyrinthitis is an inflammation of the labyrinth in the inner ear, often secondary to otitis media. It is characterized by the sudden onset of severe vertigo, nausea, vomiting, and possible hearing loss, nystagmus, and tinnitus. Manifestations are treated with bed rest in a darkened environment. Meclizine or dimenhydrinate is prescribed for nausea and vertigo. Systemic antibiotic therapy can also be prescribed.

DATA COLLECTION

RISK FACTORS

Middle-ear disorders
- Recurrent colds and otitis media
- Enlarged adenoids
- Trauma
- Changes in air pressure (scuba diving, flying)

Inner-ear disorders
- Viral or bacterial infection
- Damage due to ototoxic medications

EXPECTED FINDINGS

Middle ear disorders
- Hearing loss
- Feeling of fullness or pain in the ear
- Red, inflamed ear canal and tympanic membrane (TM)
- Bulging TM
- Fluid or bubbles behind TM
- Diffuse appearance of or inability to visualize normal light reflex
- Fever

Inner ear disorders
- Hearing loss
- Tinnitus
- Dizziness or vertigo
- Vomiting
- Nystagmus
- Alterations in balance

DIAGNOSTIC PROCEDURES

Audiometry

Audiometry is a noninvasive test of hearing ability, including frequency, pitch, and intensity. The client indicates when a tone is heard through earphones. Nurses might collaborate with an audiologist for this and other diagnostic procedures. Qᴛᴄ

Tympanogram

Tympanogram measures the mobility of the TM and middle ear structures relative to sound (effective in diagnosing middle ear disease).

Weber and Rinne tests

Weber and Rinne tests use tuning forks to determine whether hearing loss is present.

Otoscopy

An otoscope is used to examine the external auditory canal, TM, and malleus bone visible through the TM.

NURSING ACTIONS
- Otoscopic examination is done if audiometry results indicate possible impairment or if a client reports ear pain.
- After selection of a properly sized speculum, an otoscope is introduced into the external ear.
- If the ear canal curves, pull up and back on the auricle of adults, and down and back on the auricle of children, to straighten out the canal and enhance visualization.
- The TM should appear a pearly gray color and intact. It should provide complete structural separation of the outer and middle ear structures.
- The light reflex should appear visible from the center of the TM anteriorly (5 o'clock right ear; 7 o'clock left ear). **(14.1)**
- In the presence of fluid or infection in the middle ear, the TM becomes inflamed and can bulge from the pressure of the exudate. This also displaces the light reflex, causing it to look diffuse or completely obscured, which is a significant diagnostic finding.
- Avoid touching the lining of the ear canal, which causes pain due to sensitivity.

CLIENT EDUCATION: To see the TM clearly, the auricle might need to be firmly pulled.

Electronystagmography (ENG)

ENG detects involuntary eye movements (nystagmus) in order to collect data for disease of the vestibular system of the ear. Electrodes are taped near the eyes, and movements of the eyes are recorded when the ear canal is stimulated with cold/warm water instillation. A specialist can interpret and record the client's eye movements as either normal or abnormal.

NURSING ACTIONS
- Intraprocedure, the nurse should ask simple questions (name recall, math problems) to ensure the client remains alert.
- Maintain the client on bed rest and NPO postprocedure until vertigo subsides. Qs

CLIENT EDUCATION
- The client's preparation includes fasting immediately before the procedure and restricting caffeine, alcohol, sedatives, and antihistamines for several days prior to the test.
- Reinforce teaching that client may experience vertigo, vomiting, nausea, and nystagmus, which is a normal response during testing.
- This test is not performed on clients who have a pacemaker. (Pacemaker signals inhibit sensitivity of ENG.)

Caloric testing

- Caloric testing is often completed concurrently with ENG.
- Water (warmer or cooler than body temperature) is instilled in the ear in an effort to induce nystagmus.
- The eyes' response to the instillation of cold and warm water is diagnostic of vestibular disorders.

NURSING ACTIONS: The client should follow the same restrictions as those for an ENG.

CLIENT EDUCATION: Inform the client of the above restrictions.

PATIENT-CENTERED CARE

NURSING CARE

- Monitor functional ability and balance. Take fall risk precautions as necessary. Qs
- Evaluate the client's home situation. Collaborate with home health to determine home safety and falls risks, as needed.
- Encourage a client who has balance or functional limitations to rise slowly and use assistance and assistive devices as needed.
- Ototoxic medications can cause tinnitus and sensorineural hearing loss, especially at high doses or with prolonged treatment. Older adult clients are at greater risk for ototoxicity. Monitor blood levels of ototoxic medication, and reinforce teaching with clients about adverse effects. Routine audiometry is indicated with use of ototoxic IV antibiotics. Ototoxic medications include the following.
  - **Antibiotics:** gentamicin, erythromycin
  - **Diuretics:** furosemide, ethacrynic acid
  - **NSAIDs:** aspirin, ibuprofen
  - **Chemotherapeutic agents:** cisplatin
- Assist with ENG and caloric testing as needed.
- Administer antivertigo and antiemetic medications as needed.

14.1 Light reflex

otoscope

tympanic membrane

short process of malleus

pars flaccida

long process of malleus

pars tensa

annulus

umbo

light reflex

light reflex

left tympanic membrane   right tympanic membrane

MEDICATIONS

Meclizine

Meclizine has antihistamine and anticholinergic effects and is used to treat the vertigo that accompanies inner ear problems.

NURSING ACTIONS: Observe for sedation, and take appropriate precautions to ensure safe ambulation. Qs

CLIENT EDUCATION: Warn the client about the sedative effects of meclizine. (Avoid driving or operating heavy machinery.) Adverse effects include dry mouth, blurry vision, constipation, and urinary retention.

Antiemetics

- Ondansetron is one of several antiemetics used to treat nausea and vomiting associated with vertigo.
- Contraindicated for clients who have certain cardiac rhythm disorders. Qs

CLIENT EDUCATION: Report dizziness or rash.

Diphenhydramine and dimenhydrinate

Antihistamines are effective in the treatment of vertigo and nausea that accompany inner ear problems.

NURSING ACTIONS
- Observe for urinary retention.
- Observe for sedation, and take appropriate precautions to ensure safe ambulation. Qs

CLIENT EDUCATION
- Warn the client about the sedative effects. (Avoid driving or operating heavy machinery.)
- Dry mouth is expected.

Scopolamine

- Anticholinergics, such as scopolamine, are effective in the treatment of nausea that accompanies inner ear problems.
- It is available transdermal, oral, or subcutaneously and is used for motion sickness.
- Contraindicated in clients who have angle-closure glaucoma.

NURSING ACTIONS
- Observe for urinary retention, constipation, and disorientation.
- Observe for sedation, and take appropriate precautions to ensure safe ambulation. Qs
- Monitor clients who have open-angle glaucoma for increasing eye pressure.

CLIENT EDUCATION
- Warn the client about the sedative effects. (Avoid driving or operating heavy machinery.)
- Inform client that dry mouth is expected and possibility of experiencing blurry vision.

Diazepam

Diazepam is a benzodiazepine that has antivertigo effects.

NURSING ACTIONS
- Observe for sedation, and take appropriate precautions to ensure safe ambulation. Qs
- Restrict use in clients who have closed-angle glaucoma.
- For older adult clients, use the smallest effective dose (prevent oversedation, ataxia). G

CLIENT EDUCATION
- Diazepam has sedative effects. Avoid driving or operating heavy machinery.
- The addictive properties and appropriate use of the medication

INTERPROFESSIONAL CARE

Vestibular rehabilitation is an option for clients who experience frequent episodes of vertigo or are incapacitated due to vertigo. A team of providers treats the cause and teaches the client exercises that can help him adapt to and minimize the effects of vertigo. The client can receive a combination of biofeedback, physical therapy, and stress management. Educate the client about positions to avoid and positional exercises that can terminate an attack of vertigo. Qᴛᴄ

THERAPEUTIC PROCEDURES

Vertigo-reducing activities

CLIENT EDUCATION
- How to prevent stimulation/exacerbation of vertigo
- Restrict movement of the head and to change positions slowly.
- Avoid caffeine and alcohol.
- Rest in a quiet, darkened environment when vertigo is severe.
- Use assistive devices (cane, walker) as needed for safe ambulation to assist with balance. Qs
- Maintain a safe environment free of clutter.
- Take a diuretic, if prescribed, to decrease the amount of fluid in semicircular canals.
- Space intake of fluids evenly throughout the day.
- Decrease intake of salt and sodium-containing foods (processed meats, MSG).
- Resume these precautions if vertigo returns.
- Wear a medical alert bracelet.

SURGICAL INTERVENTIONS
- **Pressure point treatment** involves inserting a tympanostomy tube, which applies micropulses at intervals to relieve the vertigo of Ménière's disease by displacing fluid of the inner ear. Qᴱᴮᴾ
- **Myringotomy** is an incision to the tympanic membrane to drain fluid from the middle ear to prevent ear drum perforation in otitis media. For persistent otitis media, a pressure-equalizing tube or grommet can be inserted to temporarily take the place of the Eustachian tube. It stays in place for 6 to 18 months.

Stapedectomy

A stapedectomy is a surgical procedure of the middle ear in which the stapes is removed and replaced with a prosthesis.
- The procedure is done through the external ear canal and TM.
- The TM is repaired, and sterile ear packing is placed postoperatively.
- The procedure is done when otosclerosis has developed and the bones of the middle ear fuse together.
- Otosclerosis is one of the causes of conductive hearing loss in older adults. G

NURSING ACTIONS
- Collect data for facial nerve damage.
- Intervene for vertigo, nausea, and vomiting (common findings following the procedure).

Cochlear implant for sensorineural hearing loss

- Available for clients who have no hearing at all.
- Cochlear implants consist of a microphone that picks up sound, a speech processor, a transmitter and receiver that convert sounds into electric impulses, and electrodes that are attached to the auditory nerve. **(14.2)**
- The implant's transmitter is located outside the head, behind the ear, and connects via a magnet to the receiver located immediately below it, under the skin.
- Young children and adults who lost their hearing after speech development adapt to cochlear implants more quickly than those who were born totally deaf.
- Intensive and prolonged language training is necessary for individuals who did not develop speech.

NURSING ACTIONS: Follow pre-, intra- and postoperative outpatient surgery guidelines.

CLIENT EDUCATION

- Inform the client that immediately after surgery, the unit is not turned on.
- The external unit is applied and the speech processor is programmed 2 to 6 weeks after surgery.
- Reinforce with the client on precautions to prevent infection.
- Reinforce with the client to avoid MRIs.
- Refer the client to speech therapy.

Labyrinthectomy

A labyrinthectomy is a surgical treatment for vertigo that involves removal of the labyrinthine portion of the inner ear.

NURSING ACTIONS: The client will have severe nausea and vertigo postoperatively. Take appropriate safety precautions and give antiemetics as needed. Q EBP

CLIENT EDUCATION: Expect hearing loss in the affected ear.

CLIENT EDUCATION FOLLOWING MIDDLE EAR SURGERY

- Avoid air travel for 2 to 3 weeks.
- Avoid straining or coughing, and blow nose gently with the mouth open for 2 to 3 weeks following surgery.
- Keep ear canal clean and dry. Avoid washing hair or showering for several days to 1 week.
- When able to shower, loosely place a cotton ball with petroleum jelly into the ear canal to prevent water from entering.
- Expect some temporary hearing loss in the affected ear due to presence of fluid or packing.
- Report drainage from the ear canal to the provider.

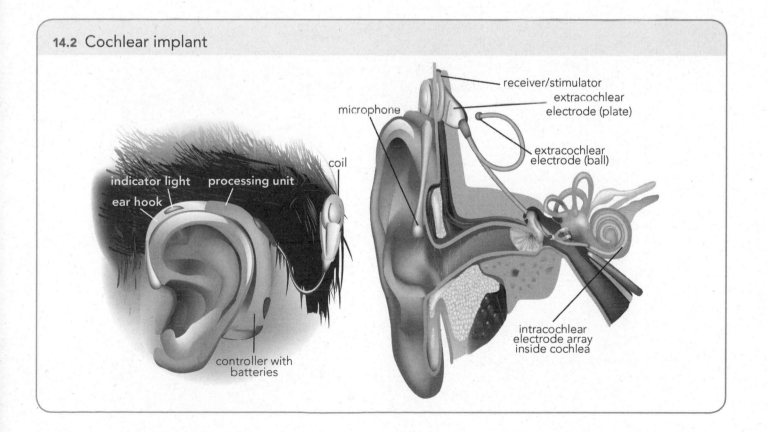

14.2 Cochlear implant

receiver/stimulator
extracochlear electrode (plate)
microphone
extracochlear electrode (ball)
coil
indicator light
processing unit
ear hook
intracochlear electrode array inside cochlea
controller with batteries

Application Exercises

1. A nurse is performing an otoscopic examination of a client. Which of the following is an unexpected finding?

    A. Pearly, gray tympanic membrane (TM)

    B. Malleus visible behind the TM

    C. Presence of soft cerumen in the external canal

    D. Fluid bubble seen behind the TM

2. A nurse is reviewing the health record of a client who has severe otitis media. Which of the following are expected findings? (Select all that apply.)

    A. Enlarged adenoids

    B. Report of recent colds

    C. Client prescription for daily furosemide

    D. Light reflex visible on otoscopic exam in the affected ear

    E. Ear pain relieved by meclizine

3. A nurse in a clinic is caring for a client who has been experiencing mild to moderate vertigo due to benign paroxysmal vertigo for several weeks. Which of the following actions should the nurse recommend to help control the vertigo? (Select all that apply.)

    A. Reduce exposure to bright lighting.

    B. Move head slowly when changing positions.

    C. Do not eat fruit high in potassium.

    D. Plan evenly spaced daily fluid intake.

    E. Avoid fluids containing caffeine.

4. A nurse is caring for a client who has suspected Ménière's disease. Which of the following is an expected finding?

    A. Purulent lesion in the external ear canal

    B. Feeling of pressure in the ear

    C. Bulging red bilateral tympanic membranes

    D. Unilateral hearing loss

5. A nurse is reinforcing discharge teaching with a client following middle ear surgery. Which of the following statements by the client indicates understanding of the teaching?

    A. "I should restrict rapid movements and avoid bending from the waist for several weeks."

    B. "I should wait until the day after surgery to wash my hair."

    C. "I will remove the dressing behind my ear in 7 days."

    D. "My hearing should be back to normal right after my surgery."

PRACTICE Active Learning Scenario

A nurse in a clinic is reinforcing preoperative teaching for an adult client who will receive a cochlear implant. What should the nurse include in the discussion? Use the ATI Active Learning Template: Therapeutic Procedure to complete this item.

DESCRIPTION OF PROCEDURE: Describe a cochlear implant.

INDICATIONS: Describe the indication for a cochlear implant.

NURSING INTERVENTIONS: List at least four.

Application Exercises Key

1. A. A pearly, gray TM is an expected finding during an otoscopic examination.

   B. Visualization of the malleus behind the TM is an expected finding during an otoscopic examination.

   C. Cerumen of various colors, depending on the client's skin color or ethnic background, is an expected finding in the external ear canal.

   D. **CORRECT:** Fluid behind the TM indicates the possibility of otitis media and is not an expected finding.

   Ⓝ *NCLEX® Connection: Reduction of Risk Potential, Diagnostic Tests*

2. A. **CORRECT:** Enlarged tonsils and adenoids are a finding associated with a middle ear infection.

   B. **CORRECT:** Frequent colds are findings associated with a middle ear infection.

   C. Furosemide is an ototoxic medication and can cause sensorineural hearing loss, but taking furosemide does not cause a middle ear disorder.

   D. Light reflexes are absent or in altered positions in a client who has a middle ear disorder.

   E. **CORRECT:** Meclizine is prescribed to relieve vertigo for inner ear disorders but does not relieve the pain of a middle ear infection.

   Ⓝ *NCLEX® Connection: Physiological Adaptation, Basic Pathophysiology*

3. A. **CORRECT:** Remaining in a darkened, quiet environment can reduce vertigo, particularly when it is severe.

   B. **CORRECT:** Moving slowly when standing or changing positions can reduce vertigo.

   C. The client who has vertigo should avoid foods containing high levels of sodium to reduce fluid retention, which can cause vertigo.

   D. **CORRECT:** The client should plan to evenly space fluid intake throughout the day to prevent excess fluid accumulation in the semicircular canals.

   E. **CORRECT:** The client should avoid fluids containing caffeine or alcohol to minimize vertigo.

   Ⓝ *NCLEX® Connection: Reduction of Risk Potential, Potential for Alterations in Body Systems*

4. A. Ménière's disease is an inner ear disorder. A purulent lesion in the external ear canal is not an expected finding.

   B. A feeling of pressure in the ear can occur with otitis media, but is not an expected finding in Ménière's

   C. Ménière's disease is an inner ear disorder. Bulging red bilateral tympanic membranes is a finding associated with a middle ear infection.

   D. **CORRECT:** Unilateral sensorineural hearing loss is an expected finding in Ménière's disease.

   Ⓝ *NCLEX® Connection: Physiological Adaptation, Basic Pathophysiology*

5. A. **CORRECT:** The client should avoid rapid movements and bending from the waist for 3 weeks following ear surgery.

   B. The client should avoid showering and washing hair for at least several days up to 1 week following ear surgery. The ear must remain dry during this time.

   C. Middle ear surgery is performed through the tympanic membrane, and the client will have a dry dressing within the ear canal. There is no external excision.

   D. Decreased hearing is expected following middle ear surgery due to presence of a dressing within the ear canal and possible drainage.

   Ⓝ *NCLEX® Connection: Reduction of Risk Potential, Potential for Complications from Surgical Procedures and Health Alterations*

PRACTICE Answer

Using the ATI Active Learning Template: Therapeutic Procedure

DESCRIPTION OF PROCEDURE: A cochlear implant consists of a microphone to pick up sound, a speech processor, a transmitter and receiver to convert sounds into electrical impulses, and electrodes that are attached to the auditory nerve. The implant's transmitter is placed outside the head, behind the ear, via a magnet that attaches to the receiver located under the skin below it.

INDICATIONS: A cochlear implant is performed for sensorineural hearing loss.

NURSING INTERVENTIONS
- Pre- and postoperative teaching is completed.
- Intraoperative care is provided in an outpatient setting.
- Reinforce client education.
  - The unit is not turned on immediately after surgery.
  - The external unit is applied and the speech processor is programmed 2 to 6 weeks after surgery.
  - The client should take measures to prevent infection.
  - The client who has a cochlear implant should avoid having an MRI.

Ⓝ *NCLEX® Connection: Reduction of Risk Potential, Potential for Complications from Surgical Procedures and Health Alterations*

When reviewing the following chapters, keep in mind the relevant topics and tasks of the NCLEX outline, in particular:

Pharmacological Therapies

ADVERSE EFFECTS/CONTRAINDICATIONS/SIDE EFFECTS/INTERACTIONS: Monitor the client for actual and potential adverse effects of medications (prescribed, over-the-counter and/or herbal supplements).

EXPECTED ACTIONS/OUTCOMES: Apply knowledge of pathophysiology when addressing the client's pharmacological agents.

MEDICATION ADMINISTRATION: Collect required data prior to medication administration.

Reduction of Risk Potential

LABORATORY VALUES: Identify laboratory values for ABGs (pH, PO_2, PCO_2, SaO_2, HCO_3), BUN, cholesterol (total), glucose, hematocrit, hemoglobin, glycosylated hemoglobin (HgbA1C), platelets, potassium, sodium, WBC, creatinine, PT, PTT and APTT, INR.

POTENTIAL FOR COMPLICATIONS OF DIAGNOSTIC TESTS/TREATMENTS/PROCEDURES: Maintain the client's tube patency (chest tube, tracheostomy tube).

THERAPEUTIC PROCEDURES: Assist with the performance of a diagnostic or invasive procedure.

Physiological Adaptation

ALTERATIONS IN BODY SYSTEMS
Provide care to a client on a ventilator.

Intervene to improve client respiratory status (breathing treatment, suctioning or repositioning).

BASIC PATHOPHYSIOLOGY: Consider general principles of the client's disease process when providing care (injury and repair, immunity, cellular structure).

MEDICAL EMERGENCIES: Respond/intervene to a client's life-threatening situation (cardiopulmonary resuscitation).

CHAPTER 15

Respiratory Diagnostic and Therapeutic Procedures

Respiratory diagnostic procedures are used to evaluate a client's respiratory status by checking indicators such as the oxygenation of the blood, lung functioning, and the integrity of the airway. Procedures nurses should be knowledgeable about include pulmonary function tests, arterial blood gases, bronchoscopy, and thoracentesis.

Chest tubes are inserted into the pleural space to drain fluid, blood, or air; reestablish a negative pressure; facilitate lung expansion; and restore normal intrapleural pressure. Chest tubes can be inserted in the emergency department, at the bedside, or in the operating room through a thoracotomy incision. Chest tubes are removed when the lungs have re-expanded or there is no more fluid drainage.

Pulmonary function tests

Pulmonary function tests (PFTs) determine lung function and breathing difficulties.
- PFTs measure lung volumes and capacities, diffusion capacity, gas exchange, flow rates, and airway resistance, along with distribution of ventilation.
- Helpful in identifying clients who have lung disease.
- Commonly performed for clients who have dyspnea.
- Can be performed before surgical procedures to identify clients who have respiratory risks.
- If client is a smoker, instruct the client not to smoke 6 to 8 hr prior to testing.
- If a client uses inhalers, withhold 4 to 6 hr prior to testing. (This can vary according to facility policy.)

Arterial blood gases

An arterial blood gas (ABG) sample reports the status of oxygenation and acid–base balance of the blood.
- An ABG measures the following.
  - **pH:** amount of free hydrogen ions in the arterial blood (H+)
  - **PaO₂:** partial pressure of oxygen
  - **PaCO₂:** partial pressure of carbon dioxide
  - **HCO₃⁻:** concentration of bicarbonate in arterial blood
  - **SaO₂:** percentage of oxygen bound to Hgb as compared with the total amount that can be possibly carried
- An RN or respiratory therapist can obtain an ABG sample by an arterial puncture or through an arterial line.

INDICATIONS

POTENTIAL DIAGNOSES
- Blood pH levels can be affected by a number of disease processes (respiratory, renal, malnutrition, electrolyte imbalance, endocrine, or neurologic).
- These assessments are helpful in monitoring the effectiveness of various treatments (such as acidosis interventions), in guiding oxygen therapy, and in evaluating client responses to weaning from mechanical ventilation.

INTERPRETATION OF FINDINGS

Blood pH levels less than 7.35 reflect acidosis, and levels greater than 7.45 reflect alkalosis. (15.1)

COMPLICATIONS

Hematoma, arterial occlusion

A hematoma occurs when blood accumulates under the skin at the IV site.

NURSING ACTIONS
- Observe for changes in temperature, swelling, color, loss of pulse, or pain.
- Notify the provider immediately if manifestations persist. Qᴛᴄ
- Apply pressure to the hematoma site.

15.1 ABG measures and expected reference ranges	
ABG MEASURE	**EXPECTED REFERENCE RANGE**
pH	7.35 to 7.45
PAO₂	80 to 100 mm Hg
PACO₂	35 to 45 mm Hg
HCO₃⁻	21 to 28 mEq/L
SAO₂	95% to 100%

Air embolism

Air enters the arterial system during catheter insertion.

NURSING ACTIONS

- Place the client on his left side in the Trendelenburg position.
- Monitor for sudden onset of shortness of breath, decrease in SaO_2 levels, chest pain, anxiety, and air hunger.
- Notify the provider immediately if manifestations occur, administer oxygen therapy, and obtain ABGs. Continue to monitor the client's respiratory status for any deterioration.

Bronchoscopy

Bronchoscopy permits visualization of the larynx, trachea, and bronchi through either a flexible fiber-optic or rigid bronchoscope.

- Bronchoscopy can be performed as an outpatient procedure, in a surgical suite under general anesthesia, or at the bedside under local anesthesia and moderate (conscious) sedation.
- Bronchoscopy can also be performed on clients who are receiving mechanical ventilation by inserting the scope through the client's endotracheal tube.

INDICATIONS

POTENTIAL DIAGNOSES

- Visualization of abnormalities such as tumors, inflammation, and strictures
- Biopsy of suspicious tissue (lung cancer): Clients undergoing a bronchoscopy with biopsy have additional risks for bleeding and perforation.
- Aspiration of deep sputum or lung abscesses for culture and sensitivity or cytology (pneumonia)

> ! Bronchoscopy is also performed for therapeutic reasons, such as removal of foreign bodies and secretions from the tracheobronchial tree, treating postoperative atelectasis, and to destroy and excise lesions.

CONSIDERATIONS

PREPROCEDURE

NURSING ACTIONS

- Check for allergies to anesthetic agents or routine use of anticoagulants.
- Ensure that a consent form is signed by the client prior to the procedure.
- Remove the client's dentures or partial plates, if applicable, prior to the procedure.
- Maintain the client on NPO status prior to the procedure, usually 4 to 8 hr, to reduce the risk of aspiration when the cough reflex is blocked by anesthesia.
- Ensure the preprocedure medications are administered (anxiolytic, atropine, viscous lidocaine, local anesthetic throat spray).

INTRAPROCEDURE

NURSING ACTIONS

- Position the client in a sitting or supine position.
- Assist in collecting and labeling specimens. Ensure prompt delivery to the laboratory.
- Monitor vital signs, respiratory pattern, and oxygenation status throughout the procedure.
- Sedation given to older adult clients who have respiratory insufficiency can precipitate respiratory arrest. ©

POSTPROCEDURE

NURSING ACTIONS

- Continuously monitor respirations, blood pressure, pulse oximetry, heart rate, and level of consciousness during the recovery period. Observe the level of consciousness while recognizing that older adult clients can develop confusion or lethargy due to the effects of medications given during the bronchoscopy.
- Observe for the level of consciousness, presence of gag reflex, and ability to swallow prior to resuming oral intake.
  - Allow adequate time for the cough and gag reflex to return prior to resuming oral intake. The gag reflex can be slower to return in older adult clients receiving local anesthesia due to impaired laryngeal reflex.
  - Once the gag reflex returns, the nurse can offer ice chips to the client and eventually fluids.
- Monitor for development of significant fever (mild fever for less than 24 hr is not uncommon), productive cough, significant hemoptysis indicative of hemorrhage (a small amount of blood-tinged sputum is expected), and hypoxemia.
- Be prepared to intervene for unexpected responses, aspiration, and laryngospasm.
- Provide oral hygiene.
- Evaluate and document the client's response to the procedure (stable vital signs, return of gag reflex).
- For older adult clients, encourage coughing and deep breathing every 2 hr. There is an increased risk of respiratory infection and pneumonia in older adult clients due to decreased cough effectiveness and decreased secretion clearance. Respiratory infections can be more severe and last longer in older adult clients. ©
- The client is not discharged from the recovery room until adequate cough reflex and respiratory effort are present.

CLIENT EDUCATION

- Gargling with salt water or using throat lozenges can provide comfort for soreness of the throat.
- Immediately report persistent cough, increased swallowing, blood tinged or purulent sputum, difficulty breathing, or chest pain.

COMPLICATIONS

Laryngospasm

- Laryngospasm is uncontrolled muscle contractions of the laryngeal cords (vocal cords) that impede the ability to inhale.
- Continuously monitor for manifestations of respiratory distress.

Pneumothorax

- Pneumothorax can occur following a rigid bronchoscopy.
- Check for diminished or absent breath sounds, changes in oxygen saturation, or sudden onset of chest pain or tightness, and obtain a follow-up chest x-ray.

Aspiration

Aspiration can occur if the client chokes on oral or gastric secretions.

NURSING ACTIONS
- Prevent aspiration by withholding oral fluids or food until the gag reflex returns (usually 2 hr). Qs
- Perform suctioning as needed.

Thoracentesis

Thoracentesis is the surgical perforation of the chest wall and pleural space with a large-bore needle. It is performed to obtain specimens for diagnostic evaluation, instill medication into the pleural space, and remove fluid (effusion) or air from the pleural space for therapeutic relief of pleural pressure.
- Thoracentesis is performed under local anesthesia by a provider at the client's bedside, in a procedure room, or in a provider's office.
- Use of an ultrasound for guidance decreases the risk of complications.

INDICATIONS

POTENTIAL DIAGNOSES

- Transudates (heart failure, cirrhosis, nephritic syndrome, hypoproteinemia)
- Exudates (inflammatory, infectious, neoplastic conditions)
- Empyema
- Pneumonia
- Blunt, crushing, or penetrating chest injuries/trauma, or invasive thoracic procedures, such as lung or cardiac surgery

CLIENT PRESENTATION

- Large amounts of fluid in the pleural space compress lung tissue and can cause pain, shortness of breath, cough, and other manifestations of pleural pressure.
- Data collection of the effusion area can reveal abnormal breath sounds, dull percussion sounds, and decreased chest wall expansion. Pain can occur due to inflammatory process.

INTERPRETATION OF FINDINGS

Aspirated fluid is analyzed for general appearance, cell counts, protein and glucose content, the presence of enzymes such as lactate dehydrogenase (LDH) and amylase, abnormal cells, and cultures.

CONSIDERATIONS

PREPROCEDURE

Percussion, auscultation, radiography, or sonography is used to locate the effusion and needle insertion site.

The nurse should, when necessary, assist the older adult client to maintain an appropriate position for the thoracentesis. Arthritis, tremors, or weakness can make it difficult for the client to remain still in the required position for the procedure. Ⓖ

NURSING ACTIONS
- Verify the client has signed the informed consent form.
- Gather all needed supplies.
- Obtain preprocedure x-ray to locate pleural effusion and to determine needle insertion site.
- Position the client sitting upright with both arms and shoulders raised and supported on pillows or on an overbed table and with feet and legs well-supported.
- Explain the procedure to the client.

CLIENT EDUCATION: Remain absolutely still (risk of accidental needle damage) during the procedure and do not cough or talk unless instructed by the provider.

INTRAPROCEDURE

NURSING ACTIONS
- Position the client in a sitting position, and leaning over the bedside table with his or her arms crossed on it.
- Assist the provider with the procedure (strict surgical aseptic technique). Qтc
- Prepare the client for a feeling of pressure with needle insertion and fluid removal.
- Monitor vital signs, skin color, respirations, and oxygen saturation throughout the procedure.
- Measure and record the amount and appearance of fluid removed from the chest.
- Label specimens at the bedside, and promptly send them to the laboratory.

  ! The amount of fluid removed is limited to 1 L at a time to prevent re-expansion pulmonary edema.

POSTPROCEDURE

NURSING ACTIONS

- Apply a dressing over the puncture site, and check the dressing for bleeding or drainage.
- Monitor vital signs and respiratory status (respiratory rate and rhythm, breath sounds, oxygenation status) every 15 minutes for the first hour and then hourly for the first several hours after the thoracentesis.
- Auscultate lungs for diminished or absent breath sounds on side of thoracentesis.
- Encourage the client to deep breathe to assist with lung expansion.
- Obtain a postprocedure chest x-ray (check resolution of effusions, rule out pneumothorax).

COMPLICATIONS

Mediastinal shift

Shift of thoracic structures to one side of the body

NURSING ACTIONS

- Monitor vital signs.
- Auscultate lungs for a decrease in or absence of breath sounds.

Pneumothorax

Pneumothorax is a collapsed lung. It can occur due to injury to the lung during the procedure.

NURSING ACTIONS

- Monitor for manifestations of pneumothorax, such as diminished breath sounds, distended neck veins, asymmetry of the chest wall, respiratory distress, sudden onset of chest pain and cyanosis.
- Monitor postprocedure chest x-ray results.
- Reinforce teaching with the client on indications of a pneumothorax, which can develop during the first 24 hr following a thoracentesis. Indications include deviated trachea, sudden onset of pain on the affected side that worsens at the end of inhalation and exhalation, affected side not moving in and out upon inhalation and exhalation, increased heart rate, rapid shallow respirations, nagging cough, or feeling of air hunger.

Bleeding

Bleeding can occur if the client is moved during the procedure or is at an increased risk for bleeding.

NURSING ACTIONS

- Monitor for coughing and hemoptysis.
- Monitor vital signs and laboratory results for evidence of bleeding (hypotension, reduced Hgb level).
- Monitor the thoracentesis site for bleeding.

Infection

Infection can occur due to the introduction of bacteria with the needle puncture.

NURSING ACTIONS

- Ensure that sterile technique is maintained.
- Monitor the client's temperature following the procedure.

Chest tube systems

A disposable three-chamber drainage system is most often used (15.2)

- First chamber: drainage collection
- Second chamber: water seal
- Third chamber: suction control (can be wet or dry)

Water seals are created by adding sterile fluid to a chamber up to the 2 cm line. While this is the minimum amount required for functioning, recommended amounts can vary by manufacturer. The water seal allows air to exit from the pleural space on exhalation and stops air from entering with inhalation.

- To maintain the water seal, keep the chamber upright and below the chest tube insertion site at all times. Routinely monitor the water level due to the possibility of evaporation. Add fluid as needed to maintain the manufacturer's recommended water seal level.
- **Wet suction:** The height of the sterile fluid in the suction control chamber determines the amount of suction transmitted to the pleural space. A suction pressure of -20 cm H_2O is commonly prescribed. The prescribed amount of suction is applied by setting the regulator on the chest tube drainage device. The application of suction results in continuous bubbling in the suction chamber. Monitor the fluid level and add fluid as needed to maintain the prescribed level of suctioning.
- **Dry suction:** When a dry suction control device is used, the provider prescribes a level of suction for the device, typically -20 cm H_2O. When connected to wall suction, the regulator on the chest tube drainage system is set to the manufacturer's recommendation.
- Tidaling (movement of the fluid level with respiration) is expected in the water seal chamber. With spontaneous respirations, the fluid level will rise with inspiration (increase in negative pressure in lung) and will fall with expiration. With positive-pressure mechanical ventilation, the fluid level will rise with expiration and fall with inspiration.
- Cessation of tidaling in the water seal chamber signals lung re-expansion or an obstruction within the system.
- Continuous bubbling in the water seal chamber indicates an air leak in the system.

Chest tube insertion

INDICATIONS

POTENTIAL DIAGNOSES

Pneumothorax: partial to complete collapse of the lung due to accumulation of air in the pleural space

Hemothorax: partial to complete collapse of the lung due to accumulation of blood in the pleural space

Postoperative chest drainage: thoracotomy or open-heart surgery

Pleural effusion: abnormal accumulation of fluid in the pleural space

Pulmonary empyema: accumulation of purulent fluid in the pleural space due to pulmonary infection, lung abscess, or infected pleural effusion

CLIENT PRESENTATION

- Dyspnea
- Distended neck veins
- Hemodynamic instability
- Pleuritic chest pain
- Cough
- Absent or reduced breath sounds on the affected side
- Hyperresonance on percussion of affected side (pneumothorax)
- Dullness or flatness on percussion of the affected side (hemothorax, pleural effusion)
- Asymmetrical chest wall motion

CONSIDERATIONS

PREPROCEDURE

- Verify that the consent form is signed.
- Reinforce client teaching. Breathing will improve when the chest tube is in place. Qᴘᴄᴄ
- Check for allergies to local anesthetics.
- Assist the client into the desired position (supine or semi-Fowler's).
- Prepare the chest drainage system prior to the chest tube insertion per the facility's protocol. (Fill the water seal chamber.)
- Administer pain and sedation medications as prescribed.
- Prep the insertion site with povidone-iodine or other facility-approved agent.

INTRAPROCEDURE

- Assist the provider with insertion of the chest tube, application of a dressing to the insertion site, and set-up of the drainage system. Qᴛᴄ
- Place the chest tube drainage system below the client's chest level with the tubing coiled on the bed. Ensure that the tubing from the bed to the drainage system is straight to promote drainage via gravity.
- The nurse should continually monitor vital signs and response to the procedure.

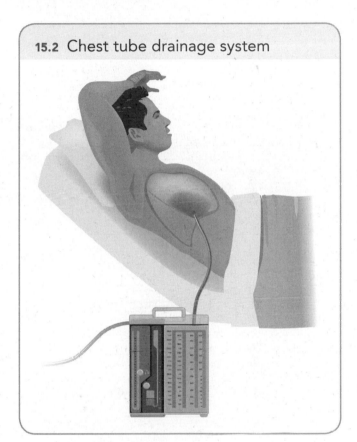

15.2 Chest tube drainage system

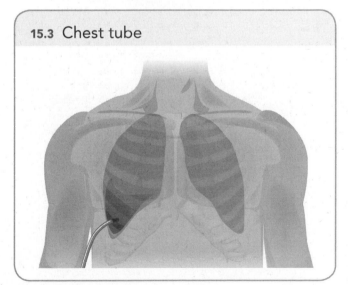

15.3 Chest tube

POSTPROCEDURE

- Check vital signs, breath sounds, SaO₂, color, and respiratory effort as indicated by the status of the client and at least every 4 hr.
- Encourage coughing and deep breathing every 2 hr.
- Keep the drainage system below the client's chest level, including during ambulation.
- Monitor chest tube placement and function. (15.3)
  - Check the water seal level every 2 hr, and add fluid as needed. The fluid level should fluctuate with respiratory effort.
  - Document the amount and color of drainage hourly for the first 24 hr and then at least every 8 hr. Mark the date, hour, and drainage level on the container at the end of each shift. Report excessive drainage (greater than 70 mL/hr) or drainage that is cloudy or red to the provider. Drainage often increases with position changes or coughing.
  - Monitor the fluid in the suction control chamber, and maintain the prescribed fluid level.
  - Ensure the regulator dial on the dry suction device is at the prescribed level.
  - Check for expected findings of tidaling in the water seal chamber and continuous bubbling only in the suction chamber.
- Routinely monitor tubing for kinks, occlusions, or loose connections.
- Monitor the chest tube insertion site for redness, pain, infection, and crepitus (air leakage in subcutaneous tissue).
- Tape all connections between the chest tube and chest tube drainage system.
- Position the client in the semi- to high-Fowler's position to promote optimal lung expansion and drainage of fluid from the lungs.
- Administer pain medications as prescribed. Qᴘᴄᴄ
- Obtain a chest x-ray to verify the chest tube's placement.
- Keep two enclosed hemostats, sterile water, and an occlusive dressing located at the bedside at all times.
- Due to the risk of causing a tension pneumothorax, chest tubes are clamped only when prescribed in specific circumstances, such as in the case of an air leak, during drainage system change, accidental disconnection of tubing, or damage to the drainage system.
- Do not strip or milk tubing; only perform this action when prescribed. Stripping creates a high negative pressure and can damage lung tissue.

COMPLICATIONS

Air leaks

Air leaks can result if a connection is not taped securely.

NURSING ACTIONS
- Monitor the water seal chamber for continuous bubbling (air leak finding). If observed, locate the source of the air leak, and intervene accordingly (tighten the connection, replace drainage system).
- Check all connections.
- Notify the charge nurse or provider if an air leak is noted. Qᴛᴄ

Accidental disconnection, system breakage, removal

These complications can occur at any time.

NURSING ACTIONS
- If the tubing separates, instruct the client to exhale as much as possible and to cough to remove as much air as possible from the pleural space.
- If the chest tube drainage system is compromised, immerse the end of the chest tube in sterile water to restore the water seal.
- If a chest tube is accidentally removed, dress the area with a sterile occlusive dressing, taped only on three sides. This allows air to escape while preventing air from entering the wound during inhalation.

Tension pneumothorax

- Sucking chest wounds, prolonged clamping of the tubing, kinks or obstruction in the tubing, or mechanical ventilation with high levels of positive end expiratory pressure (PEEP) can cause a tension pneumothorax.
- Data collection findings include tracheal deviation, absent breath sounds on one side, distended neck veins, respiratory distress, asymmetry of the chest, and cyanosis.

Chest tube removal

- Provide pain medication 30 min before removing chest tubes. Qᴇʙᴘ
- Assist the provider with sutures and chest tube removal.
- Instruct the client to take a deep breath, exhale, and bear down (Valsalva maneuver) or to take a deep breath and hold it (increases intrathoracic pressure and reduces risk of air emboli) during chest tube removal.
- Apply airtight sterile petroleum jelly gauze dressing. Secure in place with a heavyweight stretch tape.
- Obtain chest x-rays as prescribed. This is performed to verify continued resolution of the pneumothorax, hemothorax, or pleural effusion.
- Monitor for excessive wound drainage, manifestations of infection, or recurrent pneumothorax.

Application Exercises

1. A nurse is collecting data on a client following a bronchoscopy. Which of the following findings should the nurse report to the provider?

   A. Blood-tinged sputum

   B. Dry, nonproductive cough

   C. Sore throat

   D. Laryngospasm

2. A nurse is caring for a client who is scheduled for a thoracentesis. Which of the following supplies should the nurse ensure are in the client's room? (Select all that apply.)

   A. Oxygen equipment

   B. Incentive spirometer

   C. Pulse oximeter

   D. Sterile dressing

   E. Suture removal kit

3. A nurse is caring for a client following a thoracentesis. Which of the following manifestations should the nurse recognize as risks for complications? (Select all that apply.)

   A. Dyspnea

   B. Localized bloody drainage on the dressing

   C. Fever

   D. Hypotension

   E. Report of pain at the puncture site

4. A nurse is collecting data from a client who has a chest tube and drainage system in place. Which of the following findings should the nurse expect? (Select all that apply.)

   A. Continuous bubbling in the water seal chamber

   B. Gentle constant bubbling in the suction control chamber

   C. Rise and fall in the level of water in the water seal chamber with inspiration and expiration

   D. Exposed sutures without dressing

   E. Drainage system upright at chest level

5. A nurse is assisting a provider with the removal of a chest tube. Which of the following actions should the nurse instruct the client to do?

   A. Lie on his left side.

   B. Use the incentive spirometer.

   C. Cough at regular intervals.

   D. Perform the Valsalva maneuver.

PRACTICE Active Learning Scenario

A nurse is caring for a client who is scheduled for a chest tube placement. Use the ATI Active Learning Template: Therapeutic Procedure to complete this item.

NURSING INTERVENTIONS (PRE, INTRA, POST):
Include three preprocedure nursing actions.

Application Exercises Key

1. A. Blood tinged sputum is an expected finding following a bronchoscopy.

   B. A dry, nonproductive cough is an expected finding following a bronchoscopy.

   C. A sore throat is an expected finding following a bronchoscopy.

   D. **CORRECT:** Laryngospasms can indicate the client is having difficulty maintaining a patent airway. The nurse should notify the provider immediately.

   Ⓝ NCLEX® Connection: Reduction of Risk Potential, Potential for Complications of Diagnostic Tests/Treatments/Procedures

2. A. **CORRECT:** Oxygen equipment is necessary to have in the client's room if the client becomes short of breath following the procedure.

   B. An incentive spirometer is indicated for a client following thoracic surgery to promote improved oxygenation and pulmonary function.

   C. **CORRECT:** Pulse oximetry is necessary to monitor oxygen saturation level during the procedure.

   D. **CORRECT:** A sterile dressing is necessary to apply to the puncture site following the procedure.

   E. A suture removal kit is needed to remove sutures following surgery.

   Ⓝ NCLEX® Connection: Reduction of Risk Potential, Therapeutic Procedures

3. A. **CORRECT:** Dyspnea can indicate a pneumothorax or a reaccumulation of fluid. The nurse should notify the provider immediately.

   B. Localized bloody drainage contained on a dressing is an expected finding following a thoracentesis.

   C. **CORRECT:** Fever can indicate an infection. The nurse should notify the provider immediately.

   D. **CORRECT:** Hypotension can indicate intrathoracic bleeding. The nurse should notify the provider immediately.

   E. The client's report of pain at the puncture site is an expected finding following a thoracentesis.

   Ⓝ NCLEX® Connection: Reduction of Risk Potential, Potential for Complications of Diagnostic Tests/Treatments/Procedures

4. A. Continuous bubbling in the water seal chamber indicates an air leak.

   B. **CORRECT:** Gentle bubbling in the suction control chamber is an expected finding as air is being removed.

   C. **CORRECT:** A rise and fall of the fluid level in the water seal chamber upon inspiration and expiration indicates that the drainage system is functioning properly.

   D. The nurse should cover the sutures at the insertion site with an airtight dressing.

   E. The nurse should maintain the drainage system in an upright position below the level of the client's chest.

   Ⓝ NCLEX® Connection: Reduction of Risk Potential, Potential for Complications of Diagnostic Tests/Treatments/Procedures

5. A. The position the client should assume during removal of a chest tube depends upon the location of the insertion site.

   B. Use of an incentive spirometer is not indicated during chest tube removal.

   C. The nurse should instruct the client to breathe normally and remain calm during the procedure.

   D. **CORRECT:** The nurse should instruct the client to take a deep breath, exhale, and bear down (Valsalva maneuver) as the chest tube is being removed. This increases intrathoracic pressure and reduces the risk of an air embolism.

   Ⓝ NCLEX® Connection: Reduction of Risk Potential, Therapeutic Procedures

---

PRACTICE Answer

Using the ATI Active Learning Template: Therapeutic Procedure

NURSING INTERVENTIONS (PRE, INTRA, POST)
- Verify that the consent form is signed.
- Reinforce client teaching. Breathing will improve when the chest tube is in place.
- Check for allergies to local anesthetics.
- Assist the client into the desired position (supine or semi-Fowler's).
- Prepare the chest drainage system per the facility's protocol. (Fill the water seal chamber.)
- Administer pain and sedation medications as prescribed.
- Prep the insertion site with povidone-iodine or other facility-approved agent.

Ⓝ NCLEX® Connection: Reduction of Risk Potential, Potential for Complications from Surgical Procedures and Health Alterations

CHAPTER 16 ## Respiratory Management and Mechanical Ventilation

Oxygen is a tasteless and colorless gas that accounts for 21% of atmospheric air. Oxygen helps maintain adequate cellular oxygenation. It is used in the treatment of many acute and chronic respiratory problems.

Oxygen is administered in an attempt to maintain an SaO_2 of 95% to 100% by using the lowest amount of oxygen without putting the client at risk for complications.

Clients who cannot spontaneously breathe on their own require mechanical ventilation. This can include clients who need respiratory assistance due to severe respiratory disease, general anesthesia, trauma, or other illnesses.

Oxygen delivery devices

Supplemental oxygen can be delivered by a variety of methods based on the client's particular circumstances. The percentage of oxygen delivered is expressed as the fraction of inspired oxygen (FiO_2).

LOW-FLOW OXYGEN DELIVERY SYSTEMS

These deliver varying amounts of oxygen based on the method and the client's breathing pattern.

Nasal cannula

- A length of tubing with two small prongs for insertion into the nares (16.1)
- FiO_2 24% to 44% at flow rates of 1 to 6 L/min

ADVANTAGES
- Safe, easy to apply, comfortable, and well tolerated.
- The client can eat, talk, and ambulate.

DISADVANTAGES
- FiO_2 varies with the flow rate and the client's rate and depth of breathing.
- Extended use can lead to skin breakdown and drying of the mucous membranes.
- Tubing is easily dislodged.

NURSING ACTIONS
- Collect data about the patency of the nares and nasal prongs.
- Ensure that the prongs fit in the nares properly.
- Use water-soluble gel to prevent dry nares.
- Provide humidification for flow rates of 3 L/min and greater.

16.1 Nasal cannula

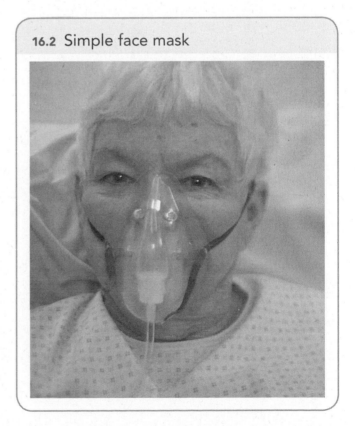

16.2 Simple face mask

Simple face mask

- Covers the client's nose and mouth. **(16.2)**
- FiO_2 35% to 50% can be achieved with flow rate of 6 to 12 L/min. (The minimum flow rate is 5 L/min to ensure flushing of CO_2 from the mask.)

ADVANTAGES: A face mask is easy to apply and can deliver oxygen quickly for short-term therapy.

DISADVANTAGES
- Flow rates of less than 5 L/min can result in rebreathing of CO_2.
- Device is poorly tolerated by clients who have anxiety or claustrophobia.
- Eating, drinking, and talking are impaired.
- Moisture and pressure can collect under the mask and cause skin breakdown.

NURSING ACTIONS
- Use caution with clients who have a high risk of aspiration or airway obstruction. **Qs**
- Check for proper fit to ensure a secure seal over the nose and mouth.
- Ensure that the client wears a nasal cannula during meals.
- Apply padding to straps if needed.

Partial nonrebreather mask

- Covers the client's nose and mouth
- FiO_2 40% to 60% at flow rates of 6 to 10 L/min

ADVANTAGES: The mask has a reservoir bag attached with no valve, which allows the client to rebreathe up to one third of exhaled air, which contains carbon dioxide, together with room air.

DISADVANTAGES
- Complete deflation of the reservoir bag during inspiration causes CO_2 buildup.
- FiO_2 varies with the client's breathing pattern.
- Mask is poorly tolerated by clients who have anxiety or claustrophobia.
- Eating, drinking, and talking are impaired.

NURSING ACTIONS
- Use with caution for clients who have a high risk of aspiration or airway obstruction. **Qs**
- Keep the reservoir bag from deflating by adjusting the oxygen flow rate to keep it inflated.
- Ensure a proper fit to ensure a secure seal over the nose and mouth.
- Check for skin breakdown beneath the edges of the mask and bridge of nose.
- Ensure that the client uses a nasal cannula during meals.

Nonrebreather mask

- Covers the client's nose and mouth **(16.3)**
- FiO_2 60% to 90% at flow rates of 10 to 15 L/min to keep the reservoir bag two-thirds full during inspiration and expiration

ADVANTAGES
- Delivers the highest O_2 concentration without intubation.
- A one-way valve situated between the mask and reservoir allows the client to inhale maximum O_2 from the reservoir bag. The two exhalation ports have flaps covering them that prevent room air from entering the mask.

16.3 Nonrebreather mask

16.4 Venturi mask

16.5 Face tent

DISADVANTAGES

- The valve and flap on the mask must be intact and functional during each breath.
- Poorly tolerated by clients who have anxiety or claustrophobia.
- Eating, drinking, and talking are impaired.

NURSING ACTIONS

- Use with caution for clients who have a high risk of aspiration or airway obstruction. Qs
- Perform an hourly data collection of the valve and flaps.
- Ensure a proper fit to ensure a secure seal over the nose and mouth.
- Check for skin breakdown beneath the edges of the mask and bridge of nose.
- Ensure that the client uses a nasal cannula during meals.

HIGH-FLOW OXYGEN DELIVERY SYSTEMS

These deliver precise amounts of oxygen when properly fitted.

Venturi mask

- Covers the client's nose and mouth (16.4)
- FiO₂ 24% to 50% at flow rates of 4 to 10 L/min via different sizes of adapters, which allow specific amounts of air to mix with oxygen

ADVANTAGES

- Delivers the most precise oxygen concentration
- Delivers consistent FiO₂ regardless of breathing pattern
- Humidification not required
- Best suited for clients who have chronic lung disease

DISADVANTAGES: Must be removed for eating, drinking, and taking medications

NURSING ACTIONS

- Collect data frequently to ensure an accurate flow rate.
- Make sure the tubing is free of kinks. Qs
- Check for skin breakdown beneath the edges of the mask, particularly on the nares.
- Ensure that the client wears a nasal cannula during meals.

Aerosol mask, face tent, tracheostomy collar

- Face tent fits loosely around the face and neck. (16.5)
- Tracheostomy collar is a small mask that covers a surgically created opening in the trachea.
- FiO₂ 24% to 100% at flow rates of at least 10 L/min. (Provide high humidification with oxygen delivery.)

ADVANTAGES

- Good for clients who do not tolerate masks well.
- Useful for clients who have facial trauma, burns, or thick secretions.

DISADVANTAGES: High humidification requires frequent monitoring.

NURSING ACTIONS

- Empty condensation from the tubing often.
- Ensure that there is adequate water in the humidification canister.
- Ensure that the aerosol mist leaves from the vents during inspiration and expiration.
- Make sure the tubing does not pull on the tracheostomy.

T-bar

FiO₂ 24% to 100% at flow rates of at least 10 L/min

ADVANTAGES: Can be used for clients who have tracheostomies, laryngectomies, or endotracheal (ET) tubes.

DISADVANTAGES: High humidification requires frequent monitoring.

NURSING ACTIONS

- Ensure that the exhalation port is open and uncovered.
- Ensure that the T-piece does not pull on the tracheostomy or ET tube.
- Ensure that the mist is evident during inspiration and expiration.
- Empty condensation from the tubing; do not get fluid into tracheostomy.
- Remove and clean T-bar device every 4 hr.

Oxygen therapy

INDICATIONS

POTENTIAL DIAGNOSES

Hypoxemia and hypoxia: Hypoxemia is an inadequate level of oxygen in the blood. Hypovolemia, hypoventilation, and interruption of arterial flow can lead to hypoxemia.

CLIENT PRESENTATION

EARLY FINDINGS

- Tachypnea
- Tachycardia
- Restlessness
- Pale skin and mucous membranes
- Elevated blood pressure
- Symptoms of respiratory distress (use of accessory muscles, nasal flaring, tracheal tugging, and adventitious lung sounds)

LATE FINDINGS

- Confusion and stupor
- Cyanotic skin and mucous membranes
- Bradypnea
- Bradycardia
- Hypotension
- Cardiac dysrhythmias

CONSIDERATIONS

PREPARATION OF THE CLIENT

- Explain all procedures to the client.
- Place the client in semi-Fowler's or Fowler's position to facilitate breathing and promote chest expansion.
- Ensure that all equipment is working properly.

ONGOING CARE

- Provide oxygen therapy at the lowest flow that will correct hypoxemia.
- Monitor respiratory rate, rhythm, and effort, and lung sounds to determine the need for supplemental oxygen.
  - Manifestations of hypoxemia are shortness of breath, anxiety, tachypnea, tachycardia, restlessness, pallor or cyanosis of the skin or mucous membranes, adventitious breath sounds, and confusion.
  - Manifestations of hypercarbia (elevated levels of CO_2) are restlessness, hypertension, and headache.
- Monitor oxygenation status with pulse oximetry and ABGs.
- Apply the oxygen delivery device. Check the fit of the mask to ensure a secure seal over the client's nose and mouth.
- Promote good oral hygiene, and provide as needed.
- Promote turning, coughing, deep breathing, use of incentive spirometer, and suctioning.
- Promote rest, and decrease environmental stimuli. Qpcc
- Provide emotional support for clients who appear anxious.
- Collect data about nutritional status. Provide supplements.
- Monitor skin integrity. Provide moisture and pressure-relief devices as indicated.
- Monitor and document the client's response to oxygen therapy.
- Titrate oxygen to maintain prescribed oxygen saturation.
- Discontinue supplemental oxygen gradually.

INTERVENTIONS

Monitor for manifestations of respiratory depression, (decreased respiratory rate, decreased level of consciousness). Notify the provider if findings are present.

Respiratory distress
- Position the client for maximum ventilation (Fowler's or semi-Fowler's position).
- Complete a focused respiratory data collection.
- Promote deep breathing, and use supplemental oxygen.
- Stay with the client, and provide emotional support to decrease anxiety.
- Promote airway clearance by encouraging coughing and oral/oropharyngeal suctioning if necessary.

COMPLICATIONS

Oxygen toxicity

- Oxygen toxicity can result from high concentrations of oxygen (typically greater than 50%), long durations of oxygen therapy (typically more than 24 to 48 hr), and the degree of lung disease.
- Oxygen toxicity can result in lung damage.
- Manifestations include a nonproductive cough, substernal pain, nasal stuffiness, nausea, vomiting, fatigue, headache, sore throat, and hypoventilation.

NURSING ACTIONS
- Use the lowest level of oxygen necessary to maintain an adequate SaO_2.
- Monitor ABGs. Notify the provider if PaO_2 is greater than the expected level of 90 mm Hg.
- Use an oxygen mask with continuous positive airway pressure (CPAP) or bi-level positive airway pressure (BiPAP) if prescribed to help decrease the amount of oxygen needed.
- Use positive end expiratory pressure (PEEP) while the client is on a mechanical ventilator to decrease the amount of needed oxygen.

Oxygen-induced hypoventilation

Oxygen-induced hypoventilation can develop in clients who have COPD and chronic hypoxemia with hypercarbia.

NURSING ACTIONS
- Monitor respiratory rate and pattern, level of consciousness, and SaO_2.
- Provide oxygen therapy at the lowest flow rate that manages hypoxemia.
- If the client tolerates it, use a Venturi mask to deliver precise oxygen levels.
- Notify the provider of impending respiratory depression, such as a decreased respiratory rate and a decreased level of consciousness.

Combustion

Oxygen is combustible.

NURSING ACTIONS
- Post "No Smoking" or "Oxygen in Use" signs to alert others of a fire hazard. Qs
- Know where the closest fire extinguisher is located.
- Reinforce teaching with the client and others about the fire hazard of smoking during oxygen use.
- Have the client wear a cotton gown because synthetic or wool fabrics can generate static electricity.
- Ensure that all electric devices (razors, televisions, radios) are working well. Frayed cords could cause a spark.
- Ensure electric machinery (monitors, suction machines) are well-grounded.
- Do not use volatile, flammable materials (alcohol, acetone) near clients who are receiving oxygen.

Noninvasive positive pressure ventilation

Continuous positive airway pressure

Provides continuous positive pressure using a leak-proof mask via noninvasive positive-pressure ventilation device.
- The continuous pressure does not change with the client's breathing.
- The device keeps the airways open throughout the respiratory cycle and improves gas exchange in the alveoli.
- The device uses room air (not oxygen) to provide pressure to improve oxygenation.
- Most effective treatment for sleep apnea because the positive pressure acts as a splint to keep the upper airway and trachea open during sleep.

Bi-level positive airway pressure

Machine cycles to provide a set positive inspiratory pressure when inspiration takes place and then during expiration to deliver a lower set end expiratory pressure.
- Requires wearing a leak-proof mask
- Most often used for clients who have COPD and who require ventilatory assistance

NURSING ACTIONS
- Check the skin around the masks for breakdown as a tight seal is required.
- Check the percentage of oxygen on the machine for both the inspiratory pressure and expiratory pressure when the client is on BiPAP.

Transtracheal oxygen therapy

- Delivers oxygen directly into the lungs per a small, flexible catheter that is passed through trachea via a small incision.
- The catheter is less visible and avoids irritation that occurs from the use of nasal prongs.

16.6 Common modes of ventilation, adjunctive therapy, and weaning modalities

Mode of ventilation

ASSIST-CONTROL (AC)
- Preset rate and tidal volume. Client initiates breath and ventilator takes over for the intubated client.
- Hyperventilation can result in respiratory alkalosis.
- Client can require sedation to decrease respiratory rate.

SYNCHRONIZED INTERMITTENT MANDATORY VENTILATION (SIMV)
- Preset rate and tidal volume for machine breaths.
- Client initiates breath and tidal volume will depend upon client's effort.
- Ventilator initiated breaths are synchronized to reduce competition between ventilator and client.
- Used as a regular mode of ventilation or a weaning mode (rate decreased to allow more spontaneous ventilation) for the intubated client.
- Can increase work of breathing, causing respiratory muscle fatigue.

INVERSE RATIO VENTILATION (IRV)
- Lengthens inspiratory phase to maximize oxygenation in the intubated client.
- Used for hypoxemia refractory to PEEP.
- Uncomfortable for clients and requires sedation and/or neuromuscular blocking agents.
- High risk of volutrauma and decreased cardiac output due to air trapping.

AIRWAY PRESSURE RELEASE VENTILATION (APRV)
- Allows alveolar gas to be expelled by the lungs own natural recoil
- Time-triggered and pressure-limited
- Breaths can be initiated spontaneously or by the ventilator
- Causes less ventilator-induced lung injury and fewer adverse effects on the cardiovascular system

INDEPENDENT LUNG VENTILATION (ILV)
- Double-lumen ET tube allows ventilation of each lung separately.
- Used for clients who have unilateral lung disease.
- Requires two ventilators, sedation and/or use of neuromuscular blocking agents.

HIGH-FREQUENCY VENTILATION
- Delivers small amount of gas at rates of 60 to 3,000 cycles/min.
- High frequency ventilation often used in children.
- Client must be sedated and/or receiving neuromuscular blocking agents.
- Breath sounds difficult to assess.

Adjunctive therapy

POSITIVE END EXPIRATORY PRESSURE (PEEP)
- Preset pressure delivered during expiration.
- Added to prescribed ventilator settings to treat persistent hypoxemia.
- Improves oxygenation by enhancing gas exchange and preventing atelectasis.
- Amount of PEEP added is typically 5 to 15 cm H_2O.

Weaning modality

PRESSURE SUPPORT VENTILATION (PSV)
- Works to keep the alveoli from collapsing during expiration.
- Allows for greater oxygenation and makes the work of breathing easier.
- Allows for lower levels of FiO_2 to be used.
- Can be used with IMV or AC modes to treat or prevent atelectasis.
- Settings 5 to 20 cm H_2O (greater than 20 cm H_2O can cause lung damage).

CONTINUOUS POSITIVE AIRWAY PRESSURE (CPAP)
- Positive pressure supplied during spontaneous breathing. No ventilator breaths delivered unless in conjunction with SIMV.
- Risks include volutrauma, decreased cardiac output and ICP.

Endotracheal tube and endotracheal intubation

INDICATIONS

- A tube is inserted through the client's nose or mouth into the trachea. This allows for emergency airway management.
- Mouth intubation is the easiest and quickest form of intubation and is often performed in the emergency department.
- Nasal intubation is performed when the client has facial or oral trauma. This route is not used if the client has a clotting problem.

PLACEMENT

- Intubation is typically performed by a nurse anesthetist, anesthesiologist, or pulmonologist.
- A chest x-ray verifies correct placement of the ET tube.
- ET tubes can be cuffed or uncuffed. The cuff on the tracheal end of an ET tube is inflated to ensure proper placement and the formation of a seal between the cuff and the tracheal wall. This prevents air from leaking around the ET tube.
- The seal ensures that an adequate amount of tidal volume is delivered by the mechanical ventilator when attached to the external end of the ET tube.
- The client is unable to talk when the cuff is inflated.

Mechanical ventilation

Mechanical ventilation provides breathing support until lung function is restored, delivering body temperature (37° C [98.6° F]), 100% humidified oxygen at FiO₂ levels 21% to 100%.
- Positive-pressure ventilators deliver air to the lungs under pressure throughout inspiration and/or expiration to keep the alveoli open during inspiration and to prevent alveolar collapse during expiration. Benefits include the following.
  - Forced/enhanced lung expansion
  - Improved gas exchange (oxygenation)
  - Decreased work of breathing
- Mechanical ventilation can be delivered via
  - ET tube
  - Tracheostomy tube
- Mechanical ventilators can be cycled based on pressure, volume, time, and flow. **(16.6)**

INDICATIONS

- To maintain a patent airway and adequate oxygen saturation of 90% or greater
- Used for clients who are unable to maintain adequate ventilation, due to respiratory, neuromuscular or neurologic problems or in the event of respiratory failure

CONSIDERATIONS

PREPARATION OF THE CLIENT

- Explain the procedure to the client.
- Establish a method for the client to communicate (asking yes/no questions, providing writing materials, using a dry-erase or picture communication board, lip reading). Qᴘᴄᴄ

ONGOING CARE

- Maintain a patent airway.
  - Check the position and placement of tube.
  - Use caution when moving the client. Qs
  - Suction oral and tracheal secretions to maintain tube patency.
  - Check that the tube is secured with tape to prevent dislodgement.
- Collect data regarding respiratory status every 1 to 2 hr: breath sounds equal bilaterally, reduced or absent breath sounds, respiratory effort, or spontaneous breaths.
- Suction the tracheal tube to clear secretions from the airway.
- Check provider's prescription each shift. Check and document ventilator settings hourly.
  - Rate, FiO₂, and tidal volume
  - Mode of ventilation
  - Use of adjuncts (PEEP, CPAP)
  - Peak inspiratory pressure (PIP)
  - Alarm settings
- Monitor ventilator alarms, which signal if the client is not receiving the correct ventilation.

  ! Never bypass or turn off ventilator alarms.

- Maintain adequate (but not excessive) volume in the cuff of the endotracheal tube.
  - Check the cuff pressure to ensure it is at the prescribed level.
  - Monitor for and report an air leak around the cuff.
- Provide medications for sedation or anxiety.
- Provide adequate nutrition.
- Administer enteral or parenteral feedings.
- Continually monitor the client during the weaning process: vital signs, respiratory rate, ease of breathing, oxygen saturation

COMPLICATIONS

Barotrauma: Monitor for manifestations such as absent breath sounds over one lung area.

Oxygen toxicity: Monitor for manifestations such as a nonproductive cough.

Impaired cardiac output: Monitor for manifestations such as a decrease in blood pressure or level of consciousness.

Infection: Monitor for manifestations such as change in color of sputum, increased WBC count, or fever.

Fluid retention: Monitor for manifestations such as an increase in body weight or peripheral edema.

Gastric distention: Monitor for manifestations such as an increased abdominal girth.

Gastrointestinal bleeding: Monitor for manifestations such as a positive stool guaiac or a decreasing hemoglobin.

PRACTICE Active Learning Scenario

A nurse is assisting with the plan of care for a client who is receiving mechanical ventilation. What actions should the nurse include to maintain the client's airway? Use the ATI Active Learning Template: Therapeutic Procedure to complete this item.

NURSING INTERVENTIONS: Describe three nursing actions to maintain the client's airway.

Application Exercises

1. A nurse is caring for a client who is experiencing respiratory distress. Which of the following early manifestations of hypoxemia should the nurse recognize? (Select all that apply.)

   A. Confusion
   B. Pale skin
   C. Bradycardia
   D. Hypotension
   E. Elevated blood pressure

2. A nurse is caring for a client who has dyspnea and will receive oxygen continuously. Which of the following oxygen devices should the nurse use to deliver a precise amount of oxygen to the client?

   A. Nonrebreather mask
   B. Venturi mask
   C. Nasal cannula
   D. Simple face mask

3. A nurse is caring for a client who has a new prescription for oxygen therapy of 4 L/min using a nasal cannula. Which of the following actions should the nurse take?

   A. Provide humidification.
   B. Remove the cannula during meal times.
   C. Establish an alternative means of communication.
   D. Lubricate the nares with 0.9% sodium chloride.

4. A nurse is assisting with the plan of care for a client who has respiratory distress. Which of the following interventions should the nurse include in the plan? (Select all that apply).

   A. Position the client on his left side.
   B. Provide emotional support to the client.
   C. Encourage the client to cough.
   D. Perform oral suctioning as needed.
   E. Have the client take short, shallow breaths.

5. A nurse is collecting data from a client who is receiving mechanical ventilation. Which of the following findings indicates that the client might have developed an infection?

   A. Decrease in blood pressure
   B. Increase in abdominal girth
   C. Change in sputum color
   D. Absent breath sounds over one lung area

Application Exercises Key

1. A. Confusion is a late manifestation of hypoxemia.

   B. **CORRECT:** Pale skin is an early manifestation of hypoxemia.

   C. Bradycardia is a late manifestation of hypoxemia.

   D. Hypotension is a late manifestation of hypoxemia.

   E. **CORRECT:** Elevated blood pressure is an early manifestation of hypoxemia.

   Ⓝ *NCLEX® Connection: Physiological Adaptation, Basic Pathophysiology*

2. A. A nonrebreather mask delivers an approximated amount of oxygen.

   B. **CORRECT:** A Venturi mask incorporates an adapter that allows a precise amount of oxygen to be delivered.

   C. A nasal cannula delivers an approximated amount of oxygen.

   D. A simple face mask delivers an approximated amount of oxygen.

   Ⓝ *Physiological Adaptation, Alterations in Body Systems*

3. A. **CORRECT:** Humidification should be provided for flow rates of 3 L/min or greater.

   B. The client is able to eat while the nasal cannula is in place.

   C. The client is able to talk and communicate while the cannula is in place.

   D. Use water-soluble gel to prevent dry nares.

   Ⓝ *NCLEX® Connection: Physiological Adaptation, Alterations in Body Systems*

4. A. The nurse should position the client in a Fowler's or semi-Fowler's position.

   B. **CORRECT:** The nurse should provide emotional support to decrease anxiety.

   C. **CORRECT:** The nurse should encourage the client to cough to promote airway clearance.

   D. **CORRECT:** The nurse should perform oral suctioning as necessary to promote airway clearance.

   E. The nurse should have the client take deep breaths to promote oxygenation.

   Ⓝ *NCLEX® Connection: Physiological Adaptation, Medical Emergencies*

5. A. A decrease in blood pressure can indicate an impaired cardiac output.

   B. An increased abdominal girth can indicate gastric distention.

   C. **CORRECT:** A change in color of sputum can be a manifestation of an infection.

   D. Absent breath sounds over one lung area can indicate barotrauma.

   Ⓝ *NCLEX® Connection: Reduction of Risk Potential, Therapeutic Procedures*

PRACTICE Answer

Using ATI Active Learning Template: Therapeutic Procedure

NURSING INTERVENTIONS
- Check that the tube is secured with tape to prevent dislodgement.
- Check the position and placement of the tube.
- Use caution when moving the client.
- Suction oral and tracheal secretions to maintain tube patency.
- Check ventilator tubing for tension or stretching whenever a client is repositioned.

Ⓝ *NCLEX® Connection: Physiological Adaptation, Alterations in Body Systems*

UNIT 3   NURSING CARE OF CLIENTS WHO
HAVE RESPIRATORY DISORDERS
SECTION: RESPIRATORY SYSTEM DISORDERS

CHAPTER 17 *Acute Respiratory Disorders*

The airway structures permit air to enter and provide for adequate oxygenation and tissue perfusion. Common acute and chronic disorders affect these airway structures.

Acute respiratory disorders include rhinitis, sinusitis, influenza, and pneumonia. A nursing priority for clients who have acute respiratory disorders is to maintain a patent airway to promote oxygenation.

Older adult clients are more susceptible to infections and have decreased pulmonary reserves due to normal lung changes, including decreased lung elasticity and thickening alveoli. ⓒ

HEALTH PROMOTION AND DISEASE PREVENTION

- Perform hand hygiene to prevent the spread of infection by bacteria and viruses.
- Get immunizations that prevent respiratory disorders. Young children, older adults, and people who have chronic illnesses or who are immunocompromised should especially get immunizations for influenza and pneumonia. Ⓠ EBP
- Limit exposure to airborne allergens, which can trigger a hypersensitivity reaction.
- Stop smoking.

RISK FACTORS

- Extremely young or advanced age ⓒ
- Recent exposure to viral, bacterial, or influenza infections
- Lack of current immunizations (pneumonia, influenza)
- Exposure to plant pollen, molds, animal dander, foods, medications, and environmental contaminants
- Tobacco smoke
- Substance use (alcohol, cocaine)
- Chronic lung disease (asthma, emphysema)
- Immunocompromised status
- Presence of a foreign body
- Conditions that increase risk of aspiration (dysphagia)
- Impaired ability to mobilize secretions (decreased level of consciousness, immobility, recent abdominal or thoracic surgery)
- Inactivity and immobility
- Mechanical ventilation (VAP)

Rhinitis

Rhinitis is an inflammation of the nasal mucosa and often the mucosa in the sinuses that can be caused by infection (viral or bacterial) or allergens.

- The common cold (coryza) is caused by viruses spread from person to person in droplets from sneezing, coughing, or direct contact.
- This disorder often coexists with other disorders, such as asthma and allergies, and is acute or chronic, nonallergic or allergic (seasonal or perennial).
- The presence of an allergen causes the release of histamine and other mediators from WBCs in the nasal mucosa. The mediators bind to blood vessel receptors, causing capillary leakage, which leads to local edema and swelling.

DATA COLLECTION

EXPECTED FINDINGS

- Excessive nasal drainage, runny nose (rhinorrhea), nasal congestion
- Purulent nasal discharge
- Sneezing and pruritus of the nose, throat, and ears
- Itchy, watery eyes
- Sore, dry throat
- Red, inflamed, swollen nasal mucosa
- Low-grade fever
- Diagnostic testing can include allergy tests to identify possible allergens.

PATIENT-CENTERED CARE

NURSING CARE

- Encourage rest and increased fluid intake (at least 2,000 mL/day).
- Encourage the use of a home humidifier or breathing steamy air after running hot shower water.
- Promote proper disposal of tissues and use of cough etiquette (sneeze or cough into tissue, elbow or shoulder and not the hands).

MEDICATIONS

Antihistamines

Block histamine to reduce edema and itching

First-generation antihistamines can cause adverse effects such as sedation, vertigo, hypertension, and urinary retention. ⓒ

First-generation: chlorpheniramine, diphenhydramine (oral agents)

Second-generation: loratadine, fexofenadine, azelastine (oral agents), olopatadine (intranasal)

Leukotriene inhibitors

Montelukast blocks leukotriene receptors, which can cause nasal congestion

- Can cause rare neuropsychiatric effects (agitation, aggression, hallucinations, suicidal behavior).
- Montelukast is often reserved for clients who do not respond to or cannot tolerate intranasal glucocorticoids or antihistamines.

Mast cell stabilizers

- Intranasal cromolyn is used to block the release of histamine to reduce edema and itching.
- Can take 1 to 2 weeks for a response.

Sympathomimetics (decongestants)

Pseudoephedrine (oral), phenylephrine (intranasal), and oxymetazoline (intranasal) constrict blood vessels and decreases edema. Use of these medications is contraindicated for clients who have hypertension, glaucoma, or benign prostatic hyperplasia.

CLIENT EDUCATION: Limit use as prescribed for 3 to 4 days to prevent rebound nasal congestion.

Intranasal glucocorticoid sprays

Fluticasone, beclomethasone, and mometasone used for prevention and treatment of seasonal and perennial rhinitis.

Can cause dryness and nosebleeds.

Anticholinergic agents

Ipratropium nasal spray inhibits secretions from the nasal mucosa.

Can cause dryness and nosebleeds.

Antipyretics/analgesics

Acetaminophen, ibuprofen for fever/pain (muscle aches or headache)

Broad-spectrum antibiotics

Amoxicillin used on a limited basis for a confirmed causative bacterial pathogen

CLIENT EDUCATION

- Review hand hygiene as a measure to prevent transmission.
- Complementary therapies (echinacea, large doses of vitamin C, zinc preparations [lozenges and nasal sprays]) might increase the immune response. Q**EBP**
- Limiting exposure to others will prevent and reduce transmission. This is especially important for vulnerable populations such as the very young, older adults, and people who are immunosuppressed. **Ⓒ**
- Advise clients that OTC decongestants which contain pseudoephedrine and ephedrine are regulated and require identification for purchase.

Sinusitis

Sinusitis, often called rhinosinusitis, is an inflammation of the mucous membranes of one or more of the sinuses, usually the maxillary or frontal sinus. Swelling of the mucosa can block the drainage of secretions, which can cause a sinus infection.

- Sinusitis often occurs after rhinitis and can be associated with a deviated nasal septum, nasal polyps, inhaled air pollutants or cocaine, facial trauma, dental infections, or loss of immune function.
- The infection is commonly caused by *Streptococcus pneumoniae*, *Haemophilus influenzae*, diplococcus, and bacteroides.

DATA COLLECTION

EXPECTED FINDINGS

- Nasal congestion
- Headache
- Facial pressure or pain (worse when head is tilted forward)
- Cough
- Bloody or purulent nasal drainage
- Tenderness to palpation of forehead, orbital, and facial areas
- Low-grade fever

DIAGNOSTIC PROCEDURES

- CT scan or sinus x-rays confirm the diagnosis, which is typically based on findings and physical assessment.
- Endoscopic sinus cavity lavage or surgery to relieve the obstruction and promote drainage of secretions may be done.

PATIENT-CENTERED CARE

NURSING CARE

- Encourage the use of steam humidification, sinus irrigation, saline nasal sprays, and hot and wet packs to relieve sinus congestion and pain.
- Reinforce with the client to increase fluid intake and rest.
- Discourage air travel, swimming, and diving.
- Encourage cessation of tobacco use in any form.
- Reinforce with the client on correct technique for sinus irrigation and self-administration of nasal sprays.

MEDICATIONS

Nasal decongestants, such as phenylephrine, are used to reduce swelling of the mucosa.

- Clients should be encouraged to begin over-the-counter decongestant use at the first manifestation of sinusitis.
- Signs of rebound nasal congestion can occur if decongestants are used for more than 3 to 4 days.

Broad-spectrum antibiotics, such as amoxicillin, are used on a limited basis for a confirmed causative bacterial pathogen.

Pain relief medications include NSAIDs, and acetaminophen

CLIENT EDUCATION

- Sinus irrigation and saline nasal sprays are an effective alternative to decongestants for relieving nasal congestion.
- Contact the provider for manifestations of a severe headache, neck stiffness (nuchal rigidity), and high fever, which can indicate complications.

COMPLICATIONS

Meningitis and encephalitis can occur if pathogens enter the bloodstream from the sinus cavity.

Influenza

Seasonal influenza, or "flu," occurs as an epidemic, usually in the fall and winter months.

- It is a highly contagious acute viral infection that occurs in children and adults of all ages.
- Influenza is caused by one of several virus families, and this can vary yearly. Adults are contagious from 24 hr before manifestations develop and up to 5 days after they begin.

Pandemic influenza refers to a viral infection among animals or birds that has mutated and is becoming highly infectious to humans. The resulting viral infection has the potential to spread globally, such as H1N1 ("swine flu") and H5N1 ("avian flu").

DATA COLLECTION

EXPECTED FINDINGS

- Severe headache and muscle aches
- Chills
- Fatigue, weakness
- Severe diarrhea and cough (avian flu)
- Fever
- Hypoxia (avian flu)
- Nausea, vomiting

DIAGNOSTIC PROCEDURES

Rapid influenza diagnostic tests: A sample is collected from the nasopharynx or throat swab.

PATIENT-CENTERED CARE

NURSING CARE

- Maintain droplet and contact precautions for hospitalized clients who have pandemic influenza.
- Provide saline gargles.
- Monitor hydration status and I&O.
- Administer fluid therapy as prescribed.
- Monitor respiratory status.

MEDICATIONS

Antivirals

- Oseltamivir and zanamivir are used for the prevention and treatment of influenza A and B.
- Antivirals such as the oral inhalant zanamivir and the oral tablet oseltamivir might shorten the duration of the influenza infection. In cases of pandemic influenza, these medications might be distributed widely among the population.
- CLIENT EDUCATION: Begin antiviral medications 36 to 48 hr after the onset of manifestations depending on the medication. When treatment is started within 12 hr of manifestations, duration is reduced by more than 3 days.

Influenza vaccines

- Trivalent vaccines are prepared yearly depending upon the suspected strain of influenza expected to appear. They include an IM or intradermal injection of inactivated influenza vaccine.
  - Vaccination is encouraged for everyone older than 6 months of age.
  - Clients who have a history of pneumonia or chronic medical conditions, those over age 65, pregnant clients, and health care providers are at higher risk and require vaccination.
  - Collect data on clients for precautions to vaccination including egg allergy, history of Guillain-Barré Syndrome, anaphylaxis after a previous dose, and acute illness.
- H1N1 vaccine is available for the general population.
- H5N1 vaccine is stockpiled for distribution if a pandemic occurs.

INTERPROFESSIONAL CARE

- Consult respiratory services for respiratory support.
- Community health officials are notified of influenza outbreaks.
- State and federal public health officials are consulted for containment and prevention directives during pandemic influenza.

CLIENT EDUCATION

- Encourage annual influenza vaccination when vaccines become available.
- Reduce the risk for spreading viruses by thoroughly washing hands and following cough etiquette.
- Avoid places where people gather. Avoid close personal contact (hand shaking, kissing, hugging).
- If flu manifestations develop, increase fluid intake, rest, and stay home from work or school.
- Avoid travel to areas where pandemic influenza is identified.
- Be aware of public health announcements and activation of the early warning system by public health officials in case of pandemic influenza.

COMPLICATIONS

Pneumonia is a complication of influenza and affects older adults and clients who are debilitated or immunocompromised. Ⓖ

Pneumonia

Pneumonia is an inflammatory process in the lungs that produces excess fluid.

- Pneumonia is triggered by infectious organisms or by the aspiration of an irritant, such as fluid or a foreign object. The inflammatory process in the lung parenchyma results in edema and exudate that fills the alveoli.
- Pneumonia can be a primary disease or a complication of another disease or condition. It affects people of all ages, but young clients, older adult clients, and clients who are immunocompromised are more susceptible.
- Immobility is a contributing factor in the development of pneumonia. Ⓖ

TYPES OF PNEUMONIA

Community-acquired pneumonia (CAP) is the most common type and often occurs as a complication of influenza.

Health care-acquired pneumonia (HAP) has a higher mortality rate and is more likely to be resistant to antibiotics. It usually takes more than 48 hr from the time the client is exposed to acquire HAP.

- **Ventilator-associated pneumonia (VAP)** occurs 48 to 72 hr after endotracheal intubation.

DATA COLLECTION

EXPECTED FINDINGS

- Anxiety
- Fatigue
- Weakness
- Chest discomfort due to coughing
- Confusion from hypoxia is a common manifestation of pneumonia in older adult clients. Ⓖ

PHYSICAL FINDINGS

- Fever
- Chills
- Flushed face
- Diaphoresis
- Shortness of breath or difficulty breathing
- Tachypnea
- Pleuritic chest pain (sharp)
- Sputum production (yellow-tinged)
- Crackles and wheezes
- Coughing
- Dull chest percussion over areas of consolidation
- Decreased oxygen saturation levels (expected reference range is 95% to 100%)
- Purulent, blood-tinged or rust-colored sputum

LABORATORY TESTS

Sputum culture and sensitivity
- Obtain specimen before starting antibiotic therapy.
- Obtain specimen by suctioning if the client is unable to cough.
- Older adult clients have a weak cough reflex and decreased muscle strength. Therefore, older adult clients have trouble expectorating, which can lead to difficulty in breathing and make specimen retrieval more difficult. Ⓖ

CBC: Elevated WBC count (might not be present in older adult clients)

ABGs: Hypoxemia (PaO₂ less than 80 mm Hg)

Blood culture: To rule out organisms in the blood

Serum electrolytes: To identify dehydration

DIAGNOSTIC PROCEDURES

Chest x-ray

- A chest x-ray will show consolidation (solidification, density) of lung tissue. (17.1)
- Chest x-ray might not indicate pneumonia for a few days after manifestations develop.
- A chest x-ray is an important diagnostic tool because the early manifestations of pneumonia are often vague in older adult clients. Ⓖ

Pulse oximetry

Clients who have pneumonia usually have oximetry levels less than the expected reference range of 95% to 100%.

PATIENT-CENTERED CARE

NURSING CARE

- Position the client to maximize ventilation (high-Fowler's = 90%) unless contraindicated.
- Encourage coughing or suction to remove secretions.
- Administer breathing treatments and medications.
- Administer oxygen therapy.
- Monitor for skin breakdown around the ears, nose, and mouth from the oxygen device.
- Encourage deep breathing with an incentive spirometer to prevent alveolar collapse.
- Determine the client's physical limitations and structure activity to include periods of rest. Qpcc
- Promote adequate nutrition and fluid intake.
  ○ The increased work of breathing requires additional calories.
  ○ Proper nutrition aids in the prevention of secondary respiratory infections.
  ○ Encourage fluid intake of 2.5 to 3 L/day to promote hydration and thinning of secretions, unless contraindicated due to another condition.
- Provide rest periods for clients who have dyspnea.
- Reassure the client who is experiencing respiratory distress.

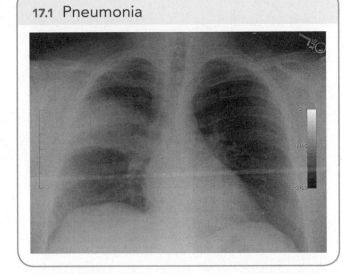

17.1 Pneumonia

MEDICATIONS

Antibiotics

- Antibiotics are given to destroy infectious pathogens. Commonly used antibiotics include fluoroquinolones, penicillins, and cephalosporins.
- Antibiotics are often initially given via IV and then switched to an oral form as the condition improves.
- It is important to obtain any culture specimens prior to giving the first dose of an antibiotic. Once the specimen is obtained, the antibiotics can be given while waiting for the results of the culture.

NURSING ACTIONS
- Observe clients taking cephalosporins for frequent stools.
- Monitor kidney function, especially older adults who are taking penicillins and cephalosporins. Ⓖ

CLIENT EDUCATION: Encourage clients to take penicillins and cephalosporins with food. Some penicillins should be taken 1 hr before meals or 2 hr after.

Bronchodilators

- Bronchodilators are given to reduce bronchospasms and reduce irritation.
- Short-acting beta₂ agonists, such as albuterol, provide rapid relief.
- Cholinergic antagonists (anticholinergic medications), such as ipratropium, block the parasympathetic nervous system, allowing for increased bronchodilation and decreased pulmonary secretions.

NURSING ACTIONS
- Albuterol: Increase fluid intake if not contraindicated. Can cause hypokalemia, insomnia, headache, or nausea. Monitor for tremors, tachycardia, hypertension, nervousness, palpations, and dry mouth.
- Ipratropium: Observe for dry mouth and difficulty with urination. Monitor heart rate. Adverse effects can include headache, blurred vision, and palpitations, which can indicate toxicity.

CLIENT EDUCATION

- Reinforce teaching on how to use a metered-dose inhaler (MDI).
- Encourage clients to suck on hard candies to moisten dry mouth while taking ipratropium. Q_{EBP}
- Encourage increased fluid intake unless contraindicated.

Anti-inflammatories

- Anti-inflammatories decrease airway inflammation.
- Glucocorticosteroids, such as fluticasone (MDI) and prednisone (oral), are prescribed to reduce inflammation. Monitor for immunosuppression, fluid retention, hyperglycemia, hypertension, hypokalemia, and poor wound healing.

NURSING ACTIONS

- Monitor for decreased immunity function and infection.
- Monitor for hyperglycemia.
- Monitor for hypertension
- Advise the client to report black, tarry stools.
- Observe for fluid retention and weight gain. This can be common.
- Monitor for electrolyte imbalance
- Monitor the client's throat and mouth for aphthous lesions (canker sores).

CLIENT EDUCATION

- Drink plenty of fluids to promote hydration.
- Take glucocorticosteroids with food.
- Avoid discontinuing glucocorticosteroids without consulting the provider.
- Use MDI.
- Rinse mouth and gargle after inhaled glucocorticoids to reduce the risk of dysphonia and candidiasis.

INTERPROFESSIONAL CARE

- Consult with respiratory services for inhalers, breathing treatments, and suctioning for airway management.
- Consult with nutritional services for weight loss or gain related to medications or diagnosis.
- Consult with rehabilitation care if the client has prolonged weakness and needs assistance with increasing level of activity.

CLIENT EDUCATION

- Continue medications for treatment of pneumonia. Q_{PCC}
- Rest as needed.
- Maintain hand hygiene to prevent infection.
- Avoid crowded areas to reduce the risk of infection. Q_{EBP}
- Teatment and recovery from pneumonia can take time.
- Receive immunizations for influenza and pneumonia.
- Stop smoking.

COMPLICATIONS

Atelectasis
- Airway inflammation and edema lead to alveolar collapse and increase the risk of hypoxemia.
- The client reports shortness of breath and exhibits findings of hypoxemia.
- The client has diminished or absent breath sounds over the affected area.
- A chest x-ray shows an area of density.

Bacteremia (sepsis): This occurs if pathogens enter the bloodstream from the infection in the lungs.

Acute respiratory distress syndrome
- Hypoxemia persists despite oxygen therapy.
- Dyspnea worsens as bilateral pulmonary edema develops that is noncardiac related.
- A chest x-ray shows an area of density with a ground-glass appearance.
- Blood gas findings demonstrate high arterial blood levels of carbon dioxide (hypercarbia) and pulse oximetry shows decreased saturation.

Application Exercises

1. A nurse is monitoring a group of clients for increased risk for developing pneumonia. Which of the following clients should the nurse expect to be at risk? (Select all that apply.)

   A. Client who has dysphagia

   B. Client who has AIDS

   C. Client who received vaccines for pneumococcus and influenza 6 months ago

   D. Client who is ambulatory after receiving a local anesthesia

   E. Client who has a closed head injury and is receiving ventilation

   F. Client who has myasthenia gravis

2. A nurse in a clinic is caring for a client whose partner states the client woke up this morning, did not recognize him, and did not know where she was. The client reports chills and chest pain that is worse upon inspiration. Which of the following actions is the nursing priority?

   A. Obtain baseline vital signs and oxygen saturation.

   B. Obtain a sputum culture.

   C. Obtain a complete history from the client.

   D. Provide a pneumococcal vaccine.

3. A nurse is caring for a client who has pneumonia. Data collection findings include temperature 37.8° C (100° F), respirations 30/min, blood pressure 130/76 mm Hg, heart rate 100/min, and SaO₂ 91% on room air. Which of the following actions is the nurse's priority?

   A. Administer antibiotics.

   B. Administer oxygen therapy.

   C. Perform a sputum culture.

   D. Administer an antipyretic medication to promote client comfort.

4. A nurse in a clinic is collecting data on a client who has sinusitis. Which of the following techniques should the nurse use to identify manifestations of this disorder?

   A. Percussion of posterior lobes of lungs

   B. Auscultation of the trachea

   C. Inspection of the conjunctiva

   D. Palpation of the orbital areas

5. A nurse is reinforcing teaching with a client about influenza. Which of the following client statements indicates an understanding of the teaching

   A. "I should wash my hands after blowing my nose to prevent spreading the virus."

   B. "I need to avoid drinking fluids if I develop symptoms."

   C. "I need a flu shot every 2 years because of the different flu strains."

   D. "I should cover my mouth with my hand when I sneeze."

PRACTICE Active Learning Scenario

A nurse in a clinic is discussing health promotion and disease management with a client who has rhinitis. What should the nurse include in this discussion? Use the ATI Active Learning Template: System Disorder to complete this item.

RISK FACTORS: Identify three risk factors for rhinitis.

EXPECTED FINDINGS: Describe at least four.

CLIENT EDUCATION: Describe two client self-care activities.

MEDICATIONS: Identify two over-the-counter medications the client can use.

Application Exercises Key

1. A. **CORRECT:** The client who has difficulty swallowing is at increased risk for pneumonia due to aspiration.

   B. **CORRECT:** The client who has AIDS is immunocompromised, which increases the risk of opportunistic infections, such as pneumonia.

   C. The client who has recently been vaccinated in the past few months has a decreased risk of aquiring pneumonia.

   D. A client who is ambulatory and has received local anesthesia has a decreased risk to acquire pneumonia.

   E. **CORRECT:** Mechanical ventilation is invasive and increases the risk of pneumonia.

   F. **CORRECT:** A client who has myasthenia gravis has generalized weakness and can have difficulty clearing airway secretions, which increases the risk of pneumonia.

   Ⓝ *NCLEX® Connection: Health Promotion and Maintenance, Health Promotion/Disease Prevention*

2. A. **CORRECT:** The first action the nurse should take using the nursing process is to collect data on the client. The data collected will help the nurse assist in developing a plan of care for the client.

   B. The nurse should obtain a sputum culture to determine the causative organism and sensitivity for antibiotic therapy. However, there is another action the nurse should take first.

   C. The nurse should obtain a complete history from the client to assist the nurse in determining the plan of care. However, there is another action the nurse should take first.

   D. The nurse should provide a pneumococcal vaccination to decrease the risk of pneumonia in the future. However, there is another action the nurse should take first.

   Ⓝ *NCLEX® Connection: Reduction of Risk Potential, Changes/Abnormalities in Vital Signs*

3. A. The nurse should administer antibiotics as prescribed to eradicate the infection. However, there is another action the nurse should take first.

   B. **CORRECT:** The first action the nurse should take when using the airway, breathing, circulation approach to client care is administer oxygen to the client to reduce hypoxia and improve oxygenation.

   C. The nurse should obtain a sputum culture as prescribed to determine the causative organism. The nurse should obtain the sputum culture prior to administering antibiotics, to ensure accurate results. However, there is another action the nurse should take first.

   D. The nurse should administer an antipyretic medication as prescribed to promote comfort. However, there is another action the nurse should take first.

   Ⓝ *NCLEX® Connection: Reduction of Risk Potential, Potential for Complications of Diagnostic Tests/Treatments/Procedures*

4. A. Lung percussion is not an effective technique to identify manifestations of sinusitis; it is used to identify pneumonia.

   B. Auscultation of the trachea is not an effective technique to identify manifestations of sinusitis; it is used to identify bronchitis.

   C. Inspection of the conjunctiva is not an effective technique to identify manifestations of sinusitis; it is used to identify anemia.

   D. **CORRECT:** Palpation of the orbital, frontal, and facial areas will elicit a report of tenderness from a client who has sinusitis.

   Ⓝ *NCLEX® Connection: Reduction of Risk Potential, Diagnostic Tests*

5. A. **CORRECT:** Hand hygiene decreases the risk of the client spreading influenza viruses. The client should wash his hands after blowing his nose to prevent spreading the virus.

   B. The client should increase fluid intake if influenza manifestations develop to maintain hydration and to promote expectoration of mucous.

   C. Influenza vaccines are administered yearly. The client should receive a vaccination yearly.

   D. Cough etiquette includes the client to sneeze into the shoulder or elbow rather than the hands.

   Ⓝ *NCLEX® Connection: Health Promotion and Maintenance, Health Promotion/Disease Prevention*

PRACTICE Answer

Using the ATI Active Learning Template: System Disorder

RISK FACTORS
- Recent exposure to viral, bacterial, or influenza infections
- Lack of current immunization status (pneumonia, influenza)
- Exposure to plant pollen, molds, animal dander, foods, medications, and environmental contaminants
- Tobacco smoke
- Substance use (alcohol, cocaine)
- Presence of a foreign body
- Inactivity and immobility

EXPECTED FINDINGS
- Excessive nasal drainage, runny nose (rhinorrhea), nasal congestion
- Purulent nasal drainage
- Sneezing and pruritus of the nose, throat, and ears
- Itchy, watery eyes
- Sore, dry throat
- Red, inflamed, swollen nasal mucosa
- Low-grade fever

CLIENT EDUCATION
- Rest, increased fluid intake (at least 2,000 mL/day)
- Use of a home humidifier or breathing steamy air after running hot shower water
- Proper disposal of tissues and use of cough etiquette

MEDICATIONS: Chlorpheniramine, pseudoephedrine, loratadine, cromolyn, phenylephrine, antipyretics

Ⓝ *NCLEX® Connection: Physiological Adaptation, Alterations in Body Systems*

CHAPTER 18 *Asthma*

Asthma is a chronic inflammatory disorder of the airways that results in intermittent and reversible airflow obstruction of the bronchioles. The obstruction occurs either by inflammation or airway hyperresponsiveness.

Asthma can occur at any age. The cause is unknown. Manifestations include mucosal edema, bronchoconstriction, and excessive mucus production. (18.1)

HEALTH PROMOTION AND DISEASE PREVENTION

- Stop smoking.
- Use protective equipment (mask) and ensure proper ventilation while working in environments that contain carcinogens or particles in the air. Qs
- Older adults and all clients who have asthma should receive influenza and pneumonia vaccines. ©
- Recognize and avoid triggering agents.
  - Environmental factors, such as changes in temperature (especially warm to cold) and humidity
  - Air pollutants
  - Strong odors (perfume)
  - Seasonal allergens (grass, tree, weed pollens) and perennial allergens (mold, feathers, dust, roaches, animal dander, foods treated with sulfites)
  - Stress and emotional distress
  - Medications (aspirin, NSAIDs, beta blockers, cholinergics)
  - Enzymes, including those in laundry detergents
  - Chemicals (household cleaners)
  - Sinusitis with postnasal drip
  - Viral respiratory tract infection
- Self-administer medications (nebulizers, inhalers).
- Use a peak flow-meter.
- Maintain a balance between exercise and rest.
- Practice infection prevention techniques.
- Maintain regular exercise as part of asthma therapy.
  - Promotes ventilation and perfusion.
  - Maintains cardiac health.
  - Enhances skeletal muscle strength.
  - Clients might require pre-medication before exercise.
- Wash bed linens with hot water to eliminate dust mites.

M◇ *Online Video: Asthmatic Breathing –*
Metered-Dose Inhaler

DATA COLLECTION

Diagnosis is based on manifestations and classified into one of the following four categories.
- **Mild intermittent:** Manifestations occur less than once per week.
- **Mild persistent:** Manifestations arise more than once per week but not daily.
- **Moderate persistent:** Manifestations occur daily, more than once per week, or are present at night at least once per week.
- **Severe persistent:** Manifestations occur continually, along with frequent exacerbations that limit physical activity and quality of life.

Obtain history regarding current and previous asthma exacerbations. Qpcc
- Onset and duration
- Precipitating factors (stress, exercise, exposure to irritant)
- Changes in medication regimen
- Medications that relieve symptoms
- Other medications taken
- Self-care methods used to relieve symptoms (relaxation techniques)

RISK FACTORS

- Older adult clients have decreased pulmonary reserves due to physiologic lung changes that occur with the aging process. ©
  - Older adult clients are more susceptible to infections.
  - The sensitivity of beta adrenergic receptors decreases with age. As the beta receptors age and lose sensitivity, they are less able to respond to agonists, which relax smooth muscle and can result in bronchospasms.
- Family history of asthma
- Smoking
- Secondhand smoke exposure
- Environmental allergies
- Exposure to chemical irritants or dust
- Gastroesophageal reflux disease

EXPECTED FINDINGS

- Dyspnea
- Chest tightness
- Anxiety or stress

PHYSICAL FINDINGS
- Coughing
- Wheezing
- Mucus production
- Use of accessory muscles
- Prolonged exhalation
- Poor oxygen saturation (low SaO_2)
- Barrel chest or increased chest diameter

LABORATORY TESTS

Arterial blood gases

Hypoxemia (PaO_2 less than 80 mm Hg)

Hypocapnia/hypocarbia ($PaCO_2$ less than 35 mm Hg: early in attack)

Hypercapnia/hypercarbia ($PaCO_2$ greater than 45 mm Hg: later in attack)

Sputum cultures

Bacteria can indicate infection. Ⓠ

DIAGNOSTIC PROCEDURES

- Pulmonary function tests (PFTs) are used to diagnose asthma and its severity.
  - Total lung capacity (TLC) is the amount of air the lung can retain following maximal inspiration.
  - Tidal volume is the amount of air inspired or exhaled during each breath.
  - Functional residual capacity is the residual amount of air left in the lungs at the end of expiration.
  - Residual volume is the residual amount of air left in the lungs after maximal expiration.
  - Forced vital capacity (FVC) is the volume of air exhaled from full inhalation to full exhalation.
  - Forced expiratory volume in the first second (FEV1) is the volume of air blown out as hard and fast as possible during the first second of the most forceful exhalation after the greatest full inhalation.
  - Peak expiratory flow is the fastest airflow rate reached during exhalation.
  - A decrease in FEV1 by 15% to 20% below the expected value is common in clients who have asthma. An increase in these values by 12% following the administration of bronchodilators is diagnostic for asthma.
- A chest x-ray is used to diagnose changes in chest structure over time.

PATIENT-CENTERED CARE

NURSING CARE

- Position the client to maximize ventilation (high-Fowler's). Ⓠ EBP
- Administer oxygen therapy as prescribed.
- Monitor cardiac rate and rhythm for changes during an acute attack (can be irregular, tachycardic, or with PVCs).
- Monitor IV access.
- Maintain a calm and reassuring demeanor.
- Provide rest periods for older adult clients who have dyspnea. Design room and walkways with opportunities for rest. Incorporate rest into ADLs. Ⓖ
- Encourage prompt medical attention for infections and recommended vaccinations.
- Administer medications as prescribed.

MEDICATIONS

Many asthma medications are administered by inhalation.

Metered-dose inhaler (MDI): Hand-held device consisting of a pressured canister that delivers a specific amount of medication in aerosol form, requiring hand-breath coordination.

- Spacers when added to the MDI: Break up and slow down the medication particles, which increases the amount of medication delivered to the lungs, instead of the oropharyngeal mucosa.

Respimat: Like an MDI, but creates fine mist particles resulting in more medication being delivered to the lungs.

Dry powder inhaler (DPI): A dry micronized powder is delivered to the lungs and is breath-activated, which does not require hand-breath coordination.

Nebulizer: A machine is used to convert a drug solution into a mist and delivered through a mouthpiece or mask.

Bronchodilators

Inhaled

- **Short-acting beta₂ agonists,** such as albuterol, provide rapid relief of acute symptoms and prevent exercise-induced asthma.
- **Long-acting beta₂ agonists,** such as salmeterol, combined with a glucocorticoid, for prophylactic prevention of bronchospasms.
- **Anticholinergic medications,** such as ipratropium, block the parasympathetic nervous system. This allows for the sympathetic nervous system effects of increased bronchodilation and decreased pulmonary secretions.

Oral/IV: Methylxanthines, such as aminophylline, are available in both oral and IV dosing.

NURSING ACTIONS

- Albuterol: Monitor for tremors and tachycardia.
- Salmeterol: Monitor for tachycardia, muscle tremors, and hypokalemia.
- Ipratropium: Observe for dry mouth and monitor heart rate. Adverse effects can include headache, blurred vision, and palpitations, which can indicate toxicity
- Aminophylline: Monitor for irritability, restlessness, tremors, tachycardia, nausea, and diarrhea.

CLIENT EDUCATION

- Ipratropium: Suck on hard candies to help relieve dry mouth; increase fluid intake; and report headache, blurred vision, or palpitations, which can indicate toxicity of ipratropium. Monitor heart rate.
- Salmeterol: Use to prevent an asthma attack and not at the onset of an attack.

Anti-inflammatory agents

These medications decrease airway inflammation and are for prophylactic prevention of bronchospasms.

If bronchodilator and anti-inflammatory are prescribed separately for inhalation administration at the same time, administer the bronchodilator first in order to increase the absorption of the anti-inflammatory agent. Examples include albuterol/ipratropium and salmeterol/fluticasone.

Glucocorticosteroids
- **Inhaled:** fluticasone, budesonide
- **Oral:** prednisone, methylprednisolone
  - NURSING ACTIONS
    - Monitor for manifestations of an infection (sore throat, fever.)
    - Observe for fluid retention and weight gain
    - Monitor for hyperglycemia, hypertension, hypokalemia, and poor wound healing.
    - Monitor for electrolyte imbalance.
    - Monitor the throat and mouth for aphthous lesions (canker sores).
    - Can promote bone loss; advise clients to increase weight bearing exercises and increase intake of calcium and vitamin D.

Mast cell stabilizers (inhaled), such as cromolyn
- Can take 2 or more weeks for therapeutic response.

Combination agents: Leukotriene antagonists (oral), such as montelukast
- Can cause rare neuropsychiatric effects (agitation, aggression, hallucinations, suicidal behavior).
- Can cause headache, dizziness, nausea, vomiting, diarrhea, fatigue, or abdominal pain.

Others
- Immunomodulators (injection), such as omalizumab
  - NURSING ACTIONS
    - Monitor for anaphylaxis.
    - Associated with an increased risk of heart attack.
    - Administer subcutaneously every 2 to 4 weeks.
- Phosphodiesterase 4 inhibitors (roflumilast, cilomilast)
  - Prescribed as a maintenance medication.
  - Increase risk of adverse psychiatric effects with roflumilast.
  - Nausea associated with cilomilast.

CLIENT EDUCATION
- Report black, tarry stools.
- Drink plenty of fluids to promote hydration.
- Take prednisone with food.
- Use this medication to prevent asthma, not for the onset of an attack.
- Avoid people who have respiratory infections.
- Use good mouth care.
- Do not discontinue this type of medication suddenly.
- Practice proper use of MDI.
- Rinse mouth and gargle after inhaled glucocorticoids to minimize dysphonia and candidiasis.

18.1 Normal and asthmatic bronchioles

normal bronchiole   asthmatic bronchiole

INTERPROFESSIONAL CARE
- Consult with respiratory services for inhalers and breathing treatments for airway management.
- Contact nutritional services for weight loss or gain related to medications or diagnosis.
- Consult with rehabilitation care if the client has prolonged weakness and needs assistance with increasing level of activity.

COMPLICATIONS

Respiratory failure

Persistent hypoxemia related to asthma can lead to respiratory failure.

NURSING ACTIONS
- Monitor oxygenation levels and acid–base balance.
- Prepare for intubation and mechanical ventilation.

Status asthmaticus Qs

This is a life-threatening episode of airway obstruction that is often unresponsive to treatment. It involves extreme wheezing, labored breathing, use of accessory muscles, distended neck veins, and creates a risk for cardiac and/or respiratory arrest.

NURSING ACTIONS
- Prepare for emergency intubation.
- Administer IV fluids, oxygen, bronchodilators, and epinephrine. Initiate systemic steroid therapy.

Application Exercises

1. A nurse is collecting data from a client who is having an acute asthma attack. Which of the following findings should indicate to the nurse that the client's respiratory status is declining? (Select all that apply.)

    A. SaO_2 95%

    B. Wheezing

    C. Retraction of sternal muscles

    D. Pink mucous membranes

    E. Premature ventricular complexes (PVCs)

2. A nurse is collecting data from a client who is being admitted to an acute care facility. The client has an SaO_2 of 91%, exhibits audible wheezes, and is using accessory muscles when breathing. Which of the following classes of medications should the nurse expect to administer?

    A. Antibiotic

    B. Beta blocker

    C. Antiviral

    D. $Beta_2$ agonist

3. A nurse is reinforcing discharge teaching with a client who has a new prescription for prednisone to treat asthma. Which of the following client statements indicates an understanding of the teaching?

    A. "I will decrease my fluid intake while taking this medication."

    B. "I will expect to have black, tarry stools."

    C. "I will take my medication with meals."

    D. "I will monitor for weight loss while on this medication."

4. A nurse is collecting data from a client who has a history of asthma. Which of the following factors should the nurse identify as a risk for asthma?

    A. Gender

    B. Environmental allergies

    C. Alcohol use

    D. Race

5. A nurse is reinforcing teaching with a client on the purpose of taking inhaled albuterol. Which of the following client statements indicates an understanding of the teaching?

    A. "This medication can decrease my immune response."

    B. "I take this medication to stop an asthma attack."

    C. "I need to take this medication with food."

    D. "This medication has a slow onset to treat my symptoms."

PRACTICE Active Learning Scenario

A nurse is caring for a client who has asthma and a prescription for prednisone. Use the ATI Active Learning Template: Medication to complete this item.

NURSING INTERVENTIONS: Include at least three.

Application Exercises Key

1. A. Oxygen saturation 95% is an expected finding and does not indicate respiratory distress.

   B. **CORRECT:** Wheezing is a manifestation of bronchoconstriction and is an indication that the client's respiratory status is declining.

   C. **CORRECT:** Retraction of sternal muscles is a manifestation of bronchoconstriction and is an indication that the client's respiratory status is declining.

   D. Pink mucous membranes are an expected finding and does not indicate respiratory distress.

   E. **CORRECT:** PVCs are a manifestation of hypoxemia and an indication that the client's respiratory status is declining.

   Ⓝ *NCLEX® Connection: Physiological Adaptation, Basic Pathophysiology*

2. A. An antibiotic is administered to treat a bacterial infection.

   B. A beta blocker is administered to treat dysrhythmias, heart disease, or hypertension.

   C. An antiviral medication is administered to treat a virus.

   D. **CORRECT:** The nurse should expect to administer a beta$_2$ agonist, which causes dilation of the bronchioles and improves oxygen exchange.

   Ⓝ *NCLEX® Connection: Pharmacological Therapies, Expected Actions/Outcomes*

3. A. The client should drink plenty of fluids while taking prednisone. This medication can cause the client to have a dry mouth or to become thirsty.

   B. The client should inform the provider of any black, tarry stools. This medication can increase bleeding tendency. Black stools is a manifestation of bleeding.

   C. **CORRECT:** The client should take this medication with food. Taking prednisone on an empty stomach can cause gastrointestinal distress.

   D. The client should monitor his mouth for canker sores. This medication can cause bleeding of the gums and soreness in the mouth. It also decreases immune function.

   Ⓝ *NCLEX® Connection: Pharmacological Therapies, Medication Administration*

4. A. Gender is not a risk factor associated with asthma.

   B. **CORRECT:** Environmental allergies are a risk factor associated with asthma. A client who has environmental allergies might have other allergic manifestations (rhinitis, skin rash).

   C. Alcohol use is not a risk factor associated with asthma.

   D. Race is not a risk factor associated with asthma.

   Ⓝ *NCLEX® Connection: Health Promotion and Maintenance, Health Promotion/Disease Prevention*

5. A. A bronchodilator does not decrease the body's immune response. However, an anti-inflammatory medication can cause this effect.

   B. **CORRECT:** Inhaled albuterol is a short-acting beta$_2$ agonist used to abort an ongoing asthma attack or to prevent exercise-induced bronchospasms.

   C. An inhaled bronchodilator does not need to be taken with food. However, an anti-inflammatory medication can cause gastrointestinal distress and should be taken with food.

   D. A short-acting inhaled bronchodilator, such as albuterol, has a fast onset to relieve bronchospasms.

   Ⓝ *NCLEX® Connection: Pharmacological Therapies, Expected Actions/Outcomes*

PRACTICE Answer

Using the ATI Active Use the ATI Active Learning Template: Medication

NURSING INTERVENTIONS

- Monitor for manifestations of an infection such as sore throat or fever.
- Monitor for hyperglycemia.
- Advise the client to report black, tarry stools.
- Observe for fluid retention and weight gain.
- Monitor the throat and mouth for aphthous lesions (canker sores).
- Advise client to increase weight bearing exercises and increase intake of calcium and vitamin D.

Ⓝ *NCLEX® Connection: Pharmacological Therapies, Medication Administration*

CHAPTER 20

UNIT 3 NURSING CARE OF CLIENTS WHO HAVE RESPIRATORY DISORDERS
SECTION: RESPIRATORY SYSTEM DISORDERS

CHAPTER 19 # Chronic Obstructive Pulmonary Disease

Chronic obstructive pulmonary disease (COPD) encompasses two diseases: emphysema and chronic bronchitis. Most clients who have emphysema also have chronic bronchitis. COPD is irreversible and typically affects middle-age to older adults. ©

Emphysema is characterized by the loss of lung elasticity and hyperinflation of lung tissue. Emphysema causes destruction of the alveoli, leading to a decreased surface area for gas exchange, carbon dioxide retention, and respiratory acidosis.

Chronic bronchitis is an inflammation of the bronchi and bronchioles due to chronic exposure to irritants.

HEALTH PROMOTION AND DISEASE PREVENTION

- Promote smoking cessation.
- Avoid exposure to secondhand smoke.
- Use protective equipment, such as a mask, and ensure proper ventilation while working in environments that contain carcinogens or particles in the air.
- Influenza and pneumonia vaccinations are important for all clients who have COPD, especially older adults. ©

DATA COLLECTION

RISK FACTORS

- Older adult clients have a decreased pulmonary reserve due to normal lung changes.
- Cigarette smoking is the primary risk factor for the development of COPD.
- Alpha$_1$ antitrypsin (AAT) deficiency
- Exposure to environmental factors (air pollution, secondhand smoke, occupational exposure to dust and particulate matter)

EXPECTED FINDINGS

Chronic dyspnea

PHYSICAL FINDINGS
- Dyspnea upon exertion
- Productive cough that is most severe upon rising in the morning (chronic bronchitis)
- Hypoxemia
- Crackles and wheezes
- Use of accessory muscles
- Barrel chest or increased chest diameter (emphysema) **(19.1)**
- Thin extremities and enlarged neck muscles
- Clubbing of fingers and toes (late stages)
- Pallor and cyanosis of nail beds and mucous membranes (late stages)
- Decreased oxygen saturation levels (expected reference range is 95% to 100%)
- Red-blue color to the skin (chronic bronchitis)
- Pink undertones to skin (emphysema)
- Repeated respiratory infections (bronchitis)
- Prolonged expiratory effort
- Tripod positioning
- Weight loss (emphysema)

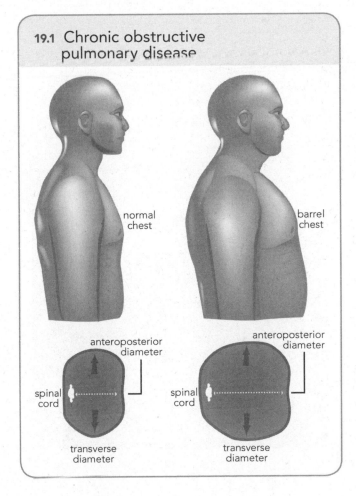

19.1 Chronic obstructive pulmonary disease

normal chest

barrel chest

anteroposterior diameter

spinal cord

transverse diameter

anteroposterior diameter

spinal cord

transverse diameter

LABORATORY TESTS

- Increased hematocrit level is due to low oxygenation levels.
- Sputum cultures and WBC counts are used to diagnose acute respiratory infections.

Arterial blood gases (ABGs)
- Hypoxemia (PaO_2 less than 80 mm Hg)
- Hypercapnia ($PaCO_2$ greater than 45 mm Hg)
- Acidosis (pH less than 7.35)

DIAGNOSTIC PROCEDURES

Pulmonary function tests

- These tests are used for diagnosis, as well as determining the effectiveness of therapy.
- Comparisons of forced expiratory volume (FEV) to forced vital capacity (FVC) are used to classify COPD as mild to very severe.

Imaging

Computed tomography: Used as a diagnostic tool to determine the presence of emphysema

Chest x-ray
- Reveals hyperinflation of alveoli and flattened diaphragm in the late stages of emphysema (19.2)
- Often not useful for the diagnosis of early or moderate disease

Pulse oximetry

Clients who have COPD usually have oxygen levels less than the expected reference range of 95% to 100%.

19.2 X-ray of lungs with emphysema

Alpha₁ antitrypsin levels

Used to assess for deficiency in AAT, an enzyme produced by the liver that helps regulate other enzymes (which help break down pollutants) from attacking lung tissue.

Peak expiratory flow meter

- Determines effectiveness of therapy.
- Decreased levels from client baseline can indicate the need for additional respiratory treatments.

PATIENT-CENTERED CARE

NURSING CARE

- Position the client to maximize ventilation (high-Fowler's). Q꜀ᴮᴾ
- Reinforce teaching of smoking cessation strategies.
- Encourage effective coughing, or suction to remove secretions.
- Encourage deep breathing and use of an incentive spirometer.
- Administer breathing treatments and medications.
- Provide oral care after treatments with nebulizer or MDI.
- Administer oxygen.
- Monitor for skin breakdown around the nose and mouth from the oxygen device.
- Apply and monitor use of continuous positive airway pressure (CPAP) device
- Instruct the client to practice breathing techniques to control dyspneic episodes. Q꜀ᴮᴾ
  - For diaphragmatic (abdominal) breathing
    - Lie on back with knees bent.
    - Take deep breaths in, pushing abdomen outward.
    - Rest a hand over the abdomen to create resistance.
    - If the client's hand on the abdomen rises and lowers upon inhalation and exhalation, the breathing is being performed correctly.
  - For pursed-lip breathing
    - Inhale through the nose.
    - Form the mouth as if preparing to whistle.
    - Exhale through the lips/mouth taking twice as long as inhalation.
    - Do not puff the cheeks.
    - Take breaths deep and slow.
  - For huff coughing
    - Lean forward at the waist while inhaling deeply.
    - Exhale quickly with a "huff" sound.
- Administer chest physiotherapy.
- Provide percussion using cupped hand to break secretions loose.
- Use postural drainage to assist in moving secretions to larger airways where they can be expectorated.

- Promote adequate nutrition.
  - Monitor weight, serum albumin, and electrolytes.
  - Encourage fluids to promote adequate hydration.
  - Provide fluids between and at the end of meals to prevent early satiety.
  - Dyspnea decreases energy available for eating. Encourage soft, high-calorie, high-protein foods.
  - Avoid lying down for 1 hr after eating.
  - Recommend four to six small meals per day to reduce fatigue and fullness.
  - Provide between meal-supplements.
  - Reinforce teaching to avoid gas-forming foods to prevent bloating.
- Monitor weight and note any changes.
- Increase fluid intake. Encourage the client to drink 2 to 3 L/day to liquefy mucus.
- **Exercise conditioning** includes improving pulmonary status by strengthening the condition of the lungs by exercise.
  - The client walks daily at a self-paced rate until symptoms of dyspnea occur, allowing rest periods, and then resuming walking.
  - The client walks 20 min/day, two to three times per week.
  - Determine the client's physical limitations, and structure activity to include periods of rest.
  - Provide rest periods for older adult clients who have dyspnea. Design the room and walkways with opportunities for relaxation. Ⓖ
- Provide emotional support to the client and family. Talk about disease and lifestyle changes.
- Collaborate with discharge planner or social worker to arrange for home care services such as portable oxygen.
- Encourage verbalization of feelings. Ⓠᴘᴄᴄ
- Reinforce teaching about manifestations of upper respiratory infections and when to contact the provider.

MEDICATIONS

Bronchodilators (inhalers)

Short-acting beta₂ adrenergic agonists, such as albuterol, provide rapid relief by producing bronchodilation and increasing ciliary activity and clearance of mucus.

Long-acting beta-adrenergic agonists, such as salmeterol, result in bronchodilation by relaxing bronchial smooth muscles. These medications are not used for quick relief.

Cholinergic antagonists (anticholinergic medications), such as ipratropium, block the parasympathetic nervous system. This allows for the sympathetic nervous system effects of increased bronchodilation and decreased pulmonary secretions. These medications are long-acting and are used to prevent bronchospasms.

Methylxanthines, such as theophylline, relax smooth muscles of the bronchi. These medications require close monitoring of serum medication levels due to narrow therapeutic ranges. Use only when other treatments are ineffective.

NURSING ACTIONS
- Monitor serum levels for toxicity for clients taking theophylline. Adverse effects include tachycardia, nausea, and diarrhea.
- Watch for tremors and tachycardia for clients taking albuterol.
- Observe for dry mouth for clients taking ipratropium.
- Monitor heart rate. Palpitations can occur, which can indicate toxicity of ipratropium.

CLIENT EDUCATION
- Suck on hard candies to help moisten dry mouth while taking ipratropium.
- Increase fluid intake, and report headaches or blurred vision.

Anti-inflammatory agents

These medications decrease airway inflammation.
- **Glucocorticoids**, such as budesonide, provide long-term control by suppressing airway inflammation.
- **Leukotriene antagonists**, such as montelukast; **mast cell stabilizers**, such as cromolyn; and **monoclonal antibodies**, such as omalizumab, can be used.
- **Phosphodiesterase type 4 inhibitors**, such as roflumilast, decrease inflammation and mucus production while suppressing cough.
- Omalizumab can cause anaphylaxis.

NURSING ACTIONS
- Watch for a decrease in immune function.
- Monitor for hyperglycemia, hypokalemia, and poor wound healing.
- Observe for fluid retention and weight gain. This is common with glucocorticoid medications
- Check the throat and mouth for aphthous lesions (canker sores) and candida (yeast) infections.
- Monitor for weight loss and depression in clients taking roflumilast.

CLIENT EDUCATION
- Report black, tarry stools.
- Drink plenty of fluids to promote hydration.
- Take oral glucocorticoids with food.
- Use medication to prevent and control bronchospasms.
- Avoid people who have respiratory infections.
- Use good mouth care.
- Use medication as a prophylactic for COPD symptoms.
- Do not discontinue medication suddenly.

Mucolytic agents

These agents help thin secretions, making them easier for the client to expel.
- Nebulizer treatments include acetylcysteine and dornase alfa.
- Guaifenesin is an oral agent that can be taken.

THERAPEUTIC PROCEDURES

- Chest physiotherapy uses percussion and vibration to mobilize secretions.
- Raising the foot of the bed slightly higher than the head can facilitate optimal drainage and removal of secretions by gravity.

INTERPROFESSIONAL CARE

- Consult respiratory services for inhalers, breathing treatments, and suctioning for airway management.
- Contact nutritional services for weight loss or gain related to medications or diagnosis.
- Consult rehabilitative care if the client has prolonged weakness and needs assistance with increasing activity level.
- Consult case manager or social worker for home care needs.
- COPD is debilitating for older adult clients. Referrals to assistance programs, such as food delivery services, can be indicated. Ⓖ
- Set up referral services, including home care services such as portable oxygen.

CLIENT EDUCATION

- Provide support to the client and family.
- Eat high-calorie, high-protein foods to promote energy. Ⓠᴘᴄᴄ
- Rest as needed.
- Use hand hygiene to prevent infection.
- Take medications (inhalers, oral medications) as prescribed.
- Stop smoking if needed.
- Obtain immunizations, such as influenza and pneumonia, to decrease the risk of infection.
- Use oxygen as prescribed. Inform other caregivers not to smoke around the oxygen due to flammability.
- Avoid crowds during respiratory illness outbreaks, such as influenza.

COMPLICATIONS

Respiratory infection

Can result from increased mucus production and poor oxygenation levels

NURSING ACTIONS
- Administer oxygen therapy.
- Monitor oxygenation levels.
- Administer antibiotics and other medications.

CLIENT EDUCATION
- Avoid crowds and people who have respiratory infections.
- Obtain pneumonia and influenza immunizations.

Right-sided heart failure (cor pulmonale)

- Air trapping, airway collapse, and stiff alveoli lead to increased pulmonary pressures.
- Blood flow through the lung tissue is difficult. This increased workload leads to enlargement and thickening of the right atrium and ventricle.

MANIFESTATIONS
- Low oxygenation levels
- Cyanotic lips
- Enlarged and tender liver
- Distended neck veins
- Dependent edema
- Weight gain

NURSING ACTIONS
- Monitor respiratory status and administer oxygen therapy.
- Monitor heart rate and rhythm.
- Administer medications.
- Administer IV fluids and diuretics to maintain fluid balance.

Application Exercises

1. A nurse is reinforcing discharge teaching with a client who has COPD and a new prescription for albuterol. Which of the following client statements indicates understanding of the teaching?

   A. "This medication can increase my blood sugar levels."

   B. "This medication can decrease my immune response."

   C. "I can have an increase in my heart rate while taking this medication."

   D. "I can have mouth sores while taking this medication."

2. A nurse is preparing to administer a dose of prednisone to a client who has COPD. The nurse should monitor for which of the following adverse effects of this medication? (Select all that apply.)

   A. Hypokalemia

   B. Tachycardia

   C. Fluid retention

   D. Nausea

   E. Black, tarry stools

3. A nurse is assisting with the discharge of a client who has COPD. Upon discharge, the client is concerned that he will never be able to leave his house now that he is on continuous oxygen. Which of the following is an appropriate response by the nurse?

   A. "There are portable oxygen delivery systems that you can take with you."

   B. "When you go out, you can remove the oxygen and then reapply it when you get home."

   C. "You probably will not be able to go out as much as you used to."

   D. "Home health services will come to you so you will not need to get out."

4. A nurse is reinforcing teaching with a client about the use of an incentive spirometer. Which of the following client statements indicates understanding of the teaching?

   A. "I will place the adapter on my finger to read my blood oxygen saturation level."

   B. "I will lie on my back with my knees bent."

   C. "I will rest my hand over my abdomen to create resistance."

   D. "I will take in a deep breath and hold it before exhaling."

5. A nurse is reinforcing teaching with a client about how to perform pursed-lip breathing. Which of the following should the nurse include in the instruction?

   A. "Inhale quickly through the mouth."

   B. "Place your hand over your stomach."

   C. "Take a deep breath in through your nose."

   D. "Puff your cheeks upon exhalation."

PRACTICE Active Learning Scenario

A nurse is reinforcing discharge instructions with a client who has a new prescription for ipratropium. Use the ATI Active Learning Template: Medication to complete this item.

NURSING INTERVENTIONS: List at least three.

Application Exercises Key

1. A. Anti-inflammatory agents, such as corticosteroids, can cause hyperglycemia.

   B. Anti-inflammatory agents can decrease the immune response.

   C. **CORRECT:** Bronchodilators, such as albuterol, can cause tachycardia.

   D. Anti-inflammatory agents can cause mouth sores.

   Ⓝ *NCLEX® Connection: Pharmacological Therapies, Adverse Effects/ Contraindications/Side Effects/Interactions*

2. A. **CORRECT:** The nurse should observe for hypokalemia. This is an adverse effect of prednisone.

   B. Tachycardia is an adverse effect of bronchodilators.

   C. **CORRECT:** The nurse should observe for fluid retention. This is an adverse effect of prednisone.

   D. Nausea is an adverse effect of bronchodilators.

   E. **CORRECT:** The nurse should monitor for black, tarry stools. This is an adverse effect of prednisone.

   Ⓝ *NCLEX® Connection: Pharmacological Therapies, Adverse Effects/ Contraindications/Side Effects/Interactions*

3. A. **CORRECT:** The nurse should inform the client that there are portable oxygen systems that he can use to leave the house. This should alleviate the client's anxiety.

   B. The nurse should tell the client use oxygen at all times to prevent becoming hypoxic.

   C. The nurse should encourage the client to return to his daily routine, but include periods of rest.

   D. The nurse should encourage the client to return to his daily routine. Home health services promote a client's independence.

   Ⓝ *NCLEX® Connection: Reduction of Risk Potential, Potential for Alterations in Body Systems*

4. A. The client should place an adapter on her finger to read the blood oxygen saturation level while performing a pulse oximetry reading.

   B. The client who practices diaphragmatic or abdominal breathing should lie on her back with knees bent.

   C. The client who practices diaphragmatic or abdominal breathing should rest her hand over her abdomen to determine if the breathing is done correctly.

   D. **CORRECT:** The client who is using the spirometer should slowly inhale with her lips forming a seal around the mouthpiece. As the client inhales, the spirometer indicator will rise. The client should hold her breath for a period of 2 to 6 seconds to promote lung expansion.

   Ⓝ *NCLEX® Connection: Reduction of Risk Potential, Therapeutic Procedures*

5. A. The client should inhale deeply through the nose and exhale through the lips. Exhalation should be longer than inhalation to expel carbon dioxide.

   B. The client should place her hand on her stomach while performing diaphragmatic or abdominal breathing. This allows resistance to be met and serves as a guide that the client is inhaling and exhaling correctly.

   C. **CORRECT:** The client should take a deep breath in through her nose while performing pursed-lip breathing. This controls the client's breathing.

   D. The client should not puff her cheeks upon exhalation. This does not allow the client to optimally exhale the carbon dioxide from her lungs.

   Ⓝ *NCLEX® Connection: Reduction of Risk Potential, Therapeutic Procedures*

PRACTICE Answer

Using ATI Active Learning Template: Medication

NURSING INTERVENTIONS
- Inform the client that dry mouth can occur when taking this medication.
- Encourage the client to suck on hard candies to help moisten dry mouth while taking ipratropium.
- Encourage the client to increase fluid intake, and to report headaches or blurred vision.
- Monitor heart rate. Palpitations can occur, which can indicate toxicity of ipratropium.

Ⓝ *NCLEX® Connection: Pharmacological Therapies, Medication Administration*

CHAPTER 20 *Tuberculosis*

Tuberculosis (TB) is an infectious disease caused by *Mycobacterium tuberculosis*. TB is transmitted through aerosolization (airborne route).

Once inside the lung, the body encases the TB bacillus with collagen and other cells. This can appear as a Ghon tubercle on a chest x-ray.

Only a small percentage of people infected with TB develop an active form of the infection. The TB bacillus can lie dormant for many years before producing the disease.

TB primarily affects the lungs but can spread to any organ. The risk of transmission decreases after 2 to 3 weeks of antituberculin therapy.

HEALTH PROMOTION AND DISEASE PREVENTION

- Screen clients who live in high-risk areas for tuberculosis on a yearly basis.
- Screen family members of clients who have tuberculosis.
- Early detection and treatment are vital. TB has a slow onset, and the client might not be aware until the symptoms and disease are advanced. TB diagnosis should be considered for any client who has a persistent cough, chest pain, weakness, weight loss, anorexia, hemoptysis, dyspnea, fever, night sweats, or chills.
- Increasing the percentage of clients who complete treatment for TB should be a goal.
- Individuals who have been exposed to TB but have not developed the disease can have latent TB. This means that *Mycobacterium tuberculosis* is in the body, but the body has been able to fight off the infection. If not treated, it can lie dormant for several years and then become active as the individual ages or becomes immunocompromised. ©

DATA COLLECTION

RISK FACTORS

- Frequent and close contact with an untreated individual
- Lower socioeconomic status and homelessness
- Immunocompromised status (HIV, chemotherapy, kidney disease, diabetes mellitus, Crohn's disease)
- Poorly ventilated, crowded environments (prisons, long-term care facilities)
- Older adults
- Recent travel to countries where TB is endemic
- Immigration (especially from Mexico, Philippines, Vietnam, China, Japan, and Eastern Mediterranean countries)
- Substance use
- Health care occupation that involves performance of high-risk activities (respiratory treatments, suctioning, coughing procedures)

EXPECTED FINDINGS

- Persistent cough lasting longer than 3 weeks
- Purulent sputum, possibly blood-streaked
- Fatigue and lethargy
- Weight loss and anorexia
- Night sweats and low-grade fever in the afternoon

PHYSICAL FINDINGS: Older adult clients often present with atypical symptoms of the disease (altered mentation or unusual behavior, fever, anorexia, weight loss). ©

LABORATORY TESTS

A client will have a positive intradermal TB test within 2 to 10 weeks of exposure to the infection.

QuantiFERON-TB Gold

Blood test that detects interferon-gamma release assays (IGRAs) in fresh heparinized whole blood from sensitized people
- Diagnostic for infection, whether active or latent.
- Results are available within 24 hr.

DIAGNOSTIC PROCEDURES

Mantoux test (20.1)

- Read within 48 to 72 hr.
- An intradermal injection of an extract of the tubercle bacillus is made.
- An induration (palpable, raised, hardened area) of 10 mm or greater in diameter indicates a positive skin test.
- An induration of 5 mm is considered a positive test for immunocompromised clients.
- A positive Mantoux test indicates that the client has developed an immune response to TB. It does not confirm that active disease is present. Clients who have been treated for TB can have a positive reaction. Q EBP

20.1 Mantoux test

20.2 N95 mask

- Individuals who have latent TB can have a positive Mantoux test and can receive treatment to prevent development of an active form of the disease.
- Clients who have received a Bacillus Calmette-Guerin vaccine within the past 10 years can have a false-positive Mantoux test. These clients need a chest x-ray or QuantiFERON-TB Gold test to evaluate the presence of active TB infection.
- Test clients who are immunocompromised (such as those who have HIV) and older adult clients for TB. Test clients starting immunosuppressive therapy (such as tumor necrosis factor antagonists) for TB prior to starting treatment.

CLIENT EDUCATION: Return for a reading of the injection site by a health care personnel within 48 to 72 hr.

Chest x-ray

Prescribed to detect active lesions in the lungs

Acid-fast bacilli smear and culture

- A positive acid-fast test suggests an active infection.
- The diagnosis is confirmed by a positive culture for *Mycobacterium tuberculosis*.

NURSING ACTIONS
- Obtain three early-morning sputum samples.
- Wear personal protective equipment when obtaining specimens.
- Obtain samples in a negative airflow room.

PATIENT-CENTERED CARE

NURSING CARE

- Administer heated and humidified oxygen therapy as prescribed.
- Prevent infection transmission.
  - Wear an N95 HEPA filter or powered air purifying respirator when caring for clients who are hospitalized with TB. (20.2)
  - Place the client in a negative-airflow room, and implement airborne precautions.
  - Use barrier protection when the risk of hand or clothing contamination exists.
  - Have the client wear a surgical mask if transportation to another department is necessary. The client should be transported using the shortest and least busy route.
  - Reinforce teaching with the client to cough and expectorate sputum into tissues that are disposed of by the client into provided plastic bags or no-touch receptacles.
- Administer prescribed medications.
- Promote adequate nutrition.
  - Encourage fluid intake and a well-balanced diet for adequate caloric intake.
  - Encourage foods that are rich in protein, iron, and vitamins C and B.
- Provide emotional support.
- Test exposed family members for TB.

MEDICATIONS

Due to the resistance that is developing against the antituberculin medications, combination therapy for active TB consists of at least four medications. For latent TB infection (LTBI) two or more medications at a time is recommended.

- Because these medications are taken for 6 to 12 months, medication noncompliance is a significant contributing factor in the development of resistant strains of TB.
- The current four-medication regimen includes isoniazid, rifampin, pyrazinamide, and ethambutol.

CLIENT EDUCATION: Complete a series of prescribed medication.

Isoniazid

Isoniazid (INH) is bactericidal and inhibits growth of mycobacteria by preventing synthesis of mycolic acid in the cell wall.

NURSING ACTIONS
- Monitor for hepatotoxicity (jaundice, anorexia, malaise, fatigue, nausea) and neurotoxicity (such as tingling of the hands and feet).
- Vitamin B_6 (pyridoxine) is used to prevent neurotoxicity from isoniazid.
- Monitor liver function laboratory tests prior to and monthly after starting INH.

CLIENT EDUCATION
- Take this medication on an empty stomach.
- Do not drink alcohol while taking isoniazid, because it can increase the risk for hepatotoxicity. Qs
- Report any manifestations of hepatotoxicity.

Rifampin

Rifampin (RIF) is a bacteriostatic and bactericidal antibiotic that inhibits DNA-dependent RNA polymerase activity in susceptible cells.

NURSING ACTIONS
- Observe for hepatotoxicity.
- Monitor liver function laboratory tests prior to and at least monthly after starting RIF.

CLIENT EDUCATION
- Urine and other secretions will be orange.
- Immediately report yellowing of the skin, pain or swelling of joints, loss of appetite, or malaise.
- This medication can interfere with the efficacy of oral contraceptives.

Pyrazinamide

Pyrazinamide (PZA) is bacteriostatic and bactericidal. Its exact mechanism of action is unknown.

NURSING ACTIONS
- Observe for hepatotoxicity.
- Monitor clients who have a history of gout, as the medication will cause nongouty polyarthralgias.
- Obtain liver enzymes at baseline and every 2 weeks after starting PZA.

CLIENT EDUCATION
- Drink a glass of water with each dose and increase fluids during the day to help prevent gout and kidney problems.
- Immediately report yellowing of the skin, pain or swelling of joints, loss of appetite, or malaise.
- Avoid using alcohol while taking pyrazinamide.

Ethambutol

Ethambutol (EMB) is bacteriostatic and works by suppressing RNA synthesis, subsequently inhibiting protein synthesis.

NURSING ACTIONS
- Obtain baseline visual acuity tests, and complete monthly after starting treatment.
- Determine color discrimination ability.
- This medication should not be given to children younger than 8 years old.
- Stop medication immediately if ocular toxicity occurs.

CLIENT EDUCATION: Report changes in vision immediately. Qebp

Streptomycin sulfate

Streptomycin sulfate is an aminoglycoside antibiotic. It potentiates the efficacy of macrophages during phagocytosis.

NURSING ACTIONS
- Due to its high level of toxicity, this medication should be used only in clients who have multidrug-resistant TB (MDR-TB).
- Streptomycin can cause ototoxicity, so monitor hearing function and tolerance often.
- Report significant changes in urine output and renal function studies.

CLIENT EDUCATION
- Drink at least 2 L fluid daily.
- Notify the provider if hearing declines.

INTERPROFESSIONAL CARE

- Contact social services if the client will need assistance in obtaining prescribed medications.
- Refer the client to a community clinic as needed for follow-up appointments to monitor medication regimen and status of disease.
- Directly observed therapy, in which a health care professional watches the client swallow the medication, is frequently used for noncompliant clients.

CLIENT EDUCATION

- TB is often treated in the home setting. Qᴘᴄᴄ
- Airborne precautions are not needed in the home setting, because family members have already been exposed.
- Continue medication therapy for its full duration of 6 to 12 months (up to 2 years for MDR-TB). Failure to take the medications can lead to a resistant strain of TB.
- Continue with follow-up care for 1 full year.
- Sputum samples are needed every 2 to 4 weeks to monitor therapy effectiveness. Clients are no longer considered infectious after three consecutive negative sputum cultures, and can return to employment.
- Use proper hand hygiene.
- Cover mouth and nose when coughing or sneezing.
- Dispose of contaminated tissues in plastic bags.
- Wear a mask when in public places or in contact with crowds.

COMPLICATIONS

Miliary TB

The organism invades the bloodstream and can spread to multiple body organs with complications including the following.

- Headaches, neck stiffness, and drowsiness (can be life-threatening)
- Pericarditis: Dyspnea, swollen neck veins, pleuritic pain, and hypotension due to an accumulation of fluid in pericardial sac that inhibits the heart's ability to pump effectively

NURSING ACTIONS: Treatment is the same as for pulmonary TB.

Application Exercises

1. A home health nurse is reinforcing teaching with a client who has active tuberculosis. The provider has prescribed isoniazid 250 mg PO daily, rifampin 500 mg PO daily, pyrazinamide 750 mg PO daily, and ethambutol 750 mg PO daily. Which of the following statements indicates the client understands the teaching? (Select all that apply.)

   A. "I can substitute one medication for another if I run out, because they all fight infection."

   B. "I will wash my hands each time I cough."

   C. "I will wear a mask when I am in a public area."

   D. "I am glad I don't have to have any more sputum specimens."

   E. "I don't need to worry where I go once I start taking my medications."

2. A nurse is reinforcing teaching with a client who has tuberculosis. Which of the following statements should the nurse include in the teaching?

   A. "You will need to continue to take the multimedication regimen for 4 months."

   B. "You will need to provide sputum samples every 4 weeks to monitor the effectiveness of the medication."

   C. "You will need to remain hospitalized for treatment."

   D. "You will need to wear a mask at all times."

3. A nurse is caring for a client who has a new diagnosis of tuberculosis and has been placed on a multimedication regimen. Which of the following instructions should the nurse give the client related to ethambutol?

   A. "Your urine can turn a dark orange."

   B. "Monitor for weight gain."

   C. "Watch for any changes in vision."

   D. "Take vitamin B₆ daily."

4. A nurse is preparing to administer isoniazid to a client who has tuberculosis. The nurse should instruct the client to report which of the following findings as an adverse effect of the medication?

   A. Orange urine

   B. Joint pain

   C. Tingling in the hands

   D. Constipation

5. A nurse is providing information about tuberculosis to a group of clients at a local community center. Which of the following manifestations should the nurse include in the teaching? (Select all that apply.)

   A. Persistent cough

   B. Weight gain

   C. Fatigue

   D. Night sweats

   E. Purulent sputum

PRACTICE Active Learning Scenario

A nurse is caring for a client who has tuberculosis. Use the ATI Active Learning Template: System Disorder to complete this item.

PATHOPHYSIOLOGY RELATED TO CLIENT PROBLEM

NURSING CARE: Include three nursing interventions.

COMPLICATIONS: Identify one potential complication.

1. A. The client should not replace one medication for another. It is important that the client adhere to the multimedication regimen prescribed to treat tuberculosis.

    B. **CORRECT:** The client should wash her hands each time she coughs to prevent spreading the infection.

    C. **CORRECT:** The client should wear a mask while in public areas to prevent spreading the infection. The client has active TB, which is transmitted through the airborne route.

    D. The client will need to collect sputum cultures every 2 to 4 weeks until three consecutive sputum cultures have come back negative.

    E. The client should continue to avoid crowded areas if possible and take preventative measures, such as wearing a mask when going out.

    Ⓝ *NCLEX® Connection: Physiological Adaptation, Alterations in Body Systems*

2. A. The client who has tuberculosis needs to continue taking the multimedication regimen for 6 to 12 months.

    B. **CORRECT:** The client who has tuberculosis needs to provide sputum samples every 2 to 4 weeks to monitor the effectiveness of the medication.

    C. The client who has tuberculosis is often treated in the home setting.

    D. The client who has tuberculosis needs to wear a mask when in public areas.

    Ⓝ *NCLEX® Connection: Physiological Adaptation, Alterations in Body Systems*

3. A. The client who is receiving rifampin should expect to see urine turn a dark orange.

    B. The client who is taking ethambutol can have nausea and vomiting but not weight gain.

    C. **CORRECT:** The client who is receiving ethambutol will need to watch for visual changes due to optic neuritis, which can result from taking this medication.

    D. The client who is taking isoniazid should take vitamin B$_6$ daily and observe for signs of hepatotoxicity.

    Ⓝ *NCLEX® Connection: Pharmacological Therapies, Adverse Effects/ Contraindications/Side Effects/Interactions*

4. A. Orange urine is an adverse effect of rifampin.

    B. Experiencing pain in the joints is an adverse effect of rifampin.

    C. **CORRECT:** Tingling of the hands is an adverse effect of isoniazid.

    D. Isoniazid can cause nausea and vomiting, but not constipation.

    Ⓝ *NCLEX® Connection: Pharmacological Therapies, Adverse Effects/ Contraindications/Side Effects/Interactions*

5. A. **CORRECT:** A persistent cough is a manifestation of tuberculosis.

    B. Weight loss is a manifestation of tuberculosis.

    C. **CORRECT:** Fatigue is a manifestation of tuberculosis.

    D. **CORRECT:** Night sweats is a manifestation of tuberculosis.

    E. **CORRECT:** Purulent sputum is a manifestation of tuberculosis.

    Ⓝ *NCLEX® Connection: Physiological Adaptation, Basic Pathophysiology*

PRACTICE Answer

Using the ATI Active Learning Template: System Disorder

PATHOPHYSIOLOGY RELATED TO CLIENT DIAGNOSIS: Tuberculosis (TB) is an infectious disease caused by *Mycobacterium tuberculosis*. TB is transmitted through aerosolization (airborne route). Once inside the lung, the body encases the TB bacillus with collagen and other cells. This can appear as a Ghon tubercle on a chest x-ray. Only a small percentage of people infected with TB develop an active form of the infection. The TB bacillus can lie dormant for many years before producing the disease. TB primarily affects the lungs but can spread to any organ.

NURSING CARE

- Administer heated and humidified oxygen therapy as prescribed.
- Prevent infection transmission.
- Wear an N95 or HEPA respirator when caring for clients who are hospitalized with TB.
- Place the client in a negative airflow room, and implement airborne precautions.
- Use barrier protection when the risk of hand or clothing contamination exists.
- Have the client wear a surgical mask if transportation to another department is necessary.

- Transport the client using the shortest and least busy route.
- Reinforce teaching with the client to cough and expectorate sputum into tissues that are disposed of by the client into provided sacks.
- Administer medications as prescribed.
- Promote adequate nutrition.
- Encourage fluid intake and a well-balanced diet for adequate caloric intake.

COMPLICATIONS

- Miliary TB
  - The organism invades the bloodstream and can spread to multiple body organs.
  - Complications include the following.
    - Headaches, neck stiffness, and drowsiness (can be life-threatening)
    - Pericarditis: dyspnea, swollen neck veins, pleuritic pain, and hypotension due to an accumulation of fluid in the pericardial sac that inhibits the heart's ability to pump effectively
  - Treatment is the same as for pulmonary TB.

Ⓝ *NCLEX® Connection: Physiological Adaptation, Basic Pathophysiology*

UNIT 3   NURSING CARE OF CLIENTS WHO
HAVE RESPIRATORY DISORDERS
SECTION: RESPIRATORY EMERGENCIES

CHAPTER 21 *Pulmonary Embolism*

A pulmonary embolism (PE) occurs when a substance (solid, gaseous, or liquid) enters venous circulation and forms a blockage in the pulmonary vasculature. (21.1)

Emboli originating from venous thromboembolism, also known as deep-vein thrombosis (DVT), are the most common cause. Tumors, bone marrow, amniotic fluid, air, and foreign matter also can become emboli. Increased hypoxia to pulmonary tissue and impaired blood flow can result from a large embolus. PE is a medical emergency.

Prevention, rapid recognition, and treatment of a PE are essential for a positive outcome.

HEALTH PROMOTION AND DISEASE PREVENTION

- Do not smoke.
- Maintain an appropriate weight for height and body frame.
- Consume a healthy diet and engage in physical activity.
- Prevent DVT by doing leg exercises, wearing compression stockings, and avoiding sitting for long periods of time.

DATA COLLECTION

RISK FACTORS

- Long-term immobility
- Oral contraceptive use and estrogen therapy
- Pregnancy
- Tobacco use
- Hypercoagulability (elevated platelet count)
- Obesity
- Surgery (especially orthopedic surgery of the lower extremities or pelvis)
- Central venous catheters
- Heart failure or chronic atrial fibrillation
- Autoimmune hemolytic anemia (sickle cell)
- Long bone fractures
- Cancer
- Trauma
- Age Ⓒ
  - Older adult clients have decreased pulmonary reserves due to normal lung changes, including decreased lung elasticity and thickening alveoli. Older adult clients can decompensate more quickly.
  - Certain pathological conditions and procedures that predispose clients to DVT formation (peripheral vascular disease, hypertension, hip and knee arthroplasty) are more prevalent in older adults.
  - Many older adult clients experience decreased physical activity levels, thus predisposing them to DVT formation and pulmonary emboli.

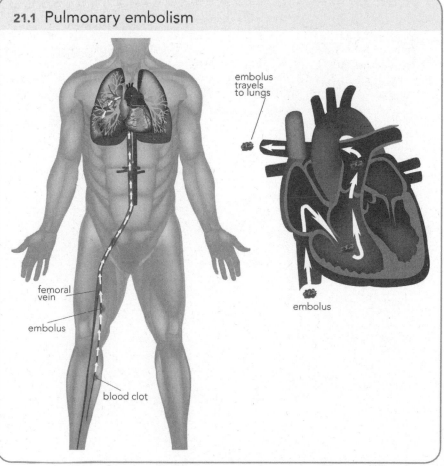

21.1 Pulmonary embolism

embolus travels to lungs

femoral vein

embolus

blood clot

embolus

EXPECTED FINDINGS

- Anxiety
- Feelings of impending doom
- Pressure in chest
- Pain upon inspiration and chest wall tenderness
- Dyspnea and air hunger
- Cough
- Hemoptysis

PHYSICAL FINDINGS
- Pleurisy
- Pleural friction rub
- Tachycardia
- Hypotension
- Tachypnea
- Adventitious breath sounds (crackles) and cough
- Heart murmur in S_3 and S_4
- Diaphoresis
- Low-grade fever
- Decreased oxygen saturation levels (expected reference range is 95% to 100%), low SaO_2, cyanosis
- Petechiae (red dots under the skin) over chest and axillae
- Pleural effusion (fluid in the lungs)
- Distended neck veins
- Syncope
- Cyanosis

LABORATORY TESTS

ABG analysis

- $PaCO_2$ levels are low (expected reference range is 35 to 45 mm Hg) due to initial hyperventilation (respiratory alkalosis).
- As hypoxemia progresses, respiratory acidosis occurs.
- Further progression leads to metabolic acidosis due to buildup of lactic acid from tissue hypoxia.

CBC analysis

To monitor hemoglobin and hematocrit

D-dimer

Elevated above expected reference range in response to clot formation and release of fibrin degradation products (expected reference range is 0.43 to 2.33 mcg/mL).

DIAGNOSTIC PROCEDURES

Chest x-ray, computed tomography scan

These provide initial identification of a PE. A computed tomography (CT) scan is most commonly used. A chest x-ray can show a large PE.

Ventilation-perfusion scan

Ventilation-perfusion (V/Q) scan images show circulation of air and blood in the lungs and can detect a PE.

Pulmonary angiography

- This is the gold standard and most thorough test to detect a PE, but it is invasive and costly. A catheter is inserted into the vena cava to visually see a PE.
- Pulmonary angiography is a higher-risk procedure than a V/Q scan.

NURSING ACTIONS
- Verify that informed consent has been obtained.
- Monitor status (vital signs, SaO_2, anxiety, bleeding with angiography) during and after the procedure.

PATIENT-CENTERED CARE

NURSING CARE

- Administer oxygen therapy to relieve hypoxemia and dyspnea. Position the client to maximize ventilation (high-Fowler's = 90°).
- Maintain IV access.
- Administer medications as prescribed.
- Monitor respiratory status at least every 30 min. Qpcc
  - Auscultate lung sounds.
  - Measure rate, rhythm, and ease of respirations.
  - Inspect skin color and capillary refill.
  - Examine for position of trachea.
- Monitor cardiac status. Qpcc
  - Compare blood pressure in both arms.
  - Palpate pulse quality.
  - Check for dysrhythmias on cardiac monitor.
  - Examine the neck for distended neck veins.
  - Inspect the thorax for petechiae.
- Provide emotional support and comfort to control client anxiety.
- Monitor changes in level of consciousness and mental status.

MEDICATIONS

Anticoagulants

Heparin, enoxaparin, warfarin, and fondaparinux are used to prevent clots from getting larger or additional clots from forming.

NURSING ACTIONS
- Check for contraindications (active bleeding, peptic ulcer disease, history of stroke, recent trauma).
- Monitor bleeding times: prothrombin time (PT) and international normalized ratio (INR) for warfarin, partial thromboplastin time (aPTT) for heparin, and complete blood count (CBC). Qᴱᴮᴾ
- Monitor for side effects of anticoagulants (thrombocytopenia, anemia, hemorrhage).

Direct factor Xa inhibitor

Rivaroxaban binds directly with the active center of factor Xa, which inhibits the production of thrombin.

NURSING ACTIONS
- Check for bleeding from any site. Clients have experienced epidural hematomas, as well as intracranial, retinal, adrenal, and GI bleeds.
- Due to risk for spinal or epidural hematoma, medication should be discontinued for 18 hr prior to removing an epidural catheter, and wait another 6 hr to restart.

Thrombolytic therapy

- Alteplase, reteplase, and tenecteplase are used to dissolve blood clots and restore pulmonary blood flow.
- Similar side effects and contraindications as anticoagulants.

NURSING ACTIONS
- Check for contraindications (bleeding disorders, uncontrolled hypertension, active bleeding, peptic ulcer disease, history of stroke, recent trauma or surgery, pregnancy).
- Monitor for evidence of bleeding, thrombocytopenia, and anemia.
- Monitor blood pressure, heart rate, respirations, and oxygen saturation per facility protocol before, during, and after administration of medication. Qˢ

INTERPROFESSIONAL CARE

- Cardiology and pulmonary services should be consulted to manage and treat PE.
- Respiratory services should be consulted for oxygen therapy, breathing treatments, and ABGs.
- Radiology should be consulted for diagnostic studies to determine PE.
- If the client is homebound, set up home care services to perform weekly blood draws.
- Set up referral services to supply portable oxygen for clients who have severe dyspnea.

THERAPEUTIC PROCEDURES

Embolectomy

Surgical removal of embolus

NURSING ACTIONS
- Prepare the client for the procedure (NPO status, informed consent).
- Monitor postoperatively (vital signs, SaO_2, incision drainage, pain management).

Vena cava filter

Insertion of a filter in the vena cava to prevent further emboli from reaching the pulmonary vasculature

NURSING ACTIONS
- Prepare the client for the procedure (NPO status, informed consent).
- Monitor postoperatively (vital signs, SaO_2, incision drainage, pain management).

CLIENT EDUCATION

- Practice strategies for treatment and prevention of PE. Qᴾᶜᶜ
  - Do not smoke.
  - Avoid long periods of immobility.
  - Engage in physical activity such as walking.
  - Wear compression stockings to promote circulation.
  - Avoid crossing legs.
- Monitor intake of foods high in vitamin K (green, leafy vegetables) if taking warfarin. Vitamin K can reduce the anticoagulant effects of warfarin.
- Adhere to a schedule for monitoring PT and INR, follow instructions regarding medication dosage adjustments (for clients on warfarin), and adhere to weekly blood draws.
- There is an increased risk for bruising and bleeding.
  - Avoid taking aspirin products, unless specified by the provider.
  - Check the mouth and skin daily for bleeding and bruising.
  - Use electric shavers and soft-bristled toothbrushes.
  - Avoid blowing the nose hard, and gently apply pressure if nosebleeds occur.
- Use measures to prevent PE when traveling.
  - Arise from a sitting position for 5 min out of every hour.
  - Wear support stockings.
  - Remain hydrated by drinking plenty of water.
  - Perform active ROM exercises when sitting.

COMPLICATIONS

Decreased cardiac output

Blood volume is decreased.

NURSING ACTIONS
- Monitor for hypotension, tachycardia, cyanosis, jugular venous distention, and syncope.
- Check for the presence of S_3 or S_4 heart sounds.
- Maintain IV access.
- Monitor urinary output (should be 30 mL/hr or more).
- Enusre IV fluids (crystalloids) are administered to replace vascular volume.
- Continuously monitor the ECG.

Hemorrhage

Risk for bleeding increases due to anticoagulant therapy.

NURSING ACTIONS
- Check for oozing, bleeding, or bruising from injection and surgical sites at least every 2 hr.
- Monitor cardiovascular status (blood pressure, heart rate and rhythm).
- Monitor CBC (hemoglobin, hematocrit, platelets) and bleeding times (PT, aPTT, INR).
- Ensure IV fluids and blood products are administered as required.
- Test stools, urine, and vomit for occult blood.
- Monitor for internal bleeding (measure abdominal girth and abdominal or flank pain) at least every 8 hr.

Application Exercises

1. A nurse is caring for a group of clients. Which of the following clients are at risk for a pulmonary embolism? (Select all that apply.)

   A. A client who has a BMI of 30

   B. A client who is postmenopausal

   C. A client who has a fractured femur

   D. A client who is a marathon runner

   E. A client who has chronic atrial fibrillation

2. A nurse is collecting data on a client who has a pulmonary embolism. Which of the following manifestations should the nurse expect to find? (Select all that apply.)

   A. Bradypnea

   B. Pleural friction rub

   C. Hypertension

   D. Petechiae

   E. Tachycardia

3. A nurse is reviewing prescriptions for a client who has acute dyspnea and diaphoresis. The client states she is anxious and is unable to get enough air. Vital signs are heart rate 117/min, respirations 38/min, temperature 38.4° C (101.2° F), and blood pressure 100/54 mm Hg. Which of the following nursing actions is the priority?

   A. Notify the provider.

   B. Ensure access to heparin via IV infusion.

   C. Administer oxygen therapy.

   D. Obtain a spiral CT scan.

4. A nurse is caring for a client who has a pulmonary embolism and a new prescription for heparin therapy. Which of the following statements by the client should indicate an immediate concern for the nurse?

   A. "I am allergic to morphine."

   B. "I take antacids several times a day for a stomach ulcer."

   C. "I had a blood clot in my leg several years ago."

   D. "It hurts to take a deep breath."

5. A nurse is caring for a client who is to receive thrombolytic therapy. Which of the following factors should the nurse recognize as a contraindication to the therapy?

   A. Hip arthroplasty 2 weeks ago

   B. Elevated sedimentation rate

   C. Incident of exercise-induced asthma 1 week ago

   D. Elevated platelet count

PRACTICE **Active Learning Scenario**

A nurse is caring for a client who has a pulmonary embolism. Use the ATI Active Learning Template: System Disorder to complete this item.

PATHOPHYSIOLOGY RELATED TO CLIENT PROBLEM

NURSING CARE: Describe three nursing interventions.

MEDICATIONS: Identify two.

Application Exercises Key

1. A. **CORRECT:** The client who has a BMI of 30 is considered obese and is at increased risk for a blood clot.

   B. A client who is postmenopausal has decreased estrogen levels and is not at risk for developing a pulmonary embolism.

   C. **CORRECT:** A fractured bone, particularly in a long bone such as the femur, increases the risk of fat emboli.

   D. The client who is a marathon runner has increased blood flow and circulation of his body, which decreases the risk for developing a pulmonary embolism.

   E. **CORRECT:** The client who has turbulent blood flow in the heart, such as with atrial defibrillation, is at increased risk of a blood clot.

   ⓝ *NCLEX® Connection: Health Promotion and Maintenance, Health Promotion/Disease Prevention*

2. A. The nurse should expect the client to have tachypnea, which is a manifestation associated with a pulmonary embolism.

   B. **CORRECT:** The nurse should expect the client to have a pleural friction rub.

   C. The nurse should expect the client to have hypotension.

   D. **CORRECT:** The nurse should expect the client to have petechiae.

   E. **CORRECT:** The nurse should expect the client to have tachycardia.

   ⓝ *NCLEX® Connection: Physiological Adaptation, Basic Pathophysiology*

3. A. The nurse should notify the provider about the condition. However, another action is the priority.

   B. The nurse should ensure access to IV heparin as a treatment to prevent growth of the existing clot and to prevent additional clots from forming. However, another action is the priority.

   C. **CORRECT:** When using the airway, breathing, circulation (ABC) priority approach to care, the priority finding is related to the respiratory status. Meeting oxygenation needs by administering oxygen therapy is the priority action.

   D. The nurse should obtain a spiral CT scan to detect the presence and location of the blood clot. However, another action is the priority

   ⓝ *NCLEX® Connection: Physiological Adaptation, Medical Emergencies*

4. A. The nurse should document the client's allergy to morphine to manage the client's discomfort due to a blood clot. However, another action is the priority.

   B. **CORRECT:** The greatest risk to the client is the possibility of bleeding from a peptic ulcer. The priority intervention is to notify the provider of the finding.

   C. The nurse should know the client's history of a blood clot to provide preventative measures. However, another action is the priority.

   D. The nurse should expect the client who has a pulmonary embolism to report pain with breathing. However, another action is the priority.

   ⓝ *NCLEX® Connection: Pharmacological Therapies, Adverse Effects/ Contraindications/Side Effects/Interactions*

5. A. **CORRECT:** The client who has undergone a major surgical procedure within the last 3 weeks should not receive thrombolytic therapy because of the risk of hemorrhage from the surgical site.

   B. An elevated sedimentation rate does not place the client at risk for hemorrhage.

   C. An incident of exercise-induced asthma does not place the client at risk for hemorrhage, nor is it contraindicated with this type of medication.

   D. An elevated platelet count does not place the client at risk for hemorrhage when receiving this medication.

   ⓝ *NCLEX® Connection: Pharmacological Therapies, Adverse Effects/ Contraindications/Side Effects/Interactions*

PRACTICE Answer

Using the ATI Active Learning Template: System Disorder

PATHOPHYSIOLOGY RELATED TO CLIENT PROBLEM: A pulmonary embolism occurs when a substance (solid, gaseous, or liquid) enters venous circulation and forms a blockage in the pulmonary vasculature. Emboli originating from deep-vein thrombosis are the most common cause. Tumors, bone marrow, amniotic fluid, and foreign matter can also become emboli.

NURSING CARE
- Administer oxygen therapy as prescribed to relieve hypoxemia and dyspnea.
- Position the client to maximize ventilation (high-Fowler's).
- Maintain IV access.
- Administer medications as prescribed.
- Provide emotional support and comfort to control client anxiety.
- Monitor changes in level of consciousness and mental status.

MEDICATIONS
- Anticoagulants: enoxaparin, heparin, warfarin
- Thrombolytic therapy: alteplase, reteplase, tenecteplase

ⓝ *NCLEX® Connection: Physiological Adaptation, Alterations in Body Systems*

UNIT 3   NURSING CARE OF CLIENTS WHO
HAVE RESPIRATORY DISORDERS
SECTION: RESPIRATORY EMERGENCIES

CHAPTER 22 *Pneumothorax,*
Hemothorax,
and Flail Chest

A **pneumothorax** is the presence of air or gas in the pleural space that causes lung collapse. **(22.1)**

A tension pneumothorax occurs when air enters the pleural space during inspiration through a one-way valve and is not able to exit upon expiration. The trapped air causes pressure on the heart and the lung. As a result, the increase in pressure compresses blood vessels and limits venous return, leading to a decrease in cardiac output. Death can result if not treated immediately. As a result of a tension pneumothorax, air and pressure continue to rise in the pleural cavity, which causes a mediastinal shift.

A spontaneous pneumothorax can occur when there has been no trauma. A small bleb on the lung ruptures and air enters the pleural space.

A **hemothorax** is an accumulation of blood in the pleural space. **(22.2)**

A **flail chest** occurs when at least two neighboring ribs, usually on one side of the chest, sustain multiple fractures causing instability of the chest wall and paradoxical chest wall movement. This results in significant limitation in chest wall expansion.

Pneumothorax and hemothorax

DATA COLLECTION

RISK FACTORS

- Blunt chest trauma
- Penetrating chest wounds
- Closed/occluded chest tube
- Older adult clients have decreased pulmonary reserves due to normal lung changes, including decreased lung elasticity and thickening alveoli. Ⓖ

CHRONIC OBSTRUCTIVE PULMONARY DISEASE (COPD)

EXPECTED FINDINGS

- Anxiety
- Pleuritic pain

PHYSICAL FINDINGS
- Manifestations of respiratory distress (tachypnea, tachycardia, hypoxia, cyanosis, dyspnea, use of accessory muscles)
- Tracheal deviation to the unaffected side (tension pneumothorax)
- Reduced or absent breath sounds on the affected side
- Asymmetrical chest wall movement
- Hyperresonance on percussion due to trapped air (pneumothorax)
- Dull percussion (hemothorax)
- Subcutaneous emphysema (air accumulating in subcutaneous tissue)

LABORATORY TESTS

ABGs: Hypoxemia (PaO_2 less than 80 mm Hg)

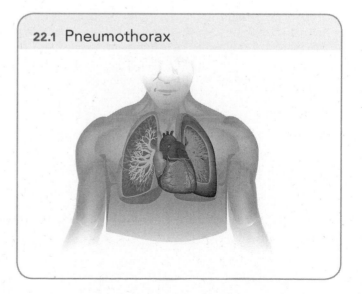

22.1 Pneumothorax

DIAGNOSTIC PROCEDURES

Chest x-ray

Used to confirm pneumothorax or hemothorax

Thoracentesis

Thoracentesis can be used to confirm hemothorax. Thoracentesis is the surgical perforation of the chest wall and pleural space with a large-bore needle.

NURSING ACTIONS
- Ensure that informed consent has been obtained.
- Make sure the client understands the importance of remaining still during the procedure (no moving, coughing, or deep breathing).
- Assist with client positioning and specimen transport.
- Monitor status (vital signs, SaO₂, injection site).
- Assist the client to the edge of the bed and to lean over a bedside table.
- Inform the client he will feel discomfort when local anesthetic solution is injected. When the needle is inserted into the lung, some pressure can be felt, but no pain.

PATIENT-CENTERED CARE

NURSING CARE
- Administer oxygen therapy.
- Auscultate heart and lung sounds and monitor vital signs every 4 hr.
- Check ABGs, SaO₂, CBC, and chest x-ray results.
- Position the client to maximize ventilation (high-Fowler's = 90°).
- Provide emotional support to the client and family.
- Monitor chest tube drainage. **Q**EBP
- Administer medications as prescribed.
- Encourage prompt medical attention when evidence of infection occurs.
- Instruct the client to deep breathe to promote lung expansion.
- Set up referral services (home health, respiratory services) to provide portable oxygen if needed. **Q**TC
- Reinforce teaching with the client and family about the illness, and encourage them to express their feelings.

MEDICATIONS

Benzodiazepines (sedatives)

Lorazepam or midazolam can be used to decrease anxiety.

NURSING ACTIONS
- Monitor vital signs. (Benzodiazepines can cause hypotension and respiratory distress.)
- Monitor for paradoxical effects (euphoria, rage).

CLIENT EDUCATION: Medications have amnesic effects and cause drowsiness.

Opioid agonists (pain medications)
- Morphine sulfate and fentanyl are opioid agents used to treat moderate to severe pain. These medications act on the mu and kappa receptors that help alleviate pain.
- Activation of these receptors produces analgesia (pain relief), respiratory depression, euphoria, sedation, and decrease in gastrointestinal motility.

NURSING ACTIONS
- Use cautiously for clients who have asthma or emphysema, due to the risk of respiratory depression.
- Check the client's pain level every 4 hr.
- Remind clients who are receiving a fentanyl patch that the initial patch takes several hours to take effect. A short-acting pain medication is administered for breakthrough pain.
- Monitor clients, especially older adults, for manifestations of respiratory depression. If respirations are 12/min or less, stop the medication and notify provider immediately.
- Monitor vital signs for hypotension and bradypnea.
- Observe for nausea and vomiting.
- Check the level of sedation (drowsiness, level of consciousness).
- Monitor for constipation.
- Encourage fluid intake and activity related to a decrease in gastric motility.
- Monitor I&O and fluid retention (common in clients who have an enlarged prostate).

CLIENT EDUCATION
- Clients who do not have fluid restrictions due to other conditions should drink plenty of fluids to prevent constipation.
- Use a patient-controlled analgesia (PCA) pump if applicable. The client is the only person who should push the medication administration button. The safety lockout mechanism on the PCA prevents overdosing of medication.
- If the client is receiving ventilation, the nursing considerations and client education can vary.

22.2 Hemothorax

blood in pleural space

INTERPROFESSIONAL CARE

Respiratory services should be consulted for ABGs, breathing treatments, and suctioning for airway management.

Pulmonary services may be consulted for chest tube management and pulmonary care.

Pain management services may be consulted if pain persists or is uncontrolled.

Rehabilitation care may be consulted if the client has prolonged weakness and needs assistance with an increasing level of activity.

THERAPEUTIC PROCEDURES

Chest tube insertion

Chest tubes are inserted in the pleural space to drain fluid, blood, or air; re-establish a negative pressure; facilitate lung expansion; and restore normal intrapleural pressure.

NURSING ACTIONS
- Verify informed consent has been signed, gather supplies, monitor status (vital signs, SaO_2, chest tube drainage), report abnormalities to the provider, and administer pain medications.
- Continually monitor vital signs and the client's response to the procedure.
- Monitor chest tube placement, function, and dressing.

CLIENT EDUCATION

- Take rest periods as needed.
- Use proper hand hygiene to prevent infection.
- Get immunizations for influenza and pneumonia.
- Recovery from a pneumothorax/hemothorax can be lengthy.
- Do not smoke.
- Follow-up care is important. Report the following to the provider.
  - Upper respiratory infection
  - Fever
  - Cough
  - Difficulty breathing
  - Sharp chest pain

COMPLICATIONS

Decreased cardiac output

- The amount of blood pumped by the heart decreases as intrathoracic pressure rises.
- Hypotension develops.

NURSING ACTIONS
- Assist with the care of the client receiving IV fluids and blood products.
- Monitor heart rate and rhythm.
- Monitor I&O (chest tube drainage).

Respiratory failure

Inadequate gas exchange due to lung collapse

NURSING ACTIONS
- Assist in preparing for mechanical ventilation.
- Monitor respiratory status.

Flail chest

Flail chest is the inability of the injured side of the chest to expand adequately upon inhalation and contract upon exhalation. One side of the chest is typically affected due to multiple rib fractures.

DATA COLLECTION

RISK FACTORS

Multiple rib fractures from blunt chest trauma (often caused by motor-vehicle crash or as a result of cardiopulmonary resuscitation on older adults)

EXPECTED FINDINGS

- Unequal chest expansion (the unaffected side of the chest will expand, while the affected side can appear to diminish in size or remain stationary)
- Paradoxical chest wall movement (inward movement of segment during inspiration, outward movement of segment during expiration)
- Tachycardia
- Hypotension
- Dyspnea
- Cyanosis
- Anxiety
- Chest pain

PATIENT-CENTERED CARE

NURSING CARE

- Administer humidified oxygen.
- Monitor vital signs and SaO_2.
- Review findings of pulmonary function tests, periodic chest x-rays, and ABGs.
- Auscultate lung sounds, color, and capillary refill.
- Promote lung expansion by encouraging deep breathing and proper positioning.
- Assist with the care of suctioning trachea and endotracheal tube as needed.
- Administer pain medication. PCA or epidural block is commonly used.
- Ensure access to IV fluids as prescribed.
- Monitor I&O.
- Offer support and reassurance by explaining all procedures.

Application Exercises

1. A nurse is collecting data on a client following a gunshot wound to the chest. For which of the following findings should the nurse monitor to detect a pneumothorax? (Select all that apply.)

   A. Tachypnea

   B. Deviation of the trachea

   C. Bradycardia

   D. Decreased use of accessory muscles

   E. Pleuritic pain

2. A nurse is reviewing the prescriptions for a client who has a pneumothorax. Which of the following actions should the nurse perform first?

   A. Check the client's pain.

   B. Obtain a large-bore IV needle for decompression.

   C. Administer lorazepam.

   D. Prepare for chest tube insertion.

3. A nurse is reinforcing discharge instructions for a client who experienced a pneumothorax. Which of the following statements should the nurse use when teaching the client?

   A. "Notify your provider if you experience weakness."

   B. "You should be able to return to work in 1 week."

   C. "You need to wear a mask when in crowded areas."

   D. "Notify your provider if you experience a productive cough."

4. A nurse is collecting data on a client who has a suspected flail chest. Which of the following findings should the nurse expect? (Select all that apply.)

   A. Bradycardia

   B. Cyanosis

   C. Hypotension

   D. Dyspnea

   E. Paradoxic chest movement

PRACTICE Active Learning Scenario

A nurse is reinforcing teaching with a newly licensed nurse regarding care for a client who has a hemothorax. What should be included in the teaching? Use the ATI Active Learning Template: System Disorder to complete this item.

ALTERATION IN HEALTH (DIAGNOSIS)

NURSING CARE: Describe three nursing interventions.

MEDICATIONS: Describe two medications used for hemothorax

Application Exercises Key

1. A. **CORRECT:** The client who has a pneumothorax can experience tachypnea related to respiratory distress caused by the injury.

    B. **CORRECT:** The client who has a pneumothorax can experience deviation of the trachea as tension increases within the chest.

    C. The client who has a pneumothorax can experience tachycardia related to respiratory distress and pain.

    D. The client who has a pneumothorax can experience an increase in the use of accessory muscles as respiratory distress occurs.

    E. **CORRECT:** The client who has a pneumothorax can experience pleuritic pain related to the inflammation of the pleura of the lung caused by the injury.

    Ⓝ *NCLEX® Connection: Physiological Adaptation, Basic Pathophysiology*

2. A. The nurse should check the client's pain and administer pain medication. However, another action is the priority.

    B. **CORRECT:** The priority action the nurse should take when using the airway, breathing, circulation (ABC) approach to client care is to establish and maintain the client's respiratory function. Obtaining a large-bore IV needle for decompression is the priority action.

    C. The nurse can administer benzodiazepine to treat anxiety. However, another action is the priority.

    D. The nurse should gather supplies to prepare for chest tube insertion. However, another action is the priority.

    Ⓝ *NCLEX® Connection: Physiological Adaptation, Alterations in Body Systems*

3. A. Weakness is an expected finding following recovery from a pneumothorax.

    B. The client should expect a lengthy recovery following a pneumothorax.

    C. The client should wear a mask if immunosuppressed.

    D. **CORRECT:** The client should notify the provider of a productive or persistent cough. This can indicate need for treatment of a respiratory infection.

    Ⓝ *NCLEX® Connection: Reduction of Risk Potential, Potential for Complications from Surgical Procedures and Health Alterations*

4. A. The client will have tachycardia as a manifestation indicative of flail chest due to inadequate oxygenation.

    B. **CORRECT:** The client can have cyanosis as a manifestation indicative of flail chest due to inadequate oxygenation.

    C. **CORRECT:** The client can have hypotension as a manifestation indicative of flail chest.

    D. **CORRECT:** The client can have dyspnea as a manifestation indicative of flail chest. This is due to injury and the client's inability to effectively inhale and exhale.

    E. **CORRECT:** The client can have paradoxic chest movement as a manifestation indicative of flail chest. This is due to injury to the chest and the inability to inhale and exhale.

    Ⓝ *NCLEX® Connection: Physiological Adaptation, Basic Pathophysiology*

PRACTICE Answer

Using the ATI Active Learning Template: System Disorder

ALTERATION IN HEALTH (DIAGNOSIS): Hemothorax is an accumulation of blood in the pleural space.

NURSING CARE
- Administer oxygen therapy.
- Document ventilator settings hourly if the client is receiving ventilation.
- Monitor ABGs, SaO_2, CBC, and chest x-ray findings.
- Position the client to maximize ventilation (high-Fowler's).
- Provide emotional support to the client and family.
- Monitor chest tube drainage.
- Administer medications as prescribed.
- Encourage prompt medical attention when manifestations of infection occur.
- Auscultate heart and lung sounds and monitor vital signs every 4 hr.

MEDICATIONS
- Benzodiazepines (sedatives): Lorazepam or midazolam can be used to decrease anxiety.
- Opioid agonists (pain medications): Morphine sulfate and fentanyl are opioid agents used to treat moderate to severe pain. These medications act on the mu and kappa receptors that help alleviate pain.

Ⓝ *NCLEX® Connection: Physiological Adaptation, Alterations in Body Systems*

CHAPTER 23 *Respiratory Failure*

Respiratory failure includes acute respiratory failure (ARF), acute respiratory distress syndrome (ARDS), and severe acute respiratory syndrome (SARS). Because older adult clients have decreased pulmonary reserves due to normal lung changes, including decreased lung elasticity and thickening alveoli, they can decompensate more quickly. ©

Acute respiratory failure

Failure to adequately ventilate or oxygenate leads to ARF.
- Ventilatory failure is due to a mechanical abnormality of the lungs or chest wall, impaired muscle function (especially the diaphragm), or a malfunction in the respiratory control center of the brain.
- Oxygenation failure can result from a lack of perfusion to the pulmonary capillary bed (pulmonary embolism) or a condition that alters the gas exchange medium (pulmonary edema, pneumonia).
- Both inadequate ventilation and oxygenation can occur in clients who have diseased lungs (asthma, emphysema, cystic fibrosis). Diseased lung tissue can cause oxygenation failure and increased work of breathing, eventually resulting in respiratory muscle fatigue and ventilatory failure. Combined failure leads to more profound hypoxemia than either ventilatory failure or oxygenation failure alone.

Acute respiratory distress syndrome

ARDS is a state of acute respiratory failure with a mortality rate of about 60%.
- A systemic inflammatory response injures the alveolar-capillary membrane. It becomes permeable to large molecules, and the lung space fills with fluid.
- A reduction in surfactant weakens the alveoli, which causes collapse or filling of fluid, leading to worsening edema.

Severe acute respiratory syndrome

SARS is the result of a viral infection from a mutated strain of the coronaviruses, a group of viruses that also cause the common cold.
- The virus invades the pulmonary tissue, which leads to an inflammatory response.
- The virus spreads easily through airborne droplets from sneezing, coughing, or talking.
- The virus does not spread to the bloodstream because it flourishes at temperatures slightly below normal core body temperature.

DATA COLLECTION

RISK FACTORS

Acute respiratory failure

Ventilatory failure
- COPD
- Pulmonary embolism
- Pneumothorax
- Flail chest
- ARDS
- Asthma ℚEBP
- Pulmonary edema
- Fibrosis of lung tissue
- Neuromuscular disorders (multiple sclerosis, Guillain-Barré syndrome), spinal cord injuries, and cerebrovascular accidents that impair the client's rate and depth of respiration
- Elevated intracranial pressure (closed-head injuries, cerebral edema, hemorrhagic stroke)

Oxygenation failure
- Pneumonia
- Hypoventilation
- Hypovolemic shock
- Pulmonary edema
- Pulmonary embolism
- ARDS
- Low hemoglobin
- Low concentrations of oxygen (carbon monoxide poisoning, high altitude, smoke inhalation)

Combined ventilatory and oxygenation failure
- Decreased gas exchange results in poor diffusion of oxygen into arterial blood with carbon dioxide retention
- Hypoventilation (poor respiratory movement)
- Chronic bronchitis
- Asthma attack
- Emphysema

Cardiac failure

Acute respiratory distress syndrome
- Can result from localized lung damage or from the effects of other systemic problems
- Aspiration
- Pulmonary emboli (fat, amniotic fluid)
- Pneumonia and other pulmonary infections
- Sepsis
- Near-drowning accident
- Trauma
- Transfusion
- Damage to the central nervous system
- Smoke or toxic gas inhalation
- Drug use/overdose (heroin, opioids, salicylates)

Severe acute respiratory syndrome
- Exposure to an infected individual
- Immunocompromise (chemotherapy, AIDS)

EXPECTED FINDINGS

- Shortness of breath
- Dyspnea with or without exertion
- Orthopnea (difficulty breathing lying flat)
- Rapid, shallow breathing
- Cyanotic, mottled, dusky skin Q𝐏𝐂𝐂
- Tachycardia
- Hypotension
- Substernal or suprasternal retractions
- Decreased SaO_2 (less than 90%)
- Adventitious breath sounds (wheezing, rales)
- Cardiac arrhythmias
- Confusion
- Lethargy

Acute respiratory failure

- Dyspnea
- Orthopnea
- Cyanosis
- Pallor
- Hypoxemia
- Tachycardia
- Confusion
- Irritability or agitation
- Restlessness
- Hypercarbia (high levels of carbon dioxide in the blood)

Acute respiratory distress syndrome

- Dyspnea
- Bilateral noncardiogenic pulmonary edema
- Reduced lung compliance
- Dense patchy bilateral pulmonary infiltrates
- Severe hypoxemia despite administration of 100% oxygen

LABORATORY TESTS

ABGs to confirm and monitor ARF, ARDS, and SARS
- PaO_2 less than 60 mm Hg and oxygen saturation less than 90% on room air (hypoxemia)
- $PaCO_2$ greater than 50 mm Hg and pH less than 7.30 (hypoxemia, hypercarbia)

Acute respiratory failure

ABGs to confirm and monitor combined ventilatory and oxygenation failure
- Room air, PaO_2 less than 60 mm Hg (hypoxemic/ oxygenation failure), **or** $PaCO_2$ greater than 45 mm Hg in conjunction with pH less than 7.35 (hypercapnic/ ventilatory failure)
- **And** SaO_2 less than 90% in both cases

DIAGNOSTIC PROCEDURES

Chest x-ray Q𝐄𝐁𝐏

Results can include:
- Pulmonary edema (ARF, ARDS)
- Cardiomegaly (ARF)
- Diffuse infiltrates and white-out or ground-glass appearance (ARDS)
- Infiltrates (SARS)

NURSING ACTIONS
- Assist with client positioning before and after the x-ray.
- Interpret and communicate the results to the appropriate personnel in a timely manner.

Electrocardiogram (ECG)

To rule out cardiac involvement

Hemodynamic monitoring

Continuous hemodynamic monitoring is important for fluid management.

PATIENT-CENTERED CARE

NURSING CARE

- Maintain a patent airway and monitor respiratory status every hour and more often as needed.
- Mechanical ventilation is often required with positive-end expiratory pressure (PEEP) or continuous positive airway pressure (CPAP) to prevent alveolar collapse during expiration. Follow facility protocol for monitoring and documenting ventilator settings.
- Oxygenate before suctioning secretions to prevent further hypoxemia.
- Suction the client as needed.
- Observe and document sputum color, amount, and consistency.
- Check lung sounds per facility protocol.
- Obtain ABGs as prescribed.
- Maintain continuous ECG monitoring for changes that can indicate increased hypoxemia, especially when repositioning and applying suction.
- Continually monitor vital signs, including SaO_2. Check pain level.
- Position the client to facilitate ventilation and perfusion.
- Prevent infection.
  - Perform frequent hand hygiene.
  - Use appropriate suctioning technique.
  - Provide oral care every 2 hr and as needed.
  - Wear protective clothing (gown, gloves, mask) when appropriate.

- Promote nutrition.
  - Check bowel sounds.
  - Monitor elimination patterns.
  - Obtain daily weights. Qs
  - Monitor and record I&O.
  - Administer enteral and parenteral feedings.
  - Prevent aspiration with enteral feedings (elevate the head of the bed 30° to 45°).
  - Confirm nasogastric (NG) tube placement prior to feeding.
- Provide emotional support to the client and family.
  - Encourage verbalization of feelings.
  - Provide alternative communication means (dry erase board, pen and paper).

MEDICATIONS

Benzodiazepines

- Lorazepam
- Midazolam

ACTIONS: Reduces anxiety and resistance to ventilation and decreases oxygen consumption

NURSING ACTIONS
- Monitor respirations.
- Monitor blood pressure and SaO₂.
- Use cautiously in conjunction with opioid narcotics.

General anesthesia

Propofol

ACTIONS
- Induces and maintains anesthesia
- Sedates clients who are to be placed on mechanical ventilation

NURSING ACTIONS
- Contraindicated for clients who have hyperlipidemia and egg allergies.
- Administer only to clients who are intubated and ventilated.
- Clients require intensive care monitoring.

Corticosteroids

- Cortisone acetate
- Methylprednisolone sodium succinate
- Dexamethasone sodium phosphate

ACTIONS: Reduces WBC migration, decreases inflammation, and helps stabilize the alveolar-capillary membrane during ARDS

NURSING ACTIONS
- Discontinue medication gradually.
- Administer with an antiulcer medication to prevent peptic ulcer formation.
- Monitor weight and blood pressure.
- Monitor glucose and electrolytes.
- Advise the client to take oral doses with food and avoid stopping the medication suddenly.

Opioid analgesics

- Morphine sulfate
- Fentanyl

ACTIONS: Provides pain management

NURSING ACTIONS
- Monitor respiratory rate.
- Monitor blood pressure, heart rate, and SaO₂.
- Monitor ABGs. (Hypercapnia can result from depressed respirations.)
- Use cautiously in conjunction with hypnotic sedatives.
- Assess pain level and response to medication.
- Have naloxone and resuscitation equipment available for severe respiratory depression in clients who are not receiving ventilation.

Neuromuscular blocking agents

Vecuronium

ACTIONS
- Facilitates ventilation and decreases oxygen consumption
- Often used with painful ventilatory modes (inverse ratio ventilation and PEEP)

NURSING ACTIONS
- Administer only to clients who are intubated and ventilated.
- Clients require intensive care monitoring.

Antibiotics sensitive to cultured organisms

Vancomycin

ACTIONS: Treats identified organisms

NURSING ACTIONS
- Culture sputum prior to administration of first dose.
- Monitor for a hypersensitivity reaction.
- Give IV doses slowly (over at least 60 min) to avoid red man syndrome.
- Monitor the IV site for infiltration.
- Do not give with other medications.
- Monitor coagulopathy and renal function.
- Advise client to take oral doses with food and finish the prescribed dose.

INTERPROFESSIONAL CARE

Respiratory therapy
- The respiratory therapist typically manages the ventilator, adjusts the settings, and provides chest physiotherapy to improve ventilation and chest expansion.
- The respiratory therapist also can suction the endotracheal tube and administer inhalation medications, such as bronchodilators.

Physical therapy for extended ventilatory support and rehabilitation

Nutritional therapy
- Enteral or parenteral feeding
- Nutritional support following extubation

THERAPEUTIC PROCEDURES

Intubation and mechanical ventilation

Artificial airway insertion with mechanical ventilation

NURSING ACTIONS
- Monitor ECG, SaO$_2$, lung sounds, and color.
- Provide reassurance to calm the client.
- Have suction equipment, manual resuscitation bag, and face mask available at all times.
- Suction secretions as needed.
- **Preintubation**
  - Oxygenate with 100% oxygen.
  - Assist ventilation with manual resuscitation bag and face mask.
  - Have emergency resuscitation equipment readily available.
- **Postintubation**
  - Check, bilateral lung sounds, symmetrical chest movement, and chest x-ray to confirm placement of the endotracheal tube. Q^{PCC}
  - Secure the endotracheal tube per facility guidelines.
  - Check the balloon cuff for air leaks periodically.
- **PEEP**
  - Positive air pressure at the end of expiration keeps the alveoli expanded.
  - The PEEP ventilator setting increases oxygenation and improves lung expansion.
- Explain all procedures to the client.
- Reassure and calm the client.
- Explain to the client and family that the client will be unable to speak while the endotracheal tube is in place.

Kinetic therapy

A kinetic bed that rotates laterally alters client positioning to reduce atelectasis and improve ventilation.

NURSING ACTIONS
- Begin slowly and gradually to increase the degree of rotation as tolerated.
- Monitor ECG, SaO$_2$, breath sounds, and blood pressure.
- Stop rotation if the client becomes distressed.
- Provide routine skin care to prevent breakdown.

COMPLICATIONS

ENDOTRACHEAL TUBE

Trauma

Trauma during intubation or long-term intubation can cause damage to trachea and vocal cords.

NURSING ACTIONS: Consider a tracheostomy for long-term ventilation.

Altered position of endotracheal tube

NURSING ACTIONS
- Check tube positioning every 1 to 2 hr and as needed.
- Monitor lung sounds, SaO$_2$, and chest movement. After moving, transferring, or turning the client, recheck lung sounds.
- Secure endotracheal tube per facility guidelines to maintain tube placement.

Aspiration pneumonia

NURSING ACTIONS
- Check the cuff on the endotracheal tube for leaks.
- Monitor suction contents for gastric secretions.
- Verify NG tube placement.

Infection

NURSING ACTIONS
- Prevent infection by using proper hand hygiene and suctioning technique.
- Check color, amount, and consistency of secretions.

Blocked endotracheal tube

Indicated by high-pressure alarm on ventilator

NURSING ACTIONS: Suction secretions to relieve a mucous plug or insert an oral airway to prevent biting on the tube.

MECHANICAL VENTILATION

Increased intrathoracic pressure

- PEEP increases intrathoracic pressure, which can cause a decreased blood return to the heart, decreased cardiac output, and hypotension.
- Decreased cardiac output can activate the renin-angiotensin-aldosterone system, leading to fluid retention and/or decreased urine output.

NURSING ACTIONS: Monitor I&O, weight, and hydration status.

CLIENT EDUCATION: Avoid using the Valsalva maneuver (straining with bowel movement), because it can further increase intrathoracic pressure.

Barotrauma

Ventilation with positive pressure causes damage to the lungs (pneumothorax, subcutaneous emphysema).

NURSING ACTIONS
- Monitor oxygenation status and chest x-ray.
- Monitor for subcutaneous emphysema (crackles or air movement felt under skin).
- Document all ventilator changes.
- A high-pressure ventilator alarm can indicate pneumothorax.

Immobilization

Can result in muscle atrophy, pneumonia, and pressure sores

NURSING ACTIONS
- Reposition and suction every 2 hr and as needed.
- Provide routine skin care.
- Implement range-of-motion exercises to prevent muscle atrophy.

PRACTICE Active Learning Scenario

A nurse is reviewing the plan of care for a client who has acute respiratory distress syndrome (ARDS). What should be included in the plan of care? Use the ATI Active Learning Template: System Disorder to complete this item.

RISK FACTORS: Describe three conditions related to ARDS.

NURSING CARE: Describe three nursing actions to maintain oxygenation.

COMPLICATIONS: Identify two complications of ARDS.

Application Exercises

1. A nurse is assisting in the care of a client who has ARDS with absent breath sounds in the lower lobes and dyspnea. Which of the following actions should the nurse take first?

   A. Obtain a chest x-ray.

   B. Prepare for chest tube insertion.

   C. Administer oxygen via a high-flow mask.

   D. Ensure IV access.

2. A nurse is reinforcing teaching with the family of a client who has acute respiratory distress syndrome (ARDS) and is receiving vecuronium. Which of the following statements by a family member should the nurse identify as understanding of the teaching?

   A. "This medication is given to treat infection."

   B. "This medication is given to facilitate ventilation."

   C. "This medication is given to decrease inflammation."

   D. "This medication is given to reduce anxiety."

3. A nurse is reviewing the health records of five clients. Which of the following clients are at risk for developing acute respiratory distress syndrome? (Select all that apply.)

   A. A client who experienced a near-drowning incident

   B. A client following coronary artery bypass graft surgery

   C. A client who has a hemoglobin of 15.1 mg/dL

   D. A client who has dysphagia

   E. A client who experienced a drug overdose

4. A nurse is assisting with the plan of care for a client who has severe acute respiratory distress system (SARS). Which of the following interventions should the nurse recommend? (Select all that apply.)

   A. Administer antibiotics.

   B. Provide supplemental oxygen.

   C. Administer antiviral medications.

   D. Administer of bronchodilators.

   E. Maintain ventilatory support.

5. A nurse at a long-term care facility is collecting data from a client who as a history of asthma and has developed pneumonia. Which of the following findings indicate the client is developing respiratory failure? (Select all that apply.)

   A. Irritability

   B. Flushed skin

   C. Orthopnea

   D. Heart rate 55/min

   E. Dyspnea

Application Exercises Key

1. A. The nurse should obtain a chest x-ray to determine the level of injury to the lungs. However, there is another action the nurse should take first.

   B. The nurse should prepare the client for chest tube insertion to facilitate lung expansion and restore normal intrapleural pressure. However, there is another action the nurse should take first.

   C. **CORRECT:** The first action the nurse should take when using the airway, breathing, and circulation approach to client care is to administer oxygen via high-flow mask to provide the client oxygen to restore optimal breathing.

   D. The nurse should ensure IV access to medications. However, there is another action the nurse should take first.

   Ⓝ *NCLEX® Connection: Physiological Adaptation, Alterations in Body Systems*

2. A. Antibiotics treat infection that can be associated with respiratory disorders.

   B. **CORRECT:** Vecuronium is a neuromuscular blocking agent given to facilitate ventilation, especially with ventilator settings that could be painful. It also helps decrease oxygen consumption.

   C. Corticosteroids treat inflammation and stabilize the alveolar-capillary membrane to improve ARDS.

   D. Benzodiazepines treat anxiety for clients who have respiratory disorders. They also decrease the body's demand for oxygen.

   Ⓝ *NCLEX® Connection: Physiological Adaptation, Alterations in Body Systems*

3. A. **CORRECT:** A client who experienced a near-drowning incident is at risk for developing ARDS due to trauma to the lungs and cerebral edema.

   B. **CORRECT:** A client following coronary artery bypass graft surgery is at risk for developing ARDS due to trauma to the chest.

   C. Hemoglobin 15.1 mg/dL is within the expected reference range. A client who has low hemoglobin is at risk for developing ARDS.

   D. **CORRECT:** A client who has dysphagia is at risk for developing ARDS due to difficulty swallowing and risk for aspiration.

   E. **CORRECT:** A client who experienced a drug overdose is at risk for developing ARDS due to damage to the central nervous system.

   Ⓝ *NCLEX® Connection: Health Promotion and Maintenance, Health Promotion/Disease Prevention*

4. A. Antibiotics treat bacterial infections and are not effective for treating SARS, which is a viral illness.

   B. **CORRECT:** Providing supplemental oxygen should be included in the plan of care for SARS. Oxygen reverses severe hypoxemia.

   C. There are no effective antiviral medications against the coronavirus that causes SARS.

   D. **CORRECT:** Administration of bronchodilators should be included in the plan of care for SARS. Bronchodilators vasodilate the airway.

   E. **CORRECT:** Maintaining ventilatory support should be included in the plan of care for SARS. The client can require intubation to maintain a patent airway.

   Ⓝ *NCLEX® Connection: Physiological Adaptation, Alterations in Body Systems*

5. A. **CORRECT:** The nurse should identify irritability as a finding associated with respiratory failure, as it results from a lack of oxygen.

   B. The nurse should expect the client to have pale skin, with possible areas of cyanosis when experiencing respiratry failure.

   C. **CORRECT:** The nurse should expect the client to experience difficulty breathing while lying flat when experiencing respiratory failure. The client will likely be restless and want to sit up to relieve the work of breathing.

   D. A heart rate of 55/min is below the expected reference range. The nurse should expect the client to be tachycardic when experiencing respiratory failure.

   E. **CORRECT:** The nurse should expect the client to exhibit dyspnea, or shortness of breath, when experiencing respiratory failure.

   Ⓝ *NCLEX® Connection: Physiological Adaptation, Basic Pathophysiology*

PRACTICE Answer

Using the ATI Active Learning Template: System Disorder

RISK FACTORS

- Can result from localized lung damage or from the effects of other systemic problems
- Aspiration
- Pulmonary emboli (fat, amniotic fluid)
- Pneumonia and other pulmonary infections
- Sepsis
- Near-drowning accident
- Trauma
- Damage to the central nervous system
- Smoke or toxic gas inhalation
- Drug use/overdose (heroin, opioids, salicylates)

NURSING CARE

- Maintain a patent airway and monitor respiratory status every hour as needed.
- Suction the client as needed.
- Auscultate lung sounds.
- Observe and document sputum color, amount, and consistency.
- Oxygenate before suctioning secretions to prevent further hypoxemia.
- Assist with monitoring clients prescribed mechanical ventilation PEEP often can prevent alveolar collapse during expiration.
- Monitor for pneumothorax. (A high PEEP can cause the lungs to collapse.)
- Obtain ABGs as prescribed and following each ventilator setting adjustment.
- Maintain continuous ECG monitoring for changes that can indicate increased hypoxemia, especially when repositioning and applying suction.
- Continually monitor vital signs, including SaO_2.
- Position the client to facilitate ventilation and perfusion.

COMPLICATIONS

- Endotracheal tube
  - Trauma during intubation or long-term intubation
  - Can cause damage to trachea and vocal cords
  - Consider a tracheostomy for long-term ventilation.
- Aspiration pneumonia nursing actions
  - Check the cuff on the endotracheal tube for leaks.
  - Check suction contents for gastric secretions.
  - Verify NG tube placement.
- Infection nursing actions
  - Prevent infection by using proper hand hygiene and suctioning technique.
  - Monitor color, amount, and consistency of secretions.
- Blocked endotracheal tube
  - The high-pressure alarm on the ventilator can indicate a blocked endotracheal tube.
  - Suction secretions to relieve a mucous plug or insert an oral airway to prevent biting on the tube.
- Altered position of endotracheal tube nursing actions
  - Check tube positioning every 1 to 2 hr and as needed.
  - Monitor breath sounds, SaO_2, and chest movement.
  - Secure endotracheal tube per institution's guidelines to maintain tube placement.
- Mechanical ventilation
  - Increased intrathoracic pressure
  - PEEP increases intrathoracic pressure, which can cause a decreased blood return to the heart, decreased cardiac output and/or hypotension.
  - Decreased cardiac output can activate the renin-angiotensin-aldosterone system, leading to fluid retention and/or decreased urine output.
  - Monitor I&O, weight, and hydration status.
  - Advise the client to avoid using the Valsalva maneuver (straining with bowel movement), because it can further increase intrathoracic pressure.
- Barotrauma: Ventilation with positive pressure causes damage to the lungs (pneumothorax, subcutaneous emphysema).

Ⓝ *NCLEX® Connection: Physiological Adaptation, Alterations in Body Systems*

NCLEX® Connections

When reviewing the following chapters, keep in mind the relevant topics and tasks of the NCLEX outline, in particular:

Pharmacological Therapies

ADVERSE EFFECTS/CONTRAINDICATIONS/ SIDE EFFECTS/INTERACTIONS
Identify a contraindication to the administration of a prescribed or over-the-counter medication to the client.

Withhold a medication dose if the client experiences adverse effects of the medication.

MEDICATION ADMINISTRATION
Collect required data prior to medication administration.

Assist in preparing the client for insertion of a central line.

Administer intravenous piggyback (secondary) medications.

Reduction of Risk Potential

CHANGES/ABNORMALITIES IN VITAL SIGNS:
Compare vital signs to the client's baseline vital signs.

DIAGNOSTIC TESTS
Perform an electrocardiogram (ECG).

Reinforce client teaching about a diagnostic test.

POTENTIAL FOR ALTERATIONS IN BODY SYSTEMS
Perform circulatory checks.

Reinforce client teaching on methods to prevent complications associated with activity level/diagnosed illness/disease (such as foot care for a client with diabetes mellitus).

Physiological Adaptation

ALTERATIONS IN BODY SYSTEMS
Recognize and report basic abnormalities on a client's cardiac monitor strip.

Perform a check of the client's pacemaker.

BASIC PATHOPHYSIOLOGY: Identify signs and symptoms related to an acute or chronic illness.

MEDICAL EMERGENCIES: Reinforce teaching of emergency intervention explanations with the client.

UNEXPECTED RESPONSES TO THERAPIES: Intervene in response to the client's unexpected negative response to therapy (such as unexpected bleeding).

CHAPTER 24

CHAPTER 24 *Cardiovascular Diagnostic and Therapeutic Procedures*

Cardiovascular diagnostic procedures evaluate the functioning of the heart by monitoring for enzymes in the blood; using ultrasound to visualize the heart; determining the heart's response to exercise; and using catheters to determine blood volume, perfusion, fluid status, how the heart is pumping, and degree of artery blockage.

Cardiovascular diagnostic procedures that nurses should be familiar with include cardiac enzymes and lipid profile, echocardiogram, stress testing, hemodynamic monitoring, angiography, and vascular access.

Cardiac enzymes and lipid profile

Cardiac enzymes are released into the bloodstream when the heart muscle suffers ischemia. A lipid profile provides information regarding cholesterol levels and is used for early detection of heart disease.

Cardiac enzymes are specific markers in diagnosing a myocardial infarction (MI).

INDICATIONS

- Angina
- MI
- Heart disease
- Hyperlipidemia

CONSIDERATIONS

PREPROCEDURE: Reinforce teaching about the purpose of the test to the client. Qᴘᴄᴄ

INTRAPROCEDURE: Obtain a blood specimen via venipuncture.

POSTPROCEDURE: Report lab findings to the charge nurse. The provider will review the results and determine the need for treatment.

INTERPRETATION OF FINDINGS

24.1 Cardiac enzymes

EXPECTED REFERENCE RANGE	ELEVATED LEVELS FIRST DETECTABLE FOLLOWING MYOCARDIAL INJURY	EXPECTED DURATION OF ELEVATED LEVELS
Creatine kinase MB isoenzyme **more sensitive to myocardium**		
0% of total CK (30 to 170 units/L)	2 to 6 hr Peaks in 18 hour	2 to 3 days
Troponin T		
Less than 0.1 ng/mL	2 to 3 hr	10 to 14 days
Troponin I		
Less than 0.03 ng/mL	2 to 3 hr	7 to 10 days
Myoglobin		
Less than 90 mcg/L	3 hr	24 hr

24.2 Cardiac tests

EXPECTED REFERENCE RANGE	PURPOSE
Cholesterol (total)	
Less than 200 mg/dL	Screening for heart disease
LDL	
Less than 130 mg/dL	"Bad" cholesterol Transports cholesterol to the body's cells from the liver
Triglycerides	
MALES: 40 to 160 mg/dL FEMALES: 35 to 135 mg/dL	Evaluates the client's risk for heart disease
HDL	
FEMALES: greater than 55 mg/dL MALES: greater than 45 mg/dL	"Good" cholesterol Protects coronary arteries from heart disease by transporting cholesterol from the body's cells to the liver

Echocardiogram

An echocardiogram is an ultrasound of the heart. It is used to diagnose valve disorders and cardiomyopathy.

INDICATIONS

- Cardiomyopathy
- Heart failure
- Angina
- MI
- Heart valve disease
- Atrial-ventricular septal defects

CONSIDERATIONS

PREPROCEDURE: Reinforce teaching with the client regarding the reason for the test. This is a noninvasive procedure and takes up to 1 hr. Qpcc

INTRAPROCEDURE: Instruct the client to lie supine or on the left side and remain still.

POSTPROCEDURE: The provider reviews the client's test results and discusses a plan for follow-up care.

Stress testing

The client exercises the cardiac muscle by walking on a treadmill. This provides information regarding the workload of the heart. The test is discontinued once the heart rate reaches a certain rate.

Clients who are disabled or physically challenged can become too tired, and can be unable to finish the test. The provider can prescribe the test to be done as a pharmacological (chemical) stress test.

INDICATIONS

- Angina
- Heart disease
- Cardiac rehabilitation
- Dysrhythmia

CONSIDERATIONS

PREPROCEDURE

- Assist the provider in obtaining a signed informed consent form.
- Inform the client that they will be walking on a treadmill, so comfortable athletic shoes and clothing are recommended. Qpcc

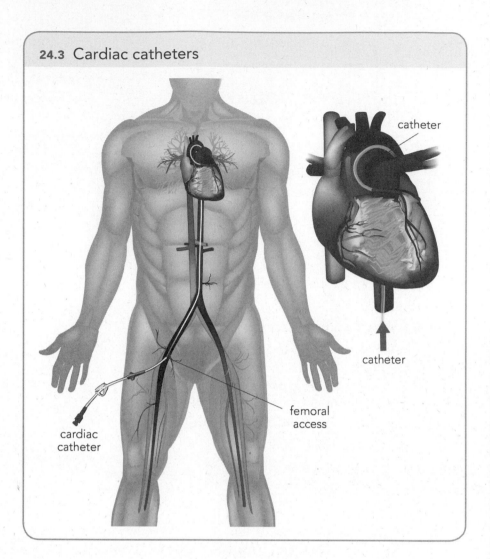

24.3 Cardiac catheters

catheter

catheter

femoral access

cardiac catheter

- Reinforce teaching with the client if a pharmacological stress test is prescribed. A medication (dipyridamole, adenosine, dobutamine) is administered to stress the heart instead of walking on the treadmill.
- Instruct the client to fast 2 to 4 hr before the procedure, or according to facility policy, and to avoid tobacco, alcohol, and caffeine before the test. Qs
- Instruct the client to get adequate rest the night before the procedure.
- Inform the client that a provider will be present during the testing.

INTRAPROCEDURE

- Apply a 12-lead ECG to monitor the client's heart rate during the test. Monitor for dysrhythmias throughout the procedure.
- Reinforce to the client to report any chest pain, shortness of breath, or dizziness during the procedure.

POSTPROCEDURE

- Monitor the client by 12-lead ECG.
- Check blood pressure frequently until the client is stable.
- The provider reviews findings with the client.

Angiography

A coronary angiogram, also called a cardiac catheterization, is an invasive diagnostic procedure used to evaluate the presence and degree of coronary artery blockage.

- Angiography is also done on the lower extremities to determine blood flow and areas of blockage.
- Angiography involves the insertion of a catheter into a femoral, radial, or brachial vessel and threading it into the right or left side of the heart. Coronary artery narrowings and occlusions are identified by the injection of contrast media under fluoroscopy. **(24.3)**

INDICATIONS

- Identify unstable angina and ECG changes (T wave inversion, ST segment elevation, depression).
- Confirm and determine the location and extent of heart disease.

CONSIDERATIONS

PREPROCEDURE

NURSING ACTIONS

- Maintain NPO status for at least 8 hr due to the risk for aspiration when lying flat for the procedure.
- Obtain vital signs and mark peripheral pulses.
- Ensure the consent form is signed.
- Reinforce teaching with the client and family regarding the procedure.
- Collect data regarding iodine/shellfish allergy (contrast media).
- Administer medications as prescribed (methylprednisolone, diphenhydramine).

CLIENT EDUCATION

- The client will be awake and sedated during procedure. A local anesthetic is used.
- A small incision is made, often in the groin, to insert the catheter. The client can feel warmth and flushed when the dye is inserted.
- After the procedure, keep the affected leg straight for a minimum of 2 hr. Pressure (a sandbag) can be placed on the incision to prevent bleeding.

POSTPROCEDURE

NURSING ACTIONS

- Check vital signs every 15 min × 4, every 30 min × 2, every hour × 4, and then every 4 hr. (Follow facility protocol.)
- Collect data regarding the capillary refill and neurovascular status at the same interval.
- Inspect the insertion site at the same intervals for
  - Bleeding and hematoma formation.
  - Thrombosis. (Document pedal pulse, color, temperature.)
- Maintain bed rest in a supine position with extremity straight for prescribed time.
  - A vascular closure device can be used to hasten hemostasis following catheter removal.
  - Older adult clients can have arthritis, which can make lying in bed for 4 to 6 hr after the procedure painful. The provider can prescribe medication to relax the client. ©
- Administer antiplatelet or thrombolytic agents as prescribed to prevent clot formation and restenosis.
  - Aspirin
  - Clopidogrel, ticlopidine
  - Heparin
  - Low molecular weight heparin (enoxaparin)
- Ask the charge nurse to administer anxiolytics and analgesics as needed.
- Monitor urine output and encourage fluids for hydration because contrast media acts as an osmotic diuretic.

CLIENT EDUCATION

- Immediately report bleeding from the insertion site, chest pain, shortness of breath, and changes in the color or temperature of the extremity.
- Clients who have stent placement will receive anticoagulation therapy for 6 to 8 weeks.
  - Take the medication at the same time each day.
  - Schedule regular laboratory tests to determine therapeutic levels.
  - Avoid activities that could cause bleeding. (Use soft toothbrush. Wear shoes when out of bed.)
- Adhere to these lifestyle guidelines.
  - Manage weight.
  - Consume a low-fat/low-sodium diet.
  - Exercise regularly.
  - Stop smoking.
  - Decrease alcohol intake.

COMPLICATIONS

Hematoma formation

Blood clots can form near the insertion site.

NURSING ACTIONS

- Inspect the groin at prescribed intervals and as needed.
- Hold pressure for uncontrolled oozing/bleeding.
- Monitor peripheral circulation.
- Notify the provider if changes occur.

Application Exercises

1. A nurse is reinforcing teaching with a client who is scheduled for an angiography. Which of the following statements should the nurse include in the teaching?

   A. "You should have nothing to eat or drink for 4 hours prior to the procedure."

   B. "You will be given general anesthesia during the procedure."

   C. "You should not have this procedure done if you are allergic to eggs."

   D. "You will need to keep your affected leg straight following the procedure."

2. A nurse is reviewing a client's laboratory test results. The nurse should identify that which of the following results indicates the client is at risk for heart disease? (Select all that apply.)

   A. Cholesterol (total) 245 mg/dL

   B. HDL 90 mg/dL

   C. LDL 140 mg/dL

   D. Triglycerides 125 mg/dL

   E. Troponin I 0.02 ng/mL

3. A nurse is assisting in the care of a client who began having chest pain 2 hr ago. Which of the following laboratory findings should the nurse identify as an indication the client has sustained injury to the heart?

   A. Troponin T 0.8 ng/mL

   B. Creatine kinase (MB) 100 units/L

   C. Myoglobin 80 mcg/L

   D. Triglycerides 120 mg/dL

4. A nurse is reinforcing teaching with a client who is scheduled for an echocardiogram. Which of the following statements should the nurse include in the teaching?

   A. "You may experience a warm feeling when the dye is injected."

   B. "The test will require 2 hours to complete."

   C. "You will be placed onto your right side during the procedure."

   D. "The test allows us to see how your heart valves work."

5. A nurse is reinforcing teaching with a client who is scheduled for a stress test. Which of the following statements should the nurse include in the teaching?

   A. "You should not have anything to eat or drink for 8 hours prior to the test."

   B. "You will exercise your heart by walking on a treadmill."

   C. "A chest x-ray will be obtained following the test."

   D. "The test will be delayed if your troponin I level is less than 0.5 ng/mL."

PRACTICE Active Learning Scenario

A nurse is assisting with the plan of care for a client who is scheduled for a stress test. What information should be included in the review? Use the ATI Active Learning Template: Diagnostic Procedure to complete this item.

DESCRIPTION OF THE PROCEDURE

INDICATIONS: List at least two.

NURSING INTERVENTIONS (PRE, INTRA, POST)
▪ Describe at least four preprocedure actions.
▪ Describe at least two intraprocedure actions.

Application Exercises Key

1. A. The nurse should instruct the client to remain NPO for at least 8 hr prior to the procedure to decrease the risk for aspiration while lying flat during the angiography.

   B. The nurse should instruct the client that he is awake and sedated during the procedure and that a local anesthetic is used at the catheter insertion site.

   C. The nurse should check the client for an allergy to iodine/shellfish due to the use of contrast dye. An allergy to eggs is not a contraindication to angiography.

   D. **CORRECT:** The nurse should instruct the client of the need to remain on bed rest in the supine position with the affected leg straight for a prescribed amount of time. This positioning decreases the client's risk for bleeding and hematoma formation at the catheter insertion site.

   Ⓝ *NCLEX® Connection: Reduction of Risk Potential, Diagnostic Tests*

2. A. **CORRECT:** A client who has a total cholesterol level greater than 200 mg/dL is at increased risk for heart disease.

   B. An HDL level greater than 55 mg/dL for a female client or greater than 45 mg/dL for a male client decreases the risk for heart disease.

   C. **CORRECT:** A client who has an LDL level greater than 130 mg/dL is at increased risk for heart disease.

   D. A triglyceride level between 35 and 135 mg/dL for a female client or 40 to 160 mg/dL for a male client is within the expected reference range and does not indicate an increased risk for heart disease.

   E. Troponin I level is monitored to detect cardiac injury due to an MI rather than to identify a client's risk for heart disease. A troponin I level less than 0.03 ng/mL is within the expected reference range.

   Ⓝ *NCLEX® Connection: Reduction of Risk Potential, Laboratory Values*

3. A. **CORRECT:** A client who has a troponin T level greater than 0.1 ng/mL has sustained myocardial injury.

   B. A creatine kinase (MB) of 100 units/L is within the expected reference range. The creatine kinase levels begins to rise at 2 hr and peaks within 18 hr following injury.

   C. Myoglobin is a cardiac marker that begins to increase 3 hr following injury. However, a myoglobin level of 80 mcg/L is within the expected reference range.

   D. Elevated triglyceride levels indicate the client is at risk for heart disease, but it is not indicative of myocardial injury. The client's triglyceride level is within the expected reference range.

   Ⓝ *NCLEX® Connection: Reduction of Risk Potential, Laboratory Values*

4. A. Clients undergoing a cardiac catheterization can experience a warm feeling when the dye is injected. However, no dye is used for an echocardiogram.

   B. An echocardiogram is completed within 1 hr.

   C. Clients undergoing an echocardiogram are placed supine and on the left side in order to bring the heart closest to the thoracic cage.

   D. **CORRECT:** An echocardiogram is an ultrasound test that is used to evaluate the heart's position and the function of the valves.

   Ⓝ *NCLEX® Connection: Reduction of Risk Potential, Diagnostic Tests*

5. A. The nurse should reinforce that the client should avoid eating 2 to 4 hr prior to taking stress test to avoid nausea and vomiting.

   B. **CORRECT:** The stress test is performed with the client walking on a treadmill or receiving medication to stimulate the heart.

   C. Throughout the testing, the client is monitored using continuous electrocardiogram monitoring. Chest x-ray is not used as a part of a stress test.

   D. Troponin T level is a cardiac marker than indicates myocardial damage. A troponin T level greater than 0.3 ng/mL would be an indication for canceling the stress test.

   Ⓝ *NCLEX® Connection: Reduction of Risk Potential, Diagnostic Tests*

PRACTICE Answer

Using the ATI Active Learning Template: Diagnostic Procedure

DESCRIPTION OF THE PROCEDURE: The cardiac muscle is exercised by walking on a treadmill. This provides information regarding the workload of the heart.

INDICATIONS
- Angina
- Heart failure
- Myocardial infarction
- Dysrhythmia

NURSING ACTIONS (PRE, INTRA, POST)
- Preprocedure
  - Ensure that a signed informed consent form is obtained.
  - Reinforce teaching with the client that he will walk on a treadmill. Comfortable athletic shoes and clothing are recommended.
  - Reinforce teaching with the client that a pharmacological stress test can be prescribed if the client cannot walk on the treadmill and complete the test. A medication such as dipyridamole, adenosine, or dobutamine is administered to stress the heart.
  - Reinforce teaching with the client to fast 2 to 4 hr before the procedure or according to facility policy and to avoid tobacco, alcohol, and caffeine before the test.
  - Reinforce teaching with the client to get adequate rest the night before the test.

- Intraprocedure
  - Monitor heart rate and rhythm with a 12-lead ECG during the test.
  - Reinforce teaching with the client to report any chest pain, shortness of breath, or dizziness during the test.

Ⓝ *NCLEX® Connection: Reduction of Risk Potential, Diagnostic Tests*

CHAPTER 25   *Electrocardiography and Dysrhythmia Monitoring*

Cardiac electrical activity can be monitored by using an electrocardiogram (ECG). The heart's electrical activity can be monitored by a standard 12-lead ECG (resting ECG), ambulatory ECG (Holter monitoring), continuous cardiac monitoring, or telemetry.

Cardiac monitoring is used to diagnose dysrhythmias, chamber enlargement, myocardial ischemia, injury, or infarction and to monitor the effects of electrolyte imbalances or medication administration.

Cardiac dysrhythmias are the result of electrical disturbances in the heart or an alteration of the heart muscle itself (beat formation, beat conduction, or myocardial response to beat).

Nurses should be familiar with cardioversion and defibrillation procedures for treating dysrhythmias. (25.1)

25.1 ECG strip

Name:
ID:
Patient ID:
Incident:
Age: Sex:

12-Lead 2

PR 0 138s
QT/QTc
P-QRS-T Axes

HR 62 bpm
9:00:00
QRS 0 112s
0.398s/0.395s
27° 80° 49°

Normal ECG
Normal sinus rhythm

x1.0 .05-158Hz 25mm/sec

Electrocardiography

Electrocardiography uses an electrocardiograph to record the electrical activity of the heart over time. The electrocardiograph is connected by wires (leads) to skin electrodes placed on the chest and limbs of a client.

- Continuous cardiac monitoring requires the client to be in close proximity to the monitoring system.
- Telemetry allows the client to ambulate while maintaining proximity to the monitoring system.
- Inform clients receiving continuous ECG monitoring that the monitoring will not detect shortness of breath, chest pain, or other manifestations of acute coronary syndrome. Instruct the client to report new or worsening sensations. Qs

INDICATIONS

Dysrhythmias
- Sinus bradycardia and tachycardia
- Atrioventricular (AV) blocks
- Atrial fibrillation
- Atrial flutter
- Junctional rhythms
- Ventricular asystole
- Premature atrial complexes (PACs) and premature ventricular complexes (PVCs)
- Supraventricular tachycardia
- Ventricular tachycardia
- Ventricular fibrillation

Electrolyte disturbances
- Hypokalemia and hyperkalemia
- Hypocalcemia and hypercalcemia
- Hypomagnesemia and hypermagnesemia

Medications
- Toxicities
- Digoxin, calcium channel blockers, beta adrenergic blockers

CLIENT PRESENTATION

- Cardiovascular disease
- Myocardial infarction (MI)
- Hypoxia
- Acid-base imbalances
- Electrolyte disturbances
- Kidney failure, liver, or lung disease
- Heart failure
- Metabolic disorders
- Pericarditis or endocarditis
- Drug or alcohol use
- Hypovolemia
- Shock
- Open heart surgery
- Increased intracranial pressure

CONSIDERATIONS

PREPROCEDURE

NURSING ACTIONS
Prepare the client for a 12-lead ECG, if prescribed. **(25.2)**
- Position the client in a supine position with chest exposed.
- Wash the client's skin to remove oils.
- If the area on which the electrode is to be placed has hair on it, clip—do not shave—the area to provide skin adherence and electrical conduction.
- Attach one electrode to each of the client's extremities by applying electrodes to flat surfaces above the wrists and ankles and the other six electrodes to the chest, avoiding chest hair. (Chest hair might need to be shaved.)

INTRAPROCEDURE

NURSING ACTIONS
- Reinforce teaching with the client to remain still and breathe normally while the 12-lead ECG is performed.
- Monitor for manifestations of dysrhythmia (chest pain, decreased level of consciousness, shortness of breath) and hypoxia.

POSTPROCEDURE

NURSING ACTIONS
- Remove leads from the client, print the ECG report, and notify the provider.
- Apply an ambulatory or Holter monitor if the client is on a telemetry unit or needs continuous cardiac monitoring.
- Continue to monitor for dysrhythmia.

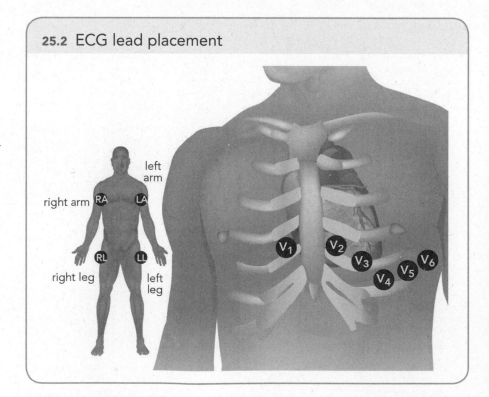

25.2 ECG lead placement

left arm
right arm   RA   LA
RL   LL
right leg   left leg

V1 V2 V3 V4 V5 V6

Dysrhythmias

- Dysrhythmias are classified by the following.
  - Site of origin: sinoatrial (SA) node, atria, atrioventricular (AV) node, or ventricle
    - Electrophysiological study is performed to determine the area of the heart causing the dysrhythmia.
    - Ablation of the area is possible. **(25.3)**
  - Effect on the rate and rhythm of the heart: bradycardia, tachycardia, heart block, premature beat, flutter, fibrillation, or asystole
- Dysrhythmias can be benign or life-threatening.
- The life-threatening effects of dysrhythmias are generally related to decreased cardiac output and ineffective tissue perfusion.
- Cardiac dysrhythmias are a primary cause of death in clients suffering acute MI and other sudden death disorders.

- Rapid recognition and treatment of serious dysrhythmias is essential to preserve life. Treatment is based on the cardiac rhythm, which can require cardioversion, defibrillation or pacemaker insertion, and medications. **(25.4)**
- Manifestations of dysrhythmia in the older adult might be present only with increased activity. ⓒ
- Increased incidence of chronic diseases and medication use in older adults increases the risk for drug interactions that can affect the cardiovascular system. ⓒ
- Risks for heart disease, hypertension, dysrhythmias, and atherosclerosis increase with age.
- Treatment of dysrhythmias follows Advanced Cardiac Life Support (ACLS) evidence-based protocols. Ⓠ**EBP**

25.3 Dysrhythmias

ATRIAL FIBRILLATION

PREMATURE ATRIAL COMPLEXES

PREMATURE VENTRICULAR COMPLEXES

VENTRICULAR TACHYCARDIA

25.4 Dysrhythmia treatments

	MEDICATION	ELECTRICAL MANAGEMENT
Bradycardia (any rhythm less than 60/min) Treat if the client is symptomatic	Atropine and isoproterenol	Pacemaker
Atrial fibrillation	Adenosine, digoxin	Synchronized cardioversion
Supraventricular tachycardia **Ventricular tachycardia with pulse**	Amiodarone, disopyramide, quinidine, procainamide, diltiazem and verapamil	Synchronized cardioversion
Ventricular tachycardia without pulse or ventricular fibrillation	Amiodarone, lidocaine, bretylium, sotalol and epinephrine	Defibrillation

Cardioversion and defibrillation

Cardioversion is the delivery of a direct countershock to the heart synchronized to the QRS complex. Defibrillation is the delivery of an unsynchronized, direct countershock to the heart. Defibrillation stops all electrical activity of the heart, allowing the SA node to take over and reestablish a perfusing rhythm.

INDICATIONS

Cardioversion: Elective or emergency treatment of atrial dysrhythmias, supraventricular tachycardia, and ventricular tachycardia with a pulse. Cardioversion is the treatment of choice for clients who are symptomatic.

Defibrillation: Ventricular fibrillation or pulseless ventricular tachycardia.

CONSIDERATIONS

PREPROCEDURE

Clients who have atrial fibrillation of unknown duration must receive adequate anticoagulation for 4 to 6 weeks prior to cardioversion therapy to prevent dislodgement of thrombi into the bloodstream.

NURSING ACTIONS
- Reinforce teaching about the procedure to the client, and obtain consent.
- Administer oxygen.
- Document preprocedure rhythm.
- Have emergency equipment available.

INTRAPROCEDURE

NURSING ACTIONS
- All staff must stand clear of the client, equipment connected to the client, and the bed when a shock is delivered.
- Perform CPR for cardiac asystole or other pulseless rhythms.
- Assist with immediate defibrillation of the client for ventricular fibrillation.

POSTPROCEDURE

NURSING ACTIONS
- After cardioversion or defibrillation, monitor vital signs, check airway patency, and obtain an ECG.
- Provide the client and family with reassurance and emotional support.
- Document the following.
  - Postprocedure rhythm
  - Number of defibrillation or cardioversion attempts, energy settings, time, and response
  - Client's condition and state of consciousness following the procedure
  - Skin condition under the electrodes
- Reinforce teaching with the client and family how to determine the pulse.

CLIENT EDUCATION: Report palpitations or irregularities.

COMPLICATIONS

Embolism

Cardioversion can dislodge blood clots, potentially causing the following.

- Pulmonary embolism (evidenced by dyspnea, chest pain, air hunger, decreasing SaO_2)
- Cerebrovascular accident (evidenced by decreased level of consciousness, slurred speech, muscle weakness/paralysis)
- MI (evidenced by chest pain and ST segment depression or elevation)

NURSING ACTIONS: Provide therapeutic anticoagulation for clients who have dysrhythmias. Monitor for cardiopulmonary complications.

Decreased cardiac output and heart failure

Cardioversion can damage heart tissue and impair heart function.

NURSING ACTIONS

- Monitor for manifestations of decreased cardiac output (hypotension, syncope, increased heart rate) and heart failure (dyspnea, productive cough, edema, venous distention).
- Provide prescribed medications to increase output (inotropic agents) and decrease cardiac workload.

> **PRACTICE** Active Learning Scenario
>
> A nurse is assisting in the planning of a staff in-service regarding electrocardiography. What information should the nurse recommend be included in this discussion? Use the ATI Active Learning Template: Therapeutic Procedure to complete this item.
>
> **DESCRIPTION OF PROCEDURE:** Describe electrocardiography and describe the difference between continuous cardiac monitoring and telemetry.
>
> **INDICATIONS:** List four dysrhythmias that can be identified.
>
> **NURSING INTERVENTIONS (PRE, INTRA, POST):** Identify at least two preprocedure, one intraprocedure, and two postprocedure.

Application Exercises

1. A nurse is caring for a group of clients. Which of the following clients is at risk for development of a dysrhythmia? (Select all that apply.)
    - A. A client who has metabolic alkalosis
    - B. A client who has a serum potassium level of 4.3 mEq/L
    - C. A client who has an SaO_2 of 96%
    - D. A client who has COPD
    - E. A client who underwent stent placement in a coronary artery

2. A nurse is assisting in the care of a client who underwent defibrillation. Which of the following should be included in the documentation of this procedure? (Select all that apply.)
    - A. Follow-up ECG
    - B. Energy settings used
    - C. IV fluid intake
    - D. Urinary output
    - E. Skin condition under electrodes

3. A nurse is caring for a client who is on telemetry. The nurse recognizes the client's heart rate is 46/min and notifies the provider. The nurse should anticipate that which of the following management strategies will be used for this client?
    - A. Defibrillation
    - B. Pacemaker insertion
    - C. Synchronized cardioversion
    - D. Administration of amiodarone PO

4. A nurse is observing a cardioversion procedure and hears the team leader call out, "Stand clear." The purpose of this action is to alert personnel of which of the following?
    - A. The cardioverter is being charged to the appropriate setting.
    - B. They should initiate CPR due to pulseless electrical activity.
    - C. They cannot be in contact with equipment connected to the client.
    - D. A time-out is being called to verify correct protocols.

5. A nurse is reinforcing teaching with a client scheduled for cardioversion. Which of the following client statements should the nurse identify as an indication the teaching has been understood?
    - A. "I should stop taking my warfarin 1 week prior to the procedure."
    - B. "I will receive an electrocardiogram following the procedure."
    - C. "Mechanical ventilation will be required during the procedure."
    - D. "Palpitations are an expected effect following the procedure."

Application Exercises Key

1. A. **CORRECT:** A client who has an acid-base imbalance, such as metabolic alkalosis, is at risk for a dysrhythmia.

   B. A serum potassium of 4.3 mEq/L is within the expected reference range and does not increase the risk of a dysrhythmia.

   C. SaO₂ of 96% is within the expected reference range and does not increase the risk of a dysrhythmia.

   D. **CORRECT:** A client who has lung disease, such as COPD, is at risk for a dysrhythmia.

   E. **CORRECT:** A client who has cardiac disease and underwent a stent placement is at risk for a dysrhythmia.

   Ⓝ *NCLEX® Connection: Health Promotion and Maintenance, Health Promotion/Disease Prevention*

2. A. **CORRECT:** The ECG rhythm is documented following the procedure.

   B. **CORRECT:** Energy settings used during the procedure are documented.

   C. IV fluid intake is not documented during defibrillation.

   D. Urinary output is not documented during defibrillation.

   E. **CORRECT:** The condition of the client's skin where electrodes were placed is documented.

   Ⓝ *NCLEX® Connection: Physiological Adaptation, Alterations in Body Systems*

3. A. Defibrillation is used when a client has ventricular fibrillation or pulseless ventricular tachycardia.

   B. **CORRECT:** A client who has bradycardia is a candidate for a pacemaker to increase heart rate.

   C. Synchronized cardioversion is used when a client has a dysrhythmia (atrial fibrillation, supraventricular tachycardia, ventricular tachycardia with pulse).

   D. The administration of amiodarone PO is used in clients who have ventricular arrhythmias or supraventricular tachycardia.

   Ⓝ *NCLEX® Connection: Physiological Adaptation, Alterations in Body Systems*

4. A. The cardioverter is charged prior to the delivery of the shock during cardioversion.

   B. The team leader calls out "Initiate CPR" when members of the team are to begin CPR.

   C. **CORRECT:** A safety concern for personnel performing cardioversion is to "stand clear" of the client and equipment connected to the client when a shock is delivered to prevent them from also receiving a shock.

   D. A time-out is called by personnel during a procedure to verify that proper protocols are being followed.

   Ⓝ *NCLEX® Connection: Reduction of Risk Potential, Therapeutic Procedures*

5. A. The client who is scheduled for cardioversion should take an anticoagulant medication for 4 to 6 weeks prior to the procedure to prevent the development of an embolism.

   B. **CORRECT:** Following the procedure, the nurse should ensure the client's airway remains patent, obtain an ECG, and monitor vital signs.

   C. The client who is to receive cardioversion will be placed on oxygen via nasal cannula.

   D. The nurse should reinforce teaching that palpitations or irregular heart rhythms are an adverse effect following cardioversion and should be reported to the provider.

   Ⓝ *NCLEX® Connection: Reduction of Risk Potential, Therapeutic Procedures*

PRACTICE Answer

Using the ATI Active Learning Template: Therapeutic Procedure

DESCRIPTION OF PROCEDURE

- Electrocardiography is the use of an electrocardiograph to record the electrical activity of the heart over time by connecting wires (leads) to skin electrodes placed on the chest and limbs.
- Continuous monitoring requires the client to be in close proximity to the monitoring system. Telemetry allows the client to ambulate.

INDICATIONS

- Sinus bradycardia and tachycardia
- Atrioventricular (AV) blocks
- Atrial fibrillation
- Atrial flutter
- Junctional rhythms
- Ventricular asystole
- Premature atrial complexes (PACs) and premature ventricular complexes (PVCs)
- Supraventricular tachycardia
- Ventricular tachycardia
- Ventricular fibrillation
- Electrolyte disturbances

NURSING INTERVENTIONS (PRE, INTRA, POST)

Preprocedure
- Position the client in a supine position with chest exposed.
- Wash the skin to remove oils.
- Attach one electrode to each of the client's extremities by applying electrodes to flat surfaces above the wrists and ankles and the other six electrodes to the chest, avoiding chest hair, which might need to be shaved.

Intraprocedure
- Instruct the client to remain still and breathe normally.
- Monitor for manifestations of dysrhythmia (chest pain, decreased level of consciousness, shortness of breath) and hypoxia.

Postprocedure
- Remove leads, print ECG report, and notify the provider.
- Apply an ambulatory or Holter monitor if the client is on the telemetry unit or needs continuous monitoring.
- Continue monitoring for manifestations of dysrhythmia and hypoxia.

Ⓝ *NCLEX® Connection: Reduction of Risk Potential, Diagnostic Tests*

UNIT 4 **NURSING CARE OF CLIENTS WHO HAVE CARDIOVASCULAR DISORDERS**
SECTION: DIAGNOSTIC AND THERAPEUTIC PROCEDURES

CHAPTER 26 *Invasive Cardiovascular Procedures*

Cardiovascular procedures include invasive methods used to improve blood flow for occluded arteries and veins.

Invasive cardiovascular procedures are indicated after noninvasive interventions have been tried (diet, exercise, medications). Invasive cardiovascular procedures include percutaneous coronary intervention (PCI), coronary artery bypass grafts (CABG), and peripheral bypass grafts.

Percutaneous coronary intervention

PCI is a nonsurgical procedure performed to open coronary arteries through one of the following means.
- **Atherectomy**: Used to break up and remove plaques within cardiac vessels
- **Stent**: Placement of a mesh-wire device to hold an artery open and prevent restenosis
- **Percutaneous transluminal coronary angioplasty**: Inserting a balloon-tipped angiocatheter into a coronary artery that is obstructed, inflating the balloon to dilate the arterial lumen and the adhering plaque, thus widening the arterial lumen and increasing blood flow through the obstructed area
  ○ Can include placement of a stent, which remains in the artery as a support to keep the vessel unobstructed
  ○ Also referred to simply as angioplasty

INDICATIONS

- On an elective basis to treat coronary artery disease when there is occlusion of one or two coronary arteries. The area of occlusion is confined, not scattered, and easy to access (proximal).
- Can reduce ischemia during the occurrence of an acute myocardial infarction (MI) by opening coronary arteries and restoring perfusion. It is usually performed within 3 hr of the onset of manifestations of impaired perfusion.
- As an alternative to coronary artery bypass graft.
- Used with stent placement to prevent artery reocclusion and to dilate the coronary artery.

CLIENT PRESENTATION

- Chest pain can occur with or without exertion.
- Substernal or epigastric pain can radiate to the jaw, left arm, through the back, or to the left shoulder.
- Manifestations can increase in cold weather or with exercise.
- Other manifestations can include dyspnea, nausea, fatigue, diaphoresis, tachycardia, and hypotension.
- The client can describe the pain as crushing, pressure, or a tightness that is not relieved with rest.
- Female clients can present differently than male clients, with atypical manifestations (fatigue, weakness that interferes with activities, sharp pain).
- Older adult clients can have manifestations such as indigestion, nausea, dyspnea, and confusion and might not experience chest pain or discomfort. ©
- ECG changes can include ST elevation, depression, or nonspecific ST changes.
- Other findings can include bradycardia, tachycardia, hypotension, elevated blood pressure, vomiting, and mental disorientation.
- The client's skin can appear pale, ashen, cool, or clammy.
- The client can have a syncopal episode.
- Laboratory findings can include elevations of troponin I and troponin T as well as creatinine kinase within 2 hr of onset of manifestations.

CONSIDERATIONS

PREPROCEDURE

NURSING ACTIONS
- Ensure that the client signs the consent form.
- Maintain NPO status for at least 8 hr if possible (risk for aspiration when lying flat for the procedure).
- Ensure the client and family understand the procedure.
- Record height, weight, and vital signs.
- Mark pedal pulses and document the quality and strength of pedal pulses.
- Check the client for an iodine/shellfish allergy (contrast dye used instead of contrast media for consistency).
- Check kidney function prior to introduction of contrast dye.
- Review client medications. If the client is taking metformin, withhold the medication prior to the procedure and up the 3 days following the procedure.
- Administer premedications as prescribed (antiplatelet or cardiac medications).

CLIENT EDUCATION: The client might be awake and sedated for the procedure, which lasts 1 to 2 hr. A local anesthetic might be administered. A small incision is made, often in the groin, to insert the catheter. The client might feel warmth, flushing, and a metallic taste when the dye is inserted. After the procedure, the client will be asked to keep the affected leg straight. Pressure (a sandbag) might be placed on the incision to prevent bleeding.

POSTPROCEDURE

NURSING ACTIONS

- Check vital signs every 15 min × 4, every 30 min × 2, every hour × 4, and then every 4 hr (or per facility protocol). Report tachycardia or a decrease in systolic blood pressure.
- Inspect the insertion site (and under the buttocks if the femoral artery at the groin was accessed) at the same intervals for bleeding and hematoma formation.
- Keep a pressure dressing in place at the groin site.
- Check for manifestations of thrombosis.
- Check and document pedal or radial pulse, capillary refill, color, and temperature of extremity at the same intervals as vital signs. Report any changes from preprocedure data findings.
- Maintain bed rest in a supine position with leg or arm straight for prescribed time.
  - Older adult clients might have arthritis, which can make lying in bed for 4 to 6 hr after the procedure painful. Ⓖ
  - Conduct continuous cardiac monitoring for dysrhythmias and report any ECG changes or client report of chest pain. (Reperfusion following angioplasty might cause dysrhythmias.)
- Administer antiplatelet or thrombolytic agents as prescribed to prevent clot formation and restenosis.
  - Aspirin
  - Clopidogrel, tirofiban
  - Heparin
  - Enoxaparin
- Administer anxiolytics and analgesics as needed.
- Monitor urine output and the administration of IV fluids for hydration. Contrast dye acts as an osmotic diuretic.

CLIENT EDUCATION

- Avoid strenuous exercise for prescribed period of time.
- Immediately report bleeding from insertion site, chest pain, shortness of breath, and changes in color or temperature of the extremity.
- Restrict lifting (less than 5 lb) for prescribed period of time.
- A client who had a stent placement receives anticoagulation therapy for 6 to 8 weeks.
  - Take medication at the same time each day.
  - Have regular laboratory tests to determine therapeutic levels.
  - Avoid activities that could cause bleeding (use a soft toothbrush, wear shoes when out of bed, use an electric razor).
- Follow lifestyle guidelines (manage weight, consume a low-fat/low-cholesterol diet, exercise regularly, stop smoking, stress reduction, and decrease alcohol intake).

COMPLICATIONS

Artery dissection

- Perforation of an artery by the catheter might cause cardiac tamponade or require emergency bypass surgery.
- Artery dissection findings include severe hypotension and tachycardia.

Cardiac tamponade

- Cardiac tamponade can result from fluid accumulation in the pericardial sac.
- Findings include hypotension, jugular venous distention (distended neck veins), muffled heart sounds, and paradoxical pulse (decrease of 10 mm Hg or more in systolic blood pressure and weakened peripheral pulses during inspiration).

NURSING ACTIONS

- Notify the provider immediately. Qs
- Monitor the administration of IV fluids to manage hypotension as prescribed.
- Obtain a chest x-ray or ECG to confirm findings.
- Prepare the client for pericardiocentesis or return to surgical suite (informed consent, gather materials, administer medications as appropriate). Monitor heart rhythm for reoccurrence of findings after the procedure.

Hematoma formation near insertion site

Manifestations can include swelling at the insertion site, bluish discoloration of the periwound skin, and a change in sensation or temperature of the extremity.

NURSING ACTIONS

- Monitor for sensation, color, capillary refill, and peripheral pulses in the extremity distal to the insertion site.
- Inspect groin or wrist for development of a hematoma at prescribed intervals and as needed.
- Hold pressure for uncontrolled oozing/bleeding.
- Notify the provider.

Allergic reaction related to the contrast dye

Manifestations can include chills, fever, rash, wheezing, tachycardia, and bradycardia.

NURSING ACTIONS

- Monitor for an allergic reaction.
- Have resuscitation equipment readily available.
- Administer diphenhydramine or epinephrine if prescribed.

External bleeding at the insertion site

NURSING ACTIONS

- Monitor insertion site for bleeding or swelling (under buttocks if access site is groin area).
- Apply pressure to site.
- Keep client's leg or arm straight.
- Notify the provider if evidence of excessive bleeding.

Embolism

Plaque or a clot can become dislodged.

NURSING ACTIONS
- Monitor for chest pain, dyspnea, or change in level of consciousness after the procedure.
- Monitor vital signs and SaO_2.

Retroperitoneal bleeding

Bleeding in the retroperitoneal space (abdominal cavity behind the peritoneum) can occur due to femoral artery puncture.

NURSING ACTIONS
- Monitor for flank pain and hypotension.
- Notify the provider immediately.
- Monitor administration of IV fluids and blood products.

CLIENT EDUCATION
- Pressure will be applied to the insertion site.
- Keep the leg straight and limit activity as prescribed.
- Report chest pain, shortness of breath, or cardiac manifestations.

Restenosis of treated vessel

Clot formation can occur in the coronary vessel immediately or several days after the procedure.

NURSING ACTIONS
- Monitor ECG patterns and for report of chest pain.
- Notify the provider immediately.
- Prepare the client for return to the cardiac catheterization laboratory.

CLIENT EDUCATION: Notify the provider of cardiac manifestations and to take medications as prescribed.

Acute kidney injury

Damage to the kidney can result from use of contrast agent, which is nephrotoxic.

NURSING ACTIONS
- Monitor urine output, BUN, creatinine, and electrolytes.
- Promote adequate hydration (oral and IV).
- Administer acetylcysteine to protect the kidneys before and after the procedure.

Coronary artery bypass grafts

CABG is an invasive surgical procedure that aims to restore vascularization of the myocardium. (26.1)
- Performed to bypass an obstruction in one or more of the coronary arteries, CABG does not alter the atherosclerotic process but improves the quality of life for clients restricted by painful coronary artery disease.
- The internal mammary artery in the chest and the greater saphenous vein from the leg are the most popular blood vessels used for the bypass grafts.
- Older adult clients are more likely to experience transient neurological changes, toxic effects from cardiac medications, and dysrhythmias. The recovery time is prolonged in the older adult client due to the stressors placed on the body and a slowed rate of healing. Ⓖ
- Less invasive revascularization procedures have been developed to reduce risk and improve client outcomes (off-pump coronary artery bypass, robotic heart surgery, minimally invasive direct coronary artery bypass). These procedures have characteristics similar to traditional CABG.

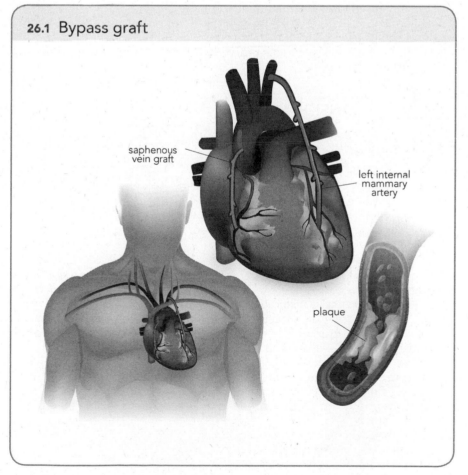

26.1 Bypass graft

saphenous vein graft

left internal mammary artery

plaque

INDICATIONS

POTENTIAL DIAGNOSES

- Over 50% blockage of left main coronary artery with anginal episodes (blockage inaccessible to angioplasty and stenting)
- Significant two-vessel disease with unstable angina
- Triple-vessel disease with or without angina
- Persistent ischemia or likely MI following coronary angiography, PCI, or stent placement
- Heart failure or cardiogenic shock with acute MI or ischemia (might not be reasonable for clients who have poor ejection fractions)
- Coronary arteries that are unable to be accessed or treated by angioplasty and stent placement (narrow or calcified)
- Coronary artery disease nonresponsive to medical management

CLIENT PRESENTATION

- Chest pain can occur with or without exertion.
- Pain can radiate to jaw, left arm, through the back, or to the shoulder.
- Effects can increase in cold weather or with exercise.
- Other findings can include dyspnea, nausea, fatigue, and diaphoresis.
- ECG changes can include ST elevation, depression, or nonspecific ST changes.
- Other findings can include bradycardia, tachycardia, hypotension, elevated blood pressure, vomiting, and mental disorientation.

CONSIDERATIONS

PREPROCEDURE

NURSING ACTIONS

- A CABG might be an elective procedure or done as an emergency. When planned, preparation begins before the client comes to the facility for the procedure.
- Verify that the client has signed the informed consent form.
- Confirm that recent chest x-ray, ECG, and laboratory reports are available if needed.
- Obtain vital signs.
- Administer preoperative medications as prescribed.
  - Anxiolytics (lorazepam, diazepam)
  - Prophylactic antibiotics
  - Anticholinergics, such as scopolamine, to reduce secretions
- Provide safe transport of the client to the operating suite.
- Monitor heart rate and rhythm, oxygenation, and other vital indicators.
- Monitor the client and family anxiety levels surrounding the procedure. Encourage clients to verbalize feelings. Qpcc

CLIENT EDUCATION Qpcc

- Coughing and deep breathing after the procedure is important to prevent complications.
- Splint the incision when coughing and deep breathing.
- Use arm and leg exercises to prevent complications.
- Report pain to the nursing staff. The majority of pain stems from the harvest site for the vein.
- Expect the following postoperatively.
  - Endotracheal tube and mechanical ventilator for airway management for several hours following surgery
  - Inability to talk while endotracheal tube is in place
  - Sternal incision and possible leg incision
  - Early ambulation to prevent complications
  - Administration of analgesics for pain control
  - One to two mediastinal chest tubes
  - Indwelling urinary catheter
  - Pacemaker wires
  - Hemodynamic monitoring devices (pulmonary artery catheter, arterial line)
- Alter or discontinue regular medications as prescribed by the provider.
  - Medications frequently discontinued for CABG
    - Diuretics 2 to 3 days before surgery
    - Aspirin and other anticoagulants 1 week before surgery
  - Medications often continued for CABG
    - Potassium supplements
    - Scheduled antidysrhythmics, such as amiodarone
    - Scheduled antihypertensives (metoprolol, a beta blocker; diltiazem, a calcium-channel blocker)
    - Insulin (clients who have diabetes mellitus and are insulin-dependent usually receive half the regular insulin dose)

POSTPROCEDURE

NURSING ACTIONS

- Maintain patent airway and adequate ventilation. Qs
  - Monitor respiratory rate and effort.
  - Auscultate breath sounds. Report crackles.
  - Monitor SaO_2.
- Encourage the client to splint the incision while deep breathing and coughing.
- Consult respiratory services to aid in recovery and client education.
- Consult case management services to initiate discharge planning: need for home oxygen therapy, transfer to tertiary care facility.
- Continually monitor heart rate and rhythm. Treat dysrhythmias per protocol.
- Maintain an adequate circulating blood volume.
  - Monitor blood pressure.
  - Monitor skin temperature and peripheral pulses.

- Monitor chest tube patency and drainage.
  - Measure drainage at least once an hour.
  - Volume exceeding 150 mL/hr could be an indication of possible hemorrhage and should be reported to the surgeon.
  - Monitor hemoglobin and hematocrit values. Report excessive blood loss or falling values.
  - Avoid dependent loops in tubing to facilitate drainage.
- Monitor and control pain.
  - Determine source of pain (angina, incisional pain).
    - Anginal pain often radiates and is unaffected by breathing. Report anginal pain immediately to provider.
    - Incisional pain is localized, sharp, aching, burning, and often worsens with deep breathing.
- Administer analgesics as prescribed (morphine, fentanyl).
  - Pain will stimulate the sympathetic nervous system, resulting in increased heart rate and systemic vascular resistance.
  - Provide frequent and adequate doses to control pain. Maintain around-the-clock administration. Document effectiveness of analgesia.
- Monitor fluid and electrolyte status.
  - Fluid administration is determined by blood pressure, chest tube blood loss, and urine output. Report urinary output of less than 30 mL/hr for 2 consecutive hours.
  - Monitor for electrolyte imbalances, especially hypokalemia and hyperkalemia. Report significant changes.
  - Obtain daily weight.
- Prevent and monitor for infection.
  - Practice proper hand hygiene.
  - Use surgical aseptic technique during procedures such as dressing changes.
  - Administer antibiotics.
  - Monitor WBC counts, incisional redness and drainage, and fever.
  - Monitor the client's temperature.
- Encourage the client to verbalize feelings.
- Discuss home environment and social supports. Consult case management to assist with home planning needs. Qpcc

CLIENT EDUCATION
- Monitor and report manifestations of infection (fever, incisional drainage, redness).
- To treat angina:
  - Maintain a fresh supply of sublingual nitroglycerin.
  - Store nitroglycerin in a light-resistant container.
  - Discontinue activity and rest with the onset of pain. Follow directions for treating anginal pain.
  - Older female clients might show milder manifestations (dyspnea, indigestion). Ⓖ
- Adhere to the pharmacological regimen.
- Clients who have diabetes mellitus should closely monitor blood glucose levels.

- Consume a heart-healthy diet (low fat, low cholesterol, high fiber, low salt).
- Quit smoking if applicable.
- Engage in physical activity. Consult the cardiac rehabilitation program or a physical therapist to devise a specific program.
- Remain home during the first week after surgery and resume normal activities slowly.
  - Week 2: possible return to work part time, increase in social activities
  - Week 3: lifting up to 15 lb (avoidance of heavier lifting for 6 to 8 weeks)
- Resume sexual activity based on the advice of the provider. Walking one block or climbing two flights of stairs without manifestations of coronary distress generally indicates that it is safe to resume normal sexual activity.

COMPLICATIONS

Pulmonary complications

Include the primary complication of atelectasis, as well as pneumonia and pulmonary edema

NURSING ACTIONS
- Turn the client every 2 hr, and advance him out of bed as soon as possible.
- Monitor breath sounds, SaO_2, ABGs, and urine output. Obtain chest x-ray as indicated.

CLIENT EDUCATION: Coughing, deep breathing, and use of an incentive spirometer is encouraged. Increasing activity reduces postoperative complications.

Electrolyte disturbances

Potassium and magnesium depletion is common.

NURSING ACTIONS: Monitor ECG and electrolytes.

Neurologic deficits

Transient hypertension, hypotension, or a blood clot might cause an intraoperative cerebrovascular accident.

NURSING ACTIONS
- Check neurologic status, including pupils, level of consciousness, and sensory and motor function.
- Maintain pressure within prescribed parameters.
- Explain procedures to the client.

CLIENT EDUCATION: Memory loss and neurological deficits might be temporary.

Peripheral bypass grafts

Bypass graft surgery aims to restore adequate blood flow to the areas affected by peripheral artery disease.

- A peripheral bypass graft involves suturing graft material or autogenous saphenous veins proximal and distal to occluded area of an artery. This procedure improves blood supply to the area normally served by the blocked artery.
- If bypass surgery fails to restore circulation, the client might need to undergo amputation of the limb.

INDICATIONS

- Acute circulatory compromise in limb
- Severe pain at rest that interferes with ability to work

CLIENT PRESENTATION

- Numbness or burning pain to the lower extremity with exercise; might stop with rest (intermittent claudication)
- Numbness or burning pain to the lower extremity at rest; might wake the client at night; might be relieved by lowering the extremity below the level of the heart
- Legs often feel cold or numb as well as painful.
- Decreased or absent pulses to feet
- Dry, hairless, shiny skin on calves
- Muscles might atrophy with advanced disease.
- Skin might be cold and dark-colored.
- Feet and toes might be mottled and dusky, and toenails might be thick.
- Skin might become reddened (rubor) when extremity is dropped to a dependent position, and pale when extremity is elevated.
- Ulcers or lesions might be noted on toes (arterial ulcers) or ankles (venous ulcers).

CONSIDERATIONS

PREPROCEDURE

NURSING ACTIONS
- Collect data regarding the client and family's understanding of the procedure.
- Verify that the client has signed the informed consent form.
- Collect data regarding client allergies.
- Document baseline vital signs and peripheral pulses.
- Administer prophylactic antibiotic therapy as prescribed.
- Instruct the client to maintain NPO status for at least 8 hr prior to surgery.
- Provide information about postoperative pain management, and reinforce deep breathing/incentive spirometer exercises.

CLIENT EDUCATION
- Do not cross the legs or wear knee-high stockings.
- An arterial line might be inserted for blood and blood pressure.
- Pedal pulses will be checked frequently.

POSTPROCEDURE

NURSING ACTIONS
- Monitor vital signs every 15 min for 1 hr and then hourly (or per facility policy).
- Follow standing orders to maintain blood pressure within the prescribed range. Hypotension might reduce blood flow to graft, and hypertension might cause bleeding.
- Check the operative limb every 15 min for 1 hr and then hourly after that, paying particular attention to the following.
  - Incision site for bleeding.
  - Peripheral pulses, capillary refill, skin color/temperature, and sensory and motor function for manifestations of bypass graft occlusion. In clients who have dark skin, check nail beds and soles of feet to detect early cyanosis.
  - Site is marked with an indelible marker.
- Monitor administration of IV fluids.
- Identify the type of pain experienced by the client. Qs
  - Throbbing pain is experienced due to an increase in blood flow to extremity.
  - Ischemic pain is often difficult to relieve with opioid administration.
- Administer analgesics (morphine sulfate, fentanyl). Check effect of analgesics on pain.
- Administer antibiotics as prescribed.
- Use surgical aseptic technique for dressing changes.
- Monitor incision sites for evidence of infection (erythema, tenderness, drainage).
- Administer anticoagulant therapy (warfarin, heparin, enoxaparin) to prevent reocclusion.
- Administer antiplatelet therapy (clopidogrel, tirofiban, aspirin).
- Help the client turn, cough, and deep breathe every 2 hr.
- Maintain bed rest for 18 to 24 hr. The leg should be kept straight during this time.
- Assist the client to get out of bed and ambulate. Encourage the use of a walker initially.
- Discourage the client from sitting for long periods of time.
- Apply antiembolic stockings to promote venous return.
- Set up a progressive exercise program that includes walking. Consider a physical therapy consult.
- Reinforce activity restrictions.

CLIENT EDUCATION Qpcc
- Abstain from tobacco products. Consider a nicotine-cessation program.
- Avoid crossing the legs or wearing constricting knee socks.
- Avoid elevating the legs above heart level.
- Avoid risk factors for atherosclerosis (smoking, sedentary lifestyle, uncontrolled diabetes mellitus).
- Practice techniques of foot inspection and care.
  - Keep feet dry and clean.
  - Avoid extreme temperatures.
  - Use lotion.
  - Avoid socks with tight cuffs.
  - Wear clean white cotton socks and always wear comfortable shoes.

COMPLICATIONS

Graft occlusion

The graft might occlude due to reduced blood flow and clot formation. Occurs primarily in first 24 hr after the procedure.

NURSING ACTIONS
- Notify the provider immediately for changes in pedal pulse, extremity color, or temperature.
- Prepare the client for thrombectomy or thrombolytic therapy.
- Monitor for bleeding with thrombolytics.
- Monitor coagulation studies.
- Monitor for anaphylaxis.

Compartment syndrome

Pressure from tissue swelling or bleeding within a compartment or a restricted space causes reduced blood flow to the area. Untreated, the affected tissue will become cyanotic and die.

NURSING ACTIONS
- Monitor for worsening pain, numbness, swelling, and tense or taut skin at graft site or in distal extremity.
- Collect data regarding capillary refill distal to the graft.
- Report unusual findings to the provider immediately.
- Prepare the client for a fasciotomy to relieve compartmental pressure.

Infection

Infection of the surgical site can result in loss of the graft and increased ischemia.

NURSING ACTIONS
- Monitor the wound for evidence of infection (increased redness, swelling, tenderness, drainage).
- Monitor WBC count and temperature.
- Collect specimens (wound or blood cultures).
- Administer antibiotic therapy as prescribed.
- Use surgical aseptic technique for dressing changes.

CLIENT EDUCATION: Notify the provider of decreased sensation, increased ischemic pain, redness, or swelling at the incisional site or in the affected limb.

PRACTICE Active Learning Scenario

A nurse is contributing to the plan of care for a client who is returning to the unit following angioplasty. What should the nurse include in the plan of care? Use the ATI Active Learning Template: Therapeutic Procedure to complete this item.

NURSING INTERVENTIONS: Describe five postprocedure nursing actions.

POTENTIAL COMPLICATIONS:
- Describe at least two.
- Describe at least two actions related to each of these complications.

Application Exercises

1. A nurse is caring for a client following peripheral bypass graft surgery of the left lower extremity. Which of the following findings pose an immediate concern? (Select all that apply.)

   A. Trace of bloody drainage on dressing

   B. Capillary refill of affected limb of 6 seconds

   C. Mottled appearance of the limb

   D. Throbbing pain of affected limb that is decreased following IV bolus analgesic

   E. Pulse of 2+ in the affected limb

2. A nurse is caring for a client following an angioplasty through the femoral artery. While turning the client, the nurse discovers blood underneath the client's lower back. Which of the following complications should the nurse suspect?

   A. Retroperitoneal bleeding

   B. Cardiac tamponade

   C. Bleeding from the incisional site

   D. Heart failure

3. A nurse is collecting data from a client who will undergo peripheral bypass graft surgery on the left leg. Which of the following findings should the nurse expect?

   A. Rubor of the affected leg when elevated

   B. 3+ dorsal pedal pulse in left foot

   C. Thin, peeling toenails of left foot

   D. Report of intermittent claudication in the affected leg

4. A nurse is contributing to the plan of care for a client who has transferred from the coronary care unit following coronary artery bypass graft surgery. Which of the following interventions should the nurse include?

   A. Provide percussion chest physiotherapy to loosen pulmonary secretions.

   B. Report urinary output less than 300 mL in 8 hr.

   C. Limit administration of opioid analgesics for pain ratings greater than 7 out of 10.

   D. Instruct the client to splint chest when deep breathing.

5. A nurse is reinforcing discharge teaching with a client following an atherectomy using the right femoral artery as an access. Which of the following client statements indicates an understanding of the teaching?

   A. "I should expect moderate swelling of the insertion site on my right groin."

   B. "I will limit fluid intake for the first 24 hours following the procedure."

   C. "I should restrict lifting to 5 pounds."

   D. "I can resume high-impact aerobic exercises right away."

Application Exercises Key

1. A. A trace of bloody drainage on the dressing is an expected finding and does not require immediate concern.

    B. **CORRECT:** Capillary refill greater than 4 seconds is outside the expected reference range and should be reported to the provider.

    C. **CORRECT:** Mottled appearance of the affected extremity indicates poor tissue perfusion and should be reported to the provider.

    D. Pain that is decreased following IV bolus analgesia is an expected finding and does not require immediate concern.

    E. Pulse of 2+ in the affected extremity is an expected finding and does not require immediate concern.

    Ⓝ *NCLEX® Connection: Reduction of Risk Potential, Potential for Complications from Surgical Procedures and Health Alterations*

2. A. Retroperitoneal bleeding is internal bleeding.

    B. Cardiac tamponade includes manifestations of bleeding in the pericardial sac, which is internal.

    C. **CORRECT:** Bleeding is occurring from the incision site and then draining under the client. The nurse should check the incision for hematoma, apply pressure, monitor the client, and notify the provider.

    D. Heart failure does not including findings of blood underneath the lower back.

    Ⓝ *NCLEX® Connection: Reduction of Risk Potential, Potential for Complications of Diagnostic Tests/Treatments/Procedures*

3. A. Reddening (rubor) of a leg affected by peripheral artery disease occurs when it is placed in a dependent position.

    B. Pulses are decreased or absent in the feet in cases of peripheral artery disease.

    C. Toenails are thickened in cases of peripheral artery disease.

    D. **CORRECT:** A client who has peripheral artery disease might report that numbness or burning pain in the extremity ceases with rest (intermittent claudication).

    Ⓝ *NCLEX® Connection: Physiological Adaptation, Basic Pathophysiology*

4. A. Chest physiotherapy is administered to clients who have chronic lung diseases such as COPD. Percussion and vibration is contraindicated for a client who is postoperative following thoracic surgery, as these procedures can increase pain and cause trauma to the thoracic cage.

    B. The nurse should report a urinary output of less than 30 mL/hr for 2 consecutive hours, as this can indicate a decrease in kidney function.

    C. Postoperative pain control management should include opioid analgesics around the clock rather than limited to treating pain when it becomes severe.

    D. **CORRECT:** Instructing the client to splint the chest when deep breathing and coughing will decrease the pain associated with expansion of the thoracic cage with inspiration and the increased intrathoracic pressure with coughing for the client who is postoperative following a CABG.

    Ⓝ *NCLEX® Connection: Reduction of Risk Potential, Potential for Complications from Surgical Procedures and Health Alterations*

5. A. Swelling at the insertion site is an indication of bleeding or hematoma formation and should be reported to the provider immediately.

    B. The contrast agent used in percutaneous coronary interventions, such as an atherectomy, is nephrotoxic. The nurse should encourage the client to increase consumption of liquids to increase excretion of the contrast agent.

    C. **CORRECT:** Lifting restrictions of 5 lb (2.27 kg) can prevent increased strain on the operative site and limit the risk of bleeding or hematoma formation.

    D. The nurse should reinforce that strenuous activity such as high-impact aerobic exercises should be restricted for a period of time determined by the provider to limit the risk of bleeding and hematoma formation.

    Ⓝ *NCLEX® Connection: Reduction of Risk Potential, Potential for Complications from Surgical Procedures and Health Alterations*

PRACTICE Answer

Using ATI Active Learning Template: Therapeutic Procedure

NURSING INTERVENTIONS

- Check vital signs every 15 min × 4, every 30 min × 2, every hour × 4, and then every 4 hr (or per facility protocol).
- Inspect the groin site with vital signs.
- Keep a pressure dressing in place at the groin site.
- Maintain bed rest in supine position with leg straight for prescribed time.
- Conduct continuous cardiac monitoring for dysrhythmia.
- Administer antiplatelet or thrombolytic agents as prescribed.
- Administer anxiolytics and analgesics as prescribed.
- Monitor urine output and the administration IV fluids for hydration.

POTENTIAL COMPLICATIONS

- Cardiac tamponade: Notify the provider; monitor the administration of IV fluids to manage hypotension; obtain chest x-ray or echocardiogram; prepare the client for pericardiocentesis.
- Hematoma formation: Monitor sensation, color, capillary refill, and pulse in extremity distal to insertion site; hold pressure for uncontrolled oozing/bleeding; notify the provider.
- Allergic reaction: Monitor the client; have resuscitation equipment available; administer diphenhydramine or epinephrine as needed.
- External bleeding: Monitor insertion site for bleeding or swelling; apply pressure to insertion site; keep client's leg or arm straight.
- Embolism: Monitor for chest pain; monitor for dyspnea or change in level of consciousness; monitor vital signs and SaO2.
- Retroperitoneal bleeding: Monitor for flank pain and hypotension; notify the provider; monitor the administration of IV fluids and blood products as prescribed.
- Restenosis of vessel: Monitor ECG pattern and for report of chest pain; notify the provider; prepare for return to cardiac catheterization laboratory.

Ⓝ *NCLEX® Connection: Physiological Adaptation, Alterations in Body Systems*

CHAPTER 27

CHAPTER 27 *Angina and Myocardial Infarction*

The continuum from angina to myocardial infarction (MI) is called acute coronary syndrome. Manifestations of acute coronary syndrome are due to an imbalance between myocardial oxygen supply and demand.

Angina pectoris can be an indication of an impending acute MI. Female clients and older adults do not always experience manifestations typically associated with angina or MI. They can report indigestion, nausea, vomiting, and upper back pain. Qpcc

The area of infarction in clients experiencing a myocardial infarction (MI) develops over minutes to hours. Early recognition and treatment of an acute MI is essential to prevent death. Most deaths occur within the first hour after the onset of manifestations.

Research shows improved outcomes following an MI in clients treated with aspirin, beta blockers, and angiotensin-converting enzyme (ACE) inhibitors or angiotensin receptor blockers.

When blood flow to the heart is compromised, ischemia causes chest pain. (27.1) Anginal pain is often described as a tight, squeezing, heavy pressure, or constricting feeling in the chest. The pain can radiate to the jaw, neck, shoulders, or arm. (27.2) Pain unrelieved by rest or nitroglycerin and lasting for more than 15 min differentiates MI from angina. (27.3)

An abrupt interruption of oxygen to the heart muscle produces myocardial ischemia. Ischemia can lead to tissue necrosis (infarction) if blood supply and oxygen are not restored. Ischemia is reversible. An infarction results in permanent damage. When the cardiac muscle suffers ischemic injury, cardiac enzymes are released into the bloodstream, providing specific markers of MI.

27.1 Myocardial infarction

27.2 Anginal pain

Possible areas of referred pain:
Jaw, chest, shoulders, neck, arms

HEALTH PROMOTION AND DISEASE PREVENTION

- Maintain an exercise routine to remain physically active. Consult with a provider before starting any exercise regimen.
- Have cholesterol level and blood pressure checked regularly.
- Consume a diet low in saturated fats and sodium. Consult with a provider regarding diet restrictions.
- Promote cessation of all forms of tobacco use.

DATA COLLECTION

Types of angina

Stable (exertional) angina occurs with exercise or emotional stress and is relieved by rest or nitroglycerin.

Unstable (preinfarction) angina occurs with exercise or at rest, but increases in occurrence, severity, and duration over time.

Variant (Prinzmetal's) angina is due to a coronary artery spasm, often occurring during periods of rest.

RISK FACTORS

- Male or postmenopausal client
- Ethnic background
- Sedentary lifestyle
- Hypertension
- Tobacco use
- Hyperlipidemia
- Obesity
- Excessive alcohol consumption
- Metabolic disorders (diabetes mellitus, hyperthyroidism)
- Methamphetamine or cocaine use
- Stress (with ineffective coping skills)
- An increased risk of coronary artery disease exists for older adult clients who are physically inactive, have one or more chronic diseases (hypertension, heart failure, diabetes mellitus), or have lifestyle habits (smoking and diet) that contribute to atherosclerosis. Atherosclerotic changes related to aging predispose the heart to poor blood perfusion and oxygen delivery. Ⓖ
- Incidence of cardiac disease increases with age, especially in the presence of hypertension, diabetes mellitus, hypercholesterolemia, elevated homocysteine, and highly sensitive C-reactive protein (HS-CRP).

EXPECTED FINDINGS

- Anxiety, feeling of impending doom
- Chest pain: substernal or precordial
  - Can radiate down the shoulder or arm
  - Can present as jaw pain
  - Can be described as a crushing or aching pressure
- Nausea
- Dizziness

PHYSICAL FINDINGS
- Pallor and cool, clammy skin
- Tachycardia and heart palpitations
- Tachypnea and dyspnea (shortness of breath)
- Diaphoresis
- Vomiting
- Decreased level of consciousness
- Possible dysrhythmias

LABORATORY TESTS

Cardiac enzymes released with cardiac muscle injury
- **Myoglobin:** Earliest marker of injury to cardiac or skeletal muscle. Levels no longer evident after 24 hr.
- **Creatinine kinase-MB:** Peaks around 24 hr after onset of chest pain. Levels no longer evident after 3 days.
- **Troponin I or T:** Any positive value indicates damage to cardiac tissue and should be reported.
  - **Troponin I:** Levels no longer evident after 7 to 10 days.
  - **Troponin T:** Levels no longer evident after 10 to 14 days.

DIAGNOSTIC PROCEDURES

Refer to **CHAPTER 24: CARDIOVASCULAR DIAGNOSTIC AND THERAPEUTIC PROCEDURES**.

Electrocardiogram (ECG)

Recording of electrical activity of the heart over time

NURSING ACTIONS
- Identify changes on serial ECGs.
- Angina: ST depression and/or T-wave flattening or inversion indicates presence of ischemia.
- MI: T-wave inversion indicates ischemia; ST-segment elevation indicates injury; abnormal Q-wave indicates necrosis.

Stress test

Also known as exercise electrocardiography. Client tolerance of activity is tested using a treadmill, bicycle, or medication to evaluate response to increased heart rate.

Thallium scan

Assesses for ischemia or necrosis. Radioisotopes cannot reach areas with decreased or absent perfusion, and the areas appear as "cold spots."

CLIENT EDUCATION: Avoid smoking and consuming caffeinated beverages 4 hr prior to the procedure. These can affect the test.

Cardiac catheterization

- A coronary angiogram, also called a cardiac catheterization, is an invasive diagnostic procedure used to evaluate the presence and degree of coronary artery blockage.
- Angiography involves the insertion of a catheter into a femoral (sometimes a brachial) vessel and threading it into the right or left side of the heart. Coronary artery narrowing and occlusions are identified by the injection of contrast media under fluoroscopy.

NURSING ACTIONS
- Ensure the client understands the procedure prior to signing informed consent. Qpcc
- Ensure that the client remains NPO 8 hr prior to procedure.
- Ensure that the client and family understand the procedure.
- Check for iodine/shellfish allergy (contrast media).

MI CLASSIFICATION

MIs are classified based on the following.
- Affected area of the heart: anterior, lateral, inferior, or posterior
- ECG changes produced: ST elevation myocardial infarction vs. non–ST elevation myocardial infarction
- Time frame within the progression of the infarction: acute, evolving, old

PATIENT-CENTERED CARE

NURSING CARE

- Monitor the following.
  - Vital signs every 5 min until stable, then every hour
  - Skin color, temperature, and moisture; capillary refill; oxygen saturation levels
  - Serial ECG, continuous cardiac monitoring
  - Location, precipitating factors, severity, quality, and duration of pain
  - Hourly urine output: greater than 30 mL/hr indicates adequate kidney perfusion
  - Laboratory data: cardiac enzymes, electrolytes, ABGs
- Administer oxygen 2 to 4 L/min.
- Obtain and maintain IV access.
- Promote energy conservation. Cluster nursing interventions for uninterrupted rest periods.

27.3 Distinguishing characteristics

Stable angina

Precipitated by exertion or stress

Relieved by rest or nitroglycerin

Manifestations last less than 15 min

Not associated with nausea, epigastric distress, dyspnea, anxiety, diaphoresis

Myocardial infarction

Can occur without cause, often in the morning after rest

Pain is relieved only by opioids; not relieved by rest or NTG

Manifestations last more than 20 min

Associated with nausea, epigastric distress, dyspnea, anxiety, diaphoresis

---

MEDICATIONS

Vasodilators

Nitroglycerin prevents coronary artery vasospasm and reduces preload and afterload, decreasing myocardial oxygen demand and increases blood flow to the ischemic heart muscle.
- Used to treat angina and help control blood pressure.
- Used cautiously with other antihypertensive medications.
- Can cause orthostatic hypotension.

CLIENT EDUCATION FOR CHEST PAIN
- Stop activity and rest.
- Place a nitroglycerin tablet under the tongue to dissolve (quick absorption).
- If pain is unrelieved in 5 min, call 911 or be driven to an emergency department.
- The client can take up to two more doses of nitroglycerin at 5-min intervals.
- A headache is a common adverse effect of this medication.
- Change positions slowly.

Analgesics

Morphine sulfate is an opioid analgesic used to treat moderate to severe pain. Analgesics act on the mu and kappa receptors that help alleviate pain. Activation of these receptors produces analgesia (pain relief), respiratory depression, euphoria, sedation, and decreases in myocardial oxygen consumption and gastrointestinal (GI) motility.

> ! Use cautiously with clients who have asthma or emphysema due to the risk of respiratory depression.

NURSING ACTIONS
- For the client having chest pain, monitor pain every 5 to 15 min.
- Watch for manifestations of respiratory depression, especially in older adults. If respirations are 12/min or less, stop medication and notify the provider immediately. ©
- Monitor vital signs for hypotension and decreased respirations.
- Check for nausea and vomiting.

CLIENT EDUCATION

- If nausea and vomiting persist, notify a nurse.
- Use the PCA pump, if applicable. The client is the only person who should push the medication administration button. The safety lockout mechanism on the PCA pump prevents overdosing of the medication.

Beta blockers

- Metoprolol has antidysrhythmic and antihypertensive properties that decrease the imbalance between myocardial oxygen supply and demand by reducing afterload and slowing heart rate.
- In an acute MI, beta blockers decrease infarct size and improve short- and long-term survival rates.

NURSING ACTIONS

- Beta blockers can cause bradycardia and hypotension. Hold the medication if the apical pulse rate is less than 60/min, and notify the provider. Qs
- Avoid giving to clients who have asthma. Cardioselective beta blockers (which affect only beta$_1$ receptors), such as metoprolol, are preferred because they minimize the effects on the respiratory system.
- Use with caution in clients who have heart failure.
- Monitor for decreased level of consciousness, crackles in the lungs, and chest discomfort.

CLIENT EDUCATION

- Change positions slowly.
- Notify the provider immediately of shortness of breath, edema, weight gain, cough or if heart rate drops below 60/min.

Thrombolytic agents

- Alteplase and reteplase are used to break up blood clots.
- Thrombolytic agents have similar adverse effects and contraindications as anticoagulants.
- For best results, give within 6 hr of infarction.

NURSING ACTIONS

- Monitor for contraindications (active bleeding, peptic ulcer disease, history of stroke, recent trauma).
- Monitor for effects of bleeding (mental status changes, hematuria).
- Monitor bleeding times: PT, aPTT, INR, fibrinogen levels, CBC.
- Monitor for the same adverse effects as anticoagulants (thrombocytopenia, anemia, hemorrhage).
- Ensure streptokinase is administered slowly to prevent hypotension.
- Remind the client of the risk for bruising and bleeding while on this medication.

Antiplatelet agents

- Aspirin and clopidogrel prevent platelets from forming together, which can produce arterial clotting.
- Aspirin prevents vasoconstriction. Due to this and antiplatelet effects, it should be administered with nitroglycerin at the onset of chest pain. It is given to clients with suspected MI in the emergency department. QEBP
- Antiplatelet agents can cause GI upset.

- Contraindicated in clients who have known bleeding disorders, history of stroke, uncontrolled hypertension, pregnancy, or recent trauma.
- Use cautiously with clients who have a history of GI ulcers.
- Tinnitus (ringing in the ears) can be a finding of aspirin toxicity.

NURSING ACTIONS: Remind the client of the risk for bruising and bleeding while on this medication.

CLIENT EDUCATION

- Use aspirin tablets with enteric coating and take with food.
- Report ringing in the ears.

Anticoagulants

Heparin and enoxaparin are used to prevent clots from becoming larger or other clots from forming.

NURSING ACTIONS

- Check for contraindications (active bleeding, peptic ulcer disease, history of stroke, recent trauma).
- Monitor platelet levels and bleeding times (PT, aPTT, INR, CBC).
- Monitor for adverse effects of anticoagulants (thrombocytopenia, anemia, hemorrhage).
- Remind the client of the risk for bruising and bleeding while on this medication.

Glycoprotein IIB/IIIA inhibitors

Eptifibatide is used to prevent binding of fibrinogen to platelets, in turn blocking platelet aggregation. In combination with aspirin therapy, IIB/IIIA inhibitors are standard therapy. This medication can cause active bleeding.

NURSING ACTIONS: Monitor platelet levels.

CLIENT EDUCATION: Report evidence of bleeding during medication therapy.

INTERPROFESSIONAL CARE

- Pain management services can be consulted if pain persists or is uncontrolled.
- Cardiac rehabilitation care can be consulted if the client has prolonged weakness and needs assistance with increasing level of activity.
- Nutritional services can be consulted for diet modification to promote food choices low in sodium and saturated fat.

THERAPEUTIC PROCEDURES

- Percutaneous transluminal coronary angioplasty (PTCA)
- Coronary artery bypass graft (CABG)

CLIENT EDUCATION

- Cardiac rehabilitation should be consulted for a specific exercise program related to the heart.
- Nutritional services, such as a dietitian, can be consulted for diet modification or weight management.

- Monitor and report indications of infection (fever, incisional drainage, redness).
- Avoid straining, strenuous exercise, or emotional stress when possible.
- Sexual activity can be restricted.
- Regarding response to chest pain, follow instructions on use of sublingual nitroglycerin.
- Quit smoking.
- Remain active and exercise regularly.

COMPLICATIONS

Acute MI

A complication of angina not relieved by rest or nitroglycerin

NURSING ACTIONS
- Administer oxygen.
- Notify the provider immediately.

Heart failure/cardiogenic shock

Injury to the left ventricle can lead to decreased cardiac output, impaired tissue perfusion, and heart failure. Progressive heart failure can lead to cardiogenic shock.
- This is a serious complication of pump failure, commonly following an MI of 40% blockage.
- Manifestations are those of impaired tissue perfusion: tachycardia; hypotension; low urinary output; decreased level of consciousness; respiratory distress (crackles, tachypnea); cool, clammy skin; decreased peripheral pulses; chest pain.

NURSING ACTIONS
- Administer oxygen. Intubation and ventilation can be required.
- Assist with the emergency management of the client.

Ventricular aneurysms/rupture

- Can be due to necrosis from MI and replacement of necrotic muscle with scar tissue
- Usually affects the left ventricle due to significantly greater work load
- Can present as sudden chest pain, dysrhythmias, and severe hypotension

NURSING ACTIONS
- Administer oxygen.
- Notify the provider immediately.

Dysrhythmias

- An inferior wall MI can lead to an injury to the AV node, resulting in bradycardia and second-degree AV heart block.
- An anterior wall MI can lead to an injury to the ventricle, resulting in premature ventricular contractions, bundle branch block, or complete heart block.

NURSING ACTIONS
- Monitor ECG and vital signs.
- Administer oxygen.
- Assist with administration of antidysrhythmic medications.
- Prepare for cardiac pacemaker if needed.

Application Exercises

1. A nurse is assisting with admission of a client who has a suspected myocardial infarction (MI) and a history of angina. Which of the following findings will help the nurse distinguish angina from an MI?

   A. Stable angina can be relieved with rest and nitroglycerin.

   B. The pain of an MI resolves in less than 15 min.

   C. The type of activity that causes an MI can be identified.

   D. Stable angina can occur for longer than 30 min.

2. A nurse is reviewing the laboratory findings of a client who has myocardial infarction (MI) and reports that dyspnea began 2 weeks ago. Which of the following cardiac enzymes would confirm the MI occurred 14 days ago?

   A. CK-MB

   B. Troponin I

   C. Troponin T

   D. Myoglobin

3. A nurse is assisting with the care of a client who asks why her provider prescribed a daily aspirin. Which of the following is an appropriate response by the nurse?

   A. "Aspirin reduces the formation of blood clots that could cause a heart attack."

   B. "Aspirin relieves the pain due to myocardial ischemia."

   C. "Aspirin dissolves clots that are forming in your coronary arteries."

   D. "Aspirin relieves headaches that are caused by other medications."

4. A nurse is reinforcing teaching with a client who has angina about a new prescription for metoprolol. Which of the following statements by the client indicates understanding of the teaching?

   A. "I should place the tablet under my tongue."

   B. "I should have my clotting time checked weekly."

   C. "I will report any ringing in my ears."

   D. "I will call my doctor if my pulse rate is less than 60."

5. A nurse is assisting with a community education program on recommended lifestyle changes to prevent angina and myocardial infarction. Which of the following changes should the nurse recommend be made first?

   A. Diet modification

   B. Relaxation exercises

   C. Tobacco cessation

   D. Exercise routine

PRACTICE Active Learning Scenario

A nurse is reinforcing teaching with a client who has new diagnosis of angina about coronary syndrome. What information should the nurse include in the teaching? Use the ATI Active Learning Template: System Disorder to complete this item.

RISK FACTORS: Describe five.

CLIENT EDUCATION: Describe at least two teaching points the nurse can use to help the client decrease his risk of having angina or an MI.

EXPECTED FINDINGS
- List five subjective findings.
- Describe four physical findings.

Application Exercises Key

1. A. **CORRECT:** Stable angina can be relieved by rest and nitroglycerin.

   B. Pain associated with an MI usually lasts longer than 20 min and requires opioid analgesics for relief.

   C. There is no specific type of activity that causes an MI. It can occur following rest.

   D. The pain of stable angina usually occurs for 15 min or less.

   Ⓝ *NCLEX® Connection: Physiological Adaptation, Basic Pathophysiology*

2. A. The creatinine kinase MB levels are no longer evident after 3 days.

   B. Troponin I levels are no longer evident after 7 to 10 days.

   C. **CORRECT:** The Troponin T level will still be evident 10 to 14 days following an MI.

   D. Myoglobin levels are no longer evident after 24 hr.

   Ⓝ *NCLEX® Connection: Reduction of Risk Potential, Laboratory Values*

3. A. **CORRECT:** Aspirin decreases platelet aggregation that can cause a myocardial infarction.

   B. One aspirin per day is not sufficient to alleviate ischemic pain.

   C. Aspirin does not dissolve clots.

   D. Aspirin can be taken on a PRN basis for analgesia. However, the provider prescribes a daily aspirin for a different therapeutic effect.

   Ⓝ *NCLEX® Connection: Pharmacological Therapies, Expected Actions/Outcomes*

4. A. Lopressor is administered orally, not sublingually.

   B. Lopressor does not affect bleeding or clotting time. The client should have CBC and blood glucose checked periodically.

   C. Ringing in the ears is not an adverse effect of the medication. Dry mouth and mucous membranes can occur.

   D. **CORRECT:** The client is advised to notify the provider if bradycardia (heart rate less than 60/min) occurs.

   Ⓝ *NCLEX® Connection: Pharmacological Therapies, Medication Administration*

5. A. The nurse should recommend changing the diet to decrease consumption of sodium and saturated fat. However, there is another change the client should make first.

   B. The nurse should recommend using relaxation exercise to cope with stress. However, there is another change the client should make first.

   C. **CORRECT:** According to the airway, breathing, and circulation (ABC) priority-setting framework, the first change the nurse should recommend is to stop using tobacco products. Nicotine causes vasoconstriction, elevates blood pressure, and narrows coronary arteries.

   D. The nurse should recommend an exercise routine to remain physically active. However, there is another change the client should make first.

   Ⓝ *NCLEX® Connection: Health Promotion and Maintenance, Lifestyle Choices*

PRACTICE Answer

Using the ATI Active Learning Template: System Disorder

RISK FACTORS
- Male or postmenopausal clients
- Sedentary lifestyle
- Hypertension
- Substance use (tobacco, cocaine, methamphetamine, excessive alcohol)
- Hyperlipidemia
- Obesity
- Metabolic disorders (diabetes mellitus, hyperthyroidism)
- Stress (with ineffective coping skills)

CLIENT EDUCATION
- Have routine cholesterol, blood pressure, and blood sugar screenings.
- Participate in regular physical activity for exercise and stress reduction.

EXPECTED FINDINGS
- Subjective findings: Feeling of impending doom; chest pain, pressure, or crushing radiating to the arm or jaw; nausea; dizziness; anxiety
- Physical findings: Pale, cool, clammy skin; tachycardia; tachypnea; diaphoresis

Ⓝ *NCLEX® Connection: Physiological Adaptation, Alterations in Body Systems*

CHAPTER 28 *Heart Failure and
Pulmonary Edema*

Heart failure occurs when the heart muscle is unable to pump effectively, resulting in inadequate cardiac output, myocardial hypertrophy, and pulmonary/systemic congestion. The heart is unable to maintain adequate circulation to meet tissue needs.

Heart failure is the result of an acute or chronic cardiopulmonary problem, such as systemic hypertension, myocardial infarction (MI), pulmonary hypertension, dysrhythmias, valvular heart disease, pericarditis, or cardiomyopathy. (28.1)

Pulmonary edema is a severe, life-threatening accumulation of fluid in the alveoli and interstitial spaces of the lung that can result from severe heart failure.

ACC and AHA staging heart failure

American College of Cardiology (ACC) and American Heart Association (AHA) developed evidence-based guidelines for staging and managing heart failure in comparison with the NYHA system.

A: High risk for developing heart failure without structural heart disease or clinical manifestations

B: Cardiac structural abnormalities or remodeling but no heart failure clinical manifestations

C: Current or prior clinical manifestations of heart failure

D: Refractory end-stage heart failure

Low-output heart failure

Low-output heart failure can initially occur on either side of the heart.
- Left-sided heart (ventricular) failure results in inadequate left ventricle (cardiac) output and consequently in inadequate tissue perfusion.
  - Systolic heart (ventricular) failure (ejection fraction below 40%, pulmonary and systemic congestion)
  - Diastolic heart (ventricular) failure (inadequate relaxation or "stiffening" prevents ventricular filling)
- Right-sided heart (ventricular) failure results in inadequate right ventricle output and systemic venous congestion (peripheral edema).

High-output heart failure

An uncommon form of heart failure is high-output failure, in which cardiac output is normal or above normal.

Heart failure

NYHA functional classification scale

The severity of heart failure is graded on the New York Heart Association's (NYHA) functional classification scale indicating the level of activity it takes to adversely affect the client (chest pain or shortness of breath).

CLASS I: Client exhibits no clinical manifestations with activity.

CLASS II: Client has clinical manifestations with ordinary exertion.

CLASS III: Client displays clinical manifestations with minimal exertion.

CLASS IV: Client has clinical manifestations at rest.

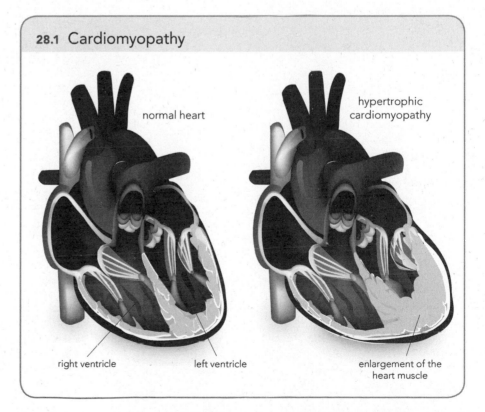

28.1 Cardiomyopathy

normal heart

hypertrophic cardiomyopathy

right ventricle

left ventricle

enlargement of the heart muscle

HEALTH PROMOTION AND DISEASE PREVENTION

- Maintain an exercise routine to remain physically active, and consult with the provider before starting any exercise regimen.
- Consume a diet low in sodium, along with fluid restrictions, and consult with the provider regarding diet specifications.
- Refrain from smoking.
- Follow medication regimen, and follow up with the provider as needed.

DATA COLLECTION

RISK FACTORS

- Systolic blood pressure is elevated in older adults, putting them at risk for coronary artery disease and heart failure. ⊜
- Some medications can increase the risk of heart failure or worsen manifestations in older adult clients.

Left-sided heart (ventricular) failure

- Hypertension
- Coronary artery disease, angina, MI
- Valvular disease (mitral and aortic)

Right-sided heart (ventricular) failure

- Left-sided heart (ventricular) failure
- Right ventricular MI
- Pulmonary problems (COPD, pulmonary fibrosis)

High-output heart failure

- Increased metabolic needs
- Septicemia (fever)
- Anemia
- Hyperthyroidism

Cardiomyopathy

- Coronary artery disease
- Infection or inflammation of the heart muscle
- Various cancer treatments
- Prolonged alcohol use
- Heredity

EXPECTED FINDINGS

The presence of other chronic illnesses (lung disease, kidney failure) can mask the presence of heart failure in older adult clients. ⊜

Left-sided failure

- Dyspnea, orthopnea (shortness of breath while lying down), nocturnal dyspnea
- Fatigue
- Displaced apical pulse (hypertrophy)
- S_3 heart sound (gallop)

- Pulmonary congestion (dyspnea, cough, bibasilar crackles)
- Frothy sputum (can be blood-tinged)
- Altered mental status
- Manifestations of organ failure, such as oliguria (decrease in urine output)

Right-sided failure

- Jugular vein distention
- Ascending dependent edema (legs, ankles, sacrum)
- Abdominal distention, ascites
- Fatigue, weakness
- Nausea and anorexia
- Polyuria at rest (nocturnal)
- Liver enlargement (hepatomegaly) and tenderness
- Weight gain

Cardiomyopathy (leading to heart failure)

Blood circulation to the lungs is impaired when the cardiac pump is compromised.

FOUR TYPES
- Dilated (most common)
- Hypertrophic
- Restrictive

MANIFESTATIONS
- Fatigue, weakness
- Heart failure (left with dilated type, right with restrictive type)
- Dysrhythmias (heart block)
- S_3 gallop
- Cardiomegaly (enlarged heart), more severe with dilated type
- Angina (hypertrophic type)

LABORATORY TESTS

B-type natriuretic peptides (BNP)

In clients who have dyspnea, elevated BNP confirms a diagnosis of heart failure rather than a problem originating in the respiratory system. BNP levels direct the aggressiveness of treatment interventions.
- Less than 100 pg/mL indicates no heart failure.
- Greater than 100 pg/mL suggests heart failure is present.

DIAGNOSTIC PROCEDURES

Hemodynamic monitoring

- Heart failure generally results in increased central venous pressure, increased pulmonary wedge pressure, increased pulmonary artery pressure, and decreased cardiac output. See **CHAPTER 26: INVASIVE CARDIOVASCULAR PROCEDURES** for detailed information related to hemodynamic monitoring.
- Mixed venous oxygen saturation (SvO_2) is directly related to cardiac output. A drop in SvO_2 indicates worsening cardiac function.

Ultrasound

Two-or three-dimensional ultrasound (also called cardiac ultrasound or echocardiogram) is used to measure the systolic and diastolic functioning of the heart.

Left ventricular ejection fraction (EF): The volume of blood pumped from the left ventricle into the arteries upon each beat. Expected reference range is 55% to 70%. An EF of 40% or less indicates heart failure.

Right ventricular EF: The volume of blood pumped from the right ventricle to the lungs upon each beat. Expected reference range is 45% to 60%.

Transesophageal echocardiography (TEE)

Uses a transducer placed in the esophagus behind the heart to obtain a detailed view of cardiac structures. The nurse prepares the client for a TEE in the same manner as for an upper endoscopy.

Chest x-ray

Can reveal cardiomegaly and pleural effusions.

ECG, cardiac enzymes, electrolytes, and ABGs

Electrocardiogram (ECG), cardiac enzymes, electrolytes, and ABGs are used to assess factors contributing to heart failure and the impact of heart failure.

PATIENT-CENTERED CARE

NURSING CARE

- Monitor daily weight and I&O.
- Monitor for shortness of breath and dyspnea on exertion.
- Administer oxygen as prescribed.
- Monitor vital signs and hemodynamic pressures.
- Position the client to maximize ventilation (high-Fowler's).
- Check ABGs, electrolytes (especially potassium if on diuretics), SaO₂, and chest x-ray findings.
- Monitor for findings of medication toxicity (digoxin toxicity).
- Encourage bed rest until the client is stable.
- Encourage energy conservation by assisting with care and ADLs.
- Maintain dietary restrictions as prescribed (restricted fluid intake, restricted sodium intake).
- Provide emotional support to the client and family.

MEDICATIONS

Herbal medications can stimulate the cardiovascular system. Obtain a list of herbal supplements the client takes, and advise the client of potential contraindications. Q_{EBP}

Diuretics

Diuretics are used to decrease preload.

Loop diuretics (furosemide, bumetanide)

Thiazide diuretics, such as hydrochlorothiazide

Potassium-sparing diuretics, such as spironolactone

Loop and thiazide diuretics can cause hypokalemia, and potassium supplementation can be required.

CLIENT EDUCATION: When taking loop or thiazide diuretics, ingest foods and drinks that are high in potassium to counter the effects of hypokalemia. Q_S

Afterload-reducing agents

Afterload-reducing agents help the heart pump more easily by altering the resistance to contraction. These are contraindicated for clients who have kidney impairment.

Angiotensin-converting enzyme (ACE) inhibitors (enalapril, captopril)

Angiotensin receptor II blockers (losartan)

Calcium channel blockers (diltiazem, nifedipine)

Phosphodiesterase-3 inhibitors (milrinone)

NURSING ACTIONS
- Monitor clients taking ACE inhibitors for hypotension following the initial dose.
- ACE inhibitors can cause angioedema (swelling of the tongue and throat), decreased sense of taste, or skin rash.
- Monitor for increased levels of potassium.

CLIENT EDUCATION (ACE INHIBITORS)
- This medication can cause a dry cough.
- Notify the provider if a rash or a decreased sense of taste develops.
- Notify the provider if swelling of the face or extremities occurs.
- Blood pressure needs to be monitored for 2 hr after the initial dose to detect hypotension.

Inotropic agents

Inotropic agents (digoxin, dopamine, dobutamine, milrinone) are used to increase contractility and thereby improve cardiac output.

NURSING ACTIONS
- For a client taking digoxin, take the apical heart rate for 1 min. Hold the medication if apical pulse is less than 60/min, and notify the provider.
- Observe for nausea and vomiting.
- Dopamine, dobutamine, and milrinone are administered via IV by an RN. The ECG, blood pressure, and urine output must be closely monitored.

CLIENT EDUCATION
Clients who are self-administering digoxin should:
- Count pulse for 1 min before taking the medication. If the pulse rate is irregular or outside the limitations set by the provider (usually less than 60/min or greater than 100/min), hold the dose and contact the provider. Qs
- Take the digoxin dose at the same time each day.
- Do not take digoxin at the same time as antacids. Separate the two medications by at least 2 hr.
- Report indications of toxicity, including fatigue, muscle weakness, confusion, and loss of appetite.
- Regularly have digoxin and potassium levels checked.

Beta adrenergic blockers (beta blockers)

Medications such as atenolol and metoprolol can be used to improve the condition of the client who has sustained increased levels of sympathetic stimulation and catecholamines. This includes clients who have chronic heart failure.

NURSING ACTIONS
- Monitor blood pressure, pulse, activity tolerance, and orthopnea.
- Check orthostatic blood pressure readings.

CLIENT EDUCATION
- Weigh daily.
- Regularly check blood pressure.
- Follow the provider's instructions for increasing medication dosage.

Vasodilators

Nitroglycerin and isosorbide prevent coronary artery vasospasm and reduce preload and afterload, decreasing myocardial oxygen demand.
- Vasodilators are given to treat angina and help control blood pressure.
- Use cautiously with other antihypertensive mediations.
- Vasodilators can cause orthostatic hypotension.

CLIENT EDUCATION
- A headache is a common adverse effect of this medication.
- Sit and lie down slowly.

Human B-type natriuretic peptides

hBNPs, such as nesiritide, are used to treat acute heart failure by causing natriuresis (loss of sodium and vasodilation). They are administered via IV by an RN.
- hBNPs can cause hypotension, as well as a number of cardiac effects, including ventricular tachycardia and bradycardia.
- BNP levels will increase while on this medication.

NURSING ACTIONS: Monitor ECG, blood pressure, and other parameters.

CLIENT EDUCATION
- The client can experience low blood pressure without associated manifestations.
- Sit and lie down slowly.

Anticoagulants

Anticoagulants, such as warfarin, can be prescribed if the client has a history of thrombus formation.

NURSING ACTIONS
- Monitor for contraindications (active bleeding, peptic ulcer disease, history of cerebrovascular accident, recent trauma).
- Monitor bleeding times (PT, aPTT, INR, CBC).

CLIENT EDUCATION
- There is a risk for bruising and bleeding while on this medication.
- Have blood monitored routinely to check bleeding times.

INTERPROFESSIONAL CARE

Cardiology and pulmonary services should be consulted to manage heart failure.

Respiratory services should be consulted for inhalers, breathing treatments, and suctioning for airway management.

Cardiac rehabilitation services can be consulted if the client has prolonged weakness and needs assistance with increasing level of activity.

Nutritional services can be consulted for diet modification to promote low-sodium, low-saturated fat food choices.

THERAPEUTIC PROCEDURES

Ventricular assist device (VAD)

A VAD is a mechanical pump that assists a heart that is too weak to pump blood through the body. It is used in clients who are eligible for heart transplants and are awaiting a heart transplant or those who have severe end-stage heart failure and are not candidates for heart transplants. Heart transplantation is the treatment of choice for clients who have severe dilated cardiomyopathy.

NURSING ACTIONS
- Prepare the client for the procedure (NPO status, informed consent).
- Monitor postoperatively: vital signs, SaO_2, incision drainage, pain management.

Heart transplantation

- Heart transplantation is a possible option for clients who have end-stage heart failure. Immunosuppressant therapy is required post-transplantation to prevent rejection.
- Eligibility for transplantation depends on several factors, including life expectancy, age, psychosocial status, and absence of drug and alcohol use disorders.

NURSING ACTIONS
- Prepare the client for the procedure (NPO status and informed consent). Laboratory reports and results of diagnostic testing should be available as prescribed.
- Monitor postoperatively: vital signs, SaO₂, incision drainage, pain management.
- Monitor for complications. Organ transplant recipients are at risk for infection, thrombosis, and rejection.

CLIENT EDUCATION
- Take medications as prescribed.
- Take diuretics in the early morning and early afternoon.
- Maintain fluid and sodium restriction: a dietary consult can be useful.
- Increase dietary intake of potassium (cantaloupe, bananas) if the client is taking potassium-losing diuretics, such as loop and thiazide diuretics.
- Check weight daily at the same time, and notify the provider for a weight gain of 2 lb in 24 hr or 5 lb in 1 week.
- Schedule regular follow-up visits with the provider.
- Get vaccinations (pneumococcal and yearly influenza vaccines).

COMPLICATIONS

Acute pulmonary edema

A life-threatening medical emergency

EXPECTED FINDINGS: Anxiety, tachycardia, acute respiratory distress, dyspnea at rest, change in level of consciousness, ascending fluid level within lungs (crackles, cough productive of frothy, blood-tinged sputum).

NURSING ACTIONS
- Administer medications to improve cardiac output.
- Instruct the client about measures to improve tolerance to activity, such as alternating periods of activity with periods of rest.
- Prompt response to this emergency includes the following.
  - Positioning the client in high-Fowler's position
  - Administration of oxygen, positive airway pressure, and/or intubation and mechanical ventilation
  - Administration of IV morphine (to decrease anxiety, respiratory distress, and venous return)
  - IV administration of rapid-acting loop diuretics, such as furosemide
  - Effective intervention should result in diuresis (carefully monitor output), reduction in respiratory distress, improved lung sounds, and adequate oxygenation.

Cardiogenic shock

This is a serious complication of pump failure that occurs commonly following an MI and injury to greater than 40% of the left ventricle.

EXPECTED FINDINGS: Tachycardia; hypotension; diminished urinary output; altered level of consciousness; respiratory distress (crackles, tachypnea); cool, clammy skin; decreased peripheral pulses; chest pain

NURSING ACTIONS
- Monitor breath sounds. Monitor for crackles or wheezing.
- Monitor heart sounds.
- Prompt response to this emergency includes the following.
  - Administration of oxygen, intubation, and mechanical ventilation can be required.
  - Administration of IV morphine, diuretics, or nitroglycerin to decrease preload.
  - Administration of IV vasopressors and/or positive inotropes to increase cardiac output and maintain organ perfusion.
  - Continuous hemodynamic monitoring.

Pericardial tamponade

Cardiac tamponade can result from fluid accumulation in the pericardial sac.

EXPECTED FINDINGS: Hypotension, jugular venous distention, muffled heart sounds, paradoxical pulse (variance of 10 mm Hg or more in systolic blood pressure between expiration and inspiration)

NURSING ACTIONS: Notify the provider immediately.

Pulmonary edema

Cardiogenic factors are the most common cause of pulmonary edema. It is a complication of various heart and lung diseases and usually occurs from increased pulmonary vascular pressure secondary to severe cardiac dysfunction.

Noncardiac pulmonary edema can occur due to acute glomerulonephritis, inhalation of irritating gases, rapid administration of IV fluids, and acute respiratory distress syndrome.

Neurogenic pulmonary edema develops following a head injury.

OLDER ADULTS: Increased risk for pulmonary edema occurs related to decreased cardiac output and heart failure ©
- Increased risk for fluid and electrolyte imbalances occurs when the older adult client receives treatment with diuretics.
- IV infusions must be administered at a slower rate to prevent circulatory overload.

HEALTH PROMOTION AND DISEASE PREVENTION

- Maintain an exercise routine to remain physically active, and consult with the provider before starting any exercise regimen.
- Consume a diet low in sodium along with fluid restrictions, and consult with the provider regarding diet specifications.
- Refrain from smoking.
- Follow medication regimen, and follow up with the provider as needed.

DATA COLLECTION

RISK FACTORS

- Acute MI Q EBP
- Fluid volume overload
- Hypertension
- Valvular heart disease
- Postpneumonectomy
- Postevacuation of pleural effusion
- Acute respiratory failure
- Left-sided heart failure
- Acute glomerulonephritis
- Trauma
- Sepsis
- Drug overdose

EXPECTED FINDINGS

- Anxiety
- Inability to sleep
- Persistent cough with pink, frothy sputum (cardinal finding)
- Tachypnea, dyspnea, and orthopnea
- Hypoxemia (SaO_2 expected reference range greater than 95%)
- Cyanosis (later stage)
- Crackles
- Tachycardia
- Reduced urine output
- Confusion, stupor

PATIENT-CENTERED CARE

NURSING CARE

- Monitor vital signs every 15 min until stable.
- Monitor I&O.
- Check ABGs, electrolytes (especially potassium if on diuretics), SaO_2, and chest x-ray findings.
- Maintain a patent airway. Suction as needed.
- Position the client in high-Fowler's position with feet and legs dependent or sitting on the side of the bed to decrease preload.
- Administer oxygen using a high-flow rebreather mask. Continuous positive airway pressure or intubation/ventilation can become necessary. Be prepared to intervene quickly.
- Restrict fluid intake (slow or discontinue infusing IV fluids).
- Monitor hourly urine output. Watch for intake greater than output, or urine less than 30 mL/hr.
- Provide emotional support for the client and family.
- Instruct the client on effective breathing techniques.
- Instruct the client on medications.

MEDICATIONS

Rapid-acting diuretics (furosemide, bumetanide) promote fluid excretion.

Morphine decreases sympathetic nervous system response and anxiety and promotes mild vasodilation.

Vasodilators (nitroglycerin, sodium nitroprusside) decrease preload and afterload.

Inotropic agents (digoxin, dobutamine) improve cardiac output.

Antihypertensives (ACE inhibitors, beta blockers) decrease afterload.

CLIENT EDUCATION

- Continue to take medications even if feeling better.
- Report manifestations of adverse effects of medications to the provider.
- Consume a low-sodium diet and restrict fluid intake.
- Measure weight daily at the same time. Notify the provider of a gain of more than 2 lb in 1 day or 5 lb in 1 week.
- Report swelling of feet or ankles or any shortness of breath or angina.

Application Exercises

1. A nurse is caring for a client who has heart failure and reports increased shortness of breath. The nurse increases the client's oxygen per protocol. Which of the following actions should the nurse take first?

   A. Weigh the client.

   B. Assist the client into high-Fowler's position.

   C. Auscultate lungs sounds.

   D. Check oxygen saturation with pulse oximeter.

2. A nurse is reinforcing teaching with a client who has heart failure about the need to limit sodium in the diet to 2,000 mg daily. Which of the following foods should the nurse recommend for the client? (Select all that apply.)

   A. 1 slice cheddar cheese

   B. 1 medium beef hot dog

   C. 3 oz Atlantic salmon

   D. 3 oz roasted chicken breast

   E. 2 oz lean baked ham

3. A nurse is assisting with the admission data collection of a client who has suspected pulmonary edema. Which of the following manifestation are expected findings? (Select all that apply.)

   A. Tachypnea

   B. Persistent cough

   C. Increased urinary output

   D. Thick yellow sputum

   E. Orthopnea

4. A nurse is reinforcing discharge teaching with a client who has heart failure and is encouraged to increase potassium in his diet. Which of the following food selections should the nurse include as having the highest source of potassium?

   A. 1 medium apple

   B. 1 medium baked potato

   C. 1 slice toast with 1 tbsp peanut butter

   D. 1 large scrambled egg

5. A nurse is reinforcing discharge teaching with a client who has heart failure and a fluid restriction of 2,000 mL/day. The client asks the nurse how to determine the amount of fluids he is allowed. Which of the following statements is an appropriate response by the nurse?

   A. "Pour the amount of fluid you drink into an empty 2-liter bottle to keep track of how much you drink."

   B. "Each glass contains 8 ounces. There are 30 milliliters per ounce, so you can have a total of 8 glasses or cups of fluid each day."

   C. "This is the same as 2 quarts, or about the same as two pots of coffee."

   D. "Take sips of water or ice chips so you will not take in too much fluid."

PRACTICE Active Learning Scenario

A nurse is assisting with a presentation about heart failure to a group of clients. What should the nurse include in this presentation? Use the ATI Active Learning Template: System Disorder to complete this item.

ALTERATION IN HEALTH (DIAGNOSIS): Describe the difference between left- and right-sided heart failure.

LABORATORY TESTS: Describe one and its importance.

DIAGNOSTIC PROCEDURES: Describe two.

MEDICATIONS: Describe two groups of medications and an example of one medication for each group.

Application Exercises Key

1. A. Weighing the client can provide the nurse with information about possible fluid retention. However, another action is the priority

   B. **CORRECT:** Using the airway, breathing, and circulation (ABC) priority approach to client care, the first action the nurse should take is to assist the client into high-Fowler's position. This opens the client's airway for maximum use of lung space and muscles associated with breathing, decreases venous return to the heart (preload), and helps relieve lung congestion.

   C. Auscultating lung sounds can provide the nurse with information about the client's breathing pattern. However, another action is the priority.

   D. Checking oxygen saturation will provide the nurse with data to adjust oxygen therapy. However, another action is the priority.

   Ⓝ *NCLEX® Connection: Physiological Adaptation, Alterations in Body Systems*

2. A. **CORRECT:** One slice cheddar cheese contains 180 mg sodium.

   B. A medium beef hot dog contains 557 mg sodium. Foods should be less than 300 mg per serving for a 2,000 mg sodium-restricted diet.

   C. **CORRECT:** Three ounces Atlantic salmon contains 37 mg sodium.

   D. **CORRECT:** Three ounces roasted chicken breast contains 62 mg sodium.

   E. Two ounces lean baked ham contains 782 mg sodium.

   Ⓝ *NCLEX® Connection: Basic Care and Comfort, Nutrition and Oral Hydration*

3. A. **CORRECT:** Tachypnea is an expected finding in a client who has pulmonary edema.

   B. **CORRECT:** A persistent cough with pink, frothy sputum is an expected finding in a client who has pulmonary edema.

   C. Decreased urinary output is an expected finding in a client who has pulmonary edema.

   D. Pink, frothy sputum is an expected finding in a client who has pulmonary edema.

   E. **CORRECT:** Orthopnea is an expected finding in a client who has pulmonary edema.

   Ⓝ *NCLEX® Connection: Physiological Adaptation, Basic Pathophysiology*

4. A. One medium apple contains 195 mg potassium. The nurse should recommend a different food because another choice contains more potassium.

   B. **CORRECT:** A medium baked potato is the best food source of potassium because it contains 926 mg potassium per serving.

   C. One slice toast with 1 tbsp peanut butter contains 148 mg potassium per serving. The nurse should recommend a different food because another choice contains more potassium.

   D. One large egg scrambled contains 81 mg potassium per serving. The nurse should recommend a different food because another choice contains more potassium.

   Ⓝ *NCLEX® Connection: Basic Care and Comfort, Nutrition and Oral Hydration*

5. A. **CORRECT:** Pouring the amount of fluid consumed into an empty 2 L bottle provides a visual guide for the client as to the amount consumed and how to plan daily intake.

   B. Glasses and cups vary in size and can contain more than 8 oz.

   C. Offering a vague frame of reference does not assist with accurate fluid measurement.

   D. Suggesting that the client take sips of water or ice chips does not assist with accurate fluid measurement.

   Ⓝ *NCLEX® Connection: Basic Care and Comfort, Nutrition and Oral Hydration*

PRACTICE Answer

Using the ATI Active Learning Template: System Disorder

ALTERATION IN HEALTH (DIAGNOSIS):
Left-sided heart failure results in inadequate output from the left ventricle, leading to poor tissue perfusion. Systolic failure includes an ejection fraction less than 40% with pulmonary and systemic congestion. Diastolic failure includes stiffening or inadequate relaxation of the ventricle. Right-sided heart failure results in inadequate output from the right ventricle, leading to systemic venous congestion and peripheral edema.

LABORATORY TESTS: B-type natriuretic peptides (BNP) confirms a diagnosis of heart failure.

DIAGNOSTIC PROCEDURES
• Hemodynamic monitoring
• Ultrasound
• Chest x-ray
• Electrocardiogram

MEDICATIONS
• Diuretics: furosemide, bumetanide, hydrochlorothiazide, spironolactone
• Afterload-reducing agents: enalapril, captopril, losartan, diltiazem, nifedipine, milrinone

Ⓝ *NCLEX® Connection: Physiological Adaptation, Alterations in Body Systems*

CHAPTER 29

Valvular Heart Disease and Inflammatory Disorders

Valvular heart disease and inflammatory conditions of the heart (pericarditis, myocarditis, rheumatic endocarditis, infective endocarditis) can result in dysfunction that affects clients' ability to meet tissue and oxygen demands.

Valvular Heart Disease

Valvular heart disease describes an abnormality or dysfunction of any of the heart's four valves: mitral and aortic (left side), tricuspid (rare, can occur as a result of endocarditis or IV drug use), and pulmonic (right side). It affects the efficiency of the heart as a pump and reduces stroke volume. Over time, there can be remodeling of the heart itself (hypertrophy), heart failure, and pulmonary complications.

With age, fibrotic thickening occurs in the mitral and aortic valves. The aorta is stiffer in older adult clients, increasing systolic blood pressure and stress on the mitral valve. **(29.1)** Ⓖ

HEALTH PROMOTION AND DISEASE PREVENTION

- Prevent and treat bacterial infections.
- Encourage clients to consume a diet low in sodium and to follow prescribed fluid restrictions to prevent heart failure.
- Control chronic illnesses (diabetes mellitus, hypertension, hypercholesterolemia, metabolic syndrome).
- Encourage increased activity and exercise to boost low-density lipoprotein (LDL) levels.

DATA COLLECTION

- Valvular heart disease is classified as:
  - **Stenosis:** Narrowed opening when valve leaflets fuse together that impedes blood moving forward.
  - **Insufficiency/Improper closure:** Some blood flows backward (regurgitation).
- Valvular heart disease can have congenital or acquired causes.
  - **Congenital** valvular heart disease can affect all four valves and cause either stenosis or insufficiency.
  - **Acquired** valvular heart disease is classified as one of three types.
    - **Degenerative disease:** Due to damage over time from mechanical stress, atherosclerosis, and hypertension. Most common in developed countries.
    - **Rheumatic disease:** Gradual fibrotic changes, calcification of valve cusps. Most common in developing countries.
    - **Infective endocarditis:** Infectious organisms destroy the valve. Streptococcal infections are a common cause.

RISK FACTORS

- Hypertension
- Rheumatic fever (mitral stenosis and insufficiency)
- Infective endocarditis
- Congenital malformations
- Marfan syndrome (connective tissue disorder that affects the heart and other areas of the body)
- In older adult clients, the predominant causes of valvular heart disease are degenerative calcification and atherosclerosis, papillary muscle dysfunction, and infective endocarditis. Ⓖ

EXPECTED FINDINGS

- Clients who have valvular heart disease often do not experience manifestations until late in the progression of the disease.
- A murmur is heard with turbulent blood flow. The location of the murmur and timing (diastolic versus systolic) help determine the valve involved. Murmurs are graded on a scale of I (very faint) to VI (extremely loud).
- Left-sided valve damage causes increased pulmonary artery pressure, left ventricular hypertrophy, and decreased cardiac output, resulting in orthopnea, paroxysmal nocturnal dyspnea (PND), pulmonary edema (congestion), and fatigue. **(29.2)**

DIAGNOSTIC PROCEDURES

Chest x-ray shows chamber enlargement (with stenosis and insufficiencies) and pulmonary congestion (with aortic stenosis).

12-lead electrocardiogram (ECG) shows chamber hypertrophy.

Echocardiogram shows chamber size, hypertrophy, specific valve dysfunction, ejection function, and amount of regurgitant flow.

Transesophageal echocardiography (TEE) provides a more direct view of the heart without the interference of chest wall structures.

Exercise tolerance testing/stress echocardiography is used to determine the effect of the valve problem on cardiac functioning during stress.

Radionuclide studies determine ejection fraction during activity and rest.

Angiography is used to evaluate the coronary arteries and the degree of atherosclerosis.

Cardiac catheterization can be used as a diagnostic tool in valvular disease; often combined with angiography.

PATIENT-CENTERED CARE

NURSING CARE

- Monitor weight and note recent changes.
- Monitor vital signs and report changes.
- Monitor heart rhythm (can be irregular or bradycardic; check for murmur).
- Administer oxygen and medications.
- Maintain fluid and sodium restrictions.
- Monitor I&O.
- Assist the client to conserve energy.

MEDICATIONS

Diuretics

Diuretics are used to treat heart failure by removing excessive extracellular fluid.
- Loop diuretics (furosemide)
- Thiazide diuretics (hydrochlorothiazide)
- Potassium-sparing diuretics (spironolactone)

Loop and thiazide diuretics can cause hypokalemia, and a potassium supplement might be required.

CLIENT EDUCATION: If taking loop or thiazide diuretics, ingest foods (dried fruits, nuts, spinach, citrus fruits, bananas, potatoes) and drinks that are high in potassium to counter hypokalemia effect.

Afterload-reducing agents

Afterload-reducing agents help the heart pump more easily by altering the resistance to contraction.
- Angiotensin-converting enzyme (ACE) inhibitors (enalapril, captopril, lisinopril)
- Angiotensin-receptor blockers (losartan, valsartan)
- Beta-blockers (metoprolol, carvedilol)
- Calcium-channel blockers (nifedipine, amlodipine)
- Vasodilators (isosorbide)

NURSING ACTIONS: Monitor clients taking ACE inhibitors for initial dose hypotension.

Inotropic agents

Inotropic agents, such as digoxin, are used to increase contractility and thereby improve cardiac output.

CLIENT EDUCATION
- Count pulse for 1 min before taking the medication. If the heart rate is irregular or outside of the limitations set by the provider (usually less than 60/min or greater than 100/min), hold the dose and contact the provider.
- Take the dose of digoxin at the same time every day.
- Do not take digoxin at the same time as antacids. Separate the two medications by at least 2 hr.
- Report manifestations of toxicity (fatigue, muscle weakness, confusion, visual changes, loss of appetite).

Anticoagulants

Anticoagulation therapy is used for clients who have a mechanical valve replacement, atrial fibrillation, or severe left ventricle dysfunction to reduce the risk of clot formation and emboli.

CLIENT EDUCATION: Employ measures that decrease the risk of bleeding and hemorrhage (avoid aspirin and NSAIDs, use soft-bristled toothbrush, use electric razor, clean skin gently).

THERAPEUTIC PROCEDURES

Postsurgery care is similar to coronary artery bypass surgery (care for sternal incision, activity limited for 6 weeks, report fever).

Percutaneous balloon valvuloplasty: This procedure can open aortic or mitral valves affected by stenosis. A catheter is inserted through the femoral artery and advanced to the heart. A balloon is inflated at the stenotic valve to open the fused commissures, enlarge the valve opening, and improve leaflet mobility.

Valve replacement: This procedure replaces damaged heart valves with mechanical, xenografts (from other species), allografts (from cadavers), or autografts (formed from the client's pulmonic valve and a portion of the pulmonary artery). It is often done with an open-heart approach, although minimally invasive surgery is also performed in some instances.
- Mechanical valves are more durable but require lifelong anticoagulant therapy.
- Tissue valves need to be replaced every 7 to 10 years.

Miscellaneous surgical management: Other surgeries used in the treatment of valvular disorders include chordae tendineae reconstruction, commissurotomy (relieve stenosis on leaflets), annuloplasty ring insertion (correct dilatation of valve annulus by narrowing the opening), and leaflet repair.

- Medical management is appropriate for many older adult clients; surgery is indicated when manifestations interfere with daily activities.
- The goal of surgery can be to improve the quality of life rather than to prolong life. Ⓒ

INTERPROFESSIONAL CARE

- Respiratory services for inhalers, breathing treatments, and suctioning for airway management
- Cardiology for cardiac management
- Nutritional services for weight loss or gain related to medications or diagnosis
- Rehabilitative care if the client has prolonged weakness and needs assistance with increasing level of activity

CLIENT EDUCATION

- Prophylactic antibiotic use is important before any invasive dental or respiratory procedure that might cause infection. Ⓠs
- Weigh daily and notify the provider of 3 lb (1.4 kg) gain in 1 day or 5 lb (2.3 kg) gain in 1 week.
- Coordinate activities with planned rest periods.
- Follow the prescribed exercise program.

- Disease management includes activity restrictions or lifestyle changes related to valve disease.
- Adhere to dietary restrictions, including avoidance of caffeine and alcohol. Consider nutritional consultation.
- Conserve energy.
- Clean open wounds carefully; antibiotic ointment may be used.
- Immediately report fever to the provider.
- Report petechial rash or shortness of breath to the provider.
- Read labels of over-the-counter medication to avoid those that include alcohol, ephedrine, or epinephrine (can cause dysrhythmias).
- Report heart failure manifestations to the provider immediately.

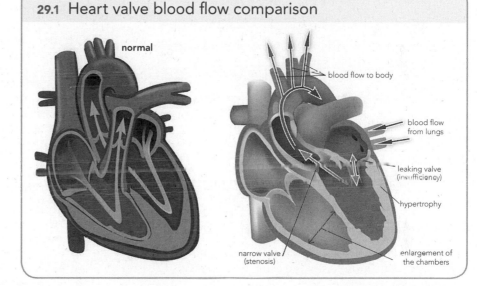

29.1 Heart valve blood flow comparison

normal

blood flow to body

blood flow from lungs

leaking valve (insufficiency)

hypertrophy

narrow valve (stenosis)

enlargement of the chambers

29.2 Left-sided valve damage

Mitral stenosis	Mitral insufficiency	Aortic stenosis	Aortic insufficiency
Apical diastolic murmur	Systolic murmur at the apex	Systolic murmur at second intercostal space, right of sternum	Diastolic murmur at third left intercostal space
Dyspnea on exertion	S_3 sounds	Dyspnea on exertion	Sinus tachycardia
Orthopnea	Fatigue and weakness	S_4 sounds	Exertional dyspnea
Atrial fibrillation	Atrial fibrillation	Angina	Pulmonary congestion
Palpitations	Dyspnea on exertion	Exertional syncope	Orthopnea
Fatigue, weakness	Orthopnea	Fatigue	Palpitations
Jugular venous distention	Atrial fibrillation	Orthopnea	Fatigue and weakness
Cyanosis	Atypical chest pain	PND	Nocturnal angina with diaphoresis
Pitting peripheral edema	Palpitations	Congestion	Widened pulse pressure
Hemoptysis	Jugular venous distention	Pulmonary edema	Bounding arterial pulse on palpation (Corrigan's pulse)
Dry cough	Pitting edema	Narrowed pulse pressure	Elevated systolic and diminished diastolic pressures
Repeated respiratory infections	Pulmonary congestion		PND
PND	Crackles in lungs		
Hepatomegaly	Possible diminished lung sounds		
	PND		
	Hepatomegaly		

COMPLICATIONS

Heart failure

- Heart failure is the inability of the heart to maintain adequate circulation to meet tissue needs for oxygen and nutrients. Ineffective valves result in heart failure.
- Monitoring the client's heart failure class (I to IV) is often the gauge for surgical intervention for valvular problems.

Inflammatory Disorders

Inflammation related to the heart is an extended inflammatory response resulting from an infection or an abnormal immune response that often leads to the destruction of healthy tissue. This primarily includes the layers of the heart.

Inflammatory disorders related to the cardiovascular system include pericarditis, myocarditis, rheumatic endocarditis, and infective endocarditis.

HEALTH PROMOTION AND DISEASE PREVENTION

- Early treatment of streptococcal infections can prevent rheumatic fever.
- Prophylactic treatments (including antibiotics for clients who have cardiac defects) can prevent infective endocarditis.
- Influenza and pneumonia immunizations are important for all clients (especially older adults) to decrease the incidence of myocarditis. Recommendations for immunizations change periodically. Check the CDC's website (www.cdc.gov) for current recommendations. ©

DATA COLLECTION

RISK FACTORS

- Congenital heart defect/cardiac anomalies
- IV substance use
- Invasive procedures or devices (dental procedures, indwelling catheters)
- Heart valve replacement
- Immunosuppression
- Rheumatic fever and other infections
- Long duration of streptococcus infection in school-age children
- Malnutrition
- Overcrowding
- Lower socioeconomic status

EXPECTED FINDINGS

Pericarditis: Inflammation of the pericardium
- Commonly follows a respiratory infection.
- Can be due to a myocardial infarction or following open-heart surgery.
- Findings include fever; chest pressure/pain aggravated by breathing (mainly inspiration), coughing, and swallowing; pericardial friction rub auscultated at left lower sternal border; shortness of breath; and relief of pain when sitting and leaning forward.

Myocarditis: Inflammation of the myocardium
- Can be due to a viral, fungal, or bacterial infection; an immune response; or a systemic inflammatory disease (Crohn's disease).
- Findings include fever, general malaise, arthralgias, tachycardia, murmur, pericardial friction rub auscultated in the lungs, cardiomegaly, chest pain, and dysrhythmias.

Rheumatic endocarditis: An infection of the endocardium due to a complication of rheumatic fever
- Preceded by group A beta-hemolytic streptococcal pharyngitis.
- Produces lesions or scars in the heart valves, causing deformity.
- Findings include fever, chest pain, joint pain, tachycardia, shortness of breath, rash on trunk and extremities, cardiac friction rub, murmur, and muscle spasms.

Infective endocarditis: Infection of the endocardium due to staphylococci, streptococci, fungi, or other infectious organisms
- Most common in clients who have structural cardiac malformations, cardiac devices (pacemaker), prosthetic heart valves, damaged cardiac tissue, or IV substance use disorder.
- Invasive procedures (dental procedures, body piercing, tattooing) can cause bacteremia, which can lead to infective endocarditis in at-risk clients.
- Untreated infections (UTI, respiratory infections)
- Findings include fever, flu-like manifestations, murmur, petechiae (on the trunk and mucous membranes), positive blood cultures, and splinter hemorrhages (red streaks under the nail beds).

Laboratory tests Q EBP

- Blood cultures detect a bacterial infection and direct the choice of antibiotic.
- An elevated WBC count can indicate bacterial infection.
- Cardiac enzymes can be elevated with pericarditis.
- Elevated ESR and CRP indicate inflammation in the body.
- Throat cultures detect a streptococcal infection, which can lead to rheumatic fever.

Inflammatory disorders

Electrocardiography (ECG) can detect a heart block, which is associated with rheumatic fever, or demonstrate ST segment elevation in almost all leads in the case of pericarditis.

Echocardiography can reveal inflamed heart layers or pericardial effusion.

Computed tomography (CT) scan or magnetic resonance imaging (MRI) can confirm pericardial effusion or thickening.

PATIENT-CENTERED CARE

NURSING CARE

- Collect data regarding heart sounds. Listen for murmur or friction rub.
- Review ABGs, SaO₂, and chest x-ray results.
- Administer oxygen.
- Monitor vital signs. Watch for fever.
- Monitor ECG, and notify the provider of changes.
- Monitor for cardiac tamponade and heart failure.
- Obtain throat cultures to identify bacteria to be treated by antibiotic therapy.
- Administer antibiotics and antipyretics.
- Determine onset, quality, duration, and severity of pain.
- Administer pain medication. Nonsteroidal anti-inflammatory drugs (NSAIDs) are often given on a regular schedule to reduce fever, inflammation, and pericardial pain.
- Encourage bed rest.
- Provide emotional support to the client and family, and encourage verbalization of feelings regarding the illness.

MEDICATIONS

Penicillin

Antibiotic to treat infection

NURSING ACTIONS
- Monitor for skin rash and hives.
- Monitor electrolyte and kidney levels.

CLIENT EDUCATION
- Report skin rash or hives.
- The medication can cause gastrointestinal (GI) distress.

Ibuprofen

NSAID to treat fever and inflammation

NURSING ACTIONS
- Do not use with clients who have peptic ulcer disease.
- Watch for indications of GI distress.
- Monitor platelets, and liver and kidney function levels.

CLIENT EDUCATION
- Take the medication with food.
- The medication can cause GI distress.
- Avoid alcohol consumption while taking the medication.

Prednisone

- Glucocorticosteroid given to treat inflammation in pericarditis not due to a bacterial infection
- Clients can have impaired wound healing when taking this medication.

NURSING ACTIONS
- Use in low doses.
- Monitor blood pressure.
- Monitor electrolytes and blood sugar levels.

CLIENT EDUCATION
- Take the medication with food.
- Avoid stopping the medication abruptly.
- Report unexpected weight gain.

Amphotericin B

Antifungal given to treat fungal infection

NURSING ACTIONS: Monitor liver and kidney function levels.

CLIENT EDUCATION: The medication can cause GI distress.

THERAPEUTIC PROCEDURES

Pericarditis

Pericardiocentesis is the insertion of a needle into the pericardium to aspirate pericardial fluid.
- This can be done in the emergency department or a procedure room and is guided by fluoroscopy or ECG.
- Pericardial fluid can be sent to the laboratory for culture and sensitivity.

NURSING ACTIONS: Monitor for reoccurrence of cardiac tamponade (drop in systolic blood pressure, decreased peripheral pulses, muffled heart sounds, distended neck veins).

Infective endocarditis

Valve debridement, draining of abscess, and repairing congenital cardiac problems are procedures involved with infective endocarditis.

NURSING ACTIONS: Monitor for indications of bleeding, infection, and alteration in cardiac output.

INTERPROFESSIONAL CARE

- Cardiology services can manage cardiac dysfunction.
- Infectious disease services can manage infection.
- Physical therapy can increase the client's level of activity once prescribed.

CLIENT EDUCATION

- Take rest periods as needed.
- Wash hands to prevent infection.
- Avoid crowded areas to reduce the risk of infection.
- Participate in cessation of tobacco use if applicable.
- Advise all providers, including dentists, of history of endocarditis so that antibiotic prophylaxis is prescribed if needed. Qs
- The importance of good oral hygiene and the prevention of infection.
- The importance of taking medications as prescribed.
- Demonstrate the administration of IV antibiotics and management before discharge.
- Express feelings about the illness.

CARE AFTER DISCHARGE

- Home health services can be indicated if the client had surgery. Qtc
- A home health service can give IV antibiotic therapy.
- Pharmaceutical services can be indicated for IV supplies and medications.
- Rehabilitation services can be indicated to help the client increase the level of activity.

COMPLICATIONS

Cardiac tamponade

Cardiac tamponade can result from fluid accumulation in the pericardial sac.

- Manifestations include dyspnea, dizziness, report of tightness in the chest, increasing restlessness, pulsus paradoxus (a decrease of 10 mm Hg or more in systolic blood pressure during inspiration), tachycardia, muffled heart sounds, and jugular venous distention.
- Hemodynamic monitoring reveals intracardiac and pulmonary artery pressures similar and elevated (plateau pressures).

NURSING ACTIONS: Notify the provider immediately.

Application Exercises

1. A nurse is reviewing the health record of a client who is being evaluated for possible valvular heart disease. Which of the following data are risk factors for this condition? (Select all that apply.)

   A. Surgical repair of an atrial septal defect at age 2

   B. Measles infection during childhood

   C. Hypertension for 5 years

   D. Weight gain of 10 lb in 1 year

   E. Diastolic murmur

2. A nurse is assisting with data collection from a client who has left-sided valvular heart disease. Which of the following findings should the nurse expect? (Select all that apply.)

   A. Dyspnea on exertion

   B. Client report of fatigue

   C. Bradycardia

   D. Pleural friction rub

   E. Peripheral edema

3. A nurse is collecting data from a client who has pericarditis. Which of the following findings should the nurse expect?

   A. Petechiae

   B. Murmur

   C. Rash

   D. Friction rub

4. A nurse is collecting data from a client who has splinter hemorrhages in the nail beds and reports a fever. The nurse should identify these findings as manifestations of which of the following disorders?

   A. Infective endocarditis

   B. Pericarditis

   C. Myocarditis

   D. Rheumatic endocarditis

5. A nurse is assisting with the admission of a client who has suspected rheumatic endocarditis. The nurse should expect a prescription for which of the following laboratory tests to assist in confirmation of this diagnosis?

   A. Arterial blood gases

   B. Serum albumin

   C. Liver enzymes

   D. Throat culture

PRACTICE Active Learning Scenario

A nurse is reinforcing discharge teaching with a client who has myocarditis. What should the nurse include in the teaching? Use the ATI Active Learning Template: System Disorder to complete this item.

CLIENT EDUCATION

- Identify at least two referral facilities and the services they can provide.
- Describe at least four actions the client should take when at home.

Application Exercises Key

1. A. **CORRECT:** A history of congenital malformations is a risk factor for valvular heart disease.

   B. Having a streptococcal infection or rheumatic fever during childhood is a risk factor for valvular heart disease.

   C. **CORRECT:** Hypertension places a client at risk for valvular heart disease.

   D. A sudden weight gain of 10 lb could indicate fluid collection related to left-sided valvular heart disease.

   E. **CORRECT:** A murmur indicates turbulent blood flow, which is often due to valvular heart disease.

   (N) *NCLEX® Connection: Health Promotion and Maintenance, Health Promotion/Disease Prevention*

2. A. **CORRECT:** Dyspnea is a manifestation of left-sided valvular heart disease.

   B. **CORRECT:** Fatigue is a manifestation of left-sided valvular heart disease.

   C. A client who has left-sided heart failure is more likely to experience tachycardia and possible atrial arrhythmias.

   D. A pleural friction rub is a manifestation of pleurisy or pneumonia.

   E. **CORRECT:** Peripheral edema is a manifestation of left-sided valvular heart disease.

   (N) *NCLEX® Connection: Physiological Adaptation, Basic Pathophysiology*

3. A. Petechiae are an expected finding in a client who has endocarditis.

   B. A murmur is an expected finding in a client who has myocarditis and endocarditis.

   C. Rash is an expected finding in a client who has rheumatic endocarditis.

   D. **CORRECT:** A friction rub can be heard during auscultation of a client who has pericarditis.

   (N) *NCLEX® Connection: Physiological Adaptation, Basic Pathophysiology*

4. A. **CORRECT:** Splinter hemorrhages in nail beds and a report of fever are findings associated with infective endocarditis.

   B. A client who has pericarditis would report chest pain.

   C. A client who has myocarditis would report a rapid heart rate.

   D. A client who has rheumatic endocarditis would report joint pain.

   (N) *NCLEX® Connection: Physiological Adaptation, Basic Pathophysiology*

5. A. Arterial blood gases are used to monitor the respiratory status of a client who has suspected rheumatic endocarditis, but they do not confirm the diagnosis.

   B. Serum albumin monitors the nutrition status of a client who has a suspected inflammatory disorder, but it does not confirm the diagnosis.

   C. Liver enzymes monitor response to antibiotic therapy, which is used to treat rheumatic endocarditis, but they do not confirm the diagnosis.

   D. **CORRECT:** A throat culture can reveal the presence of streptococcus, which is the leading cause of rheumatic endocarditis.

   (N) *NCLEX® Connection: Reduction of Risk Potential, Laboratory Values*

PRACTICE Answer

Using the ATI Active Learning Template: System Disorder

CLIENT EDUCATION

- Referral facilities
  - Home health: postoperative care, home administration of IV antibiotic therapy
  - Pharmaceutical services: IV antibiotic therapy, provision of supplies and medications
  - Rehabilitation services: assistance with monitoring and increasing activity level

- Client discharge activities
  - Rest as needed.
  - Wash hands to prevent infection.
  - Avoid crowded areas to reduce the risk of infection.
  - Maintain good oral hygiene to prevent infection.
  - Take medications as prescribed.
  - Administer and manage IV antibiotics.
  - Participate in a tobacco use cessation program.

(N) *NCLEX® Connection: Physiological Adaptation, Alterations in Body Systems*

UNIT 4   NURSING CARE OF CLIENTS WHO HAVE
CARDIOVASCULAR DISORDERS
SECTION: VASCULAR DISORDERS

CHAPTER 30 *Peripheral Vascular Diseases*

Peripheral vascular diseases include peripheral arterial disease (PAD) and peripheral venous disorders, both of which interfere with normal blood flow. PAD affects arteries (blood vessels that carry blood away from the heart), and peripheral venous disease affects veins (blood vessels that carry blood toward the heart).

Peripheral arterial disease

- PAD results from atherosclerosis that usually occurs in the arteries of the lower extremities and is characterized by inadequate flow of blood.
- Atherosclerosis is caused by a gradual thickening of the intima and media of the arteries, ultimately resulting in the progressive narrowing of the vessel lumen. Plaques can form on the walls of the arteries, making them rough and fragile.
- Progressive stiffening of the arteries and narrowing of the lumen decreases the blood supply to affected tissues and increases resistance to blood flow.
- Atherosclerosis is a type of arteriosclerosis, which means "hardening of the arteries" and alludes to the loss of elasticity of arteries over time due to thickening of their walls.
- PAD is classified as inflow (distal aorta and iliac arteries) or outflow (femoral, popliteal, and tibial arteries) and can range from mild to severe. Tissue damage occurs below the arterial obstruction.
- Buerger's disease, subclavian steal syndrome, thoracic outlet syndrome, Raynaud's disease, and popliteal entrapment are examples of PAD.

DATA COLLECTION

RISK FACTORS

- Hypertension
- Hyperlipidemia
- Diabetes mellitus
- Cigarette smoking
- Obesity
- Sedentary lifestyle
- Familial predisposition
- Female clients
- Older adult clients Ⓒ

EXPECTED FINDINGS

- Burning, cramping, and pain in the legs during exercise (intermittent claudication)
- Numbness or burning pain, primarily in the feet when in bed
- Pain that is relieved by placing legs at rest in a dependent position

PHYSICAL FINDINGS

- Bruit over femoral and aortic arteries
- Decreased capillary refill of toes (greater than 3 seconds)
- Decreased or nonpalpable pulses
- Loss of hair on lower calf, ankle, and foot
- Dry, scaly, shiny, skin
- Thick toenails
- Cold and cyanotic extremity
- Pallor of extremity with elevation
- Dependent rubor (redness) of the extremity (30.1)
- Muscle atrophy
- Ulcers and possible gangrene of toes

30.1 Rubor

DIAGNOSTIC PROCEDURES

Arteriography

- Arteriography of the lower extremities involves arterial injection of contrast medium to visualize areas of decreased arterial flow on an x-ray. Q_{EBP}
- It is usually done only to determine isolated areas of occlusion that can be treated during the procedure with percutaneous transluminal angioplasty and possible stent placement.

NURSING ACTIONS
- Observe for bleeding and hemorrhage.
- Palpate pedal pulses to identify possible occlusions.

Exercise tolerance testing

A stress test is done with or without the use of a treadmill with measurement of pulse volumes and blood pressures prior to and following the onset of manifestations or 5 min of exercise.
- Medications such as dipyridamole and adenosine may be given to mimic the effects of exercise in clients who cannot tolerate a treadmill.
- Delays in return to normal pressures and pulse waveforms indicate arterial disease.
- It is used to evaluate claudication during exercise.

Plethysmography

- Plethysmography is used to determine the variations of blood passing through an artery, thus identifying abnormal arterial flow in the affected limb.
- Blood pressure cuffs are attached to the client's upper extremities, a lower extremity, and the plethysmograph machine. Variations in peripheral pulses between the upper and lower extremity are recorded.
- A decrease in pulse pressure of the lower extremity indicates a possible blockage in the leg.

Segmental systolic blood pressure measurements

- A Doppler probe is used to take various blood pressure measurements (thigh, calf, ankle, brachial) for comparison. In the absence of PAD, pressures in the lower extremities are higher than those of the upper extremities.
- With arterial disease, the pressures in the thigh, calf, and ankle are lower.

Magnetic resonance angiography

A contrast medium, such as gadolinium, is injected to help visualize blood flow through peripheral arteries.

Ankle-brachial index (ABI)

The ankle pressure is compared to the brachial pressure. The expected finding for ABI is 0.9 to 1.3. ABI less than 0.9 in either leg is diagnostic for PAD.

Doppler-derived maximal systolic acceleration

A technique that is especially helpful for evaluating PAD in clients who have diabetes mellitus.

PATIENT-CENTERED CARE

NURSING CARE

- Encourage the client to exercise to build collateral circulation.
  - Initiate exercise gradually and increase slowly.
  - Instruct the client to walk until the point of pain, stop and rest, and then walk a little farther.
- Promote vasodilation and avoid vasoconstriction.
  - Provide a warm environment for the client.
  - Have the client wear insulated socks.
  - Tell the client to never apply direct heat, such as a heating pad, to the affected extremity because sensitivity is decreased, and this can cause a burn.
  - Instruct the client to avoid exposure to cold (causes vasoconstriction and decreased arterial flow).
  - Instruct the client to avoid stress, caffeine, and nicotine, which also cause vasoconstriction.
    - Vasoconstriction is avoided when the client abstains from smoking or chewing tobacco. Q_{EBP}
    - Vasoconstriction of vessels lasts up to 1 hr after smoking or chewing tobacco.

POSITIONING
- Instruct the client to avoid crossing the legs.
- Tell the client to refrain from wearing restrictive garments.
- Tell the client to elevate the legs to reduce swelling, but not to elevate them above the level of the heart because extreme elevation slows arterial blood flow to the feet.

MEDICATIONS

Antiplatelet medications

Aspirin, clopidogrel, pentoxifylline
Antiplatelet medications reduce blood viscosity by decreasing blood fibrinogen levels, enhancing erythrocyte flexibility, and increasing blood flow in the extremities.
- Medications such as aspirin and clopidogrel may be prescribed.
- Pentoxifylline, sometimes referred to as a hemorheologic medication, was one of the first to be used and is still used, but less commonly than other medications. It may be given to specifically treat intermittent claudication in clients who have PAD.

CLIENT EDUCATION
- The medication's effects might not be apparent for several weeks.
- Monitor for evidence of bleeding (abdominal pain; coffee-ground emesis; black, tarry stools).

Statins

Simvastatin, atorvastatin: Can relieve manifestations associated with PAD (intermittent claudication).

THERAPEUTIC PROCEDURES

Percutaneous transluminal angioplasty and laser-assisted angioplasty

- Percutaneous transluminal angioplasty is an invasive intra-arterial procedure using a balloon and stent to open and help maintain the patency of the vessel.
- Laser-assisted angioplasty is an invasive procedure in which a laser probe is advanced through a cannula to the site of stenosis. The laser is used to vaporize atherosclerotic plaque and open the artery.

NURSING ACTIONS

- The priority action is to observe for bleeding at the puncture site. Qs
- Monitor vital signs, peripheral pulses, and capillary refill.
- Keep the client on bed rest with the limb straight for 2 to 6 hr before ambulation.
- Anticoagulant therapy is used during the procedure, followed by antiplatelet therapy for 1 to 3 months.

Mechanical rotational abrasive atherectomy

Uses a rotational device to scrape plaque from the inside of the client's peripheral artery. The device is designed to cause minimal damage to the surface of the artery.

NURSING ACTIONS

- The priority action is to observe for bleeding at the puncture site. Qs
- Monitor vital signs, peripheral pulses, and capillary refill.
- Keep the client on bed rest with the limb straight for 2 to 6 hr before ambulation.
- Anticoagulant therapy is used during the procedure, followed by antiplatelet therapy for 1 to 3 months.

Arterial revascularization surgery

Used with clients who have severe claudication or limb pain at rest, or with clients who are at risk for losing a limb due to poor arterial circulation.
- Bypass grafts are used to reroute the circulation around the arterial occlusion.
- Grafts can be harvested from the client (autologous) or made from synthetic materials.

NURSING ACTIONS

- The priority action is to maintain adequate circulation in the repaired artery. The location of the pedal or dorsalis pulse should be marked, and its pulsatile strength compared with the contralateral leg on a scheduled basis using a Doppler. Qs
- Color, temperature, sensation, and capillary refill should be compared with the contralateral extremity on a scheduled basis.
- Monitor for warmth, redness, and edema of the affected limb as a result of increased blood flow.
- Monitor for pain, which can be severe due to the reestablishment of blood flow to the extremity.

- Monitor blood pressure. Hypotension can result in an increased risk of clotting or graft collapse, while hypertension increases the risk for bleeding from sutures.
- Instruct the client to limit bending of the hip and knee to decrease the risk of clot formation.
- Monitor incisions.
- Instruct the client on wound care if revascularization surgery was done.

CLIENT EDUCATION

- Avoid crossing or raising legs above the level of the heart.
- Wear loose clothing.
- Abstain from tobacco use, and avoid exposure to cold temperatures.
- Practice adequate foot care (keep feet clean and dry, wear good-fitting shoes, never go barefoot, cut toenails straight across or have the podiatrist cut nails).

COMPLICATIONS

Graft occlusion

Graft occlusion is a serious complication of arterial revascularization and often occurs within the first 24 hr following surgery.

NURSING ACTIONS

- Promptly notify the surgeon of manifestations of occlusion (absent or reduced pedal pulses, increased pain, change in extremity color or temperature). Qs
- Be prepared to assist with treatment, which can include an emergency thrombectomy (removal of a clot), local intra-arterial thrombolytic therapy with an agent such as tissue plasminogen activator, infusion of a platelet inhibitor, or a combination of these. With these treatments, monitor for indications of bleeding.

Wound or graft infection

An infection of the surgical wound or graft is a potentially life-threatening complication.

NURSING ACTIONS

- Use sterile technique when changing the surgical dressing or providing wound care.
- Indications of infection include localized induration, warmth, tenderness, erythema, edema, purulent drainage, and an elevated WBC. Promptly report findings to the provider.

Compartment syndrome

Compartment syndrome is considered a medical emergency. Tissue pressure within a confined body space can restrict blood flow, and the resulting ischemia can lead to irreversible tissue damage. **(30.2)**

NURSING ACTIONS

- Manifestations of compartment syndrome include tingling, numbness, worsening pain, edema, pain on passive movement, and unequal pulses. Immediately report findings to the provider.
- Loosen dressings.
- Prepare to assist with fasciotomy (surgical opening into the tissues), which can be necessary to prevent further injury and to save the limb.

Peripheral venous disorders

Peripheral venous disorders are problems with the veins that interfere with adequate return of blood flow from the extremities.

- There are superficial and deep veins in the lower extremities that have valves that prevent backflow of blood as it returns to the heart. The action of the skeletal muscles of the lower extremities during walking and other activities also promotes venous return.
- Three peripheral venous disorders that nurses should be familiar with are venous thromboembolism (VTE), venous insufficiency, and varicose veins.

VTE is a blood clot believed to form as a result of venous stasis, endothelial injury, or hypercoagulability. Thrombus formation can lead to a pulmonary embolism, which is a life-threatening complication. Thrombophlebitis refers to a thrombus that is associated with inflammation. **(30.3, 30.4)**

30.2 Compartment syndrome

superficial volar compartment
deep volar compartment
ulna
dorsal compartment
radius
mobile wad compartment
Fasciotomy

fibula
superficial posterior compartment
tibia
posterior compartment
lateral compartment
anterior compartment
Fasciotomy

30.3 Deep-vein thrombosis

Femoral vein
Popliteal vein
Calf swelling, deep vein thrombosis (DVT)
Tibial vein
Great saphenous vein

30.4 Thrombophlebitis

Superficial thrombophlebitis
Deep vein thrombophlebitis
Femoral vein
Great saphenous vein
Superficial veins
Blood clot

Venous insufficiency occurs secondary to incompetent valves in the deeper veins of the lower extremities, which allows pooling of blood and dilation of the veins. The veins' inability to carry fluid and wastes from the lower extremities precipitates the development of swelling, venous stasis ulcers, and in advanced cases, cellulitis.

Varicose veins are enlarged, twisted and superficial veins that can occur in any part of the body. However, they are commonly observed in the lower extremities and in the esophagus. **(30.5)**

DATA COLLECTION

RISK FACTORS

Venous thromboembolism: Associated with Virchow's triad (hypercoagulability, impaired blood flow, damage to blood vessels)

- Hip surgery, total-knee replacement, open prostate surgery
- Heart failure
- Immobility
- Pregnancy
- Oral contraceptives
- Active cancer

Venous insufficiency

- Sitting or standing in one position for a long period of time
- Obesity
- Pregnancy
- Thrombophlebitis
- Congenital absence of valves, or damaged valves

30.5 Varicose veins

Varicose veins

Incompetent venous valve

Varicose veins

- Female clients
- Older than 30 years and an occupation requiring prolonged standing
- Pregnancy
- Obesity
- Systemic diseases (heart disease)
- Family history

EXPECTED FINDINGS

Limb pain: Aching pain and feeling of fullness or heaviness in the legs after standing

PHYSICAL FINDINGS

- **Deep vein thrombosis (DVT) and thrombophlebitis**
  - Client can be asymptomatic.
  - Calf or groin pain, tenderness, and a sudden onset of edema of the extremity Q[EBP]
  - Warmth, edema, and induration and hardness over the involved blood vessel.
  - Changes in circumferences of right and left calf and thigh over time; localized edema over the affected area

  ! Shortness of breath and chest pain can indicate that the embolus has moved to the lungs (pulmonary embolism).

- **Venous insufficiency**
  - Stasis dermatitis is a brown discoloration along the ankles that extends up the calf relative to the level of insufficiency.
  - Edema
  - Stasis ulcers (typically found around ankles)
- **Varicose veins**
  - Distended, superficial veins that are visible just below the skin and are tortuous in nature
  - Clients often report muscle cramping and aches, pain after sitting, and pruritus.

LABORATORY TESTS

D-dimer test measures fibrin degradation products present in the blood produced from fibrinolysis. A positive test indicates that thrombus formation has possibly occurred.

DIAGNOSTIC PROCEDURES

DVT and thrombophlebitis

- Venous duplex ultrasonography uses high-frequency sound waves to provide a real-time picture of the blood flow through a blood vessel.
- Doppler flow study produces an audible sound when venous circulation is normal and little or no sound when veins are thrombosed.
- Impedance plethysmography can be used to determine the variations of blood passing through a vein, thus identifying abnormal venous flow in the affected limb.
- If the above tests are negative for a DVT but one is still suspected, a venogram (which uses contrast material) or magnetic resonance imaging might be needed for accurate diagnosis.

Varicose veins: Trendelenburg test

NURSING ACTIONS
- Place the client in a supine position with legs elevated.
- When the client sits up, the veins will fill from the proximal end if varicosities are present. (Veins normally fill from the distal end.)

PATIENT-CENTERED CARE

NURSING CARE

DVT and thrombophlebitis

- Encourage the client to rest.
  - Facilitate bed rest and elevation of the extremity above the level of the heart as prescribed.
  - Avoid using a knee gatch or pillow under knees.
- Apply intermittent or continuous warm moist compresses as prescribed.
- Do not massage the affected limb. Qs
- Provide thigh-high compression or antiembolism stockings.
- Prepare the client for an inferior vena cava interruption surgery (a filter traps emboli and prevents them from reaching the heart) as indicated.

Venous insufficiency

- Elevate legs for at least 20 min, four to five times a day.
- Elevate the legs above the heart when in bed.
- Instruct clients to avoid crossing legs and wearing constrictive clothing or stockings.
- Instruct clients to wear elastic compression stockings and apply them after the legs have been elevated and when swelling is at a minimum. QEBP

MEDICATIONS

DVT and thrombophlebitis: anticoagulants

Unfractionated heparin
- Given IV to prevent formation of other clots and to prevent enlargement of the existing clot.
- It has significant adverse effects and must be given in the facility. Prior to discharge, the medication will be changed to oral anticoagulation therapy with warfarin.
- NURSING ACTIONS
  - Monitor aPTT to allow for adjustments of heparin dosage.
  - Monitor platelet counts for heparin-induced thrombocytopenia. Qs
  - Ensure that protamine sulfate (the antidote for heparin) is available if needed for excessive bleeding.
  - Monitor for hazards and adverse effects associated with anticoagulant therapy.

Low-molecular-weight heparin
- Given subcutaneously and based on a client's weight.
- Enoxaparin is used for the prevention and treatment of DVT. It is usually given in the facility, but the twice-daily injections can be given in the home setting.
- NURSING ACTIONS
  - Instruct the client to observe for evidence of bleeding.
  - Instruct the client about bleeding precautions that should be taken. (Use electric instead of bladed razor. Brush teeth with a soft toothbrush.) Qs

Warfarin
- Inhibits synthesis of the four vitamin K-dependent clotting factors.
- The therapeutic effect takes 3 to 4 days to develop, so administration of the medication starts while the client is still on heparin.
- NURSING ACTIONS
  - Monitor for bleeding.
  - Monitor PT and INR.
  - Ensure that vitamin K (the antidote for warfarin) is available in case of excessive bleeding.
  - Instruct the client about food sources of vitamin K (green leafy vegetables) and to avoid fluctuations in the amount and frequency of consumption.
  - Instruct the client about observing for evidence of bleeding.
  - Instruct the client about bleeding precautions that should be taken. (Use electric instead of bladed razor. Brush teeth with soft toothbrush.)

DVT and thrombophlebitis: thrombolytic therapy

Thrombolytic therapy dissolves clots that have already developed. Therapy must be started within 5 days after the development of the clot for the therapy to be effective.

- Tissue plasminogen activator, a thrombolytic agent, and platelet inhibitors (abciximab, eptifibatide) can be effective in dissolving a clot or preventing new clots during the first 24 hr.
- Administering the medication in a manner that provides direct contact with the thrombus can be more effective and lessen the chance of bleeding.

NURSING ACTIONS
- Monitor for bleeding (intracerebral bleeding).
- Instruct the client about bleeding precautions that should be taken. (Use electric instead of bladed razor. Brush teeth with a soft toothbrush.) Qs

THERAPEUTIC PROCEDURES

DVT

Inferior vena cava filter
- Can be inserted when a client is unresponsive to medical therapy or when anticoagulation is contraindicated.
- It is inserted via the femoral vein and passed into the inferior vena cava where it traps emboli before they progress to the lungs.

Varicose veins

Sclerotherapy
- A sclerosing irritating chemical solution is injected into the varicose vein to produce localized inflammation, which will close the lumen of the vessel over time.
- For larger vessels, an incision and drainage of the trapped blood in a sclerosed vein might need to be performed 2 to 3 weeks after the injection.
- Pressure dressings are applied for approximately 1 week after each procedure to keep the vessel free of blood.
- CLIENT EDUCATION
  - Wear elastic stockings for the prescribed time.
  - Mild analgesics, such as acetaminophen, can be taken for discomfort.

Vein stripping: The removal of large varicose veins that cannot be treated with less-invasive procedures
- PREOPERATIVE NURSING ACTIONS
  - Assist the provider with vein marking.
  - Document pulses as a baseline for postoperative comparison.
- POSTOPERATIVE NURSING ACTIONS
  - Maintain elastic bandages on the legs.
  - Monitor groin and leg for bleeding through the elastic bandages.
  - Monitor extremity for edema, warmth, color, and pulses.
  - Elevate legs above the level of the heart.
  - Encourage the client to engage in range-of-motion exercises of the legs.
- CLIENT EDUCATION
  - Wear elastic stockings after bandage removal.
  - Elevate the legs when sitting, and avoid dangling them over the side of the bed.

Endovenous laser treatment: This type of treatment uses a laser fiber that is inserted into the vessel proximal to the area to be treated and then threaded to the involved area, where heat from the laser is used to close the dilated vein.

Application of radio frequency energy: This type of treatment uses a small catheter with a radio frequency electrode, instead of a laser, that is inserted into the vessel proximal to the area to be treated that scars and closes a dilated vein.

INTERPROFESSIONAL CARE

Venous insufficiency
- Care of venous stasis ulcers requires long-term management.
- Consultations with a dietitian and wound care specialist facilitate the healing process. Q꜠ᴄ

COMPLICATIONS

Ulcer formation
- Venous stasis ulcers often form over the medial malleolus. Venous ulcers are chronic, hard to heal, and often recur. They can lead to amputation or death. **(30.6)**
- Clients who have neuropathy might not feel as much discomfort from the ulcer as its appearance can warrant.

NURSING ACTIONS
- Administer and assist with treatments to improve circulation (wound vacuum, hyperbaric chamber).
- Monitor and treat pain as prescribed.
- Elevation of affected extremity
- Apply oxygen-permeable polyethylene films to superficial ulcers.
- Apply occlusive hydrocolloid dressings on deeper ulcers to promote granulation tissue and reepithelialization. Qᴇʙᴘ
- Leave a dressing on for 3 to 7 days.
- If a wound needs chemical debridement, apply prescribed topical enzymatic agents to debride the ulcer, eliminate necrotic tissue, and promote healing.
- Administer systemic antibiotics as prescribed.
- Prepare for oxygen therapy and blood gas analysis while continuing to monitor for other manifestations.
- Prepare to administer prescribed anticoagulants.

CLIENT EDUCATION
- Consume a diet high in zinc, protein, iron, and vitamins A and C.
- Use compression stockings.

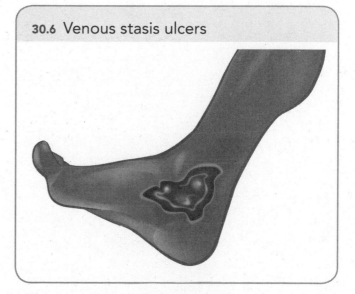

30.6 Venous stasis ulcers

Pulmonary embolism

A pulmonary embolism occurs when a thrombus is dislodged, becomes an embolus, and lodges in a pulmonary vessel. This can lead to obstruction of pulmonary blood flow, decreased systemic oxygenation, pulmonary tissue hypoxia, and death.

- Manifestations include sudden onset dyspnea, pleuritic chest pain, restlessness, apprehension, feelings of impending doom, cough, and hemoptysis.
- Findings include tachypnea, crackles, pleural friction rub, tachycardia, S_3 or S_4 heart sounds, diaphoresis, low-grade fever, petechiae over chest and axillae, and decreased arterial oxygen saturation.

NURSING ACTIONS

- Notify the provider immediately. Reassure the client. Stay with the client. Assist the client to a position of comfort with the head of the bed elevated. Qs
- Prepare for oxygen therapy and blood gas analysis while continuing to monitor for other manifestations.
- Prepare to administer prescribed anticoagulants.

Application Exercises

1. A nurse is caring for a client who has chronic venous insufficiency and a prescription for thigh-high compression stockings. Which of the following actions should the nurse take?

   A. Elevate the legs for 10 min, 2 to 3 times daily while wearing the stockings.

   B. Apply the stockings in the morning upon awakening and before getting out of bed.

   C. Roll the stockings down to the knees to relieve discomfort on the legs.

   D. Cross one leg over the other when sitting or reclining.

2. A nurse is collecting data on a client who has chronic peripheral arterial disease (PAD). Which of the following findings should the nurse expect?

   A. Edema around the ankles and feet

   B. Ulceration around the medial malleoli

   C. Brownish discoloration of the lower legs and ankles

   D. Dependent rubror with pallor following limb elevation

3. A nurse is reinforcing teaching with a client who has a new diagnosis of severe peripheral arterial disease. Which of the following instructions should the nurse include?

   A. Wear tightly fitted insulated socks with shoes when going outside.

   B. Elevate both legs above the heart when resting.

   C. Apply a heating pad to both legs for comfort.

   D. Place both legs in dependent position while sleeping.

4. A nurse is reinforcing teaching with a client who has a new prescription for clopidogrel. Which of the following instructions should the nurse include in the teaching? (Select all that apply.)

   A. Avoid consuming grapefruit while taking this medication.

   B. Monitor for black, tarry stools.

   C. Use an electric razor when shaving.

   D. Take the medication when you have pain.

   E. Limit food sources containing vitamin K while taking this medication.

5. A nurse is caring for a client who has a deep-vein thrombosis (DVT) and has been taking unfractionated heparin for 1 week. Two days ago, the provider also prescribed warfarin. The client asks the nurse about receiving both heparin and warfarin at the same time. Which of the following statements should the nurse give?

   A. "I will remind your provider that you are already receiving heparin."

   B. "Your laboratory findings indicated that two anticoagulants were needed."

   C. "It takes 3 to 4 days before the therapeutic effects of warfarin are achieved, and then the heparin can be discontinued."

   D. "Only one of these medications is being given to treat your deep-vein thrombosis."

PRACTICE Active Learning Scenario

A nurse is helping to develop a poster presentation on peripheral arterial disease (PAD) for a community health fair. What content should the nurse include on the poster? Use the ATI Active Learning Template: System Disorder to complete this item.

ALTERATION IN HEALTH (DIAGNOSIS)

RISK FACTORS: Describe at least six.

EXPECTED FINDINGS: Describe at least six findings.

CLIENT EDUCATION: Describe at least two actions by the client related to proper positioning and two actions related to promoting vasodilation.

Application Exercises Key

1. A. The nurse should tell the client who has venous insufficiency to sit with the legs elevated for at least 20 min, 4 to 5 times daily.

   B. **CORRECT:** Applying stockings in the morning upon awakening and before getting out of bed reduces venous stasis and assists in the venous return of blood to the heart. Legs are less edematous at this time.

   C. Rolling stockings down can restrict circulation and cause edema.

   D. The nurse should remind the client not to cross her legs because it further impairs venous return of blood from the legs.

   Ⓝ *NCLEX® Connection: Reduction of Risk Potential, Potential for Alterations in Body Systems*

2. A. Edema around the ankles and feet is an expected finding in a client who has venous stasis.

   B. Ulceration around the medial malleoli is an expected finding in a client who has venous stasis.

   C. Brownish discoloration of the lower legs and ankles is an expected finding in a client who has venous stasis.

   D. **CORRECT:** In a client who has chronic PAD, pallor is seen in the extremities when the limbs are elevated, and rubor occurs when they are lowered.

   Ⓝ *NCLEX® Connection: Physiological Adaptation, Basic Pathophysiology*

3. A. While insulated socks can promote warmth, they should be loose-fitting to promote circulation.

   B. The client should avoid elevating the legs above the heart while resting. This can cause a restriction in arterial blood flow to the feet.

   C. The client should not apply a heating pad to his legs due to the loss in sensation as a result of the disease. Applying direct heat to the legs can burn the client.

   D. **CORRECT:** The nurse should instruct the client to place his legs in a dependent position, such as hanging off the edge of the bed while sleeping. This can alleviate swelling and discomfort of the legs.

   Ⓝ *NCLEX® Connection: Physiological Adaptation, Alterations in Body Systems*

4. A. **CORRECT:** The nurse should instruct the client to avoid consuming grapefruit while taking clopidogrel. Grapefruit interferes with absorption of clopidogrel and can cause severe complications.

   B. **CORRECT:** The nurse should instruct the client to monitor for evidence of GI bleeding (abdominal pain; coffee-ground emesis; black, tarry stools). If this occurs, the client should report this to the provider.

   C. **CORRECT:** The nurse should warn the client to use an electric razor to prevent cuts, and that it may take a long time to stop bleeding while taking an antiplatelet medication.

   D. The nurse should inform the client to take clopidogrel routinely, as prescribed, because it can take several weeks to be effective.

   E. A client who is taking warfarin should be advised about food sources containing vitamin K.

   Ⓝ *NCLEX® Connection: Pharmacological Therapies, Medication Administration*

5. A. Warfarin is prescribed for 3 to 4 days before discontinuing IV heparin.

   B. Administration of both heparin and warfarin for DVT is part of evidence-based practice. Different laboratory values are used to monitor the effects of each medication.

   C. **CORRECT:** Warfarin depresses synthesis of clotting factors but does not have an effect on clotting factors that are present. It takes 3 to 4 days for the clotting factors that are present to decay and for the therapeutic effects of warfarin to occur.

   D. Heparin and warfarin are both effective in treating DVT.

   Ⓝ *NCLEX® Connection: Pharmacological Therapies, Expected Actions/Outcomes*

PRACTICE Answer

Using the ATI Active Learning Template: System Disorder

ALTERATION IN HEALTH (DIAGNOSIS): PAD is inadequate blood flow of the lower extremities due to atherosclerosis. The intima and media of the arteries become thickened, and plaque can form on the walls of the arteries, making them rough and fragile. The arteries progressively stiffen and the lumen narrows, decreasing blood supply to tissues and increasing resistance to blood flow. It is classified as either an inflow or outflow type of PAD.

RISK FACTORS
- Hypertension
- Hyperlipidemia
- Diabetes mellitus
- Cigarette smoking
- Obesity
- Sedentary lifestyle
- Familial predisposition
- Older adult clients
- Female clients

EXPECTED FINDINGS
- Bruits over femoral and aortic arteries
- Decreased capillary refill of toes (greater than 3 seconds)
- Decreased or nonpalpable pulses
- Loss of hair on the lower extremities
- Dry, scaly, mottled skin
- Thick toenails
- Cold, cyanotic extremity
- Pallor of extremity with elevation
- Dependent rubor
- Muscle atrophy
- Ulcers and possible gangrene of toes

CLIENT EDUCATION
- Positioning
  ○ Avoid crossing the legs.
  ○ Avoid wearing restrictive garments.
  ○ Keep legs elevated to reduce swelling, but not above the level of the heart.
- Vasodilation
  ○ Maintain a warm environment.
  ○ Wear insulated socks.
  ○ Avoid applying direct heat to the extremity.
  ○ Avoid exposure to cold.
  ○ Avoid stress, caffeine, and nicotine.

Ⓝ *NCLEX® Connection: Health Promotion and Maintenance, Health Promotion/Disease Prevention*

UNIT 4   NURSING CARE OF CLIENTS WHO HAVE
CARDIOVASCULAR DISORDERS
SECTION: VASCULAR DISORDERS

CHAPTER 31 *Hypertension*

For an adult client, hypertension occurs when systolic blood pressure is at or greater than 140 mm Hg or diastolic blood pressure is at or greater than 90 mm Hg for two or more assessments of blood pressure. For clients older than 60 years, blood pressure should be less than 150/90 mm Hg.

Essential hypertension, also called primary hypertension, accounts for most cases of hypertension. There is no known cause. Secondary hypertension can be caused by disease states, such as kidney disease, or as an adverse effect of some medications. Treatment for secondary hypertension occurs by removing the cause (adrenal tumor, medication).

Clients who have a systolic blood pressure of 120 to 139 mm Hg or a diastolic blood pressure of 80 to 89 mm Hg are considered to have prehypertension. Lifestyle changes are necessary for these clients to help prevent cardiovascular disease.

Prolonged, untreated, or poorly controlled hypertension can cause peripheral vascular disease that primarily affects the heart, brain, eyes, and kidneys. The risk of developing complications increases as blood pressure increases.

Hypertrophy of the left ventricle can develop as the heart pumps against resistance caused by hypertension.

HEALTH PROMOTION AND DISEASE PREVENTION

- Maintain body mass index less than 30.
- Clients who have diabetes mellitus should keep blood glucose within a recommended reference range.
- Limit caffeine and alcohol intake.
- Use stress-management techniques during times of stress.
- Stop smoking. Nicotine patches or engaging in a smoking cessation class are potential strategies.
- Engage in exercise that provides aerobic benefits at least three times per week.
- Limit sodium and fat intake.

DATA COLLECTION

Four bodily mechanisms regulate blood pressure.

Arterial baroreceptors are located in the carotid sinus, aorta, and left ventricle. They control blood pressure by altering the heart rate. They also cause vasoconstriction or vasodilation.

Regulation of body-fluid volume: Properly functioning kidneys retain fluid when a client is hypotensive and excrete fluid when a client is hypertensive.

Renin-angiotensin-aldosterone system: Renin is converted into angiotensin II, which causes vasoconstriction and controls aldosterone release, causing the kidneys to reabsorb sodium and inhibit fluid loss.

Vascular autoregulation maintains consistent levels of tissue perfusion.

RISK FACTORS

Essential hypertension
- Family history of hypertension
- Excessive sodium intake
- Physical inactivity
- Obesity
- Excessive alcohol consumption
- African Americans
- Smoking
- Hyperlipidemia
- Stress
- Age greater than 60 or postmenopausal

Secondary hypertension
- Kidney disease
- Cushing's disease (excessive glucocorticoid secretion)
- Primary aldosteronism (causes hypertension and hypokalemia)
- Pheochromocytoma (excessive catecholamine release)
- Brain tumors, encephalitis
- Medications (estrogen, steroids, sympathomimetics)
- Pregnancy

EXPECTED FINDINGS

Clients who have hypertension can experience few or no manifestations. Monitor for the following.

- Headaches, particularly in the morning
- Fatigue
- Irritability
- Facial flushing
- Dizziness
- Fainting
- Retinal changes, visual disturbances
- Nocturia

PHYSICAL FINDINGS

- When a blood pressure reading is elevated, take it in both arms and with the client sitting and standing.
- **Levels of hypertension** are defined by the Joint National Committee on Prevention, Detection, Evaluation, and Treatment of High Blood Pressure.
  - **Prehypertension:** systolic 120 to 139 mm Hg; diastolic 80 to 89 mm Hg
  - **Stage I hypertension:** systolic 140 to 159 mm Hg; diastolic 90 to 99 mm Hg
  - **Stage II hypertension:** systolic greater than or equal to 160 mm Hg; diastolic greater than or equal to 100 mm Hg

LABORATORY TESTS

No laboratory tests exist to diagnose hypertension. However, several laboratory tests can identify the causes of secondary hypertension and target organ damage.

- **BUN, creatinine** elevation is indicative of kidney disease.
- **Elevated serum and urinary cortisol levels** detect Cushing's disease.
- **Blood glucose and cholesterol studies** can identify contributing factors related to blood vessel changes.

DIAGNOSTIC PROCEDURES

ECG evaluates cardiac function. Tall R-waves are often seen with left-ventricular hypertrophy.

Chest x-ray can show cardiomegaly.

PATIENT-CENTERED CARE

NURSING CARE

- Discuss factors that increase the risk of hypertension and how the client can manage them.
- Provide verbal and written education to the client regarding medications and their adverse effects.
- Ensure that the client has the resources necessary to pay for and obtain prescribed antihypertensive medication.
- Instruct the client or a significant other how to monitor blood pressure at home.

MEDICATIONS

Medications are added to treat hypertension that is not responsive to lifestyle changes alone. Diuretics are often first-line medications. However, clients can require a combination of medications to control hypertension.

CLIENT EDUCATION: If taking antihypertensives, change positions slowly, and be careful when getting out of bed, driving, and climbing stairs until the medication's effects are fully known. **Qs**

Diuretics

- **Thiazide diuretics**, such as hydrochlorothiazide, inhibit water and sodium reabsorption and increase potassium excretion.
- Other diuretics can treat hypertension that is not responsive to thiazide diuretics.
  - **Loop diuretics**, such as furosemide, decrease sodium reabsorption and increase potassium excretion.
  - **Potassium-sparing diuretics**, such as spironolactone, affect the distal tubule and prevent reabsorption of sodium in exchange for potassium.

NURSING ACTIONS: Monitor potassium levels and watch for muscle weakness, irregular pulse, and dehydration. Thiazide and loop diuretics can cause hypokalemia, and potassium-sparing diuretics can cause hyperkalemia.

CLIENT EDUCATION

- Keep all appointments with the provider to monitor efficacy of pharmacological treatment and possible electrolyte imbalance (hyponatremia, hyperkalemia).
- If taking a potassium-depleting diuretic, consume potassium-rich foods, such as bananas.

Calcium-channel blockers

Verapamil, amlodipine, and diltiazem alter the movement of calcium ions through the cell membrane, causing vasodilation and lowering blood pressure.

NURSING ACTIONS
- Monitor blood pressure and pulse, and change the client's position slowly. Hypotension is a common adverse effect.
- Use calcium-channel blockers cautiously with clients who have heart failure.

CLIENT EDUCATION
- Constipation can occur with verapamil, so eat foods that are high in fiber.
- A decrease or increase in heart rate and atrioventricular (AV) block can occur. Monitor pulse and call the provider if it is irregular or lower than the established rate.
- Avoid grapefruit juice, which potentiates the medication's effects, increases hypotensive effects, and increases the risk of medication toxicity.

ANGIOTENSIN-CONVERTING ENZYME (ACE) INHIBITORS

ACE inhibitors (lisinopril, enalapril) prevent the conversion of angiotensin I to angiotensin II, which prevents vasoconstriction.

NURSING ACTIONS
- Monitor blood pressure and pulse. Hypotension is a common adverse effect.
- Monitor for evidence of heart failure, such as edema. ACE inhibitors can cause heart and kidney complications.

CLIENT EDUCATION
- Report a cough, which is an adverse effect of ACE inhibitors. Notify the provider, as the medication can be discontinued due to its persistent nature and occasional relationship to angioedema (swelling of the tissues in the throat that can progress to a life-threatening obstruction). The provider will likely discontinue the medication. Qs
- Report manifestations of heart failure (edema).

Angiotensin-II receptor antagonists

Also called angiotensin-receptor blockers (ARBs), these medications (valsartan, losartan) are a good option for clients taking ACE inhibitors who report cough or have hyperkalemia. ARBs do not require a dosage adjustment for older adult clients.

NURSING ACTIONS: Monitor for manifestations of angioedema or heart failure. Angioedema is a serious, but uncommon adverse effect.

CLIENT EDUCATION
- Change positions slowly.
- Report findings of angioedema (swollen lips or face) or heart failure (edema).
- Avoid foods that are high in potassium and have serum potassium levels monitored because ARBS can cause hyperkalemia.

Aldosterone-receptor antagonists

Aldosterone-receptor antagonists, such as eplerenone, block aldosterone action. The blocking effect of eplerenone on aldosterone receptors promotes the retention of potassium and excretion of sodium and water.

NURSING ACTIONS
- Monitor kidney function, triglycerides, sodium, and potassium levels. The risk of adverse effects increases with deteriorating kidney function. Hypertriglyceridemia, hyponatremia, and hyperkalemia can occur as the dose increases.
- Monitor potassium levels every 2 weeks for the first few months and every 2 months thereafter. The client should avoid taking potassium supplements or potassium-sparing diuretics.
- Instruct the client about potential food, medication, and herbal interactions.

CLIENT EDUCATION
- Grapefruit juice and St. John's wort can increase adverse effects.
- Do not take salt substitutes with potassium or other foods that are rich in potassium.

Beta blockers

Beta blockers (metoprolol, atenolol) are for clients who have unstable angina or MI. They decrease cardiac output and block the release of renin, subsequently decreasing vasoconstriction of the peripheral vasculature.

NURSING ACTIONS: Monitor blood pressure and heart rate. These medications can mask hypoglycemia in clients who have diabetes mellitus.

CLIENT EDUCATION
- These medications can cause fatigue, weakness, depression, and sexual dysfunction.
- Do not suddenly stop taking the medication without consulting with the provider. Stopping suddenly can cause rebound hypertension.
- Manifestations of hypoglycemia do not include tachycardia, which beta blockers suppress.

Central-alpha$_2$ agonists

Central-alpha$_2$ agonists, such as clonidine, reduce peripheral vascular resistance and decrease blood pressure by inhibiting the reuptake of norepinephrine.

NURSING ACTIONS: Monitor blood pressure and pulse. This medication is not for first-line management of hypertension.

CLIENT EDUCATION: About adverse effects include sedation, orthostatic hypotension, and impotence.

Alpha-adrenergic antagonists

Alpha-adrenergic antagonists, such as prazosin, reduce blood pressure by causing vasodilation.

NURSING ACTIONS
- Start treatment with a low dose of the medication, usually given at night.
- Monitor blood pressure for 2 hr after initiation of treatment.

CLIENT EDUCATION: Rise slowly to prevent postural hypotension. Use caution when driving until the effects of the medication are known. Qs

CLIENT EDUCATION

- Report manifestations of electrolyte imbalance (hyperkalemia, hypokalemia, hyponatremia).
- Adhere to the medication regimen, even if there are no manifestations of hypertension.
- Schedule regular provider appointments to monitor hypertension and cardiovascular status.
- Report findings and adverse effects, as they can be indicative of additional problems. Medications can often be changed to alleviate adverse effects.
- Older adult clients are more likely to experience medication interactions and orthostatic hypotension. Ⓖ
- Treatment involves making lifestyle changes.

Nutrition
- Monitor for hyperkalemia with salt substitute use.
- Consume less than 2.3 g/day of sodium.
- Consume a diet low in fat, saturated fat, and cholesterol.
- Limit alcohol intake to 2 servings per day for men and 1 serving per day for women. A serving of alcohol is equivalent to 1.5 oz 80-proof spirits, 5 oz wine, or 12 oz beer.
- Dietary approaches to stop hypertension (DASH) are effective in the prevention and treatment of hypertension. QEBP
  - The DASH diet is high in fruits, vegetables, and low-fat dairy foods.
  - Avoid foods high in sodium and fat (trans and saturated fat).
- Consume foods rich in calcium, and magnesium.
- Clients not taking a potassium-sparing medication should increase potassium consumption.

Weight reduction and maintenance
- Begin slowly and gradually advance the program with the guidance of the provider and physical therapist.
- Exercise at least three times a week in a manner that provides aerobic benefits.

Smoking cessation: Explore smoking cessation options such as nicotine replacement therapy, medications (bupropion, varenicline), and support groups. QPcc

Stress reduction: Try yoga, massage, hypnosis, or other forms of relaxation.

COMPLICATIONS

Hypertensive crisis

Hypertensive crisis often occurs when clients do not follow the medication therapy regimen and can be life-threatening.

NURSING ACTIONS
- Recognize manifestations.
  - Severe headache
  - Extremely high blood pressure (generally, systolic blood pressure greater than 240 mm Hg, diastolic greater than 120 mm Hg)
  - Blurred vision, dizziness, and disorientation
  - Epistaxis
  - Seizures
- Monitor clients receiving IV antihypertensive therapies (nitroprusside, nicardipine, labetalol).
- Before, during, and after administration of an IV antihypertensive, monitor blood pressure every 5 to 15 min.
- Check neurological status, such as pupils, level of consciousness, and muscle strength, to monitor for cerebrovascular change.
- Monitor the ECG to check cardiac status.

Application Exercises

1. A nurse is screening a client for hypertension. Which of the following actions by the client increases the risk for hypertension? (Select all that apply.)

   A. Drinking 8 oz nonfat milk daily

   B. Eating popcorn at the movie theater

   C. Walking 1 mile daily at 12 min/mile pace

   D. Consuming 36 oz beer daily

   E. Getting a massage once a week

2. A nurse in an urgent care clinic is obtaining a history from a client who has type 2 diabetes mellitus and a recent diagnosis of hypertension. This is the second time in 2 weeks that the client experienced hypoglycemia. Which of the following client data should the nurse report to the provider?

   A. Takes psyllium daily as a fiber laxative

   B. Drinks skim milk daily as a bedtime snack

   C. Takes metoprolol daily after meals

   D. Drinks grapefruit juice daily with breakfast

3. A nurse is assisting with the care of a client who is admitted to the emergency department with a blood pressure of 266/147 mm Hg. The client reports a headache and double vision. The client reports running out of diltiazem 3 days ago, and inability to purchase more. Which of the following actions should the nurse take first?

   A. Administer acetaminophen for headache.

   B. Reinforce teaching regarding the importance of not abruptly stopping an antihypertensive.

   C. Obtain IV access and ask the charge nurse to administer an IV antihypertensive.

   D. Call social services for a referral for financial assistance in obtaining prescribed medication.

4. A nurse is reinforcing teaching with a client who has a new diagnosis of hypertension and a new prescription for spironolactone 25 mg/day. Which of the following statements by the client indicates an understanding of the teaching?

   A. "I should eat a lot of fruits and vegetables, especially bananas and potatoes."

   B. "I will report any changes in heart rate to my provider."

   C. "I should replace the salt shaker on my table with a salt substitute."

   D. "I will decrease the dose of this medication when I no longer have headaches and facial redness."

5. A nurse is reinforcing discharge teaching with a client who has a prescription for furosemide 40 mg PO daily. The client should take this medication at which of the following times of day?

   A. Morning

   B. Immediately after lunch

   C. Immediately before dinner

   D. Bedtime

PRACTICE Active Learning Scenario

A nurse is helping prepare a community education presentation on hypertension. What information should the nurse include in the presentation? Use the ATI Active Learning Template: System Disorder to complete this item.

ALTERATION IN HEALTH (DIAGNOSIS): Describe hypertension to include essential, secondary, and prehypertension.

RISK FACTORS: Describe at least four risk factors each for essential and secondary hypertension.

EXPECTED FINDINGS
- Describe at least three expected subjective data findings for hypertension.
- Describe the objective data stages of hypertension.

Application Exercises Key

1. A. Consuming low-fat beverages and foods lowers the risk for developing hypertension.

    B. **CORRECT:** Popcorn at a movie theater contains a large quantity of sodium and fat, which increases the risk for hypertension.

    C. Engaging in regular exercise, such as walking, lowers the risk of developing hypertension.

    D. **CORRECT:** Consuming more than 24 oz beer per day for a male client or more than 12 oz per day for a female client increases the risk for hypertension.

    E. Stress management activities, such as a massage, lower the risk of hypertension.

    Ⓝ *NCLEX® Connection: Health Promotion and Maintenance, Health Promotion/Disease Prevention*

2. A. Adverse effects of psyllium do not include hypoglycemia.

    B. Skim milk increases blood glucose levels and lowers cholesterol.

    C. **CORRECT:** Metoprolol can mask the effects of hypoglycemia in clients who have diabetes mellitus.

    D. Grapefruit juice increases blood glucose levels.

    Ⓝ *NCLEX® Connection: Pharmacological Therapies, Adverse Effects/Contraindications/Side Effects/Interactions*

3. A. Administering acetaminophen will treat the client's pain, but there is another action that the nurse should take first.

    B. Reinforcing teaching regarding medication administration can help promote future compliance with taking medication, but there is another action that the nurse should take first.

    C. **CORRECT:** The greatest risk to the client is injury due to a blood pressure of 266/147 mm Hg, which can be life-threatening and should be lowered as soon as possible. Obtaining IV access will permit administration of an IV hypertensive, which will act more rapidly than by the oral route.

    D. Calling social services will help connect the client with financial resources, but there is another action that the nurse should take first.

    Ⓝ *NCLEX® Connection: Pharmacological Therapies, Expected Actions/Outcomes*

4. A. The nurse should instruct the client that potatoes and bananas are high in potassium, and can lead to hyperkalemia when taken with a potassium-sparing diuretic such as spironolactone.

    B. **CORRECT:** The nurse should instruct the client to monitor heart rate and report any changes to the provider.

    C. The nurse should instruct the client that salt substitutes are commonly high in potassium and can lead to hyperkalemia when taken with a potassium-sparing diuretic such as spironolactone.

    D. The nurse should instruct the client to continue taking the medication as prescribed even if there are no manifestations of hypertension.

    Ⓝ *NCLEX® Connection: Pharmacological Therapies, Medication Administration*

5. A. **CORRECT:** The client should take furosemide, a diuretic, in the morning so that the peak action and duration of the medication occurs during waking hours.

    B. Taking furosemide at this time increases the likelihood of interruption of the client's sleep due to the need to urinate.

    C. Taking furosemide at this time increases the likelihood of interruption of the client's sleep due to the need to urinate.

    D. Taking furosemide at this time increases the likelihood of interruption of the client's sleep due to the need to urinate.

    Ⓝ *NCLEX® Connection: Pharmacological Therapies, Medication Administration*

PRACTICE Answer

Using the ATI Active Learning Template: System Disorder

ALTERATION IN HEALTH (DIAGNOSIS)

- Hypertension is systolic blood pressure 140 mm Hg or greater, or diastolic blood pressure 90 mm Hg or greater for an adult client; or greater than 150/90 mm Hg for a client older than 60.
- Essential (primary) hypertension has no known cause.
- Secondary hypertension is caused by diseases such as kidney disorders, or as an adverse effect of a medication. Treatment occurs by removing the cause.
- Prehypertension is when a client has a systolic blood pressure of 120 to 139 mm Hg or a diastolic blood pressure of 80 to 89 Hg.

RISK FACTORS

- Primary hypertension: Positive family history, excessive sodium intake, physical inactivity, obesity, excessive alcohol consumption, African American, nicotine use, hyperlipidemia, stress, age greater than 60, postmenopausal
- Secondary hypertension: Kidney disease, Cushing's disease, primary aldosteronism (causes hypertension and hypokalemia), pheochromocytoma (excessive catecholamine release), brain tumors, encephalitis, and medications (estrogen, steroids, sympathomimetics)

EXPECTED FINDINGS

Subjective data: Few or no manifestations
- Can include headaches, particularly in the morning
- Dizziness, fainting, retinal changes, visual disturbances, nocturia, facial flushing

Objective data stages: Obtain blood pressure readings in both arms with the client sitting and standing.
- Prehypertension: systolic 120 to 139 mm Hg, diastolic 80 to 89 mm Hg
- Stage I: systolic 140 to 159 mm Hg, diastolic 90 to 99 mm Hg
- Stage II: systolic greater than or equal to 160 mm Hg, diastolic greater than or equal to 100 mm Hg

Ⓝ *NCLEX® Connection: Health Promotion and Maintenance, Health Promotion/Disease Prevention*

CHAPTER 32 *Aneurysms*

An aneurysm is a weakness in a section of a dilated artery that causes a widening or ballooning in the wall of the blood vessel. Aneurysms can occur in two forms: saccular (only affecting one side of the artery) or fusiform (involving the complete circumference of the artery). (32.1)

Aortic dissection (also known as a dissecting aneurysm) can occur when blood accumulates within the artery wall (hematoma) following a tear in the lining of the artery (usually due to hypertension). This is a life-threatening condition.

HEALTH PROMOTION AND DISEASE PREVENTION

- Promote smoking cessation.
- Maintain appropriate weight for height and body frame.
- Encourage a healthy diet and physical activity.
- Control blood pressure with regular monitoring and medication if needed.

DATA COLLECTION

RISK FACTORS

- Male clients
- Atherosclerosis (most common cause)
- Uncontrolled hypertension
- Tobacco use
- Hyperlipidemia
- Family history
- Blunt force trauma
- Diabetes mellitus
- History of syphilis
- With age, arterial stiffening caused by loss of elastin in arterial walls, thickening of intima of arteries, and progressive fibrosis of media occurs. Older adult clients are more prone to aneurysms and have a higher mortality rate from aneurysms than younger clients. Ⓖ

EXPECTED FINDINGS

Initially, clients are often asymptomatic.

Abdominal aortic aneurysm (AAA)

Most common, related to atherosclerosis
- Constant gnawing feeling in abdomen
- Flank or back pain
- Pulsating abdominal mass (do not palpate; can cause rupture Ⓠ𝐬)
- Bruit over the area of the aneurysm
- Elevated blood pressure (unless in cardiac tamponade or rupture of aneurysm)

Thoracic aortic aneurysm

- Severe back pain (most common)
- Hoarseness, cough, shortness of breath, and difficulty swallowing
- Decrease in urinary output (secondary to hypovolemic shock)

Aortic dissections

Often associated with Marfan syndrome
- Sudden onset of "tearing," "ripping," and "stabbing" abdominal or back pain
- Hypovolemic shock
  - Diaphoresis, nausea, vomiting, faintness, apprehension
  - Decreased or absent peripheral pulses
  - Neurological deficits
  - Hypotension and tachycardia (initial)
  - Oliguria

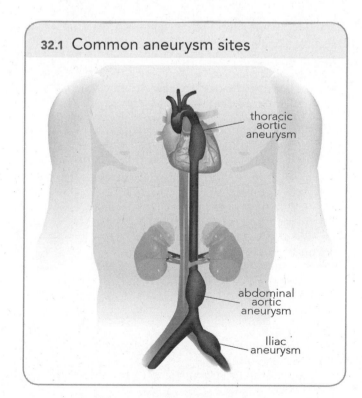

32.1 Common aneurysm sites

thoracic aortic aneurysm

abdominal aortic aneurysm

iliac aneurysm

DIAGNOSTIC PROCEDURES

Chest or abdominal x-ray: Can be used to detect the presence of an aneurysm.

Computed tomography (CT) and ultrasonography: Used to assess the size and location of aneurysms. Often repeated at periodic intervals to monitor the progression of an aneurysm.

PATIENT-CENTERED CARE

NURSING CARE

- Take vital signs every 15 min until stable, then every hour. Monitor for an increase in blood pressure.
- Check onset, quality, duration, and severity of pain.
- Check temperature, circulation, and range of motion of extremities.
- Assist with monitoring cardiac rhythm.
- Assist in monitoring ABGs, SaO₂, electrolytes, and CBC findings.
- Monitor hourly urine output. Greater than 30 mL/hr indicates adequate kidney perfusion.
- Administer oxygen.
- Assist in maintaining IV access.
- Administer medications.

> ! All aneurysms can be life-threatening and require medical attention.

MEDICATIONS

- The priority intervention is to reduce systolic blood pressure to between 90 and 120 mm Hg during an emergency. Long-term goals include maintaining systolic blood pressure at or less than 130 to 140 mm Hg. **Qs**
- Administer antihypertensive agents. Often, more than one is prescribed (beta blockers, calcium blockers).

THERAPEUTIC PROCEDURES

Abdominal aortic aneurysm resection

Excision of the aneurysm and the placement of a synthetic graft (elective or emergency)

- Elective surgery is used to manage AAA of 5.5 cm diameter or greater (2% to 5% mortality rate).
- Emergency surgery is indicated for a rupturing aneurysm.
- Risks include significant blood loss and the consequences of reduced cardiac output and tissue ischemia (myocardial infarction, acute kidney injury, respiratory distress, paralytic ileus).

NURSING ACTIONS

- Monitor for evidence of graft occlusion or rupture postoperatively.
- Monitor vital signs and circulation (pulses distal to graft) every 15 min.
- Maintain the head of the bed below 45° to prevent flexion of the graft. **QEBP**

- Report evidence of graft occlusion or rupture immediately (change in pulses, coolness of extremity below graft, white or blue extremities or flanks, severe pain, abdominal distention, decreased urine output). **Qs**
- Monitor and maintain blood pressure within the prescribed parameters. Prolonged hypotension can cause thrombi to form within the graft. Severe hypertension can cause leakage or rupture at the arterial anastomosis suture line.
- Maintain a warm environment to prevent temperature-induced vasoconstriction.
- Administer IV fluids at prescribed rates to ensure adequate hydration and kidney perfusion.
- Monitor for altered kidney perfusion and acute kidney injury caused by clamping aorta during surgery (urine output less than 30 mL/hr, weight gain, elevated BUN or serum creatinine).
- Auscultate lung sounds. Encourage coughing and deep breathing every 2 hr. Encourage splinting with coughing.
- Monitor onset, quality, duration, and severity of pain. Administer pain medication.
- Monitor bowel sounds, and observe for abdominal distention. Maintain nasogastric suction.
- Prevent thromboembolism. Maintain sequential compression devices. Encourage early ambulation. Administer antiplatelet or anticoagulant medications.
- Monitor for infection.
- Administer antibiotics to maintain adequate blood levels of the medication.

Percutaneous aneurysm repair

Insertion of endothelial stent grafts for aneurysm repair avoids abdominal incision and shortens the postoperative period (can be used to repair thoracic and abdominal aortic aneurysms).

NURSING ACTIONS: Nursing care after the procedure is similar to care following an arteriogram or cardiac catheterization (monitor pedal pulse). Refer to **CHAPTER 26: INVASIVE CARDIOVASCULAR PROCEDURES**.

Thoracic aortic aneurysm repair

Procedure is similar to thoracic surgery, such as open heart. The course of action depends on the location of the aneurysm. Cardiopulmonary bypass is commonly used for this procedure.

NURSING ACTIONS

- Nursing care after the procedure is similar to care following coronary artery bypass graft surgery. (Monitor respiratory status. Respiratory distress is common after this type of procedure.)
- Cardiac rehabilitation services are often consulted for prolonged weakness and assistance in increasing the client's level of activity.
- Nutritional services can be consulted for food choices that are low in fat and cholesterol.

CLIENT EDUCATION

- Monitor and maintain blood pressure. Stay within parameters set by the provider. Taking medications as prescribed prevents complications (rupture). Q**s**
- Follow up on scheduled CT scans to monitor aneurysm size (nonsurgical client). Collaborate with case management services to assist with transportation needs.
- Stop smoking if applicable. Q**pcc**
- Prevent infection (good hand hygiene, wound care management). Report evidence of infection following surgical intervention (wound redness, edema, drainage, elevated temperature).
- Consume a proper diet (low-fat, high-protein, vitamins A and C, zinc to promote wound healing).
- Manifestations of aneurysm rupture include abdominal fullness or pain, chest or back pain, shortness of breath, cough, difficulty swallowing, and hoarseness. Report these immediately.
- Avoid strenuous activity. Restrict heavy lifting to less than 15 lb following surgery.

INTERPROFESSIONAL CARE

- Cardiology services can assist in managing and treating hypertension.
- Radiology should be consulted for diagnostic studies to diagnose and monitor an aneurysm.
- Vascular services may be consulted for surgical intervention.

COMPLICATIONS

Rupture

- Aneurysm rupture is a life-threatening emergency, often resulting in massive hemorrhage, shock, and death.
- Treatment requires simultaneous resuscitation and immediate surgical repair.
- Older adult clients who have an aneurysm greater than 6 cm (2.4 in) along with hypertension are at greater risk of death due to spontaneous rupture than of dying during surgical repair. Ⓒ

Thrombus formation

- A thrombus can form inside the aneurysm. Emboli can be dislodged, blocking arteries distal to the aneurysm, which causes ischemia and shuts down other body systems.
- Check circulation distal to aneurysm, including pulses and color and temperature of the lower extremities. Monitor urine output.

Application Exercises

1. A nurse is assisting with the care of a client who has a possible dissecting abdominal aortic aneurysm. Which of the following actions is the priority for the nurse to take?

   A. Administer pain medication.

   B. Provide a warm environment.

   C. Administer IV fluids.

   D. Initiate a 12-lead ECG.

2. A nurse is collecting data on a client who has a new diagnosis of a thoracic aortic aneurysm. Which of the following manifestations should the nurse expect? (Select all that apply.)

   A. Cough

   B. Shortness of breath

   C. Upper chest pain

   D. Diaphoresis

   E. Altered swallowing

3. A nurse is assisting with the plan of care for a client following a surgical placement of a synthetic graft to repair an aneurysm. Which of the following interventions should be included in the plan of care? (Select all that apply.)

   A. Check pedal pulses.

   B. Monitor for an increase in pain below the graft site.

   C. Maintain the client in high-Fowler's position.

   D. Administer antiplatelet agents.

   E. Report hourly urine output of 60 mL.

4. A nurse is reinforcing teaching with a client who has a new diagnosis of an aneurysm. The client asks the nurse to explain what causes an aneurysm to rupture. Which of the following statements should the nurse give?

   A. "This happens when the wall of an artery becomes thin and flexible."

   B. "This happens when there is turbulence in blood flow in the artery."

   C. "It is due to abdominal enlargement."

   D. "It is due to hypertension."

5. A nurse is assisting with the admission of a client who has a suspected occlusion of a graft of the abdominal aorta. Which of the following manifestations should the nurse expect?

   A. Increase in urine output

   B. Bounding pedal pulse

   C. Increase in abdominal girth

   D. Redness of the lower extremities

Application Exercises Key

1. A. The nurse should administer pain medication to alleviate pain and discomfort related to the aneurysm. However, another action is the priority.

    B. The nurse should provide a warm environment due to impaired blood flow and decreasing blood pressure related to the aneurysm. However, another action is the priority.

    C. **CORRECT:** The greatest risk to this client is injury or death following hypovolemic shock; therefore, the priority is administering IV fluids. The client is at risk of inadequate circulatory volume due to impaired blood flow through major arteries.

    D. The nurse should initiate a 12-lead ECG to determine the cardiac rhythm related to the aneurysm. However, another action is the priority.

    Ⓝ *NCLEX® Connection: Physiological Adaptation, Medical Emergencies*

2. A. **CORRECT:** Cough is a manifestation of a thoracic aortic aneurysm.

    B. **CORRECT:** Shortness of breath is a manifestation of a thoracic aortic aneurysm.

    C. Report of severe back pain is a finding of thoracic aortic aneurysm.

    D. Diaphoresis is a finding of dissecting aortic aneurysm.

    E. **CORRECT:** Difficulty swallowing is a manifestation of a thoracic aortic aneurysm.

    Ⓝ *NCLEX® Connection: Physiological Adaptation, Basic Pathophysiology*

3. A. **CORRECT:** The nurse should check the pulses distal to the graft site to detect possible occlusion of the graft.

    B. **CORRECT:** The nurse should monitor for an increase of pain below the graft site. This can be an indication of graft occlusion or rupture.

    C. The head of the bed should be maintained at less than 45° to prevent flexion of the graft.

    D. **CORRECT:** The nurse should administer antiplatelet agents and anticoagulants to prevent thrombus formation.

    E. Urine output of 60 mL/hr is an expected finding.

    Ⓝ *NCLEX® Connection: Reduction of Risk Potential, Potential for Complications from Surgical Procedures and Health Alterations*

4. A. An aneurysm ruptures as a result of thickening in the intima of the artery and a lack of elasticity in the vessel wall, which is typically under pressure due to hypertension.

    B. A bruit indicates the presence of an aneurysm, not the cause of rupture.

    C. Abdominal distention can occur when an aneurysm ruptures, but it is not the cause of the rupture.

    D. **CORRECT:** Aneurysm ruptures as a result of hypertension increasing pressure within the arterial walls.

    Ⓝ *NCLEX® Connection: Physiological Adaptation, Alterations in Body Systems*

5. A. Decreased urine output is an expected finding with occlusion of a graft of the aorta.

    B. Decreased or absent pedal pulse is an expected finding with occlusion of a graft of the aorta.

    C. **CORRECT:** Abdominal distention is an expected finding with occlusion of a graft of the aorta.

    D. Pallor or cyanosis of the extremities is an expected finding with occlusion of a graft of the aorta.

    Ⓝ *NCLEX® Connection: Physiological Adaptation, Basic Pathophysiology*

PRACTICE Active Learning Scenario

A nurse is assisting the nurse manager in presenting an in-service to a group of nurses about care of the client who has an aneurysm. What information should the nurse manager include? Use the ATI Active Learning Template: System Disorder to complete this item.

RISK FACTORS: Describe three.

DIAGNOSTIC PROCEDURES: Describe two.

NURSING CARE: Describe at least four nursing actions.

PRACTICE Answer

Using the ATI Active Learning Template: System Disorder

RISK FACTORS
- Male clients
- Atherosclerosis
- Uncontrolled hypertension
- Tobacco use
- Hyperlipidemia
- Family history
- Blunt force trauma
- History of syphilis
- Age-related changes to the artery (loss of elastin, thickening of the intima, progressive fibrosis)

DIAGNOSTIC PROCEDURES
- X-rays
- CT scans
- Ultrasonography
- Transesophageal echocardiography

NURSING CARE
- Take vital signs every 15 min until stable. Then monitor for increased blood pressure hourly.
- Monitor pain (onset, quality, duration, severity).
- Check temperature, circulation, and range of motion of extremities.
- Monitor cardiac rhythm continuously.
- Monitor hemodynamic findings.
- Monitor ABGs, SaO_2, electrolytes, and CBC laboratory findings.
- Monitor hourly urine output.
- Administer oxygen.
- Assist in maintaining IV access.
- Administer medications.

Ⓝ *NCLEX® Connection: Health Promotion and Maintenance, Health Promotion/Disease Prevention*

NCLEX® Connections

When reviewing the following chapters, keep in mind the relevant topics and tasks of the NCLEX outline, in particular:

Pharmacological Therapies

MEDICATION ADMINISTRATION
Calculate and monitor intravenous (IV) flow rates.

Monitor transfusions of blood products.

Reinforce client teaching on client self–administration of medications (insulin, subcutaneous insulin pump).

Reduction of Risk Potential

LABORATORY VALUES
Compare the client's laboratory values to normal laboratory values.

Reinforce client teaching on purposes of laboratory tests.

Physiological Adaptation

ALTERATIONS IN BODY SYSTEMS: Provide care to correct the client's alteration in body system.

BASIC PATHOPHYSIOLOGY: Apply knowledge of pathophysiology to monitoring the client for alterations in body systems.

FLUID AND ELECTROLYTE IMBALANCES: Provide interventions to restore the client's fluid and/or electrolyte balance.

CHAPTER 33

CHAPTER 33 *Hematologic Diagnostic Procedures*

Hematologic diagnostic procedures evaluate blood function by testing indicators such as erythrocytes (RBCs), leukocytes (WBCs), platelets, and coagulation times. By testing the blood, diagnosis of a disease and efficacy of treatment can be determined.

Bone marrow is responsible for the production of many blood cells (RBCs, WBCs, platelets). A bone marrow biopsy provides diagnostic information about how bone marrow is functioning.

33.1 Expected reference ranges for blood diagnostic procedures

	EXPECTED REFERENCE RANGE	INTERPRETATION OF FINDINGS
RBC	Female clients: 4.2 to 5.4 million/uL Male clients: 4.7 to 6.1 million/uL	Elevated level: erythrocytosis, polycythemia vera, severe dehydration Decreased level: anemia, hemorrhage, kidney disease
WBC	5,000 to 10,000/mm³	Elevated level: infection, inflammation Decreased level: immunosuppression, autoimmune disease
MCV	80 to 95 fL	Elevated level: macrocytic (large) RBCs, megaloblastic anemia Decreased level microcytic (small) RBCs, iron deficiency anemia
MCH	27 to 31 pg/cell	Elevated/decreased level: same as above for MCV
TIBC	250 to 460 mcg/dL	Elevated level: iron deficiency anemia, polycythemia vera Decreased level: malnutrition, cirrhosis, pernicious anemia
IRON	Female clients: 60 to 160 mcg/dL Male clients: 80 to 180 mcg/dL	Elevated level: hemochromatosis, iron excess, liver disorder, or lead toxicity Decreased level: iron deficiency anemia, chronic blood loss, inadequate dietary intake of iron
PLATELETS	150,000 to 400,000 mm³	Increased level: malignancy, polycythemia vera, rheumatoid arthritis Decreased level: enlarged spleen, hemorrhage, leukemia
HGB	Female clients: 12 to 16 g/dL Male clients: 14 to 18 g/dL Older adults: levels slightly decreased	Elevated level: erythrocytosis, COPD, severe dehydration Decreased level: anemia, hemorrhage, kidney disease
HCT	Female clients: 37 to 47% Male clients: 42 to 52% Older adult: levels slightly decreased	Elevated/decreased level: same as above for Hgb
APTT	30 to 40 seconds (1.5 to 2.5 times the control value if receiving heparin therapy)	Increased time: vitamin K deficiency, disseminated intravascular coagulation (DIC), liver disease, heparin administration Decreased time: extensive cancer
PT	11 to 12.5 seconds, 85 to 100%, or 1:1.1 client-control ratio	Increased time: of clotting factors II, V, VII, or X, liver disease, warfarin therapy, disseminated intravascular coagulation Decreased time: vitamin K excess, pulmonary embolus, thrombophlebitis
INR	0.8 to 1.1 (desired goal of 2 to 3 on warfarin therapy)	Measures the mean of PT to provide a universally recognized value Elevated level: warfarin therapy Decreased level: cancer disorders
D-DIMER	Less than 0.4 mcg/mL	Positive result: disseminated intravascular coagulation, malignancy Negative result: can rule out pulmonary embolus or deep vein thrombosis
FIBRINOGEN LEVELS	200 to 400 mg/dL	Elevated level: acute inflammation, acute infection, heart disease Decreased levels: liver disease, advanced cancer, malnutrition
FIBRIN DEGRADATION PRODUCTS	Less than 10 mcg/mL	Elevated level: disseminated intravascular coagulation, massive trauma resulting in fibrinolysis Decreased level: anticoagulation therapy

Blood collection/testing

- Blood diagnostic procedures include the following. **(33.1)**
  - Serum RBC count
  - Serum WBC count
  - Mean corpuscular volume (MCV)
  - Mean corpuscular hemoglobin (MCH)
  - Total iron-binding count (TIBC)
  - Iron
  - Platelets
  - Hemoglobin (Hgb)
  - Hematocrit (Hct)
  - Coagulation studies
    - Prothrombin time (PT)
    - Partial thromboplastin time (aPTT)
    - International normalized ratio (INR)
    - D-dimer
    - Fibrinogen levels
    - Fibrin degradation products
- CBC is a series of tests that includes RBC, WBC, MCV, MCH, Hgb, and Hct.

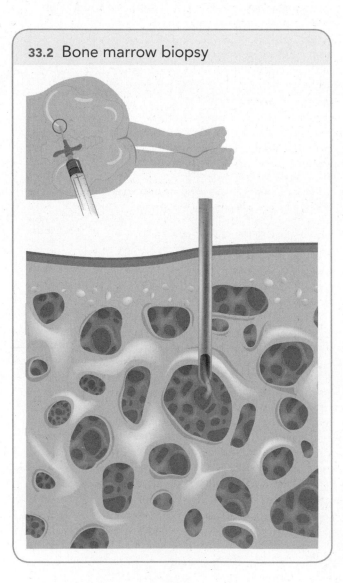

33.2 Bone marrow biopsy

CONSIDERATIONS

PREPROCEDURE

NURSING ACTIONS
- Use standard precautions and aseptic technique when collecting and handling blood for specimen collection. **Qs**
- Verify client identification
- Reinforce client education regarding test names and purposes.

INTRAPROCEDURE

NURSING ACTIONS
- Select the appropriate vial for the prescribed test.
- Collect a sufficient quantity of blood and fill to the indicated mark on the vial.
- Properly label the specimen. Deliver the specimen to the laboratory according to facility protocol for appropriate storage and analysis.
- For coagulation studies, draw blood at specific times and immediately send to the laboratory.

POSTPROCEDURE

NURSING ACTIONS
- Results of hematologic tests are usually available preliminarily within 24 to 48 hr, with final results in 72 hr.
- If results are outside of the expected reference range, it is the nurse's responsibility to report the results to the provider for further intervention.
- Adjust the dose of anticoagulant therapy based on the results and prescription. **QEBP**

Bone marrow aspiration/biopsy

- A biopsy is the extraction of a very small amount of tissue, such as bone marrow, to definitively diagnose cell type and to confirm or rule out malignancy. A bone marrow tissue sample is removed by needle aspiration for cytological (histological) examination. **(33.2)**
- Biopsies are commonly performed with local anesthesia or conscious sedation in an ambulatory setting, intraoperatively, or during endoscopic procedures.

INDICATIONS

A bone marrow biopsy is commonly performed to diagnose causes of blood disorders (anemia, thrombocytopenia); to diagnose diseases of the bone marrow, such as leukemia, and infection; or to stage lymphoma or other forms of cancer.

CONSIDERATIONS

PREPROCEDURE

NURSING ACTIONS
- Ensure that the client has provided informed consent.
- Place the client in a prone or side-lying position to expose the iliac crest for the procedure.
- Administer medication to manage discomfort and anxiety.
  - Older adult clients are at increased risk for complications associated with sedation for biopsy procedures due to chronic illnesses. ⓒ
  - Take an older adult's kidney function into consideration when using analgesics for sedation.
- Reinforce teaching about the procedure with the client.

CLIENT EDUCATION
- The biopsy site will be anesthetized with a local anesthetic. Pressure and brief pain might be felt during the aspiration.
- The test will last about 20 min.
- It is important to remain still during the procedure.

INTRAPROCEDURE

NURSING ACTIONS
- Cleanse the site with an antiseptic solution.
- Maintain sterility of equipment and supplies.
- Assist the provider with the procedure as needed.

POSTPROCEDURE

NURSING ACTIONS
- Apply pressure to the biopsy site to control bleeding.
- Place a sterile dressing over the biopsy site.
- Maintain the client on bed rest for 30 to 60 min.
- Monitor for evidence of infection (fever, increased WBCs, pain, swelling at the site) and bleeding.
- Apply ice to the biopsy site to minimize bleeding and bruising.
- Postprocedure discomfort is usually relieved by mild analgesics.
- Avoid aspirin and other medications that affect clotting.

CLIENT EDUCATION Qᴾᶜᶜ
- Report excessive bleeding and evidence of infection to the provider.
- Check the biopsy site daily. Keep the dressing clean, dry, and intact.

INTERPRETATION OF FINDINGS

After a procedure is completed, the tissue sample is sent to pathology for interpretation.

COMPLICATIONS

Infection

Infection can occur at the aspiration site.

NURSING ACTIONS: Monitor the site. Keep the dressing clean and dry.

Bleeding

Bleeding can occur from the site.

NURSING ACTIONS: Apply pressure to the site. Report bleeding to the provider immediately.

PRACTICE Active Learning Scenario

A nurse is caring for a client who is having a bone marrow biopsy. What actions should the nurse take? Use the ATI Active Learning Template: Diagnostic Procedure to complete this item.

NURSING INTERVENTIONS (PRE, INTRA, POST): Describe two for each of the pre-, intra-, and postprocedure periods.

POTENTIAL COMPLICATIONS: Identify two.

CLIENT EDUCATION: Describe two discharge teaching points.

Application Exercises

1. A nurse in a clinic is caring for a client who has suspected anemia. Which of the following laboratory test results should the nurse expect?
   - A. Iron 90 mcg/dL
   - B. RBC 6.5 million/uL
   - C. WBC 4,800 mm3
   - D. Hgb 10 g/dL

2. A nurse is caring for a client who is receiving warfarin for anticoagulation therapy. Which of the following laboratory test results indicates that the client needs an increase in the dosage?
   - A. aPTT 38 seconds
   - B. INR 1.1
   - C. PT 22 seconds
   - D. D-dimer negative

3. A nurse is reinforcing teaching with a client who is scheduled for a bone marrow biopsy of the iliac crest. Which of the following statements by the client indicates an understanding of the teaching?
   - A. "This test will be performed while I am lying flat on my back."
   - B. "I will need to stay in bed for about an hour after the test."
   - C. "This test will determine which antibiotic I should take for treatment."
   - D. "I will receive general anesthesia for the test."

Application Exercises Key

1. A. An iron level of 90 mcg/dL is within the expected reference range and is not an expected finding of anemia.

   B. RBC count of 6.5 million/uL is above the expected reference range. A decreased RBC count is an expected finding of anemia.

   C. WBC count of 4,800 mm³ is below the expected reference range and is not an expected finding of anemia.

   D. **CORRECT:** Hgb of 10 g/dL is below the expected reference range and is an expected finding of anemia.

   ⓃNCLEX® Connection: Reduction of Risk Potential, Laboratory Values

2. A. An aPTT of 38 seconds is within the expected reference range for clients not receiving heparin therapy.

   B. **CORRECT:** INR of 1.1 is within the expected reference range for a client who is not receiving warfarin. However, this value is subtherapeutic for anticoagulation therapy. The nurse should expect the client to receive an increased dosage of warfarin until the INR is 2 to 3.

   C. PT of 22 seconds is above the expected reference range for a client receiving warfarin therapy. This result indicates the client is at an increased risk for bleeding.

   D. A negative D-dimer test indicates the absence of a pulmonary embolus or deep vein thrombosis and is not used to determine the dosage needs for warfarin therapy.

   ⓃNCLEX® Connection: Reduction of Risk Potential, Laboratory Values

3. A. The client will be placed in a prone or side-lying position during the test in order to expose the iliac crest.

   B. **CORRECT:** The nurse should inform the client of the need to stay on bed rest for 30 to 60 min following the test to reduce the risk for bleeding.

   C. A culture and sensitivity test determines the type of antibiotics needed to treat an infection.

   D. The client will receive a sedative prior to the test, and a local anesthetic will be used at the site.

   ⓃNCLEX® Connection: Reduction of Risk Potential, Therapeutic Procedures

PRACTICE Answer

Using the ATI Active Learning Template: Diagnostic Procedure

NURSING INTERVENTIONS (PRE, INTRA, POST)

Preprocedure
- Ensure that the client has signed the informed consent form.
- Position the client in a prone or side-lying position.
- Administer medication to manage discomfort and anxiety.
- Reinforce teaching regarding the procedure to the client. Inform the client that she might feel pressure and brief pain during the bone marrow aspiration. Inform the client that the test will last about 20 min. Reinforce the importance of remaining still during the procedure.

Intraprocedure
- Assist with the procedure.
- Cleanse the site with an antiseptic solution.
- Maintain sterility of equipment and supplies.

Postprocedure
- Apply pressure to the biopsy site.
- Place a sterile dressing over the biopsy site.
- Monitor for evidence of infection and bleeding.
- Apply ice to the biopsy site.
- Administer mild analgesics. Avoid aspirin or medications that affect clotting.

POTENTIAL COMPLICATIONS:
Bleeding and infection

CLIENT EDUCATION
- Report excessive bleeding and evidence of infection to the provider.
- Check the biopsy site daily. Keep the dressing clean, dry and intact.

ⓃNCLEX® Connection: Reduction of Risk Potential, Potential for Complications of Diagnostic Tests/Treatments/Procedures

CHAPTER 34 *Blood and Blood Product Transfusions*

Clients can receive transfusions of whole blood or components of whole blood for replacement due to blood loss or blood disease. Blood components include packed RBCs, fresh frozen plasma, albumin, clotting factors, cryoprecipitate, and platelets.

TRANSFUSION TYPES

Standard donation: Transfusion from compatible donor blood.

Autologous transfusions: The client's blood is collected in anticipation of future transfusions (elective surgery). This blood is designated for use only by the client. Clients can donate up to 6 weeks prior to the scheduled surgery. If the client's hemoglobin and hematocrit remain stable, donation can occur weekly to arrive at the desired amount of blood for the anticipated transfusion.

Intraoperative blood salvage: Blood loss during some surgeries (trauma-related, liver transplantation) is recycled through a device that filters blood into a transfusion bag for re-infusion intraoperatively or postoperatively. Re-infusion must occur within 6 hr of salvaged blood collection.

INDICATIONS

POTENTIAL DIAGNOSES

Excessive blood loss: Packed RBCs, whole blood may be given if bleeding is acute such as hemorrhage.

Anemia (Hgb less than 6, or 6 to 10 g/dL, depending on findings): Packed RBCs

Coagulation factor deficiencies such as hemophilia: Fresh frozen plasma

Thrombocytopenia/platelet dysfunction (platelets less than 20,000 or less than 80,000 and actively bleeding): Platelets

Hemophilia A: Cryoprecipitate

CONSIDERATIONS

PREPROCEDURE

- Incompatibility is a major concern when administering blood or blood products. Preventing incompatibility requires strict adherence to blood transfusion protocols.
- Blood is typed based on the presence of antigens.

34.1 Blood type compatibility

BLOOD TYPE	ANTIGEN	ANTIBODIES AGAINST	COMPATIBLE WITH
A	A	B	A, O
B	B	A	B, O
AB	AB	None	A, B, AB, O
O	None	A, B	O

- Another consideration is the Rh factor. Clients who are Rh-negative are born without the Rh antigen in their RBCs. As a result, they do not develop antibodies unless sensitization occurs. Once this occurs, any transfusion with Rh-positive blood will cause a reaction.

NURSING ACTIONS

- Collect data from the client (medical history, history of transfusions, history of blood transfusion reactions).
- Review laboratory values (platelet count less than 20,000 and hemoglobin less than 6 g/dL).
- Verify the prescription for a specific blood product, including number of units to be infused.
- Explain the procedure to the client. Instruct the client about manifestations of transfusion reactions and to report any changes.
- Check vital signs and temperature prior to transfusion.
- Remain with the client during the initial 15 to 30 min of the transfusion. Most severe reactions occur within this time.
- Ensure the client has provided informed consent for the procedure.
- Ensure the client has a large-bore IV access. An 18- or 20-gauge needle is standard for administering blood products.
- Inspect the blood for discoloration, excessive bubbles, or cloudiness.
- Prior to the transfusion, two RNs or an RN and an LPN (depending on facility policy) must identify the correct blood product and client by looking at the hospital identification number (noted on the blood product) and the number identified on the client's identification band to make sure the numbers match.
- The nurse completing the blood product verification must be one of the nurses who administers the blood product.
- Ensure the blood administration set is primed with 0.9% sodium chloride only. Never add medications to blood products. Y-tubing with a filter is used to transfuse blood. Do not piggyback blood into any other IV line.
- OLDER ADULT CLIENTS Ⓖ
  - No larger than a 19-gauge needle is used. A 22-gauge cannula may be used due to fragile veins.
  - Older adult clients are at an increased risk for fluid overload.

INTRAPROCEDURE

NURSING ACTIONS

- Remain with the client for the first 15 to 30 min of the infusion (reactions occur most often during the first 15 min) and monitor vital signs and rate of infusion per facility policy. Qs
- Notify the provider immediately if indications of a reaction occur.
- Blood must be administered within 4 hr to decrease risk of bacterial growth.
- OLDER ADULT CLIENTS: Obtain vital signs every 15 min throughout the transfusion because changes in pulse, blood pressure, and respiratory rate can indicate fluid overload, or can be the sole indicators of a transfusion reaction. Older adult clients who have cardiac or kidney dysfunction are at an increased risk for heart failure and fluid-volume excess when receiving a blood transfusion. Ensure the blood is transfused over 2 to 4 hr. Withhold administration of other IV fluids during blood product administration to prevent fluid overload. Ⓖ

POSTPROCEDURE

NURSING ACTIONS

- Obtain vital signs upon completion of the transfusion.
- Dispose of the blood-administration set according to facility policy.
- Complete paperwork, and file in the designated location.
- Document the client's response.

TRANSFUSION REACTIONS/ ADVERSE EFFECTS

Acute hemolytic (intravascular)

ONSET: Immediate or can manifest during subsequent transfusions

FINDINGS

- Results from transfusion of a blood product that is incompatible with the client's blood type or Rh factor
- Can occur following the transfusion of as little as 10 mL of a blood product
- Can be mild or life-threatening, resulting in disseminated intravascular coagulation (DIC) or circulatory collapse
- Include chills, fever, low-back pain, tachycardia, flushing, hypotension, chest tightening or pain, tachypnea, nausea, anxiety, hemoglobinuria, and an impending sense of doom

NURSING ACTIONS

- Stop the transfusion immediately.
- Notify the provider or emergency response team.
- Remove the blood tubing from the IV access. Avoid infusing further blood products into the circulatory system.
- Ensure an infusion of 0.9% sodium chloride using new tubing is initiated.
- Monitor vital signs and fluid status.
- Send the blood bag and administration set to the lab for testing.
- Obtain blood and urine specimens per facility protocol.

Febrile (non-hemolytic)

ONSET: Commonly occurs within 2 hr of starting the transfusion

FINDINGS

- Results from the development of anti-WBC antibodies
- Can be seen when the client has received multiple transfusions
- Include chills, increase of 1° F (0.5° C) or greater from the pretransfusion temperature, flushing, hypotension, and tachycardia

NURSING ACTIONS

- Use a WBC filter for administration to prevent the reaction from occurring.
- Stop the transfusion and administer antipyretics.
- Ensure an infusion of 0.9% sodium chloride using new tubing is initiated.

Allergic

ONSET: During or up to 24 hr after transfusion

FINDINGS

- Results from a sensitivity reaction to a component of the transfused blood products.
- Findings are usually mild and include itching, urticaria, and flushing.
- The client can develop an anaphylactic transfusion reaction resulting in bronchospasm, laryngeal edema, and shock.

NURSING ACTIONS FOR A MILD REACTION

- Stop the transfusion.
- Initiate an infusion of 0.9% sodium chloride using new tubing.
- Administer an antihistamine, such as diphenhydramine.

NURSING ACTIONS FOR AN ANAPHYLACTIC REACTION

- Stop the transfusion.
- Administer epinephrine or oxygen, or initiate CPR if indicated.
- Remove the blood tubing from the client's IV access.
- Ensure an infusion of 0.9% sodium chloride using new tubing is initiated.

Bacterial

ONSET: During or up to several hours after transfusion

FINDINGS

- Include wheezing, dyspnea, chest tightness, cyanosis, hypotension, and shock
- Results from a transfusion of contaminated blood products

NURSING ACTIONS

- Stop the transfusion.
- Ensure the administration of antibiotics and an IV infusion of 0.9% sodium chloride using new tubing is initiated.
- Send a blood culture specimen to the lab for analysis.

Circulatory overload

ONSET: Can occur any time during the transfusion

FINDINGS
- Manifestations include crackles, dyspnea, cough, anxiety, jugular vein distention, and tachycardia, and can progress to pulmonary edema.
- Results from a transfusion rate that is too rapid for the client. Older adult clients or those who have a preexisting increased circulatory volume are at an increased risk. ©

NURSING ACTIONS
- Slow or stop the transfusion depending on the severity of adverse manifestations
- Position the client upright with feet lower than the level of the heart.
- Administer oxygen, diuretics, and monitor vital signs.

PRACTICE Active Learning Scenario

A nurse is caring for a client who is receiving a blood transfusion. What nursing actions should the nurse anticipate if a transfusion reaction is suspected? Use the ATI Active Learning Template: Nursing Skill to complete this item.

INDICATIONS
- Describe the four types of reactions and the time of onset.
- Describe three medications that can be administered and for which reaction.

POTENTIAL TRANSFUSION REACTIONS: Describe two nursing actions for each type of reaction.

Application Exercises

1. A nurse is assisting with the administration of a unit of packed RBCs to a client who has a Hgb of 8 g/dL. Which of the following actions should the nurse plan to take during the first 15 min of the transfusion?

   A. Verify the client has given informed consent for the transfusion.

   B. Monitor for an acute hemolytic reaction.

   C. Explain the transfusion procedure to the client.

   D. Obtain blood culture specimens to send to the lab.

2. A nurse is caring for a client who is receiving a blood transfusion. Which of the following actions should the nurse take if an allergic transfusion reaction is suspected? (Select all that apply.)

   A. Stop the transfusion.

   B. Monitor for hypertension.

   C. Maintain an IV infusion with 0.9% sodium chloride.

   D. Position the client in an upright position with the feet lower than the heart.

   E. Administer diphenhydramine.

3. A nurse is monitoring a client who began receiving a unit of packed RBCs 10 min ago. Which of the following findings should the nurse identify as an indication of a febrile transfusion reaction? (Select all that apply.)

   A. Temperature change from 37° C (98.6° F) pretransfusion to 37.2° C (99.0° F)

   B. Blood pressure 178/90 mm Hg

   C. Heart rate change from 88/min pretransfusion to 120/min

   D. Client report of itching

   E. Flushed appearance

4. A nurse is reinforcing preoperative teaching with a client who requests autologous donation in preparation for a scheduled orthopedic surgical procedure. Which of the following statements should the nurse make?

   A. "You should make an appointment to donate blood 8 weeks prior to the surgery."

   B. "If you need an autologous transfusion, the blood your brother donates can be used."

   C. "You can donate blood each week if your hemoglobin is stable."

   D. "Any unused blood that is donated can be used for other clients."

5. A newly licensed nurse is assisting a charge nurse with the administration of a blood transfusion to an older adult client. Which of the following actions by the newly licensed nurse indicates an understanding of the procedure?

   A. Ensures the insertion of an 18-gauge IV catheter in the client

   B. Verifies blood compatibility and expiration date of the blood with another PN

   C. Ensures the administration of dextrose 5% in 0.9% sodium chloride IV with the transfusion

   D. Obtains vital signs every 15 min throughout the procedure

Application Exercises Key

1. A. The nurse should verify the client has given informed consent for the transfusion prior to the initiation of the transfusion.

    B. **CORRECT:** The nurse should monitor for an acute hemolytic reaction during the first 15 min of the transfusion. This form of a reaction can occur following the transfusion of as little as 10 mL of blood product.

    C. The nurse should explain the transfusion procedure to the client prior to initiating the transfusion.

    D. The nurse should obtain blood culture specimens from the client if a bacterial reaction is suspected.

    Ⓝ *NCLEX® Connection: Pharmacological Therapies, Medication Administration*

2. A. **CORRECT:** The nurse should immediately stop the infusion if an allergic transfusion reaction is suspected.

    B. The nurse should monitor for hypotension if an allergic transfusion reaction is suspected due to the risk for shock.

    C. **CORRECT:** The nurse should maintain an infusion of 0.9% sodium chloride solution through new IV tubing if an allergic transfusion reaction is suspected.

    D. The nurse should position the client in an upright position with the feet lower than the level of the heart if a circulatory overload is suspected.

    E. **CORRECT:** The nurse should administer an antihistamine, such as diphenhydramine, if an allergic transfusion reaction is suspected.

    Ⓝ *NCLEX® Connection: Pharmacological Therapies, Adverse Effects/ Contraindications/Side Effects/Interactions*

3. A. A temperature increase of 1° F (0.5° C) is an indication of a febrile transfusion reaction.

    B. Hypotension is an indication of a febrile transfusion reaction.

    C. **CORRECT:** Tachycardia is an indication of a febrile transfusion reaction.

    D. The client's report of itching is an indication of an allergic transfusion reaction.

    E. **CORRECT:** A flushed appearance can indicate a febrile transfusion reaction.

    Ⓝ *NCLEX® Connection: Pharmacological Therapies, Adverse Effects/ Contraindications/Side Effects/Interactions*

4. A. The client should donate blood for an autologous transfusion no earlier than 6 weeks prior to surgery.

    B. An autologous donation refers to the client's donation of blood for personal use.

    C. **CORRECT:** Beginning 6 weeks prior to surgery, the client can donate blood each week for autologous transfusion if Hgb and Hct remain stable.

    D. An autologous donation is for use only by the client.

    Ⓝ *NCLEX® Connection: Reduction of Risk Potential, Therapeutic Procedures*

5. A. The nurse should ensure that the IV uses no larger than a 19-gauge needle in the older adult client.

    B. The nurse should verify the client's identity and blood compatibility, and expiration date of the blood with an RN.

    C. The nurse should ensure blood products are administered with 0.9% sodium chloride. IV solutions containing dextrose cannot be used.

    D. **CORRECT:** The nurse should check the older adult client's vital signs every 15 min throughout the transfusion to allow for early detection of fluid overload or other transfusion reaction.

    Ⓝ *NCLEX® Connection: Reduction of Risk Potential, Laboratory Values*

PRACTICE Answer

Using the ATI Active Learning Template: Nursing Skill

INDICATIONS

Types of reactions and onset
- Acute hemolytic: Immediate or during subsequent transfusions
- Febrile: Within 2 hr of starting the transfusion
- Allergic: During or up to 24 hr after transfusion
- Bacterial: During or up to 8 hr after the transfusion
- Circulatory overload: Any time during the transfusion

Medications
- Antipyretics (acetaminophen): Febrile
- Antihistamines (diphenhydramine): Mild allergic
- Antihistamines, corticosteroids, vasopressors, epinephrine: Anaphylactic
- Antibiotics: Bacterial
- Diuretics, morphine: Circulatory overload

POTENTIAL TRANSFUSION REACTIONS

Acute hemolytic
- Stop the transfusion.
- Remove the blood tubing.
- Ensure an infusion of 0.9% sodium chloride is initiated.
- Monitor vital signs and fluid status.
- Send the blood bag and administration set to the lab for testing.

Febrile
- Use a WBC filter to help prevent a febrile reaction.
- Stop the transfusion.
- Administer antipyretics.
- Ensure an infusion of 0.9% sodium chloride is initiated.

Mild allergic reaction
- Stop the transfusion.
- Ensure an infusion of 0.9% sodium chloride is initiated.
- Administer an antihistamine.

Anaphylactic reaction
- Stop the transfusion.
- Administer epinephrine and oxygen.
- Administer CPR if indicated.
- Remove the blood tubing from the client's IV access.
- Ensure an infusion of 0.9% sodium chloride is initiated.

Circulatory overload
- Slow or stop the transfusion depending on the severity.
- Position the client upright with feet lower than the level of the heart.
- Administer oxygen, diuretics, and monitor vital signs.

Bacterial
- Stop the transfusion.
- Administer antibiotics
- Ensure an infusion of 0.9% sodium chloride is initiated.
- Send blood samples to the lab for culture.

Ⓝ *NCLEX® Connection: Pharmacological Therapies, Adverse Effects/Contraindications/Side Effects/Interactions*

CHAPTER 35 *Anemias*

Anemia is an abnormally low amount of circulating RBCs, Hgb concentration, or both. It is an indicator of an underlying disease or disorder. Anemia results in diminished oxygen-carrying capacity and delivery to tissues and organs. The goal of treatment is to restore and maintain adequate tissue oxygenation.

Iron-deficiency anemia due to inadequate intake is the most common cause of anemia in children, adolescents, and pregnant clients. Iron-deficiency anemia due to blood loss (such as from a gastrointestinal ulcer) is the most common cause of anemia in women who are postmenopausal, as well as men. Clients who are menstruating can develop anemia secondary to menorrhagia.

CAUSES OF ANEMIA

- Blood loss
- Inadequate RBC production (hypoproliferative)
- Increased RBC destruction (hemolytic)
- Deficiency of necessary components (folic acid, iron, erythropoietin, vitamin B_{12})

HEALTH PROMOTION AND DISEASE PREVENTION

- Clients who are pregnant or menstruating should ensure that their diet contains adequate amounts of iron-rich foods. Otherwise, they should take an iron supplement.
- Individuals who are iron-deficient and have elevated cholesterol levels should integrate iron-rich foods that are not red or organ meats into their diets (iron-fortified cereal and breads, fish, poultry, dried peas and beans).
- Clients should regularly consume foods high in folate (spinach, lentils, bananas) and folic acid (fortified grains and juices).

DATA COLLECTION

RISK FACTORS

Acute or chronic blood loss
- Trauma
- Menorrhagia
- Gastrointestinal bleed (ulcers, tumor)
- Intra- or postsurgical blood loss or hemorrhage
- Chemical or radiation exposure

Increased hemolysis
- Defective Hgb (sickle-cell disease): RBCs become malformed during periods of hypoxia and obstruct capillaries in joints and organs (35.1)
- Impaired glycolysis
- Immune disorder or destruction (transfusion reactions, autoimmune diseases)
- Mechanical trauma to RBCs (mechanical heart valve, cardiopulmonary bypass)

Inadequate dietary intake or malabsorption
- Iron deficiency
- Vitamin B_{12} deficiency: pernicious anemia due to deficiency of intrinsic factor produced by gastric mucosa
- Folic acid deficiency
- Pica (persistent eating of substances not normally considered food [nonnutritive substances] such as soil or chalk for at least 1 month) can limit the amount of healthy food choices a client makes.

Bone-marrow suppression
- Exposure to radiation or chemicals (insecticides, solvents)
- Aplastic anemia results in a decreased number of RBCs as well as decreased platelets and WBCs.

Age
- Older adult clients are at risk for nutrition-deficient anemias (iron, vitamin B_{12}, folate). Ⓖ
- Anemia can be misdiagnosed as depression or debilitation in older adult clients.
- Gastrointestinal bleeding is a common cause of anemia in older adult clients. Check stools for occult blood.

EXPECTED FINDINGS

- Possibly asymptomatic in mild cases
- Pallor
- Fatigue
- Irritability
- Numbness and tingling of extremities
- Dyspnea on exertion
- Sensitivity to cold
- Pain and hypoxia with sickle-cell crisis

PHYSICAL FINDINGS
- Shortness of breath/fatigue, especially upon exertion
- Tachycardia and palpitations
- Dizziness or syncope upon standing or with exertion
- Pallor with pale nail beds and mucous membranes
- Nail bed deformities (spoon-shaped nails)
- Smooth, sore, bright-red tongue (vitamin B_{12} deficiency)

LABORATORY TESTS

CBC count

- RBCs are the major carriers of hemoglobin in the blood.
- Hgb transports oxygen and carbon dioxide to and from the cells and can be used as an index of the oxygen-carrying capacity of the blood.
- Hct is the percentage of RBCs in relation to the total blood volume.

RBC indices

Used to determine the type and cause of most anemias (35.2)

Mean corpuscular volume (MCV): Size of red blood cells
- Normocytic: Normal size
- Microcytic: Small cells
- Macrocytic: Large cells

Mean corpuscular hemoglobin (MCH): Determines the amount of Hgb per RBC
- Normochromic: Normal amount of Hgb per cell
- Hypochromic: Decreased Hgb per cell

Mean corpuscular hemoglobin concentration (MCHC): Indicates Hgb amount relative to the size of the cell

Iron studies

- Total iron-binding capacity (TIBC) reflects an indirect measurement of serum transferrin, a protein that binds with iron and transports it for storage.
- Serum ferritin is an indicator of total iron stores in the body.
- Serum iron measures the amount of iron in the blood. Low serum iron and elevated TIBC indicates iron-deficiency anemia.

Hemoglobin electrophoresis

- Separates normal Hgb from abnormal Hgb.
- Used to detect thalassemia and sickle-cell disease

Sickle-cell test

Evaluates the sickling of RBCs in the presence of decreased oxygen tension

Schilling test

- Measures vitamin B_{12} absorption with and without intrinsic factor
- Used to differentiate between malabsorption and pernicious anemia

DIAGNOSTIC PROCEDURES

Bone-marrow aspiration/biopsy is used to diagnose aplastic anemia (failure of bone marrow to produce RBCs as well as platelets and WBCs).

PATIENT-CENTERED CARE

NURSING CARE

- Encourage increased dietary intake of the deficient nutrient (iron, vitamin B_{12}, folic acid).
- Monitor oxygen saturation to determine a need for oxygen therapy.
- Administer medications at the proper time for optimal absorption, using a desired technique.
- Reinforce teaching with the client and family about energy conservation in the client and the risk of the client experiencing dizziness upon standing.
- Reinforce teaching with the client about the time frame for resolution.

MEDICATIONS

Iron supplements

Ferrous sulfate, ferrous fumarate, ferrous gluconate
- Oral iron supplements are used to replenish serum iron and iron stores. Iron is an essential component of Hgb, and subsequently, oxygen transport.
- Parenteral iron supplements (iron dextran) are only given for severe anemia or when oral iron supplements are ineffective or poorly tolerated by the client.

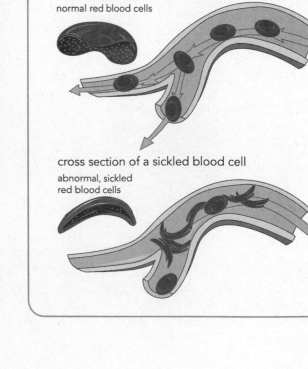

35.1 Sickled blood cells

cross section of a red blood cell
normal red blood cells

cross section of a sickled blood cell
abnormal, sickled red blood cells

35.2 RBC indices

	NORMAL MCV, MCH, MCHC	DECREASED MCV, MCH, MCHC	INCREASED MCV
CLASSIFICATION	Normocytic, normochromic anemia	Microcytic, hypochromic anemia	Macrocytic anemia
POSSIBLE CAUSES	Acute blood loss Sickle-cell disease	Iron-deficiency anemia Anemia of chronic illness Chronic blood loss	Vitamin B$_{12}$ deficiency Folic acid deficiency

NURSING ACTIONS
- Iron dextran-induced fatal anaphylactic reactions have occurred. Administer a test dose prior to administration of full dose. Have epinephrine and resuscitation equipment available.
- Administer parenteral iron using the Z-track method.

CLIENT EDUCATION
- Have hemoglobin checked in 4 to 6 weeks to determine efficacy.
- Vitamin C can increase oral iron absorption.
- Take iron supplements between meals to increase absorption, if tolerated.
- Stools can appear green to black while taking iron.

Erythropoietin (epoetin alfa)

Hematopoietic growth factor used to increase production of RBCs

NURSING ACTIONS
- Monitor for an increase in blood pressure.
- Monitor Hgb and Hct twice per week.
- Monitor for a cardiovascular event if Hgb increases too rapidly (greater than 1 g/dL in 2 weeks).

CLIENT EDUCATION: Have Hgb and Hct evaluated on a twice-per-week basis until targeted levels are reached.

Vitamin B$_{12}$ supplementation (cyanocobalamin)

- Vitamin B$_{12}$ is necessary to convert folic acid from its inactive form to its active form. All cells rely on folic acid for DNA production.
- Vitamin B$_{12}$ supplementation can be given orally if the deficit is due to inadequate dietary intake. However, if deficiency is due to lack of intrinsic factor being produced by the parietal cells of the stomach or malabsorption syndrome, it must be administered parenterally or intranasally to be absorbed.

NURSING ACTIONS
- Administer vitamin B$_{12}$ according to appropriate route related to cause of vitamin B$_{12}$ anemia (parenteral vs. oral).
- Administer parenteral forms of vitamin B$_{12}$ IM or deep subcutaneous to decrease irritation. Do not mix other medications in the syringe.

CLIENT EDUCATION
- For clients who lack intrinsic factor or have an irreversible malabsorption syndrome, this therapy must be continued for the rest of their life.
- Clients should receive vitamin B$_{12}$ injections on a monthly basis.

Folic acid supplements

Folic acid is a water-soluble B-complex vitamin. It is necessary for the production of new RBCs.

NURSING ACTIONS: Administer folic acid orally or parenterally.

CLIENT EDUCATION
- Large doses of folic acid can mask vitamin B$_{12}$ deficiency.
- Large doses of folic acid will turn urine dark yellow.

THERAPEUTIC PROCEDURES

Blood transfusions

- Blood transfusions lead to an immediate improvement in blood-cell counts and manifestations of anemia.
- Due to the risk of bloodborne infections, they are typically only used when the client has significant manifestations of anemia.

COMPLICATIONS

Heart failure

Heart failure can develop due to the increased demand on the heart to provide oxygen to tissues. A low Hct decreases the amount of oxygen carried to tissues in the body, which makes the heart work harder and beat faster (tachycardia, palpitations).

NURSING ACTIONS
- Administer oxygen, and monitor oxygen saturation.
- Monitor cardiac rhythm.
- Obtain daily weight.
- Monitor blood transfusion.
- Administer cardiac medications (diuretics, antidysrhythmics).
- Administer antianemia medications.

Application Exercises

1. A nurse is contributing to the plan of care for a client who has a Hgb of 7.5 g/dL and a Hct of 21.5%. Which of the following interventions should the nurse include? (Select all that apply.)

   A. Provide assistance with ambulation.

   B. Monitor oxygen saturation.

   C. Weigh the client weekly.

   D. Obtain stool specimen for occult blood.

   E. Schedule daily rest periods.

2. A nurse is reinforcing teaching with a client who has a new prescription for ferrous sulfate. Which of the following information should the nurse include?

   A. Stools will be dark red.

   B. Take with a glass of milk if gastrointestinal distress occurs.

   C. Foods high in vitamin C will promote absorption.

   D. Take for 14 days.

3. A nurse is reinforcing discharge teaching with a client who had a gastrectomy due to stomach cancer. Which of the following statements should the nurse make? (Select all that apply.)

   A. "You will need a monthly injection of vitamin B_{12} for the rest of your life."

   B. "Using the nasal spray form of vitamin B_{12} on a daily basis can be an option."

   C. "An oral supplement of vitamin B_{12} taken on a daily basis can be an option."

   D. "You should increase your intake of animal proteins, legumes, and dairy products to increase vitamin B_{12} in your diet."

   E. "Add soy milk fortified with vitamin B_{12} to your diet to decrease the risk of pernicious anemia."

4. A nurse is collecting data from a client who has anemia. Which of the following integumentary findings should the nurse expect?

   A. Absent turgor

   B. Spoon-shaped nails

   C. Shiny, hairless legs

   D. Yellow mucous membranes

5. A nurse in an outpatient clinic is reinforcing discharge instructions with a client who has a new prescription for erythropoietin. Which of the following statements should the nurse make?

   A. "You will need an erythrocyte sedimentation rate (ESR) test weekly."

   B. "You should have your hemoglobin level checked twice per week."

   C. "Your oxygen saturation levels should be monitored."

   D. "Your folic acid production will increase."

PRACTICE Active Learning Scenario

A nurse is helping prepare a program on anemia for a group of community residents. What should be included in this presentation? Use the ATI Active Learning Template: System Disorder to complete this item.

PATHOPHYSIOLOGY RELATED TO CLIENT PROBLEM: Describe at least three causes of the disorder.

EXPECTED FINDINGS: Identify at least six.

LABORATORY TESTS: Describe the importance of the total iron-binding capacity (TIBC) test.

Application Exercises Key

1. A. **CORRECT:** The nurse should assist the client when ambulating to prevent a fall because the client who has anemia can experience dizziness.

   B. **CORRECT:** The nurse should monitor oxygen saturation when the client has anemia due to the decreased oxygen-carrying capacity of the blood.

   C. The nurse should weigh the client daily to determine if the client is losing weight from inadequate oral intake or gaining weight, which can indicate a complication of heart failure due to lack of oxygen from low hemoglobin level.

   D. **CORRECT:** The nurse should obtain the client's stool to test for occult blood, which can identify a possible cause of anemia caused from gastrointestinal bleeding.

   E. **CORRECT:** The nurse should schedule the client to rest throughout the day because the client who has anemia can experience fatigue. Rest periods should be planned to conserve energy.

   Ⓝ *NCLEX® Connection: Reduction of Risk Potential, Potential for Alterations in Body Systems*

2. A. Stools will be dark green to black when taking iron.

   B. Milk binds with iron and decreases its absorption.

   C. **CORRECT:** Vitamin C enhances the absorption of iron by the intestinal tract.

   D. Iron therapy usually takes 4 to 6 weeks for Hgb and Hct to return to the expected reference range.

   Ⓝ *NCLEX® Connection: Pharmacological Therapies, Medication Administration*

3. A. **CORRECT:** Clients who have had a gastrectomy will require monthly injections of vitamin B_{12} for the rest of their life due to lack of intrinsic factor being produced by the parietal cells of the stomach.

   B. **CORRECT:** Cyanocobalamin nasal spray used daily is an option for a client who had a gastrectomy.

   C. The client will not be able to absorb oral vitamin B_{12} due to the lack of intrinsic factor produced by the parietal cells of the stomach.

   D. The client will not be able to absorb dietary sources of vitamin B_{12} due to the lack of intrinsic factor produced by the parietal cells of the stomach.

   E. The client will not be able to absorb dietary sources of vitamin B_{12} due to the lack of intrinsic factor produced by the parietal cells of the stomach.

   Ⓝ *NCLEX® Connection: Reduction of Risk Potential, Potential for Complications from Surgical Procedures and Health Alterations*

4. A. Absent skin turgor is an expected finding in a client who has dehydration.

   B. **CORRECT:** Deformities of the nails, such as being spoon-shaped, are expected findings in a client who has anemia.

   C. Shiny, hairless legs are expected findings in a client who has peripheral vascular disease.

   D. Yellow mucous membranes are expected findings in a client who has jaundice. The client who has anemia will have pale nail beds and mucous membranes.

   Ⓝ *NCLEX® Connection: Reduction of Risk Potential, Potential for Alterations in Body Systems*

5. A. An erythrocyte sedimentation rate test measures inflammation in the body.

   B. **CORRECT:** Hemoglobin and hematocrit are monitored twice a week to determine the effectiveness of erythropoietin until target levels are reached.

   C. The nurse should monitor the client's blood pressure for an increase and determine if the provider should prescribe an antihypertensive.

   D. The nurse should inform the client that erythropoietin promotes increased production of RBCs.

   Ⓝ *NCLEX® Connection: Pharmacological Therapies, Medication Administration*

PRACTICE Answer

Using the ATI Active Learning Template: System Disorder

PATHOPHYSIOLOGY RELATED TO CLIENT PROBLEM: Anemia is an abnormally low amount of circulating red blood cells, hemoglobin concentration, or both. It can be due to blood loss, inadequate production or increased destruction of red blood cells, and dietary deficiencies of folic acid, iron, erythropoietin, or vitamin B_{12}.

EXPECTED FINDINGS
- Shortness of breath and fatigue upon exertion
- Tachycardia, palpitations, dizziness, or syncope upon standing or with exertion
- Pallor, pale nail beds, pale mucous membranes, nail bed deformities
- Smooth, sore, bright-red tongue
- Can be asymptomatic
- Pallor, fatigue, irritability, numbness and tingling of extremities, dyspnea on exertion, sensitivity to cold
- The client who has sickle-cell crisis can experience pain and hypoxia.

LABORATORY TESTS: A TIBC test is an indirect measurement of serum transferrin, a protein that binds with iron and transports it for storage. Serum transferrin is an indicator of the total iron stores in the body.

Ⓝ *NCLEX® Connection: Physiological Adaptation, Basic Pathophysiology*

NCLEX® Connections

When reviewing the following chapters, keep in mind the relevant topics and tasks of the NCLEX outline, in particular:

Physiological Adaptation

BASIC PATHOPHYSIOLOGY: Consider general principles of client disease process when providing care (injury and repair, immunity, cellular structure).

FLUID AND ELECTROLYTE IMBALANCES: Identify signs and symptoms of the client's fluid and/or electrolyte imbalances.

MEDICAL EMERGENCIES: Reinforce teaching of emergency intervention explanations to the client.

CHAPTER 36 *Fluid Imbalances*

The body maintains homeostasis when the characteristics of body fluid remain in balance: volume, concentration (osmolality), composition (electrolyte concentration), and acidity (pH). In the healthy adult client, 55% to 60% of body weight is comprised of body fluid. This decreases to about 50% to 55% in a healthy older adult client.

Fluid moves between compartments through selectively permeable membranes by a variety of methods (diffusion, active transport, filtration, osmosis) to maintain homeostasis. Diffusion is the passive movement of electrolytes and other particles from higher concentration to lower concentration gradient. Active transport requires energy (ATP) to move electrolytes against the concentration gradient into the cell membrane. Filtration is the movement of fluids across the capillaries. Osmosis is the pulling of water into and out of the cells by osmotic pressure.

Balance is maintained through input and output. Intake is regulated by thirst, but social factors and habits also affect adequate fluid intake. Fluid output occurs in the kidneys, skin, lungs, and gastrointestinal tract. The kidneys are the major regulators of fluid output.

BODY FLUIDS

Body fluids are distributed between two compartments.

Intracellular fluid
- Two-thirds of body water
- Body fluids within the cell

Extracellular fluid
- One-third of body water
- Body fluids outside of the cell membrane
- Further divided into parts
  - **Intravascular fluid:** The liquid part of blood or the plasma
  - **Interstitial fluid:** Located between the cells and outside of the blood vessels
  - **Transcellular body fluids:** Secreted by epithelial cells (cerebrospinal, pleural, peritoneal, and synovial fluids)

CAUSES OF VOLUME IMBALANCES

Abnormal gastrointestinal losses: Vomiting, nasogastric suctioning, diarrhea

Abnormal skin losses: Diaphoresis

Abnormal kidney losses: Diuretic therapy, diabetes insipidus, kidney disease, adrenal insufficiency, osmotic diuresis

Third spacing: Peritonitis, intestinal obstruction, ascites, burns

Hemorrhage

Altered intake, such as nothing by mouth (NPO)

Fluid volume deficits

Fluid volume deficits can be divided into two main categories: volume imbalances and osmolality imbalances. When there is an issue with volume imbalance, it relates to a lack of body fluid in the extracellular compartment. Osmolality imbalances occur when there is disturbance in concentration of body fluid.

- Volume imbalances occur when too little or too much isotonic fluid is present.
- Osmolality imbalances occur when body fluid becomes either hypertonic or hypotonic. Hypernatremia (water deficit) and hyponatremia (water excess or intoxication) are good examples of this type of imbalance.

DATA COLLECTION

RISK FACTORS

Fluid loss

- Strenuous exercising
- Increased intake of caffeine and alcohol
- Living at high elevations or in dry climates
- The effect of fluid imbalance in older adults is greater due to the loss of elasticity of the skin, decrease in glomerular filtration and concentrating ability of the kidneys, loss of muscle mass (muscle tissue holds more body water), and diminished thirst reflex. Ⓖ

EXPECTED FINDINGS

Hypovolemia

VITAL SIGNS: Hyperthermia, tachycardia (in an attempt to maintain a normal blood pressure), thready pulse, hypotension, orthostatic hypotension, decreased central venous pressure, tachypnea (increased respirations to compensate for lack of fluid volume within the body), hypoxia

NEUROMUSCULOSKELETAL: Dizziness, syncope, confusion, weakness, fatigue

GASTROINTESTINAL: Thirst, dry furrowed tongue, nausea, vomiting, anorexia, acute weight loss

KIDNEYS: Oliguria (decreased production and concentration of urine)

OTHER FINDINGS: Diminished capillary refill, cool clammy skin, diaphoresis, sunken eyeballs, flattened neck veins, poor skin turgor and tenting, weight loss, low central venous pressure

Osmolality imbalances or hypernatremia

- Extreme thirst
- Skin that is dry and flushed
- Postural hypotension
- Fever
- Restlessness, confusion, agitation
- Coma and seizures can occur because onset of fluid imbalance is rapid.

LABORATORY TESTS

Hematocrit (Hct): Increased in hypovolemia

BUN: Increased (greater than 25 mg/dL) due to hemoconcentration

Urine specific gravity: Greater than 1.030

Serum sodium: Greater than 145 mEq/L

Serum osmolality: Greater than 295 mOsm/kg

PATIENT-CENTERED CARE

NURSING CARE

- Monitor I&O.
- Monitor vital signs. Check orthostatic measurements, as a client is at increased risk of falls when orthostatic hypotension present.
- Monitor for changes in mentation and confusion (an indication of worsening fluid imbalance).
- Monitor IV rehydration infusions. Monitor weight every 8 hr while fluid replacement is in progress.
- Determine level of gait stability. Encourage the client to use the call light and request assistance. Qs
- Initiate fall precautions.
- Encourage the client to change positions, rolling from side to side or standing up slowly.

INTERPROFESSIONAL CARE

Collaborate with other members of the health care team to determine adequate fluid volume replacement and oxygen management.

CLIENT EDUCATION

- Drink plenty of liquids to promote hydration, if not contraindicated.
- Causes of dehydration include nausea and vomiting.

COMPLICATIONS

Hypovolemic shock

- Occurs with significant loss of body fluid.
- The client's mean arterial pressure decreases (which slows blood flow and perfusion to tissues of the body) and the cells are no longer able to carry oxygen to the blood adequately (due to the loss of red blood cells).

NURSING ACTIONS

- Administer oxygen, and monitor oxygen saturation level. An oxygen saturation level less than 70% is a medical emergency.
- Stay with an unstable client suffering from hypovolemic shock.
- Monitor vital signs at least every 15 min.
- Check IV access. Two large-bore IV sites or a central venous catheter can be necessary for infusion of large volumes of fluids.
- Monitor fluid replacement with the following.
  - **Colloids:** whole blood, packed RBCs, plasma, synthetic plasma expanders
  - **Crystalloids:** lactated Ringer's, normal saline
- The client will require vasoconstrictors (dopamine, norepinephrine, phenylephrine), agents to improve myocardial perfusion (sodium nitroprusside), and/or positive inotropic medications (dobutamine, milrinone) and hemodynamic monitoring.

Fluid volume excesses

Overhydration occurs when there is an excess of fluids in the body. It is an indication that the intake of fluids and the excretion of fluids is not in balance. Another term for this phenomenon is hypervolemia, as there is excess fluid in the extracellular space.

- Fluid overload can also occur when the electrolytes in the body are not in balance. For example, the lack of or excess of serum sodium can result in fluid imbalance. For more information, see **CHAPTER 37: ELECTROLYTE IMBALANCES**.
- Clients who have fluid overload are at risk for developing pulmonary edema or congestive heart failure.

HEALTH PROMOTION AND DISEASE PREVENTION

- In healthy people, the body will compensate for slight changes in fluid imbalance and the excessive intake of electrolytes. In older adult clients, the risk of fluid imbalance is greater due to changes in the body with age (reduced kidney function).
- When clients have heart disease and impairment of kidney function, it is important to reinforce the following.
  - Consume a diet low in sodium. Consult with the provider regarding diet restrictions.
  - Restrict fluid intake. Consult with the provider regarding prescribed restrictions.

DATA COLLECTION

RISK FACTORS

Causes of hypervolemia
- Compromised regulatory systems (heart failure, kidney disease, cirrhosis)
- Overdose of sodium concentrated fluids
- Fluid shifts that occur following burns
- Prolonged use of corticosteroids
- Severe stress
- Hyperaldosteronism

EXPECTED FINDINGS

Fluid volume overload

VITAL SIGNS: Tachycardia, bounding pulse, hypertension, tachypnea, increased central venous pressure

NEUROMUSCULAR: Weakness due to excess fluid retained, which depletes energy and increases the workload for the body; headache; altered level of consciousness

GASTROINTESTINAL: Ascites

RESPIRATORY: Crackles, cough, increased respiratory rate, dyspnea caused by an excess of fluids within the body and lungs

OTHER INDICATIONS: Peripheral edema due to an excess of fluids within the body and lungs, resulting in weight gain, distended neck veins, and increased urine output (36.1)

LABORATORY TESTS

- Decreased Hct and Hgb
- Decreased serum and urine osmolarity
- Decreased urine sodium and specific gravity
- Decreased BUN due to plasma dilution

DIAGNOSTIC PROCEDURES

Chest x-ray reveals possible pulmonary congestion.

PATIENT-CENTERED CARE

NURSING CARE

- Monitor I&O.
- Monitor daily weight.
- Auscultate breath sounds.
- Monitor peripheral edema.
- Maintain sodium-restricted diet.
- Maintain fluid restrictions.
- Encourage rest.
- Monitor clients receiving diuretics.
- Encourage the client to discuss use of over-the-counter medications with the provider, as some of these contain sodium.

36.1 Pitting edema

- Position the client in the semi-Fowler's position, and reposition to prevent tissue breakdown in edematous skin.
- Use a pressure-reducing mattress, and check bony prominences on a regular basis.
- Monitor serum sodium and potassium levels.

INTERPROFESSIONAL CARE

- Respiratory services can assist with oxygen management.
- Pulmonology services can assist if fluid moves into lungs.

CLIENT EDUCATION

- Weigh daily. Notify the provider if there is a 1- to 2-lb gain in 24 hr, or a 3-lb gain in 1 week. After the first ½-lb weight gain, each additional pound of weight gain is equal to 500 mL retained fluid.
- Consume a low-sodium diet, read food labels to check sodium content, and keep a record of daily sodium intake. Q_{EBP}
- Restrict fluid intake. Consult with the provider regarding prescribed restrictions.

COMPLICATIONS

Pulmonary edema

- Pulmonary edema can be caused by severe fluid overload.
- Acute pulmonary edema is a medical emergency and requires prompt treatment.
- Manifestations include anxiety, tachycardia, jugular vein distention, premature ventricular contractions, dyspnea at rest, change in level of consciousness, restlessness, lethargy, ascending (fluid level within lungs), and productive cough of frothy pink-tinged sputum.

NURSING ACTIONS

- Position the client in high-Fowler's to maximize ventilation.
- Administer oxygen and positive airway pressure.
- Ask the charge nurse to administer morphine, nitrates, and diuretic if blood pressure is adequate.

Application Exercises

1. A nurse is collecting data from a client who reports nausea, vomiting, and weakness. The client has dry oral mucous membranes. Which of the following findings should the nurse identify as manifestations of fluid volume deficit? (Select all that apply.)

   A. Decreased skin turgor

   B. Concentrated urine

   C. Bradycardia

   D. Low-grade fever

   E. Tachypnea

2. A nurse is observing an older adult client who is receiving packed RBCs. Which of the following findings should the nurse identify as a manifestation of fluid volume excess and report to the charge nurse? (Select all that apply.)

   A. Dyspnea

   B. Edema

   C. Bradycardia

   D. Hypertension

   E. Weakness

3. A nurse is collecting data from a client who is dehydrated due to fluid volume deficit. Which of the following findings should the nurse expect?

   A. Moist skin

   B. Distended neck veins

   C. Increased urinary output

   D. Thready pulses

4. A nurse is caring for an older adult client in a long-term care facility who is dehydrated. Which of the following actions should the nurse take?

   A. Initiate fluid restrictions to limit the client's intake.

   B. Observe for indications of peripheral edema.

   C. Encourage the client to promote oxygenation by ambulating.

   D. Monitor for orthostatic hypotension.

PRACTICE Active Learning Scenario

A nurse is contributing the plan of care for a client who is experiencing fluid volume excess. What nursing actions should be included in the plan of care? Use the ATI Active Learning Template: System Disorder to complete this item.

NURSING CARE: Describe three actions the nurse should take.

Application Exercises Key

1. A. **CORRECT:** Decreased skin turgor is a manifestation of fluid volume deficit. Lack of fluid within the body results in dryness of the skin and decreased turgor.

   B. **CORRECT:** Concentrated urine is a manifestation of fluid volume deficit. Urine is concentrated due to a lack of fluid in the vascular system. This causes a decrease in profusion of the kidneys, resulting in increased urine specific gravity.

   C. Tachycardia is a manifestation of fluid volume deficit due to an attempt to maintain a normal blood pressure.

   D. **CORRECT:** Low-grade fever is a manifestation of fluid volume deficit. Low-grade fever is one of the body's ways to maintain homeostasis to compensate for lack of fluid within the body.

   E. **CORRECT:** Tachypnea is a manifestation of fluid volume deficit. Increased respirations are the body's way to obtain oxygen due to the lack of fluid volume within the body.

   Ⓝ *NCLEX® Connection: Physiological Adaptation, Fluid and Electrolyte Imbalances*

2. A. **CORRECT:** Dyspnea is a manifestation of fluid volume excess. Dyspnea is due to an excess of fluids within the body and lungs, and the client is struggling to breathe to obtain oxygen.

   B. **CORRECT:** Edema is a manifestation of fluid volume excess. Weight gain can be a result of edema.

   C. Tachycardia and bounding pulses are manifestations of fluid volume excess.

   D. **CORRECT:** Hypertension is a manifestation of fluid volume excess. Blood pressure rises as the heart must work harder due to the excess fluid.

   E. **CORRECT:** Weakness is a manifestation of fluid volume excess. Weakness is due to the excess fluid that is retained, which depletes energy and increases the workload for the body.

   Ⓝ *NCLEX® Connection: Pharmacological Therapies, Expected Actions/Outcomes*

3. A. The nurse should expect a client who has a fluid volume deficit to have dry skin.

   B. Distended neck veins are a manifestation of fluid volume excess.

   C. Increased urinary output is a manifestation of fluid volume excess.

   D. **CORRECT:** A weak, thready pulse is an expected manifestation of fluid volume deficit caused by low blood pressure.

   Ⓝ *NCLEX® Connection: Physiological Adaptation, Fluid and Electrolyte Imbalances*

4. A. The nurse should offer fluids when the client has manifestations of dehydration.

   B. The nurse should monitor for indications of poor skin turgor when the client has manifestations of fluid volume deficit.

   C. The nurse should keep the client in bed and assist him to the bathroom as needed because he is at risk for falling due to manifestations of dehydration.

   D. **CORRECT:** The nurse should monitor for orthostatic hypotension because the client has manifestations of dehydration due to decreased circulatory volume.

   Ⓝ *NCLEX® Connection: Physiological Adaptation, Fluid and Electrolyte Imbalances*

PRACTICE Answer

Using the ATI Active Learning Template: System Disorder

NURSING CARE
- Check ABGs, SaO₂, CBC, and chest x-ray results.
- Position the client in semi-Fowler's.
- Obtain daily weight.
- Monitor I&O.
- Administer supplemental oxygen.
- Administer diuretics (osmotic, loop).
- Limit fluid and sodium intake.
- Monitor and document presence of edema (pretibial, sacral, periorbital).
- Reposition the client at least every 2 hr.
- Support arms and legs to decrease dependent edema as needed.
- Monitor vital signs and heart rhythm.
- Auscultate lung sounds for crackles.

Ⓝ *NCLEX® Connection: Physiological Adaptation, Fluid and Electrolyte Imbalances*

CHAPTER 38

UNIT 6   NURSING CARE OF CLIENTS WHO HAVE FLUID/ELECTROLYTE/ACID-BASE IMBALANCES

CHAPTER 37

Electrolyte Imbalances

Electrolytes are molecules that dissolve in body fluids or another solvent to form ions that have an electric charge. Cations have a positive charge, and anions have a negative charge. Electrolytes are in intracellular (ICF) and extracellular (ECF) fluid compartments but with different distributions. That difference in the concentration of electrolytes in the ICF and ECF maintains cell excitability and allows for the transmission of nerve impulses.

Body fluids should be electrically neutral, with the negative and positive ions in the body fluids equal in number. Cations (magnesium, potassium, sodium, calcium ions) conduct a positive electrical current; anions (phosphorus/phosphate, sulfate, chloride, bicarbonate ions) conduct a negative electrical current.

Healthy people can develop an imbalance of electrolytes from differences in intake and output. Ill and older adult clients are at higher risk for electrolyte imbalance. Although laboratory tests can accurately reflect the electrolyte concentrations in plasma, it is not possible to measure electrolyte concentrations directly within cells.

EXPECTED REFERENCE RANGES

Sodium: 136 to 145 mEq/L

Calcium: 9.0 to 10.5 mg/dL

Potassium: 3.5 to 5.0 mEq/L

Magnesium: 1.3 to 2.1 mEq/L

Chloride: 98 to 106 mEq/L

Phosphorus: 3.0 to 4.5 mg/dL

Sodium Imbalances

- Sodium (Na^+) is the major electrolyte (cation) in ECF. It maintains ECF osmolarity, volume, and distribution as well as acid–base balance.
- The difference between ICF and ECF sodium levels is important for maintaining skeletal muscle contraction, cardiac contractility, and nerve impulse transmission.
- Water flows in the direction of sodium concentration. The ECF sodium level influences fluid balance, excretion, and movement of fluid from one body space to another.
- The kidneys regulate sodium levels with the assistance of aldosterone, antidiuretic hormone (ADH), and atrial natriuretic factor.
- Hyponatremia is a sodium level less than the expected reference range.
- Hypernatremia is a sodium level greater than the expected reference range.

Hyponatremia

Hyponatremia is a net gain of water, a loss of sodium, or an inadequate intake of sodium that results in sodium levels less than 136 mEq/L.

- Hyponatremia interferes with muscle function.
- Water moves from the ECF into the ICF, causing cells to swell (cellular edema).
- Fluid imbalance, which results in sodium loss, is the usual cause of hyponatremia.

DATA COLLECTION

RISK FACTORS

- Excessive sweating
- Diuretics
- Vomiting
- Diarrhea
- Wound drainage (especially gastrointestinal [GI], burns)
- Nasogastric tube suction of isotonic gastric contents
- Inadequate sodium intake (NPO status, low-sodium diets)
- Hypotonic fluid excess (PO ingestion including enteral feedings, IV fluids)
- Psychogenic polydipsia or excessive water intake
- Kidney disease
- Heart failure
- Liver cirrhosis
- Irrigation with hypotonic fluids, such as tap water instillation via enema
- Syndrome of inappropriate ADH secretion
- Sodium–deficient replacement fluids for GI losses
- Older age (higher incidence of chronic illnesses, use of diuretic medications, risk for insufficient sodium intake) ©

EXPECTED FINDINGS

VITAL SIGNS: Hypotension

NEUROMUSCULOSKELETAL: Headache, muscle twitching, hyperreflexia, tremors, confusion, lethargy, apprehension, anxiety, decrease in level of consciousness, decrease in sensation, seizures, coma

GASTROINTESTINAL: Increased motility, hyperactive bowel sounds, abdominal cramping, nausea, vomiting, diarrhea, anorexia

LABORATORY TESTS

Serum sodium: Less than 136 mEq/L

Serum osmolarity: Less than 285 mOsm/L

PATIENT-CENTERED CARE

NURSING CARE

- If the client can tolerate PO fluids, replace sodium with foods and fluids.
- Assist with the administration of IV fluids (lactated Ringer's or 0.9% sodium chloride).
- Restrict water intake for clients who have heart failure, kidney disease, or insufficient ADH production.
- Hypertonic sodium solution can help reduce cerebral edema.
- Some clients require diuretic therapy to eliminate excess fluid.

Acute hyponatremia

- Ensure administration of hypertonic oral and IV fluids.
- The goal is to elevate the sodium level enough to decrease neurological manifestations (lethargy, confusion, seizures).
- Encourage foods and fluids high in sodium (beef broth, tomato juice).
- Monitor I&O and daily weight.
- Monitor vital signs and level of consciousness.
- Administer diuretics.

INTERPROFESSIONAL CARE

- Nephrology can help with electrolyte and fluid replacement.
- Respiratory services can help with oxygen management.
- Nutritional services can help with high-sodium food choices and fluid restriction.

CLIENT EDUCATION

- Weigh daily and to notify the provider of a 0.5 to 0.9 kg (1 to 2 lb) gain in 24 hr, or 1.4 kg (3 lb) gain in 1 week.
- Consume a high-sodium diet, read food labels to check sodium content, and keep a daily record of sodium intake.

COMPLICATIONS

Acute hyponatremia

Complications (coma, seizures, respiratory arrest) can result from acute hyponatremia without immediate treatment.

NURSING ACTIONS
- Maintain an open airway, and monitor vital signs.
- Implement seizure precautions, and intervene if seizures occur.
- Monitor level of consciousness.

Hypernatremia

Excess sodium pulls water out of the cells, thus dehydrating them.
- Hypernatremia is a sodium level greater than 145 mEq/L.
- Hypernatremia is a serious electrolyte imbalance. It can cause significant neurological, endocrine, and cardiac disturbances.

DATA COLLECTION

RISK FACTORS

- Water deprivation (NPO)
- Hypertonic enteral feedings without adequate water supplementation
- Diabetes insipidus
- Heat stroke
- Hyperventilation
- Watery diarrhea
- Fever
- Burns
- Respiratory infection
- Oral electrolyte solutions
- Excessive sweating
- Excess IV fluids (0.9%, 3%, or 5% sodium chloride; sodium bicarbonate)
- Excessive oral intake of sodium (table salt)
- Age-related changes, specifically decreased total body water content and inadequate fluid intake due to alterations in the thirst mechanism Ⓖ

EXPECTED FINDINGS

- Thirst
- Dry, sticky mucous membranes
- Red, swollen tongue
- Hot, dry skin
- Flushing
- Oliguria
- Decrease in sweating

VITAL SIGNS: Fever, orthostatic hypotension

NEUROMUSCULOSKELETAL: Restlessness, irritability, weakness, lethargy, fatigue, muscle twitching, seizures, decrease in level of consciousness, disorientation, coma, intracranial bleeding

GASTROINTESTINAL: Diarrhea

LABORATORY TESTS

Serum sodium: Greater than 145 mEq/L

Serum osmolarity: Greater than 295 mOsm/L

PATIENT-CENTERED CARE

NURSING CARE

- Monitor level of consciousness and behavior changes, and ensure safety.
- Monitor vital signs and heart rhythm.
- Auscultate lung sounds.
- Provide oral hygiene and other comfort measures to decrease thirst.
- Monitor I&O, and report inadequate urinary output.
- Assist with administration of isotonic IV fluids (dextrose 5% in water, 0.45% sodium chloride).
- Encourage water intake, and discourage sodium intake.
- Provide water between enteral feedings.
- Administer diuretics to promote sodium excretion.

INTERPROFESSIONAL CARE

Nutritional services can help with low-sodium food choices and fluid restriction.

CLIENT EDUCATION

- Weigh daily and notify the provider of a 0.5 to 0.9 kg (1 to 2 lb) gain in 24 hr, or 1.4 kg (3 lb) gain in 1 week.
- Consume a low-sodium diet, drink water, read food labels for sodium content, and keep a record of daily sodium intake.

COMPLICATIONS

Acute hypernatremia

Complications (seizures, convulsion, death) can result from acute hypernatremia without immediate treatment.

NURSING ACTIONS
- Maintain an open airway, and monitor vital signs.
- Implement seizure precautions, and intervene if seizures occur.
- Monitor level of consciousness.

Potassium Imbalances

- Potassium (K⁺) is the major cation in ICF.
- Potassium plays a vital role in cell metabolism, transmission of nerve impulses, and the function of skeletal, smooth, and cardiac muscle tissue.
- A minor variation in the level of potassium is a significant finding.
- Hypokalemia is a potassium level less than the expected reference range.
- Hyperkalemia is a potassium level greater than the expected reference range.

Hypokalemia

Hypokalemia is the result of an increase in potassium losses or movement of potassium into the cells, resulting in a potassium level less than 3.5 mEq/L.

DATA COLLECTION

RISK FACTORS

- Overuse of potassium-wasting diuretics (such as furosemide), digoxin, or corticosteroids.
- Aldosterone excess
- GI losses (vomiting, diarrhea, prolonged nasogastric suctioning, ileostomy drainage, excessive use of laxatives or multiple tap water enemas [because tap water is hypotonic and can move from the bowel lumen into the ICF, causing water intoxication and electrolyte imbalances])
- Alkalosis
- Fistula drainage
- Excessive sweating
- Tissue repair
- Anorexia nervosa
- Polyuria
- Inadequate dietary intake of potassium
- Older age (use of diuretics and laxatives) ⑥

EXPECTED FINDINGS

Fatigue, urinary retention

VITAL SIGNS: Weak, irregular pulse

NEUROLOGIC: Lethargy, confusion

ECG: Flat or inverted T waves, prominent U waves, ST depression

GASTROINTESTINAL: Hypoactive bowel sounds, nausea, vomiting, anorexia, constipation, abdominal distention, abdominal pain, paralytic ileus

MUSCULAR: Weakness (life-threatening with respiratory muscle involvement), depressed deep-tendon reflexes, leg cramps

LABORATORY TESTS

Serum potassium: Less than 3.5 mEq/L

Arterial blood gases: Alkalosis

Urine pH: Greater than 8.0

PATIENT-CENTERED CARE

NURSING CARE

- Monitor clients receiving IV potassium for phlebitis (tissue irritant).
- Monitor I&O.
- Monitor cardiac rhythm.
- Monitor clients receiving digoxin; hypokalemia increases the risk for digoxin toxicity.
- Monitor level of consciousness, and ensure safety.
- Monitor bowel sounds and abdominal distention.
- Check hand grasps for muscle weakness.
- Check deep-tendon reflexes.
- Encourage foods high in potassium (avocados, dairy products, dried fruit, cantaloupe, bananas, meats, fish, oranges, apricot, carrots, potatoes, peas, mushrooms, tomatoes, spinach).
- Provide oral potassium supplementation.
- Reinforce teaching about the manifestations of hypokalemia.

INTERPROFESSIONAL CARE

- Nephrology can help with electrolyte and fluid management.
- Respiratory services can help with oxygen management.
- Nutritional services can help with potassium-rich food choices.
- Cardiology can help with dysrhythmia management.

CLIENT EDUCATION

- Consume potassium-rich foods.
- Prevent a decrease in potassium by avoiding the excessive use of diuretics and laxatives.

COMPLICATIONS

Respiratory failure

NURSING ACTIONS
- Maintain an open airway, and monitor vital signs.
- Monitor level of consciousness.
- Monitor for hypoxemia and hypercapnia.
- Assist with intubation and mechanical ventilation.

Cardiac arrest

NURSING ACTIONS: Perform continuous cardiac monitoring.

Hyperkalemia

Hyperkalemia is the result of an increased intake of potassium, movement of potassium out of the cells, or inadequate kidney excretion, resulting in a potassium level greater than 5.0 mEq/L.
- Hyperkalemia increases the risk for cardiac arrest.
- Hyperkalemia is rare with adequate kidney function.

DATA COLLECTION

RISK FACTORS

- Burns
- Crush injuries
- Kidney disease
- Potassium-sparing diuretics, such as spironolactone
- Excessive use of salt substitutes
- Hypoaldosteronism
- Insulin deficit
- Rapid transfusion of stored blood
- Chemotherapy
- Acidosis, diabetic ketoacidosis
- Older age (use of salt substitutes, ACE inhibitors, potassium-sparing diuretics) Ⓖ

EXPECTED FINDINGS

Fatigue

VITAL SIGNS: Slow irregular pulse, hypotension

NEUROMUSCULOSKELETAL: Restlessness, apathy, confusion, irritability, weakness to the point of paralysis, absence of reflexes, paresthesias

ECG: Heart block, peaked T waves, widened QRS, prolonged PR

GASTROINTESTINAL: Increased motility, diarrhea, hyperactive bowel sounds, nausea, abdominal cramping

LABORATORY TESTS

Serum potassium: Greater than 5.0 mEq/L

PATIENT-CENTERED CARE

NURSING CARE

- Ensure safety and prevent falls.
- Monitor I&O.
- Encourage fluid intake.
- Monitor cardiac rate and rhythm.
- Check for muscle weakness.
- Observe for GI manifestations.
- Restrict dietary potassium, including salt substitutes.
- Provide adequate carbohydrates to prevent protein depletion for energy.
- Watch potassium levels carefully for a sudden decrease.

MEDICATIONS

To increase potassium excretion

Loop diuretics (furosemide)

- Administer if kidney function is adequate.
- Loop diuretics promote excretion of potassium via the renal system.

NURSING ACTIONS
- Ensure IV access.
- Monitor weight daily.
- Observe for edema.
- Check for fluid depletion dizziness, tachycardia, and orthostatic hypotension.

CLIENT EDUCATION
- Restrict dietary potassium.
- Withhold oral potassium supplements.

Cation exchange resins

Sodium polystyrene sulfonate works as a laxative and excretes excess potassium from the body.

NURSING ACTIONS: Clients who have extremely high potassium levels might require dialysis.

CLIENT EDUCATION
- Restrict dietary potassium.
- Withhold oral potassium supplements.

INTERPROFESSIONAL CARE

- Nephrology can help with electrolyte and fluid management and determining the need for dialysis.
- Nutritional services can help with low-potassium food choices.
- Cardiology can help with dysrhythmia management.

CLIENT EDUCATION

- Consume potassium-restricted foods.
- Read food labels and avoid salt substitutes containing potassium.

COMPLICATIONS

Cardiac arrest

NURSING ACTIONS
- Perform continuous cardiac monitoring.
- Initiate cardiopulmonary resuscitation and summon the rapid response team.

Other Electrolyte Imbalances

CALCIUM: Hypocalcemia, hypercalcemia

CHLORIDE: Hypochloremia, hyperchloremia

MAGNESIUM: Hypomagnesemia, hypermagnesemia

PHOSPHORUS: Hypophosphatemia, hyperphosphatemia

Hypocalcemia

Hypocalcemia is a total calcium level less than 9.0 mg/dL.

DATA COLLECTION

RISK FACTORS

- Lactose intolerance
- Malabsorption syndromes (Crohn's disease)
- Chronic diarrhea
- End-stage kidney disease
- Parathyroidectomy
- Bariatric surgery
- Hypoparathyroidism
- Inadequate dietary intake of calcium
- Vitamin D deficiency (increasingly common due to lack of sun exposure, sunscreen use)
- Lack of weight-bearing exercise
- Pancreatitis
- Hyperphosphatemia
- Hypomagnesemia
- Thyroid cancer
- Metastatic disease
- Medications (diuretics, calcitonin)

EXPECTED FINDINGS

Tetany
- Muscle twitches
- Laryngospasm
- Frequent, painful muscle spasms at rest in the foot or calf (charley horses)
- Positive Chvostek sign (tapping on the facial nerve triggering facial twitching)
- Positive Trousseau sign (hand/finger spasms with sustained blood pressure cuff inflation)

VITAL SIGNS: Weak pulse, hypotension

NEUROLOGICAL: Confusion, anxiety, psychosis, seizures, hyperactive deep-tendon reflexes, paresthesias (especially of the fingers, toes, lips)

CARDIOVASCULAR: Dysrhythmias, prolonged QT and ST segments

GASTROINTESTINAL: Hyperactive bowel sounds, diarrhea, abdominal cramps

LABORATORY TESTS

Calcium level less than 9.0 mg/dL

PATIENT-CENTERED CARE

NURSING CARE

- Administer oral calcium supplements, plus vitamin D supplements to enhance the absorption of calcium.
- Implement seizure precautions.
- Avoid overstimulation. Keep the room quiet, limit visitors, and use soft lighting.
- Have emergency equipment readily available.
- Encourage foods high in calcium (dairy products; canned salmon; sardines; fresh oysters; dark green, leafy vegetables).
- Monitor clients receiving IV calcium gluconate or calcium chloride.

INTERPROFESSIONAL CARE

- Endocrinology can help with electrolyte and fluid management.
- Respiratory services can help with oxygen management.
- Nutritional services can help with high-calcium food choices.
- Cardiology can help with dysrhythmia management.

CLIENT EDUCATION

- Consume foods high in calcium (yogurt, milk).
- Read food labels to help increase calcium intake.

Hypomagnesemia

Hypomagnesemia is a magnesium level less than 1.3 mg/dL.

DATA COLLECTION

RISK FACTORS

- Malnutrition (insufficient magnesium intake)
- Aldosterone excess
- Diarrhea
- Nasogastric suction
- Fistula drainage
- Chronic alcohol use disorder
- Pancreatitis
- Burns
- Long-term thiazide diuretic or aminoglycoside antibiotic therapy
- Diabetic ketoacidosis
- Citrate from rapid infusion of blood products
- Steatorrhea

EXPECTED FINDINGS

VITAL SIGNS: Tachycardia, hypertension

NEUROMUSCULAR: Hyperactive deep-tendon reflexes, paresthesias, muscle tetany, leg and foot cramps, muscle twitching, tremors, seizures, positive Chvostek and Trousseau signs, insomnia, vertigo, disorientation, confusion

CARDIOVASCULAR: Dysrhythmias, prolonged PR and QT, depressed ST segments, wide QRS, flat T waves, prominent U waves

GASTROINTESTINAL: Anorexia, dysphagia

PATIENT-CENTERED CARE

NURSING CARE

- Withhold magnesium-depleting medications (loop diuretics, osmotic diuretics, aminoglycoside antibiotics).
- Administer oral or ensure the administration of IV magnesium following safety protocols.
- Implement seizure precautions, and intervene if seizures occur.
- Provide foods high in magnesium (green, leafy vegetables; meat; whole grains; seafood). Dietary changes might correct mild magnesium deficiencies.
- Monitor clients receiving digoxin. Hypomagnesemia increases the risk for digoxin toxicity.

INTERPROFESSIONAL CARE

- Endocrinology can help with electrolyte and fluid management.
- Respiratory services can help with oxygen management.
- Nutritional services can help with high-magnesium food choices.
- Cardiology can help with dysrhythmia management.

CLIENT EDUCATION

- Consume foods high in magnesium.
- Read food labels to help increase magnesium intake.

Application Exercises

1. A nurse is caring for a client who has a serum sodium level of 133 mEq/L and a serum potassium level of 3.4 mEq/L. Which of the following treatments is a risk factor for these laboratory findings?

    A. Three tap water enemas

    B. 0.9% sodium chloride IV

    C. Dextrose 5% in water with 20 mEq of K+ IV

    D. Spironolactone therapy

2. A nurse is collecting data from a client who has a serum potassium level of 5.4 mEq/L. Which of the following manifestations should the nurse expect? (Select all that apply.)

    A. ECG changes

    B. Constipation

    C. Polyuria

    D. Hypotension

    E. Tachycardia

3. A nurse is caring for a client who has a nasogastric tube with low intermittent suctioning. The nurse should monitor the client for which of the following electrolyte imbalances? (Select all that apply.)

    A. Hypercalcemia

    B. Hyponatremia

    C. Hyperphosphatemia

    D. Hypomagnesemia

    E. Hyperkalemia

4. A nurse is collecting data from a client who has hyperkalemia. Which of the following disorders is a risk factor for this electrolyte imbalance?

    A. Diabetic ketoacidosis

    B. Heart failure

    C. Aldosterone excess

    D. Excessive sweating

5. A nurse is collecting data from a client who has hypomagnesemia. Which of the following techniques should the nurse use to check for Chvostek sign?

    A. Apply a blood pressure cuff to the client's arm.

    B. Place the stethoscope's bell over the client's carotid artery.

    C. Tap lightly on the client's cheek.

    D. Ask the client to lower her chin to her chest.

PRACTICE Active Learning Scenario

A nurse is caring for a client who has hypokalemia. Use the ATI Active Learning Template: System Disorder to complete this item.

ALTERATION IN HEALTH (DIAGNOSIS)

NURSING CARE: Describe at least six actions.

INTERPROFESSIONAL CARE: Describe one action.

CLIENT EDUCATION: Describe one teaching point.

COMPLICATIONS: Describe one.

Application Exercises Key

1. A. **CORRECT:** Three tap water enemas can delete sodium and potassium. Tap water is hypotonic and can move from the bowel lumen into the ICF, causing water intoxication and electrolyte imbalances.

   B. Hypotonic IV solutions can decrease electrolyte levels, but 0.9% sodium chloride is an isotonic solution.

   C. Hypotonic IV solutions can decrease electrolyte levels, but dextrose 5% in water is an isotonic solution. With supplemental potassium, it would not cause hypokalemia.

   D. Spironolactone is a potassium-sparing diuretic. Its use can cause hyperkalemia, not hypokalemia.

   (N) *NCLEX® Connection: Physiological Adaptation, Unexpected Response to Therapies*

2. A. **CORRECT:** Changes in potassium levels can affect the heart and result in dysrhythmias and other ECG changes.

   B. Hyperkalemia causes diarrhea and abdominal cramping.

   C. Polyuria is a manifestation of hypokalemia.

   D. **CORRECT:** Hypotension is a manifestation of hyperkalemia.

   E. Hyperkalemia causes a slow, irregular pulse.

   (N) *NCLEX® Connection: Physiological Adaptation, Fluid and Electrolyte Imbalances*

3. A. Nasogastric losses due to suctioning do not increase calcium levels. A possible cause of hypercalcemia is hyperparathyroidism.

   B. **CORRECT:** Nasogastric losses are isotonic and contain sodium. Thus, nasogastric suction can cause hyponatremia.

   C. Nasogastric losses due to suctioning do not increase phosphate levels. A possible cause of hyperphosphatemia is tissue trauma.

   D. **CORRECT:** Nasogastric losses due to suctioning, diarrhea, and fistula drainage can deplete magnesium levels.

   E. Nasogastric losses due to suctioning do not increase potassium levels. A possible cause of hyperkalemia is the excessive use of salt substitutes.

   (N) *NCLEX® Connection: Reduction of Risk Potential, Potential for Complications of Diagnostic Tests/Treatments/Procedures*

4. A. **CORRECT:** Diabetic ketoacidosis, kidney disease, and crush injuries are risk factors for hyperkalemia.

   B. Heart failure is a risk factor for hyponatremia.

   C. Aldosterone excess is a risk factor for hyponatremia.

   D. Excessive sweating is a risk factor for hyponatremia.

   (N) *NCLEX® Connection: Physiological Adaptation, Basic Pathophysiology*

5. A. Applying a blood pressure cuff to the arm precedes checking for Trousseau sign.

   B. Placing the stethoscope's bell over the carotid artery helps with auscultating a carotid bruit.

   C. **CORRECT:** The nurse taps the client's cheek over the facial nerve just in front of the ear lobe to elicit Chvostek sign. A positive response is facial twitching on the same side of the face.

   D. Lowering the chin to the chest demonstrates range of motion of the neck.

   (N) *NCLEX® Connection: Reduction of Risk Potential, Diagnostic Tests*

PRACTICE Answer

Using the ATI Active Learning Template: System Disorder

ALTERATION IN HEALTH (DIAGNOSIS):
Hypokalemia is the result of an increase in potassium losses or movement of potassium into the cells, resulting in a potassium level less than 3.5 mEq/L.

NURSING CARE
- Monitor clients receiving IV potassium for phlebitis (tissue irritant).
- Monitor I&O.
- Monitor cardiac rhythm.
- Monitor clients receiving digoxin. Hypokalemia increases the risk for digoxin toxicity.
- Monitor level of consciousness, and ensure safety.
- Monitor bowel sounds and abdominal distention.
- Check hand grasps for muscle weakness.
- Check deep-tendon reflexes.
- Reinforce teaching about manifestations of hypokalemia.

INTERPROFESSIONAL CARE
- Nephrology can help with electrolyte and fluid management.
- Respiratory services can help with oxygen management.
- Nutritional services can help with potassium-rich food choices.
- Cardiology can help with dysrhythmia management.

CLIENT EDUCATION
- Consume potassium-rich foods.
- Prevent a decrease in potassium by avoiding excessive use of diuretics and laxatives.

COMPLICATIONS
- Respiratory failure
- Cardiac arrest

(N) *NCLEX® Connection: Physiological Adaptation, Fluid and Electrolyte Imbalances*

CHAPTER 38 *Acid-Base Imbalances*

For cells to function optimally, metabolic processes must maintain a steady balance between the acids and bases in the body. Acid-base balance represents homeostasis of hydrogen (H^+) ion concentration in body fluids. Hydrogen shifts between the extracellular and intracellular compartments to compensate for acid-base imbalances. Minor changes in hydrogen concentration have major effects on cellular function.

Arterial pH is an indirect measurement of hydrogen ion concentration and is a result of respiratory and kidney compensation functions. Arterial blood gases (ABGs) evaluate acid-base balance. The pH is the expression of the balance between carbon dioxide (CO_2), which the lungs regulate, and bicarbonate (HCO_3^-), a base the kidneys regulate. The greater the concentration of hydrogen, the more acidic the body fluids and the lower the pH. The lower the concentration of hydrogen, the more alkaline the body fluids and the higher the pH.

MAINTENANCE OF ACID-BASE BALANCE

Chemical, respiratory, and kidney functions maintain acid-base balance.

Chemical (bicarbonate and intracellular fluid) and protein buffers (albumin and globulins)
- First line of defense
- Either bind or release hydrogen ions
- Respond quickly to changes in pH

Respiratory buffers
- Second line of defense
- Control the level of hydrogen ions in the blood through the control of CO_2 levels
- When a chemoreceptor senses a change in the level of CO_2, it sends a signal to the brain to alter the rate and depth of respirations.
  - Hyperventilation: Decrease in hydrogen ions (helps to blow off excess hydrogen ions)
  - Hypoventilation: Increase in hydrogen ions

Kidney buffers
- Kidneys are the third line of defense.
- This buffering system is much slower to respond, but it is the most effective buffering system with the longest duration.
- Kidneys control the movement of bicarbonate in the urine. The bloodstream reabsorbs bicarbonate or the kidneys excrete it in the urine in response to blood levels of hydrogen.
- Kidneys can also produce more bicarbonate when necessary.
  - High hydrogen ions: Bicarbonate reabsorption and production
  - Low hydrogen ions: Bicarbonate excretion

COMPENSATION

Compensation is the process by which the body attempts to correct changes and imbalances in pH levels.
- Full compensation occurs when pH of blood returns to the expected reference range (7.35 to 7.45).
- If pH is not able to normalize, partial compensation has occurred.
- Acid-base imbalances are a result of insufficient compensation. Respiratory and kidney function play a large role in the body's ability to compensate effectively for acid-base alterations. Organ dysfunction negatively affects acid-base compensation.

EXAMPLES

Metabolic alkalosis, metabolic acidosis, respiratory alkalosis, and respiratory acidosis are examples of acid-base imbalances.

HEALTH PROMOTION AND DISEASE PREVENTION

- Consume a healthy diet and engage in physical activity.
- Limit the consumption of alcohol.
- Drink 6 to 8 cups of water daily.
- Maintain an appropriate weight for height and body frame.
- Refrain from smoking.

DATA COLLECTION

RISK FACTORS

Respiratory acidosis

RESULTS FROM
- Respiratory depression from opioids, poisons, anesthetics, brain injury
- Brain tumors, cerebral aneurysm, stroke or overhydration, trauma, neurological diseases (myasthenia gravis, Guillain-Barré when it affects respiratory effort)
- Inadequate chest expansion due to muscle weakness, pneumothorax/hemothorax, flail chest, obesity, sleep apnea, tumors, deformities
- Airway obstruction from neck edema, localized lymph node enlargement, foreign bodies, mucus
- Alveolar-capillary blockage from a pulmonary embolus, thrombus, acute respiratory distress syndrome, chest trauma, near-drowning, pulmonary edema, foreign-body aspiration, airway obstruction
- Inadequate mechanical ventilation
- Chronic pulmonary disease (asthma, COPD, pneumonia, cystic fibrosis)

RESULTS IN
- Increased CO_2
- Increased or normal H^+ concentration

MANIFESTATIONS
- **Vital signs:** Tachycardia (severe acidosis: bradycardia), tachypnea, hypotension
- **Neurological:** Anxiety, irritability, restlessness, somnolence, headache, dizziness, confusion, seizures, coma
- **Respiratory:** Ineffective, shallow, rapid breathing; dyspnea
- **Skin:** Warm, flushed
- **Weakness**
- **Cardiac dysrhythmias**

NURSING CARE
- Administer oxygen therapy.
- Maintain a patent airway.
- Enhance gas exchange.
  - Positioning and breathing techniques.
  - Provide ventilatory support.
  - Administer bronchodilators and mucolytics.
  - Maintain hydration.
  - Perform postural drainage.
  - Encourage deep-breathing exercises.

Respiratory alkalosis

RESULTS FROM
- Hyperventilation due to fever, respiratory infections, fear, anxiety, intracerebral trauma, salicylate toxicity, excessive mechanical ventilation
- Hypoxemia from asphyxiation, high altitudes, shock, early-stage asthma or pneumonia

RESULTS IN
- Decreased CO_2
- Decreased or normal H^+ concentration

MANIFESTATIONS
- Circumoral pallor
- Dry mouth
- Sweating
- Panic
- Spasms of hand muscles
- **Vital signs:** Tachypnea, tachycardia
- **Neurological:** Inability to concentrate, paresthesias (circumoral, extremities), tremors, blurry vision, tinnitus, loss of consciousness
- **Cardiovascular:** Palpitations
- **Respiratory:** Deep respirations, shortness of breath, chest tightness

NURSING CARE: Oxygen therapy (rebreather mask), anxiety reduction interventions, rebreathing techniques (holding the breath, breathing into and from a paper bag)

Metabolic acidosis

RESULTS FROM
- Excess production of hydrogen ions
- Diabetic ketoacidosis (DKA)
- Starvation
- Hyperkalemia
- Lactic acidosis can result from
  - Heavy exercise
  - Seizure activity
  - Hypoxia
  - Cardiac arrest
- Excessive intake of acids
  - Ethyl alcohol
  - Methyl alcohol
  - Acetylsalicylic acid (aspirin)
- Inadequate elimination of hydrogen ions
  - Kidney disease
  - Severe lung problems
- Inadequate production of bicarbonate
  - Kidney disease
  - Pancreatitis
- Impaired liver or pancreatic function: Liver failure
- Excess elimination of bicarbonate: Diarrhea

RESULTS IN
- Decreased HCO_3^-
- Increased H^+ concentration

MANIFESTATIONS

- Dysrhythmias
- **Vital signs:** Tachycardia, weak peripheral pulses, hypotension, tachypnea
- **Neurological:** Headache, drowsiness, lethargy, confusion, decreased level of consciousness, coma
- **Respiratory:** Rapid, deep (Kussmaul) respirations
- **Gastrointestinal (GI):** Nausea, vomiting, anorexia
- **Skin:** Warm, dry, flushed

NURSING CARE: Varies with causes

- If DKA, administer insulin.
- For GI losses, administer antidiarrheals and provide rehydration.
- If serum bicarbonate is low, IV sodium bicarbonate is necessary.

Metabolic alkalosis

RESULTS FROM

- Base excess
- Hypokalemia
- Oral ingestion of an excess amount of bases (antacids, sodium bicarbonate)
- Venous administration of bases (blood transfusions, total parenteral nutrition, sodium bicarbonate)
- Acid deficit
  - Loss of gastric secretions (prolonged vomiting, nasogastric suction, fistula drainage)
  - Potassium depletion (due to thiazide diuretics, laxative overuse, Cushing's syndrome, hyperaldosteronism, corticosteroids)
- Increased digoxin toxicity

RESULTS IN

- Increased HCO_3^-
- Decreased H^+ concentration

MANIFESTATIONS

- **Vital signs:** Tachycardia, normotensive or hypotensive, bradypnea
- **Neurological:** Paresthesias (circumoral, extremities), tetany, muscle weakness, irritability, lethargy, hyperreflexia, dizziness, confusion, muscle twitching, convulsions
- **Respiratory:** Depressed skeletal muscles resulting in ineffective breathing, shallow respirations, cyanosis

NURSING CARE: Varies with causes.

- For GI losses, administer antiemetics, fluids, and electrolyte replacement solutions.
- Potassium depletion requires discontinuation of causative agent.

38.1 Types of results

The following are the five classic types of ABG results demonstrating balance and imbalance.

Step 1: Look at pH	Step 2: Determine which is in the normal range		Step 3: Combine names
PH	PACO₂	HCO₃⁻	ABG RESULT
7.35 to 7.45	35 to 45	21 to 28	Homeostasis
Less than 7.35	Greater than 45	21 to 28	Respiratory acidosis
Less than 7.35	35 to 45	Less than 21	Metabolic acidosis
Greater than 7.45	Less than 35	21 to 28	Respiratory alkalosis
Greater than 7.45	35 to 45	Greater than 28	Metabolic alkalosis

DIAGNOSTIC PROCEDURES

To determine the type of imbalance **(38.1)**

STEP 1: **Look at the pH.**

- If it is below 7.35, identify it as acidosis.
- If it is above 7.45, identify it as alkalosis. ○EBP

STEP 2: **Look at the PaCO₂ and HCO₃⁻ simultaneously.**

- Determine which one is in the expected reference range.
- Conclude that the other is the indicator of imbalance.
- Identify PaCO₂ less than 35 or greater than 45 mm Hg as an indication that the problem is respiratory in origin.
- Identify HCO₃⁻ less than 21 or greater than 28 mEq/L as an indication that the problem is metabolic in origin.

STEP 3: **Combine the results of steps 1 and 2 to name the type of imbalance.**

STEP 4: **Evaluate the PaO₂ and SaO₂.** If the results are below the expected reference range, the client is hypoxic.

STEP 5: **Determine compensation.**

- **Uncompensated:** The pH and either HCO₃⁻ or PaCO₂ is outside the expected reference range.
- **Partially compensated:** The pH, HCO₃⁻, and PaCO₂ are outside the expected reference range.
- **Fully compensated:** The pH is within the expected reference range, but PaCO₂ and HCO₃⁻ are outside the expected reference range. Looking at the pH will provide a clue to which system initiated the problem, respiratory or metabolic. If the pH is below 7.40, think "acidosis," and determine which system has the acidosis value. If the pH is above 7.40, think "alkalosis," and determine which system has the alkalosis value.

PATIENT-CENTERED CARE

NURSING CARE

- For all acid-base imbalances, it is imperative to treat the underlying cause.
- Reinforce teaching about medication therapy.

INTERPROFESSIONAL CARE

- Respiratory services can help with oxygen therapy, breathing treatments, and ABGs.
- Pulmonology services can help with respiratory management.
- Assist with arrangement of referral services (home oxygen therapy).

CLIENT EDUCATION

- Adhere to the diet and dialysis regimen.
- Weigh daily and notify the provider of a 0.5 to 0.9 kg (1 to 2 lb) gain in 24 hr, or 1.4 kg (3 lb) gain in 1 week.
- Refrain from smoking.

COMPLICATIONS

Convulsions, coma, and respiratory arrest

NURSING ACTIONS
- Implement seizure precautions, and intervene if necessary.
- Provide life-support interventions if necessary.

Application Exercises

1. A nurse is caring for a client who has confusion and lethargy. The client was unresponsive at home, with an empty bottle of aspirin lying next to her bed. Vital signs are blood pressure 104/72 mm Hg, heart rate 116/min and regular, and respiratory rate 42/min with deep respirations. Which of the following arterial blood gas (ABG) results should the nurse expect?

   A. pH 7.68
   $PaCO_2$ 38 mm Hg
   HCO_3^- 28 mEq/L

   B. pH 7.48
   $PaCO_2$ 28 mm Hg
   HCO_3^- 23 mEq/L

   C. pH 7.16
   $PaCO_2$ 38 mm Hg
   HCO_3^- 18 mEq/L

   D. pH 7.58
   $PaCO_2$ 38 mm Hg
   HCO_3^- 29 mEq/L

2. A nurse is caring for a client who was in a motor-vehicle crash. The client reports chest pain and difficulty breathing. A chest x-ray indicates that the client has a pneumothorax. Which of the following ABG results should the nurse expect?

   A. pH 7.06
   $PaCO_2$ 52 mm Hg
   HCO_3^- 24 mEq/L

   B. pH 7.42
   $PaCO_2$ 38 mm Hg
   HCO_3^- 23 mEq/L

   C. pH 7.20
   $PaCO_2$ 39 mm Hg
   HCO_3^- 18 mEq/L

   D. pH 7.58
   $PaCO_2$ 38 mm Hg
   HCO_3^- 29 mEq/L

3. A nurse is checking ABG results for a client who has vomited repeatedly during the past 24 hr. Which of the following acid-base imbalances should the nurse expect?

   A. Respiratory acidosis

   B. Respiratory alkalosis

   C. Metabolic acidosis

   D. Metabolic alkalosis

4. A nurse is caring for a client who has metabolic acidosis. Which of the following components of the client's medical history should the nurse identify as a risk factor for this acid-base imbalance?

   A. Diabetic ketoacidosis

   B. Sleep apnea

   C. Asthma

   D. Pulmonary edema

5. A nurse is collecting data from a client who has pancreatitis. The client's ABGs indicate metabolic acidosis. Which of the following findings should the nurse expect? (Select all that apply.)

   A. Tachycardia

   B. Hypertension

   C. Bounding pulses

   D. Insomnia

   E. Dysrhythmias

   F. Tachypnea

PRACTICE Active Learning Scenario

A nurse is caring for a client who has liver cancer. The client's arterial blood gases indicate metabolic acidosis. Use the ATI Active Learning Template: System Disorder to complete this item.

RISK FACTORS: Include three risk factors for metabolic acidosis.

NURSING CARE: Include two nursing actions.

NURSING ACTIONS (FOR COMPLICATIONS): Identify one.

Application Exercises Key

1. A. These ABG results indicate metabolic alkalosis.

    B. These ABG results indicate respiratory alkalosis.

    C. **CORRECT:** An aspirin overdose would result in ABG results that indicate metabolic acidosis.

    D. These ABG results indicate metabolic alkalosis.

    Ⓝ *NCLEX® Connection: Reduction of Risk Potential, Laboratory Values*

2. A. **CORRECT:** A pneumothorax can cause hypoventilation and increase carbon dioxide levels, resulting in respiratory acidosis.

    B. These ABG results are within the expected reference range and reflect homeostasis.

    C. These ABG results indicate metabolic acidosis, an unlikely outcome of a pneumothorax.

    D. These ABG results indicate metabolic alkalosis, an unlikely outcome of a pneumothorax.

    Ⓝ *NCLEX® Connection: Reduction of Risk Potential, Laboratory Values*

3. A. Common causes of respiratory acidosis include pulmonary disease and airway obstruction.

    B. Common causes of respiratory alkalosis include fever and respiratory infections.

    C. Common cases of metabolic acidosis include starvation and kidney disease.

    D. **CORRECT:** Excessive vomiting causes a loss of gastric acids and an accumulation of bicarbonate in the blood, resulting in metabolic alkalosis.

    Ⓝ *NCLEX® Connection: Reduction of Risk Potential, Laboratory Values*

4. A. **CORRECT:** Metabolic acidosis results from an excess production of hydrogen ions, which occurs with diabetic ketoacidosis.

    B. Asthma can cause respiratory acidosis.

    C. Sleep apnea can cause respiratory acidosis.

    D. Pulmonary edema can cause respiratory acidosis.

    Ⓝ *NCLEX® Connection: Physiological Adaptation, Basic Pathophysiology*

5. A. **CORRECT:** Tachycardia is an expected finding of metabolic and respiratory acidosis.

    B. Hypotension is an expected finding of metabolic and respiratory acidosis.

    C. Metabolic acidosis causes weak peripheral pulsations.

    D. Drowsiness, lethargy, and decreased level of consciousness are expected findings of metabolic acidosis.

    E. **CORRECT:** Dysrhythmias are an expected finding of metabolic and respiratory acidosis.

    F. **CORRECT:** Tachypnea is an expected finding of pancreatitis, metabolic acidosis, and respiratory acidosis.

    Ⓝ *NCLEX® Connection: Physiological Adaptation, Basic Pathophysiology*

PRACTICE Answer

Using ATI Active Learning Template: System Disorder

RISK FACTORS

- Excess production of hydrogen ions
- Diabetic ketoacidosis (DKA)
- Starvation
- Hyperkalemia
- Lactic acidosis can result from
  - Heavy exercise
  - Seizure activity
  - Hypoxia
  - Cardiac arrest
- Excessive intake of acids
  - Ethyl alcohol
  - Methyl alcohol
  - Acetylsalicylic acid (aspirin)

- Inadequate elimination of hydrogen ions
  - Kidney disease
  - Severe lung problems
- Inadequate production of bicarbonate
  - Kidney disease
  - Pancreatitis
- Impaired liver or pancreatic function: Liver failure
- Excess elimination of bicarbonate: Diarrhea

NURSING CARE:
Varies with causes.
- If DKA, administer insulin.
- For GI losses, administer antidiarrheals and provide rehydration.
- If serum bicarbonate is low, IV sodium bicarbonate is necessary.

NURSING ACTIONS (FOR COMPLICATIONS)
- Implement seizure precautions, and intervene if necessary.
- Provide life-support interventions if necessary.

Ⓝ *NCLEX® Connection: Physiological Adaptation, Alterations in Body Systems*

When reviewing the following chapters, keep in mind the relevant topics and tasks of the NCLEX outline, in particular:

Basic Care and Comfort

ELIMINATION
Identify the client at risk for impaired elimination (medication, hydration status).

Monitor the client's bowel sounds.

NUTRITION AND ORAL HYDRATION: Reinforce client teaching on special diets based on the client's diagnosis/ nutritional needs and cultural considerations (high protein, kosher diet, calorie restriction).

Pharmacological Therapies

EXPECTED ACTIONS/OUTCOMES: Reinforce client teaching on actions and therapeutic effects of medications and pharmacological interactions.

MEDICATION ADMINISTRATION: Administer medication by gastrointestinal tube (G–tube, nasogastric [NG] tube, G–button, J–tube).

PHARMACOLOGICAL PAIN MANAGEMENT:
Identify the client's need for pain medication.

Reduction of Risk Potential

DIAGNOSTIC TESTS: Perform diagnostic testing (blood glucose, oxygen saturation, testing for occult blood).

THERAPEUTIC PROCEDURES
Insert, maintain, and remove nasogastric (NG) tubes.

Reinforce client teaching on treatments and procedures.

Physiological Adaptation

ALTERATIONS IN BODY SYSTEMS: Reinforce client teaching on ostomy care.

CHAPTER 39 *Gastrointestinal Diagnostic Procedures*

Gastrointestinal (GI) diagnostic procedures often involve endoscopes and x-rays to visualize parts of the GI system and to evaluate GI contents. Procedures include liver function tests, other blood tests, urine bilirubin (urobilinogen), fecal occult blood test (FOBT), stool samples, endoscopy, and GI series.

Liver function tests and other blood tests

- Liver function tests are aspartate aminotransferase (AST), alanine aminotransferase (ALT), alkaline phosphatase (ALP), bilirubin, and albumin.
- Other blood tests that provide information about the functioning of the GI system include amylase, lipase, alpha-fetoprotein, and ammonia. **(39.1)**

INDICATIONS

Suspicion of liver, pancreatic, or biliary tract disorders

CONSIDERATIONS

PREPROCEDURE: Reinforce teaching about blood sampling and what information this will provide.

POSTPROCEDURE: Explain when and how clients will receive the results.

Urine bilirubin (urobilinogen)

This urine test determines the presence of bilirubin in the urine.

INDICATIONS

Suspicion of liver or biliary tract disorders

CONSIDERATIONS

PREPROCEDURE

NURSING ACTIONS
- Use a dipstick (urine bilirubin) or a 24-hr urine collection (urobilinogen).
- Reinforce teaching about collecting urine, and provide collection containers.

POSTPROCEDURE

NURSING ACTIONS: Explain when and how clients will receive the results.

INTERPRETATION OF FINDINGS

Positive findings or elevation indicates a possible liver disorder (cirrhosis, hepatitis), biliary obstruction, hemolytic anemia, or pernicious anemia.

39.1 Blood tests: Interpretation of findings

BLOOD TEST	EXPECTED REFERENCE RANGE	INTERPRETATION OF FINDINGS
Aspartate aminotransferase	0 to 35 units/L	Elevation occurs with hepatitis or cirrhosis.
Alanine aminotransferase	4 to 36 units/L	
Alkaline phosphatase	30 to 120 units/L	Elevation indicates liver damage.
Amylase	30 to 220 units/L	Elevation occurs with pancreatitis.
Lipase	0 to 160 units/L	
Total bilirubin	0.3 to 1 mg/dL	Elevations indicate altered liver function, bile duct obstruction, or other hepatobiliary disorder.
Direct (conjugated) bilirubin	0.1 to 0.3 mg/dL	
Indirect (unconjugated) bilirubin	0.2 to 0.8 mg/dL	
Albumin	3.5 to 5 g/dL	Decrease can indicate hepatic disease.
Alpha-fetoprotein	Less than 40 mcg/L	Elevated in liver cancer, cirrhosis, hepatitis.
Ammonia	10 to 80 mcg/dL	Elevated in liver disease.

Fecal occult blood test and stool samples

Testing a stool sample can confirm the presence of blood, an increase in fat content, ova, parasites (*Giardia lamblia*), and bacteria (*Clostridium difficile*). Fecal occult blood, fecal immunochemical, and stool DNA testing can help with early detection of colorectal cancer.

INDICATIONS

CLIENT PRESENTATION
- GI bleeding
- Unexplained diarrhea

CONSIDERATIONS

PREPROCEDURE

NURSING ACTIONS
- **Occult blood**
  - Provide guaiac cards clients can mail to the provider or a specimen collection cup. Cards usually require three samples.
  - Reinforce teaching about the collection technique as well as medication restrictions (anticoagulants, NSAIDs) for 7 days before the testing starts, and dietary restrictions (vitamin C-rich foods, red meat, chicken, fish) prior to obtaining samples. Qᴘᴄᴄ
- **Stool for ova and parasites and bacteria**
  - Provide a specimen collection cup.
  - Reinforce teaching about the collection technique (time frame for submission to the laboratory, the need for refrigeration).

POSTPROCEDURE

NURSING ACTIONS: Explain when and how clients will receive results.

INTERPRETATION OF FINDINGS

- At least three instances of a positive guaiac FOBT confirms GI bleeding.
- A positive finding for blood indicates GI bleeding (ulcer, colitis, cancer).

Stool samples

- A positive finding for ova and parasites indicates a GI parasitic infection.
- A positive finding for *Clostridium difficile* indicates this opportunistic infection, which usually becomes established secondary to use of broad-spectrum antibiotics.
- Immunochemical testing can detect lower GI bleeding.
- Changes in DNA can indicate precancerous, benign, and malignant tumors.

Endoscopy

- Endoscopic procedures allow direct visualization of body cavities, tissues, and organs through the use of a flexible, lighted tube (endoscope) for diagnostic and therapeutic purposes.
- With endoscopy and in a variety of facilities, providers can perform biopsies, remove abnormal tissue, and perform minor surgery, such as cauterizing a bleeding ulcer. They can inject a contrast medium to allow visualization of structures beyond the capabilities of the scope.

GASTROINTESTINAL SCOPE PROCEDURES
- Colonoscopy
- Esophagogastroduodenoscopy (EGD)
- Endoscopic retrograde cholangiopancreatography (ERCP)
- Small bowel capsule endoscopy (M2A)
- Sigmoidoscopy

INDICATIONS

POTENTIAL DIAGNOSES: GI bleeding, ulcerations, inflammation, polyps, malignant tumors

CLIENT PRESENTATION
- Anemia (due to bleeding)
- Abdominal discomfort
- Abdominal distention or mass

CONSIDERATIONS

General endoscopic procedures

PREPROCEDURE NURSING ACTIONS
- Evaluate the client's understanding of the procedure.
- Verify that the client has signed a consent form.
- Check vital signs, and verify allergies.
- Evaluate baseline laboratory tests and report unexpected findings to the provider (CBC, electrolyte panel, BUN, creatinine, PT, aPTT, liver function studies). Evaluate chest x-ray, ECG, and ABGs.
- Evaluate the client's medical history for increased risk of complications.
- **Age** can influence the client's ability to tolerate positioning and adhere to pretest preparation. Ⓖ
- **Current health status:** Consider problems and medications that can affect tolerance of and recovery from the procedure.
- **Cognitive status:** Determine the client's understanding of the procedure and baseline mental status.
- **Support system:** Determine whether a support person will assist the client after the procedure.
- **Recent food or fluid intake** can affect the provider's ability to visualize key structures and increase the risk for complications (aspiration). Notify the provider if the client did not follow dietary restrictions.
- **Medications:** Some medications (NSAIDs, warfarin, aspirin) increase the risk for complications. Notify the provider if the client did not follow medication restrictions.

- **Previous radiographic examinations:** Any recent radiographic examinations using barium can affect the provider's ability to view key structures. Notify the provider if the client had a procedure recently that required contrast media.
- **Electrolyte and fluid status:** Imbalances due to repeated enemas can affect bowel preparation tolerance, especially in older adult clients.
- Ensure that the client followed bowel preparation instructions (laxatives, enemas). Inadequate bowel preparation can result in cancellation, delaying the examination, and subjecting the client to extended periods of being NPO or on a liquid diet.
- Ensure that the client has adhered to NPO status for the necessary time period prior to the examination.
- Reinforce instructions about medication and food restrictions.
- Provide prescriptions for bowel prep medications.
- Reinforce instructions about the number and type of enemas.

POSTPROCEDURE NURSING ACTIONS
- Monitor vital signs.
- Monitor for complications.
- Reinforce instructions about any food restrictions after a biopsy. Qᴘᴄᴄ

Colonoscopy

Insertion of a flexible fiber optic colonoscope through the anus to visualize the rectum and the sigmoid, descending, transverse, and ascending colon

ANESTHESIA: **Moderate sedation**
- Midazolam
- An opiate such as fentanyl
- An anesthetic such as propofol

POSITIONING: Left side with the knees toward the chest

PREPARATION: **Bowel prep**
- Can include laxatives (bisacodyl, polyethylene glycol)
- Clear liquid diet (no red, purple, orange fluids), NPO after midnight
- Avoidance of some medications (aspirin, anticoagulants, antiplatelet medications)
- Polyethylene glycol can cause fluid and electrolyte imbalances, especially in older adults. ⒢
- Polyethylene glycol can inhibit the absorption of some medications. Review the client's medications and consult with the provider.

POSTPROCEDURE NURSING ACTIONS
- Notify the provider of severe pain (possible perforation) or indications of hemorrhage.
- Monitor for rectal bleeding.
- Monitor vital signs and respiratory status. Maintain an open airway until the client awakens.

CLIENT EDUCATION
- Resume a usual diet.
- Increase fluid intake.
- Expect flatulence due to air instillation during the procedure.
- Do not drive or use equipment for 12 to 18 hr after the procedure.

EGD

Insertion of an endoscope through the mouth into the esophagus, stomach, and duodenum to identify or treat areas of bleeding, dilate an esophageal stricture, or diagnose gastric lesions or celiac disease.

ANESTHESIA: **Moderate sedation per IV access**
- Topical anesthetic to depress the gag reflex
- Atropine to decrease secretions

POSITIONING: Left side-lying with elevation of the head of the bed

PREPARATION: NPO 6 to 8 hr. Remove dentures prior to the procedure.

POSTPROCEDURE NURSING ACTIONS
- Monitor vital signs and respiratory status. Maintain an open airway until the client awakens.
- Notify the provider of bleeding, abdominal or chest pain, and any evidence of infection.
- Withhold fluids until the gag reflex returns. Qs
- Make sure the client tolerates oral fluids without nausea and vomiting before removing the IV catheter.

CLIENT EDUCATION
- Do not drive or use equipment for 12 to 18 hr after the procedure.
- Use throat lozenges if a sore throat or hoarse voice persists following the procedure.

Endoscopic retrograde cholangiopancreatography

Insertion of an endoscope through the mouth into the biliary tree via the duodenum allows visualization of the biliary ducts, gall bladder, liver, and pancreas. X-rays follow injection of a contrast medium into the common duct.

ANESTHESIA: **Moderate sedation per IV access**
- Topical anesthetic to depress the gag reflex
- Atropine to decrease secretions

POSITIONING: Initially semi-prone with repositioning throughout the procedure

PREPARATION
- NPO 6 to 8 hr. Remove dentures prior to the procedure.
- Explain the procedure and the need to change positions during the procedure.

POSTPROCEDURE
- Monitor vital signs and respiratory status. Maintain an open airway until the client awakens.
- Notify the provider of bleeding, abdominal or chest pain, and evidence of infection.
- Withhold fluids until the gag reflex returns.
- Make sure the client tolerates oral fluids without nausea and vomiting before removing the IV catheter.

CLIENT EDUCATION
- Do not drive or use equipment for 12 to 18 hr after the procedure.
- Use throat lozenges if a sore throat or hoarse voice persists following the procedure.

M2A

The client swallows the capsule with 8 oz water for a video enteroscopy to visualize the entire small bowel (but not the colon) over an 8-hr period.

ANESTHESIA: None

POSITIONING: Usual activity

PREPARATION
- Water only for 8 to 10 hr before the test and NPO for first 2 hr of the testing. Usual diet 4 hr after swallowing the capsule.
- The examiner marks the abdomen for the location of the sensor and places eight-lead sensors and connects them to a data recorder, which captures images of the small intestines. Q↓

POSTPROCEDURE
- After 8 hr, the client returns the recorder for downloading of the images.
- The client will evacuate the capsule in the stool.

Sigmoidoscopy

The scope is shorter than a colonoscope, allowing visualization of the anus, rectum, and sigmoid colon to test for colon cancer, investigate for GI bleeding, or diagnose or monitor inflammatory bowel disease.

ANESTHESIA: None

POSITIONING: On left side

PREPARATION
- Bowel prep, which can include laxatives, such as bisacodyl, a cleansing enema, or a sodium biphosphate enema
- Clear liquid diet at least 24 hr before the procedure
- NPO after midnight
- Avoidance of some medications (aspirin, anticoagulants, antiplatelet medications)

POSTPROCEDURE
- Monitor vital signs and respiratory status.
- Monitor for rectal bleeding.

CLIENT EDUCATION
- Resume a usual diet.
- Increase fluid intake.
- Expect flatulence due to air instillation during the procedure.

INTERPRETATION OF FINDINGS

Can indicate a need for medication or surgical removal of a lesion

COMPLICATIONS

Oversedation

Use of moderate sedation increases the risk for oversedation. Qs

MANIFESTATIONS: Difficult to arouse, poor respiratory effort, evidence of hypoxemia, tachycardia, and elevated or low blood pressure

NURSING ACTIONS
- Prepare to administer antidotes for sedatives the client receives prior to and during the procedure.
- Administer oxygen, and monitor vital signs. Maintain an open airway until the client awakens.
- Notify the provider immediately, and call for assistance.

CLIENT EDUCATION: Restrict driving and major decision-making until there are no further effects from the sedation.

Hemorrhage

MANIFESTATIONS: Bleeding, cool and clammy skin, hypotension, tachycardia, dizziness, tachypnea

NURSING ACTIONS
- Check for hemorrhage from the site. Monitor vital signs.
- Monitor diagnostic test results (particularly Hgb and Hct).
- Notify the provider immediately.

CLIENT EDUCATION: Report fever, pain, and bleeding to the provider.

Aspiration

Using moderate sedation or topical anesthesia can affect the gag reflex.

MANIFESTATIONS: Dyspnea, tachypnea, adventitious breath sounds, tachycardia, fever

NURSING ACTIONS
- Keep the client NPO until the gag reflex returns. Ensure that the client is awake and alert prior to consuming food or fluid.
- Notify the provider if there is a delay in gag-reflex return.

CLIENT EDUCATION
- Breathe deeply and cough to promote removal of secretions.
- Report any respiratory congestion or compromise to the provider.

Perforation of the gastrointestinal tract

MANIFESTATIONS: Chest or abdominal pain, fever, nausea, vomiting, abdominal distention

NURSING ACTIONS: Monitor diagnostic tests for evidence of infection, including WBC count, and notify the provider of unexpected findings.

CLIENT EDUCATION: Report fever, pain, and bleeding to the provider.

Gastrointestinal series

GI studies with or without contrast help define anatomic and functional abnormalities.

- These include radiographic imaging of the esophagus, stomach, and entire intestinal tract.
- For upper GI imaging, the client drinks a radiopaque liquid (barium). For small-bowel follow-through, the imaging traces barium through the stomach, duodenum, jejunum, and ileum to the ileocecal junction.
- A barium enema requires instilling a radiopaque liquid into the rectum and colon.

INDICATIONS

POTENTIAL DIAGNOSES: Gastric ulcers, peristaltic disorders, tumors, varices, intestinal enlargements or constrictions

CLIENT PRESENTATION: Abdominal pain, alterations in elimination habits (constipation, diarrhea), GI bleeding

CONSIDERATIONS

PREPROCEDURE

NURSING ACTIONS

- Reinforce teaching about medications, food and fluid restrictions (clear liquid and/or low residue diet, NPO after midnight), and avoiding smoking or chewing gum (increases peristalsis).
- Check the client's understanding of bowel preparation (laxatives, enemas) so feces will not distort the images.
- Barium enema studies must precede upper GI studies. Q̇EBP
- Check for contraindications for bowel preparation (possible bowel perforation or obstruction, inflammatory disease).

CLIENT EDUCATION

- Restrict food and fluids for bowel preparation.
- Visualization of the small intestine will require additional radiographs over the next 24 hr.

POSTPROCEDURE

NURSING ACTIONS

- Monitor elimination of contrast material, and administer a laxative if necessary.
- Increase fluid intake to promote elimination of contrast material.

CLIENT EDUCATION

- Monitor elimination of contrast material and report retention of contrast material (constipation) or diarrhea with weakness.
- An over-the-counter medication can be needed to prevent constipation resulting from the barium.
- Stools will be white for 24 to 72 hr until the barium clears. Report abdominal fullness, pain, or a delay in the return to brown stool.

INTERPRETATION OF FINDINGS

Unexpected findings indicate alterations in bowel shape and size, increased motility, or obstruction.

Application Exercises

1. A nurse is reinforcing teaching with a client about a bowel prep using polyethylene glycol who will undergo a colonoscopy. Which of the following instructions should the nurse reinforce?

   A. Check with the provider about taking current medications during the bowel prep.

   B. Consume the usual diet until starting the bowel prep.

   C. Expect the bowel prep to act the day after consuming it.

   D. Stop the bowel prep as soon as fecal elimination begins.

2. A nurse is having difficulty arousing a client following an esophagogastroduodenoscopy (EGD). Which of the following actions is the nurse's priority?

   A. Check the client's airway.

   B. Allow the client to sleep.

   C. Prepare to administer an antidote to the sedative.

   D. Evaluate preprocedure laboratory findings.

3. A nurse in a clinic is instructing a client about a fecal occult blood test, which requires mailing three specimens. Which of the following client statements indicates understanding of the instructions?

   A. "I will continue taking my warfarin while I complete these tests."

   B. "I'm glad I don't have to follow any special diet at this time."

   C. "This test determines if I have parasites in my bowel."

   D. "This is an easy way to screen for colon cancer."

4. A nurse is completing preprocedure instructions for a client who will undergo a sigmoidoscopy. Which of the following information should the nurse include? (Select all that apply.)

   A. "Expect more flatulence following the procedure."

   B. "Consume no fluid or food before the procedure."

   C. "You will receive moderate sedation for the procedure."

   D. "You will need repositioning throughout the procedure."

   E. "Limit your fluid intake the day after the procedure."

5. A nurse is reviewing the health record of a client who might have a tumor of the jejunum. The nurse should anticipate a prescription for which of the following tests? (Select all that apply.)

   A. Serum alpha-fetoprotein

   B. Endoscopic retrograde cholangiopancreatography (ERCP)

   C. GI x-ray with contrast

   D. Small bowel capsule endoscopy (M2A)

   E. Colonoscopy

PRACTICE Active Learning Scenario

A nurse in a clinic is reinforcing teaching with a client who will undergo a gastrointestinal series of x-rays. What should the nurse include? Use the ATI Active Learning Template: Diagnostic Procedure to complete this item.

DESCRIPTION OF THE PROCEDURE: Describe the procedure and technique.

INDICATIONS: Identify at least three potential diagnoses and two manifestations.

CLIENT EDUCATION: Describe three instructional points.

1. A. **CORRECT:** The nurse should instruct the client to check with the provider about taking current medications, because polyethylene glycol can inhibit the absorption of some medications.

   B. The nurse should instruct the client to consume a clear liquid diet prior to starting the bowel prep.

   C. The nurse should instruct the client that the actions of polyethylene glycol begin within 2 to 3 hr after consumption.

   D. The nurse should instruct the client to consume the full amount prescribed.

   Ⓝ *NCLEX® Connection: Reduction of Risk Potential, Diagnostic Tests*

2. A. **CORRECT:** When using the airway, breathing, and circulation priority-setting framework, checking and maintaining an open airway is the priority action the nurse should take.

   B. The nurse should continue to allow the client to rest to help with recovery from the procedure. However, another action is the priority.

   C. The nurse should prepare to administer an antidote to the sedative used during the procedure because oversedation could account for the inability for the client's lack of arousal. However, another action is the priority.

   D. The nurse should evaluate the preprocedure laboratory findings to see if there is a metabolic or hematologic reason for the client's lack of arousal. However, another action is the priority.

   Ⓝ *NCLEX® Connection: Reduction of Risk Potential, Potential for Complications of Diagnostic Tests/Treatments/Procedures*

3. A. Clients should stop taking anticoagulants prior to obtaining stool specimens for fecal occult blood testing because they can interfere with the results.

   B. Clients should avoid consuming red meat, chicken, and fish prior to obtaining stool specimens for fecal occult blood testing because they can interfere with the results.

   C. Fecal occult blood testing identifies blood, not parasites, present in stool.

   D. **CORRECT:** Fecal occult blood, fecal immunochemical, and stool DNA testing can help with screening for colorectal cancer.

   Ⓝ *NCLEX® Connection: Reduction of Risk Potential, Therapeutic Procedures*

4. A. **CORRECT:** The nurse should reinforce that increased flatulence can occur due to the instillation of air during the procedure.

   B. **CORRECT:** The nurse should instruct the client to remain NPO after midnight the night before the procedure.

   C. The nurse should inform the client that he will not receive sedation for a sigmoidoscopy.

   D. The nurse should inform the client that he will lie on his left side for the procedure.

   E. The nurse should instruct the client to increase, not limit, fluid intake following the procedure.

   Ⓝ *NCLEX® Connection: Reduction of Risk Potential, Potential for Complications of Diagnostic Tests/Treatments/Procedures*

5. A. Serum alpha-fetoprotein is a laboratory test that helps detect liver cancer.

   B. An ERCP helps visualize the duodenum, biliary ducts, gall bladder, liver, and pancreas.

   C. **CORRECT:** A GI x-ray with contrast involves the client drinking barium, which moves through the small intestine to its junction with the colon. This would help identify a tumor in the jejunum.

   D. **CORRECT:** M2A is a procedure for which the client swallows a capsule with water for a video enteroscopy that helps visualize the entire small intestine over 8 hr.

   E. A colonoscopy involves the use of a flexible fiber optic colonoscope, which enters through the anus, to visualize the rectum and the sigmoid, descending, transverse, and ascending colon.

   Ⓝ *NCLEX® Connection: Physiological Adaptation, Basic Pathophysiology*

PRACTICE Answer

Using the ATI Active Learning Template: Diagnostic Procedure

DESCRIPTION OF THE PROCEDURE: Gastrointestinal studies with or without contrast help define anatomic and functional abnormalities. These include radiographic imaging of the esophagus, stomach, and entire intestinal tract. For upper GI imaging, the client drinks a radiopaque liquid (barium). For small-bowel follow-through, the imaging traces barium through the small intestine to the ileocecal junction. A barium enema requires instilling a radiopaque liquid into the rectum and colon.

INDICATIONS
- Diagnoses: Gastric ulcers, peristaltic disorders, tumors, varices, intestinal enlargements or constrictions
- Manifestations: Abdominal pain, altered elimination habits (constipation, diarrhea), gastrointestinal bleeding

CLIENT EDUCATION
- Restrict food and fluids for bowel preparation.
- Visualization of the small intestine will require additional radiographs over the next 24 hr.
- Monitor elimination of contrast material and report retention of contrast material (constipation) or diarrhea with weakness.
- An over-the-counter medication can be needed to prevent constipation resulting from the barium.
- Stools will be white for 24 to 72 hr until the barium clears. Report abdominal fullness, pain, or a delay in the return to brown stool.

Ⓝ *NCLEX® Connection: Reduction of Risk Potential, Potential for Complications of Diagnostic Tests/Treatments/Procedures*

CHAPTER 40   *Gastrointestinal Therapeutic Procedures*

Gastrointestinal therapeutic procedures help to maintain nutritional intake, and treat gastrointestinal obstructions, obesity, and other disorders. Gastrointestinal therapeutic procedures include enteral feedings, total parenteral nutrition (TPN), paracentesis, nasogastric decompression, bariatric surgeries, and ostomies.

Enteral feedings

A client who is unable take adequate nutrition orally can require enteral feedings.

INDICATIONS

POTENTIAL DIAGNOSES

- Inability to eat due to a medical condition (coma, intubation)
- Pathologies that cause difficulty swallowing or increase risk of aspiration (stroke, advanced Parkinson's disease, multiple sclerosis)
- Inability to maintain adequate oral nutritional intake and need for supplementation due to increased metabolic demands (cancer therapy, burns, sepsis)

CLIENT PRESENTATION

- Malnutrition (decreased prealbumin, transferrin, or total iron-binding capacity)
- Aspiration pneumonia

COMPLICATIONS

Overfeeding

Overfeeding results from infusion of a greater quantity of feeding than can be readily digested, resulting in abdominal distention, nausea, and vomiting.

NURSING ACTIONS

- Check residual every 4 to 6 hr.
- Follow protocol for slowing or withholding feedings for excess residual volumes. Many facilities hold for residual volumes of 100 to 200 mL and then restart at a lower rate after a period of rest.
- Check pump for proper operation and ensure feeding infused at correct rate.

Diarrhea

The particular concentration of feeding or its constituents can cause diarrhea.

NURSING ACTIONS

- Slow the rate of feeding and notify the provider.
- Confer with a dietitian.
- Provide skin care and protection.
- Evaluate for *Clostridium difficile* if diarrhea continues, especially if it has a very foul odor.

Aspiration pneumonia

Aspiration of feeding can lead to pneumonia, a potentially life-threatening complication. Tube displacement is the primary cause of aspiration of feeding

NURSING ACTIONS

- Stop the feeding. **Qs**
- Turn the client to his side and suction the airway. Administer oxygen if indicated.
- Monitor vital signs for an elevated temperature.
- Auscultate breath sounds for increased congestion and diminishing breath sounds.
- Notify the provider and obtain a chest x-ray if prescribed.

Refeeding syndrome

Refeeding syndrome is a potentially life-threatening condition that occurs when enteral feeding is started in a client who is in a starvation state and whose body has begun to catabolize protein and fat for energy.

NURSING ACTIONS

- Monitor for new onset of confusion or seizures.
- Observe for shallow respirations.
- Monitor for increased muscular weakness.
- Notify the provider and obtain serum electrolytes if needed.

Total parenteral nutrition

TPN is a hypertonic IV bolus solution. The purpose of TPN administration is to prevent or correct nutritional deficiencies and minimize the adverse effects of malnourishment.

- TPN administration is usually through a central line.
  - Tunneled triple lumen catheter
  - Single- or double-lumen peripherally inserted central (PICC) line
- TPN contains complete nutrition, including calories in a high concentration (10% to 50%) of dextrose, lipids/essential fatty acids, protein, electrolytes, vitamins, and trace elements. Standard IV bolus therapy is typically no more than 700 calories/day.
- Partial parenteral nutrition, often called peripheral parenteral nutrition (PPN), is less hypertonic, intended for short-term use, and administered in a large peripheral vein. Usual dextrose concentration is 10% or less. Risks include phlebitis.

INDICATIONS

Any condition that
- Affects the ability to absorb nutrition.
- Has a prolonged recovery.
- Creates a hypermetabolic state.
- Creates a chronic malnutrition.

POTENTIAL DIAGNOSES

- Chronic pancreatitis
- Diffuse peritonitis
- Short bowel syndrome
- Gastric paresis from diabetes mellitus
- Severe burns

CLIENT PRESENTATION

- Weight loss greater than 10% of body weight and NPO or unable to eat or drink for more than 5 days
- Hypermetabolic state
- Muscle wasting, poor tissue healing, burns, bowel disease disorders, acute kidney failure

CONSIDERATIONS

PREPARATION OF THE CLIENT

Obtain baseline laboratory values, including electrolytes. Solutions are customized for each client according to daily laboratory results.

ONGOING CARE

- Titrate the flow rate to allow body adjustment (usually no more than a 10% hourly increase in rate).

  ! Never abruptly stop TPN. Speeding/slowing the rate is contraindicated. An abrupt rate change can alter blood glucose levels significantly. Qs

- Check vital signs every 4 to 8 hr.
- Maintain sterility of the TPN infusion to minimize the risk of sepsis.
  - Central lines require sterile technique for dressing changes and line manipulation
  - The pharmacy prepares TPN solution using aseptic technique with a laminar flow hood.
  - Change the tubing and solution bag every 24 hr (even if not empty).
  - TPN infusion requires filtered tubing to collect particles from the solution.
  - Do not use the line for other IV solutions (prevents contamination and interruption of the flow rate).
  - Do not add anything to the solution due to risks of contamination and incompatibility.

INTERVENTIONS

- Check capillary glucose every 4 to 6 hr for at least the first 24 hr.
- Clients receiving TPN frequently need supplemental regular insulin until the pancreas can increase its endogenous production of insulin.
- Older adult clients have an increased incidence of glucose intolerance. Ⓖ

COMPLICATIONS

Metabolic complications

Hyperglycemia, hypoglycemia, and vitamin deficiencies

NURSING ACTIONS

- Review daily laboratory tests to monitor for metabolic imbalance. TPN solutions are tailored to the client's glucose and electrolyte requirements.
- Request a prescription for a separate IV bolus, if needed, to correct fluid volume deficits.
- Monitor for hyperglycemia.

Air embolism

A pressure change during tubing changes can lead to an air embolism.

NURSING ACTIONS

- Monitor for manifestations of an air embolism (sudden onset of dyspnea, chest pain, anxiety, hypoxia).
- Clamp the catheter immediately and place the client on his left side in Trendelenburg position to trap air. Administer oxygen and notify the provider, who will have to aspirate the trapped air.

Infection

Concentrated glucose is a medium for bacteria.

NURSING ACTIONS
- Observe the central line insertion site for local infection (erythema, tenderness, exudate).
- Assist with maintaining sterility of the line and tubing.
- Observe for manifestations of systemic infection (fever, increased WBC, chills, malaise). Qpcc

> ! Do not use TPN line for other IV bolus fluids and medications. (Repeated access increases the risk for infection.)

Fluid imbalance

TPN is a hyperosmotic solution (three to six times the osmolarity of blood), which poses a risk for fluid shifts, placing client at increased risk of fluid volume excess.

OLDER ADULT CLIENTS are more vulnerable to fluid and electrolyte imbalances. Ⓖ

NURSING ACTIONS
- Monitor lungs for crackles and manifestations of respiratory distress.
- Check daily weight and I&O.
- Obtain a controlled infusion pump to administer TPN at the prescribed rate.
- Do not allow the infusion rate to be increased to catch up.
- Monitor the gradual rate increase of the solution until infusion reaches the prescribed rate.

Paracentesis

A paracentesis involves inserting a needle or trocar through the abdominal wall into the peritoneal cavity. The therapeutic goal is relief of abdominal ascites pressure.
- A paracentesis can be performed in a provider's office, outpatient center, radiology department, or acute care setting at the bed side.
- Usually performed with ultrasound as a safety precaution.
- Once drained, send the ascitic fluid for laboratory culture.

INDICATIONS

POTENTIAL DIAGNOSES

Abdominal ascites

- Ascites is an abnormal accumulation of protein-rich fluid in the abdominal cavity, most often caused by cirrhosis of the liver. The result is increased abdominal girth and distention.
- Respiratory distress indicates the need to use paracentesis to treat ascites, and improved respiratory function indicates treatment effectiveness.

CLIENT PRESENTATION

- Compromised lung expansion
- Increased abdominal girth
- Rapid weight gain

CONSIDERATIONS

PREPROCEDURE

NURSING ACTIONS
- Variables (age of the client; chronic and acute diseases) can influence ability to tolerate and recover from this procedure Ⓖ
- Review pertinent lab results (serum albumin, protein, glucose, amylase, BUN, creatinine).
- Verify that the client has signed the informed consent form prior to sedation.
- Gather equipment for the procedure.
- Have the client void, or insert an indwelling urinary catheter.
- Position the client in an upright position, either on the edge of the bed with feet supported or a high-Fowler's position in the bed. Clients who have ascites are typically more comfortable sitting up.
- Review baseline vital signs, record weight, and measure abdominal girth.
- The client can require IV bolus fluids or albumin prior to or after a paracentesis to restore fluid balance.
- Explain the procedure and its purpose to the client.

CLIENT EDUCATION
- Local anesthetics will be used at the insertion site.
- There can be pressure or pain with needle insertion.

INTRAPROCEDURE

NURSING ACTIONS
- Monitor vital signs.
- Adhere to standard precautions.
- Label laboratory specimens and send to the laboratory.
- Monitor the amount of drainage during the procedure and notifying the provider of any evidence of complications. Expected output is 4 to 6 L fluid, drained by gravity.

POSTPROCEDURE

NURSING ACTIONS
- Maintain pressure at the insertion site for several minutes. Apply a dressing to the site.
- If the insertion site continues to leak after holding pressure for several minutes, apply a dry sterile gauze dressing and replace as often as necessary.
- Check vital signs, record weight, and measure abdominal girth. Document and compare to preprocedure measurements.
- Continue to monitor vital signs and insertion site per facility protocol.
- Monitor temperature every 4 hr for a minimum of 48 hr. Fever can indicate a bowel perforation
- Determine I&O every 4 hr.

- Administer medication
  - Diuretics (spironolactone, furosemide) can be prescribed to control fluid volume.
  - Potassium supplements can be necessary when a loop diuretic such as furosemide has been administrated.
- Assist the client into a position of comfort with the head of the bed elevated to promote lung expansion.
- Document color, odor, consistency, and amount of fluid removed; location of insertion site; evidence of leakage at the insertion site; manifestations of hypovolemia; and changes in mental status.
- Continue monitoring of serum albumin, protein, glucose, amylase, electrolytes, BUN, and creatinine.

CLIENT EDUCATION
- Avoid alcohol, maintain a low-sodium diet, take prescribed medications, and monitor the puncture site for bleeding or leakage of fluid.
- Report changes in mental and cognitive status due to change in fluid and electrolyte balance.
- Change positions slowly to decrease the risk of falls, which can be related to hypovolemia from the removal of ascites fluid.

COMPLICATIONS

Hypovolemia

Albumin levels can drop dangerously low because the peritoneal fluid removed contains a large amount of protein. The removal of this protein-rich fluid can cause shifting of intravascular volume, resulting in hypovolemia.

NURSING ACTIONS
- Preventive measures include draining peritoneal fluid slowly and administration of plasma expanders, such as albumin, to counter albumin losses.
- Monitor for manifestations of hypovolemia (tachycardia, hypotension, pallor, diaphoresis, dizziness).
- Report unexpected findings to the charge nurse.

Bladder perforation

Bladder perforation is a rare but possible complication. Manifestations include hematuria, low or no urine output, suprapubic pain or distention, symptoms of cystitis, and fever. Qs

NURSING ACTIONS: If a bladder perforation is suspected, notify the provider immediately.

CLIENT EDUCATION: Report manifestations of bladder perforation.

Peritonitis

Peritonitis can occur as a result of injury to the intestines during needle insertion. Manifestations include sharp, constant abdominal pain, fever, nausea, vomiting, and diminished or absent bowel sounds.

NURSING ACTIONS: Notify the provider immediately.

CLIENT EDUCATION: Report findings listed above.

Bariatric surgery

Bariatric surgery is a treatment for morbid obesity when other weight control methods have failed. The client may try using pharmacological medication for weight loss before choosing bariatric surgery.
- **Orlistat** prevents digestion of fats. Adverse effects are oily discharge, reduced food and vitamin absorption, and decreased bile flow.
- **Lorcaserin** stimulates serotonin receptors in the hypothalamus in the brain to curb appetite. Adverse effects can be headache, dry mouth, fatigue, and nausea.
- **Phentermine-topiramate** suppresses the appetite and induces a feeling of satiety. Adverse effects include dry mouth, constipation, nausea, change in taste, dizziness, insomnia, and numbness and tingling of extremities. Contraindicated if the client has hyperthyroidism, glaucoma, or is taking an MAOI.

Bariatric surgeries include gastric restrictive and malabsorption.
- **Restrictive surgeries**, such as laparoscopic adjustable gastric band (LAGB) or laparoscopic sleeve gastrectomy (LSG), limit the amount of food eaten at one time due to decreased volume capacity. Weight loss is often regained after a period of time unless the client adheres to stringent weight loss protocols and lifestyle modifications. (40.1)
  - LAGB involves the placement of an adjustable band at the proximal portion of the stomach to restrict stomach volume to 10 to 15 mL.
  - LSG involves removal of the portion of the stomach that secretes ghrelin, a hormone that stimulates feelings of hunger. Up to 85% of the stomach is removed.
- **Vertical-banded gastroplasty** involves the creation of a new, smaller stomach pouch using staples to decrease its functional size. (40.2)
- **Malabsorption surgeries**, such as Roux-en-Y gastric bypass (RNYGB) or simply gastric bypass, interfere with the absorption of food and nutrients from the GI tract. Most clients maintain 60% to 70% of weight loss 20 years postprocedure.
  - RNYGB involves restricting the volume of the stomach to 20 to 30 mL, bypassing the majority of the stomach and the duodenum. A section of the jejunum is anastomosed to the smaller section of the stomach, bypassing the majority of the stomach. (40.3)
- Some procedures combine more than one of these approaches.

Many clients undergo plastic surgery to remove excess skin following weight loss.

INDICATIONS

DIAGNOSIS

History of morbid obesity (100% over ideal weight) with unsuccessful attempts at nonsurgical weight loss

CLIENT PRESENTATION

BMI greater than 40, or 35 with comorbidities

CONSIDERATIONS

PREPROCEDURE

NURSING ACTIONS

- Encourage the client to express emotions about eating behaviors, weight, and weight loss to identify psychosocial factors related to obesity.
- Ensure that the client understands needed diet and lifestyle changes.
- Prepare the client for postoperative course and potential complications.
- Arrange for availability of a bariatric bed and mechanical lifting devices to prevent client/staff injury. Qs
- Review pertinent lab results (CBC, electrolytes, BUN, creatinine, HbA1C, iron, vitamin B_{12}, thiamine, folate).
- Apply sequential compression stockings to help prevent deep vein thrombosis.

POSTPROCEDURE

NURSING ACTIONS

- Monitor for leak of anastomosis (increasing back, shoulder, abdominal pain; restlessness; tachycardia; oliguria) and notify the provider immediately. This is a life-threatening emergency.
- Notify the provider for suspected nasogastric (NG) tube displacement. The provider typically sutures the NG tube in place following stomach surgery. Do not attempt to manipulate the tube.
- Provide postoperative care and prevent postoperative complications.
- Monitor for the development of postoperative complications that are at increased risk due to obesity (atelectasis, thromboemboli, skin fold breakdown, incisional hernia, peritonitis).
- Monitor the airway and oxygen saturation per facility protocol. Maintain the client in a semi-Fowler's position for lung expansion.
- Monitor bowel sounds.
- Apply an abdominal binder as prescribed to prevent dehiscence if there is an abdominal incision.
- Ambulate the client as soon as possible.
- Resume fluids as prescribed. The first fluids can be restricted to 30 mL and increased in frequency and volume.
- Provide six small meals a day when the client can resume oral nutrients. Observe for indications of dumping syndrome (cramps, diarrhea, tachycardia, dizziness, fatigue).
- Collaborate with case management and mental health resources to assist with long-term behavior modification. Qᴛᴄ

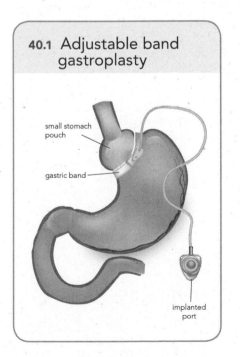

40.1 Adjustable band gastroplasty

small stomach pouch
gastric band
implanted port

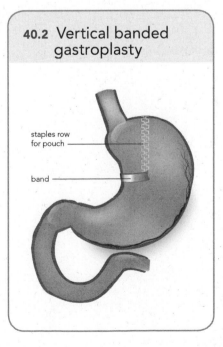

40.2 Vertical banded gastroplasty

staples row for pouch
band

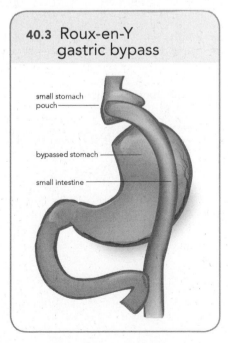

40.3 Roux-en-Y gastric bypass

small stomach pouch
bypassed stomach
small intestine

CLIENT EDUCATION

- For the first 6 weeks there are limitations on liquids or pureed foods. Do not exceed 1 cup.
- Walk daily for at least 30 min.
- Overeating can dilate the surgically created pouch causing weight to be regained.
- Take vitamin and mineral supplements.

COMPLICATIONS

Dehydration

- Warn the client to notify the surgeon about excessive thirst or concentrated urine, which can indicate dehydration.
- Work with the client to establish goals and schedule for adequate daily fluid intake.

Malabsorption/malnutrition

Because bariatric surgeries reduce the size of the stomach or bypass portions of the intestinal tract, the client takes in and absorbs fewer nutrients.

NURSING ACTIONS

- Monitor the client's tolerance of increasing amounts of food and fluids.
- Recommend a dietary referral for nutrition management.
- Encourage the client to consume meals in a low-Fowler's position and to remain in this position for 30 min after eating to delay stomach emptying and minimize dumping syndrome.

CLIENT EDUCATION

- Eat two servings of protein per day.
- Eat only nutrition-dense foods. Avoid empty calories, such as colas and fruit juice drinks.

Nasogastric decompression

Clients who have an intestinal obstruction require NG decompression using an NG tube with applied suction to relieve abdominal distention. Resolution of the obstruction indicates effectiveness of the procedure. The obstruction can be mechanical (tumors, adhesions, fecal impaction) or functional (paralytic ileus).

INDICATIONS

POTENTIAL DIAGNOSES

Any disorder that causes a mechanical or functional intestinal obstruction (surgery, trauma, GI tract infections, conditions in which peristalsis is absent)

CLIENT PRESENTATION

- Vomiting (begins with stomach contents and continues until fecal material is also being regurgitated)
- Bowel sounds absent (paralytic ileus) or hyperactive and high-pitched (obstruction)
- Intermittent, colicky abdominal pain and distention
- Hiccups
- Abdominal distention

CONSIDERATIONS

PREPROCEDURE

NURSING ACTIONS

- Gather necessary equipment and supplies.
- Instruct the client on the purpose of the NG tube and the client's role in its placement.

POSTPROCEDURE

NURSING ACTIONS

- Check and maintain proper function of the NG tube and suction equipment.
- Maintain accurate I&O.
- Monitor bowel sounds, abdominal girth, and return of flatus.
- Encourage repositioning and ambulation to help increase peristalsis.
- Monitor tube for displacement (decrease in drainage, increased nausea, vomiting, distention).
- Review pertinent lab results (electrolytes, hematocrit).
- Provide frequent oral and nares care.

CLIENT EDUCATION: Maintain NPO status.

COMPLICATIONS

Fluid/electrolyte imbalance

NURSING ACTIONS

- Monitor for fluid and electrolyte imbalance (metabolic acidosis: low obstruction; alkalosis: high obstruction).
- Monitor I&O, observing for discrepancies.

Skin breakdown

NURSING ACTIONS: Check nasal skin for irritation.

Ostomies

An ostomy is a surgical opening from the inside of the body to the outside and can be located in various areas of the body. Ostomies can be permanent or temporary.

- A stoma is the artificial opening created during the ostomy surgery. **(40.4)**
- Main types of ostomies performed in the abdominal area
  - **Ileostomy:** A surgical opening into the ileum to drain stool, which is typically frequent and liquid since large intestine is bypassed
  - **Colostomy:** A surgical opening into the large intestine to drain stool, with the ascending colon producing more liquid stools, the transverse colon producing more formed stools, and the sigmoid colon producing near-normal stool

INDICATIONS

POTENTIAL DIAGNOSES

Ileostomy: when the entire colon must be removed due to disease (Crohn's disease, ulcerative colitis).

Colostomy: when a portion of the bowel must be removed (cancer, ischemic injury) or requires rest for healing (diverticulitis, trauma).

CONSIDERATIONS

PREPROCEDURE

NURSING ACTIONS

- Determine the client's readiness for the procedure. Check visual acuity, manual dexterity, cognitive status, cultural influences, and support systems. Qᴘᴄᴄ
- Recommend a referral to the wound ostomy care nurse (WOCN) for ostomy placement marking and client teaching. Qᴛᴄ
- Work collaboratively with the WOCN to begin instructing the client and support person about ostomy care and management.

POSTPROCEDURE

NURSING ACTIONS

- Check the type and fit of the ostomy appliance. Monitor for leakage (risk to skin integrity). Fit the ostomy appliance based on the following.
  - Type and location of the ostomy
  - Visual acuity and manual dexterity of the client
- Check peristomal skin integrity and appearance of the stoma. The stoma should appear pink and moist.
- Apply skin barriers and creams (adhesive paste) to peristomal skin and allow to dry before applying a new appliance. **(40.5)**
- Evaluate stoma output. Output should be more liquid and more acidic the closer the ostomy is to the proximal small intestine. **(40.6)**

40.4 Healthy stoma

healthy stoma

- Empty the ostomy bag when it is one-fourth to one-half full of drainage.
- Check for fluid and electrolyte imbalances, particularly with a new ileostomy.
- Evaluate ability of the client or support person to perform ostomy care.
- Provide opportunities for the client to discuss feelings about the ostomy and concerns about its effect on the client's life. Encourage the client to look at and touch the stoma. Qᴘᴄᴄ
- Inform the client about ostomy support groups. Qᴛᴄ

CLIENT EDUCATION

- Dietary changes and ostomy appliances can help manage flatus and odor.
  - Foods that can cause odor: fish; eggs; asparagus; garlic; beans; and dark green, leafy vegetables
  - Foods that can decrease odor: buttermilk, cranberry juice, parsley, yogurt
  - Foods that can cause gas: dark green, leafy vegetables; beer; carbonated beverages; dairy products; and corn.
  - Chewing gum, skipping meals, and smoking can cause gas.
  - Yogurt, crackers, and toast can decrease gas.
  - Clients who have an ostomy involving the small intestine should avoid high-fiber foods for the first 2 months after surgery, chew food well, increase fluid intake, and watch for indications of blockage when slowly adding high-fiber foods to the diet.
  - Proper appliance fit and maintenance prevent odor when pouch is not open. The client can place a filter, deodorizer, or breath mint in the pouch to minimize odor while the pouch is open.

COMPLICATIONS

Stomal ischemia/necrosis

Stomal appearance should normally be pink or red and moist.

- Signs of stomal ischemia are pale pink or bluish purple color and dry appearance.

> **!** Notify the provider immediately if the stoma appears black or purple This indicates a serious lack of blood flow.

NURSING ACTIONS: Obtain vital signs, oxygen saturation, and current laboratory results. Notify the provider or surgeon of unexpected findings.

CLIENT EDUCATION: Watch for and report indications of stomal ischemia/necrosis immediately.

Intestinal obstruction

Both mechanical and functional issues can cause an intestinal obstruction.

NURSING ACTIONS
- Monitor and record output from the stoma.
- Monitor for manifestations of obstruction, including abdominal pain, hypoactive or absent bowel sounds, distention, nausea, and vomiting. Report these findings to the surgeon.

CLIENT EDUCATION: Report indications of an intestinal obstruction following discharge.

40.5 Changing an ostomy device

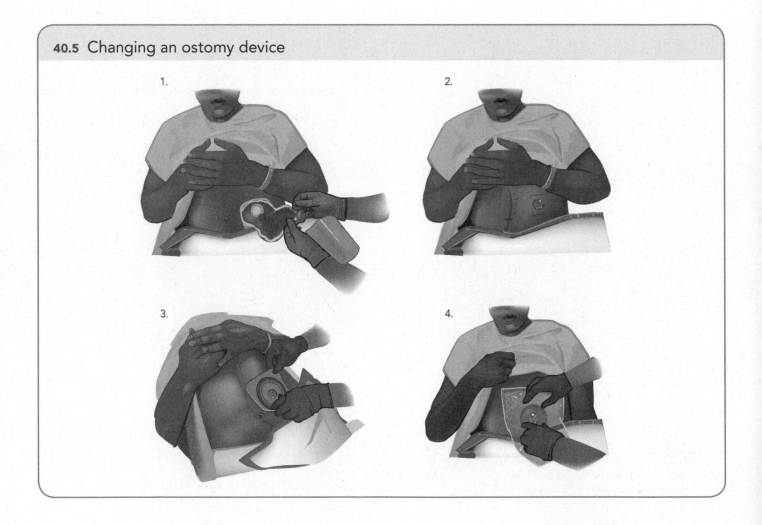

40.6 Expected output for ostomies

ILEOSTOMY	TRANSVERSE COLOSTOMY	SIGMOID COLOSTOMY
Normal postoperative output		
More than 1,000 mL/day Can be bile-colored and liquid	Small semi-liquid with some mucus 2 to 3 days after surgery Blood can be present in the first few days after surgery	Small to moderate amount of mucus with semi-formed stool 4 to 5 days after surgery
Postoperative changes in output		
After several days to weeks, the output decreases to approximately 500 to 1,000 mL/day Becomes more paste-like as the small intestine assumes the absorptive function of the large intestine	After several days to weeks, output becomes more stool-like, semi-formed, or formed	After several days to weeks, output resembles semi-formed stool
Pattern of output		
Continuous output	Unpredictable	Resumes a pattern similar to the preoperative pattern

Application Exercises

1. A nurse is monitoring a client following a paracentesis. Which of the following findings indicates bowel perforation?

   A. Report of upper chest pain

   B. Decreased urine output

   C. Pallor

   D. Temperature elevation

2. A nurse is assisting with the plan of care for a client who has a prescription for total parenteral nutrition (TPN). Which of the following interventions should the nurse include? (Select all that apply.)

   A. Measure capillary blood glucose four times daily.

   B. Administer medications through a secondary port on the TPN IV tubing.

   C. Monitor vital signs three times during the 12-hr shift.

   D. Change the TPN IV tubing every 24 hr.

   E. Obtain a daily aPTT.

3. A nurse is caring for a group of clients. Which of the following client findings should the nurse identify as an indication to recommend enteral feedings?

   A. Dysphagia secondary to Parkinson's disease

   B. Gastric paresis

   C. Short bowel syndrome

   D. Paralytic ileus

4. A nurse is providing care to a client who is 1 day postoperative following a paracentesis. The nurse observes clear, pale-yellow fluid leaking from the operative site. Which of the following is an appropriate nursing intervention?

   A. Place a clean towel near the drainage site.

   B. Apply a dry, sterile dressing.

   C. Apply direct pressure to the site.

   D. Place the client in a supine position.

5. A nurse is reinforcing discharge teaching with a client who is 3 days postoperative following a transverse colostomy. Which of the following should the nurse include in the teaching?

   A. Mucus will be present in stool for 5 to 7 days after surgery.

   B. Expect 500 to 1,000 mL semi liquid stool after 2 weeks.

   C. Stoma should be moist and pink.

   D. Empty the ostomy bag when it is three-fourths full.

Application Exercises Key

1. A. Sharp, constant abdominal pain is associated with bowel perforation.

   B. Decreased urine output is associated with bladder perforation during a paracentesis.

   C. Pallor can indicate hypovolemia related to fluid removal of ascites fluid during the procedure.

   D. **CORRECT:** Fever is an indication of bowel perforation during a paracentesis.

   Ⓝ *NCLEX® Connection: Reduction of Risk Potential, Potential for Complications of Diagnostic Tests/Treatments/Procedures*

2. A. **CORRECT:** The client is at risk for hyperglycemia during the administration of TPN and can require supplemental insulin.

   B. The nurses should not infuse other medications or fluids through the IV tubing simultaneously with TPN due to the increased risk of infection and disruption of the rate of TPN infusion.

   C. **CORRECT:** The nurse should take vital signs every 4 to 8 hr to check for fluid volume excess and infection.

   D. **CORRECT:** The nurse should have the IV tubing that is used to administer TPN changed every 24 hr.

   E. aPTT measures the coagulability of the blood, which is unnecessary during the administration of TPN.

   Ⓝ *NCLEX® Connection: Basic Care and Comfort, Nutrition and Oral Hydration*

3. A. **CORRECT:** Dysphagia, or impaired swallowing indicates a need for possible enteral nutrition. Conditions such as stroke, Parkinson's disease, or multiple sclerosis can cause dysphagia.

   B. Gastric paresis is an indication to recommend parenteral nutrition. A client who has gastric paresis has impaired gastric motility and will not be able to process enteral intake.

   C. Short bowel syndrome is an indication for parenteral nutrition. This client has the inability to absorb many nutrients through the gastrointestinal tract.

   D. Paralytic ileus is an indication to recommend parenteral nutrition. A client who has a paralytic ileus cannot move food through the gastrointestinal tract, and requires nasogastric decompression.

   Ⓝ *NCLEX® Connection: Basic Care and Comfort, Nutrition and Oral Hydration*

4. A. The nurse should apply a dressing to the operative site to prevent infection and allow for monitoring of drainage.

   B. **CORRECT:** Application of a sterile dressing will contain the drainage and allow continuous monitoring of color and quantity.

   C. Application of direct pressure can cause discomfort and potential harm to the client.

   D. The nurse should place the client with the head of the bed elevated to promote lung expansion.

   Ⓝ *NCLEX® Connection: Reduction of Risk Potential, Potential for Complications of Diagnostic Tests/Treatments/Procedures*

5. A. Mucus and blood can be present for 2 to 3 days after surgery.

   B. Output should become stool-like, semi-formed, or formed within days to weeks.

   C. **CORRECT:** A pink, moist stoma is an expected finding with a transverse colostomy.

   D. The nurse should empty or change the ostomy bag when it is one-fourth to one-half full.

   Ⓝ *NCLEX® Connection: Reduction of Risk Potential, Potential for Complications from Surgical Procedures and Health Alterations*

PRACTICE Active Learning Scenario

Using the ATI Active Learning Template: Therapeutic Procedure

DESCRIPTION OF PROCEDURE
- Vertical banded gastroplasty involves stapling a portion of the stomach to decrease its functional size.
- Adjustable banded gastroplasty involves constricting the functional size of the stomach.
- Intestinal bypass involves bypassing the stomach and part of the small intestine to decrease the absorption of nutrients and calories.

NURSING INTERVENTIONS
- Encourage client to express emotions related to weight, weight loss, and eating behaviors to identify related psychosocial concerns.
- Ensure the client understands required dietary and lifestyle changes.
- Request a bariatric bed and mechanical lifting device to prevent client/staff injury.
- Observe for leak of anastomosis, and notify provider immediately if this occurs.
- Monitor airway and oxygen saturation. Maintain client in semi-Fowler's position for lung expansion.
- Monitor bowel sounds.
- Apply abdominal binder if prescribed.
- Ambulate client as soon as possible.
- Monitor I&O.
- Monitor NG tube placement and function, as well as function of suction equipment.

CLIENT EDUCATION
- Begin taking 30 mL of fluid at a time and gradually increase in volume and frequency.
- Solid food intake includes six small meals daily.
- Volume might be limited to 1 cup of liquid or pureed foods.

Ⓝ *NCLEX® Connection: Reduction of Risk Potential, Potential for Complications from Surgical Procedures and Health Alterations*

CHAPTER 41 *Esophageal Disorders*

The esophagus is a muscular tube that leads from the throat to the stomach. It extends from the base of pharynx to the stomach. Esophageal disorders can affect any part of the esophagus.

There are two sphincters: upper esophageal (also referred to as the oropharyngeal sphincter) and lower esophageal (also referred to as the gastroesophageal sphincter). They prevent the reflux of food and fluids into the mouth or esophagus. (41.1)

Common problems in the esophagus (structural defects, inflammation, obstruction, cancer) interfere with nutrition.

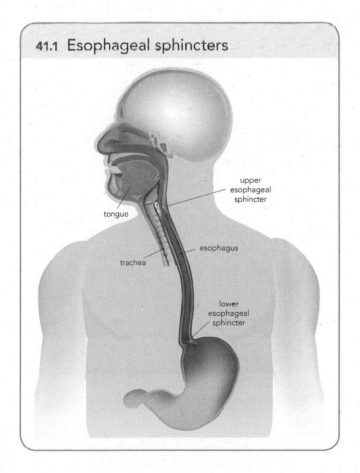

41.1 Esophageal sphincters

tongue

trachea

upper esophageal sphincter

esophagus

lower esophageal sphincter

Contractions of the esophagus propel food and fluids toward the stomach, while relaxation of the lower esophageal sphincter allows passage into the stomach. Following this, the lower esophageal sphincter (LES) contracts, preventing reflux of food back up into the esophagus.

Esophageal disorders include gastroesophageal reflux disease (GERD), hiatal hernia, and esophageal varices.

Gastroesophageal reflux disease

GERD is a common condition characterized by gastric content and enzyme backflow into the esophagus. Some backflow of stomach contents into the esophagus is expected. When the reflux is excessive due to specific conditions (incompetent LES, pyloric stenosis, hiatal hernia, excessive intra-abdominal or intragastric pressure, motility problems), the corrosive fluids irritate the esophageal tissue, causing delay in their clearance. This further exposes esophageal tissue to the acidic fluids, causing more irritation.

- The primary treatment of GERD is diet and lifestyle changes, advancing to medication use (antacids, H_2-receptor antagonists, proton pump inhibitors) and surgery. Qpcc
- Untreated GERD leads to inflammation, breakdown, and long-term complications (Barrett's esophagus, adenocarcinoma of the esophagus).

HEALTH PROMOTION AND DISEASE PREVENTION

- Maintain BMI less than 30.
- Stop smoking.
- Limit or avoid alcohol and tobacco use.
- Eat a low-fat diet.
- Avoid foods that reduce LES pressure.
- Avoid eating or drinking 2 hr before bed.
- Avoid tight-fitting clothes.
- Elevate the head of the bed 6 to 8 inches.

DATA COLLECTION

RISK FACTORS

- Obesity
- Age (delayed gastric emptying and weakened LES tone in older adult clients) Ⓖ
- Sleep apnea
- Nasogastric tube

CONTRIBUTING FACTORS

- Excessive ingestion of foods that relax the LES: fatty and fried foods, chocolate, caffeinated beverages (coffee), peppermint, spicy foods, tomatoes, citrus fruits, and alcohol
- Prolonged or frequent abdominal distention (from overeating or delayed emptying)
- Increased abdominal pressure from obesity, pregnancy, bending at the waist, ascites, or tight clothing at the waist
- Medications that relax the LES (theophylline, nitrates, calcium channel blockers, anticholinergics, diazepam)
- Increased gastric acid caused by medications (NSAIDs) or stress (environmental)
- Debilitation resulting in weakened LES tone
- Hiatal hernia (LES displacement into the thorax with delayed esophageal clearance)
- Lying flat

EXPECTED FINDINGS

- Classic report of dyspepsia after eating an offending food or fluid, and regurgitation
- Radiating pain (neck, jaw, back)
- Report of a feeling of having a heart attack
- Pyrosis (burning sensation in the esophagus)
- Dyspepsia (indigestion)
- Dysphagia or odynophagia (pain on swallowing)
- Pain that worsens with position (bending, straining, laying down)
- Pain that occurs after eating and lasts 20 min to 2 hr
- Throat irritation (chronic cough, laryngitis), hypersalivation, bitter taste in mouth (caused by regurgitation). Chronic GERD can lead to dysphagia.
- Increased flatus and eructation (burping)
- Tooth erosion
- Pain is relieved (almost immediately) by drinking water, sitting upright, or taking antacids.
- Manifestations occurring four to five times per week on a consistent basis are considered diagnostic.

PHARYNGITIS DIAGNOSTIC PROCEDURES

Esophagogastroduodenoscopy

- Esophagogastroduodenoscopy (EGD) requires moderate sedation to observe for tissue damage and to dilate strictures in the esophagus. The esophageal lining should be pink but is often red with persistent GERD. EGD can include biopsy to determine if high-grade dysplasia (HGD) is present.
- When HGD is found, there is a 30% increase in chance of developing cancer.
- EGD allows visualization of the esophagus, revealing esophagitis or Barrett's epithelium (premalignant cells).

NURSING ACTIONS: Verify gag response has returned prior to providing oral fluids or food following the procedure. Qs

Esophageal (ambulatory) pH monitoring

A small catheter is placed through the nose and into the distal esophagus, or a small capsule is attached to the esophageal wall during endoscopy. pH readings are taken in relation to food, position, and activity for 24 to 48 hr.

- Most accurate method of diagnosing GERD
- Especially helpful in diagnosis for clients who have atypical manifestations

CLIENT EDUCATION: Keep a journal of foods and beverages consumed, manifestations, and activity during the 24-hr test period.

Esophageal manometry

Esophageal manometry records lower esophageal sphincter pressure and peristaltic activity of the esophagus. The client swallows three small tubes, and pressure readings and pH levels are tested.

Barium swallow

Barium swallow identifies a hiatal hernia, strictures, or structural deviations, which would contribute to or cause GERD.

CLIENT EDUCATION: Use cathartics and increase fluid consumption to evacuate the barium from the GI tract following the procedure. Failure to eliminate the barium places the client at risk for fecal impaction.

PATIENT-CENTERED CARE

MEDICATIONS

Proton pump inhibitors (PPIs)

- Pantoprazole, omeprazole, esomeprazole, rabeprazole, and lansoprazole reduce gastric acid by inhibiting the cellular pump of the gastric parietal cells necessary for gastric acid secretion.
- Long-term use has been related to the development of community-acquired pneumonia and Clostridium difficile infections.

NURSING ACTIONS: Monitor for electrolyte imbalances and hypoglycemia in clients who have diabetes mellitus.

CLIENT EDUCATION: Long-term use of PPIs places the client at risk for fractures, especially in older adults. ©

Antacids

Aluminum hydroxide, magnesium hydroxide, calcium carbonate, and sodium bicarbonate neutralize excess acid and increase LES pressure.

NURSING ACTIONS: Ensure there are no contraindications with other prescribed medications (levothyroxine). Evaluate kidney function in clients taking magnesium hydroxide.

CLIENT EDUCATION: Take antacids when acid secretion is the highest (1 to 3 hr after eating and at bedtime), and separate from other medications by at least 1 hr.

Histamine₂ receptor antagonists

Ranitidine, famotidine, and nizatidine reduce the secretion of acid. The onset is longer than antacids, but the effect has a longer duration.

NURSING ACTIONS: Use cautiously in clients who have kidney disease.

CLIENT EDUCATION
- Take with meals and at bedtime.
- Separate dosages from antacids (1 hr before or after taking antacid).

Prokinetics

Metoclopramide increases the motility of the esophagus and stomach.

NURSING ACTIONS: Monitor clients taking metoclopramide for extrapyramidal side effects.

CLIENT EDUCATION: Report involuntary movements.

THERAPEUTIC PROCEDURES

Stretta procedure

Uses radiofrequency energy, applied by an endoscope, to decrease vagus nerve activity. This causes the LES muscle tissue to contract and tighten.

Fundoplication

Fundoplication is indicated for clients who fail to respond to other treatments. The fundus of the stomach is wrapped around and behind the esophagus through a laparoscope to create a physical barrier.

NURSING ACTIONS: Complications following fundoplication include temporary dysphagia (monitor for aspiration), gas bloat syndrome (difficulty belching to relieve distention), and atelectasis/pneumonia (monitor respiratory function).

CLIENT EDUCATION
- **Diet**
  - Avoid offending foods.
  - Avoid large meals.
  - Remain upright after eating.
  - Avoid eating before bedtime.
  - Consume four to six small meals throughout the day.
- **Lifestyle**
  - Avoid clothing that is tight-fitting around the abdomen.
  - Lose weight, if applicable.
  - Elevate the head of the bed 15.2 to 20.3 cm (6 to 8 in) with blocks.
  - Sleep on the right side.

COMPLICATIONS

Aspiration of gastric secretion

CAUSES: Reflux of gastric fluids into the esophagus can be aspirated into the trachea.

RISKS ASSOCIATED WITH ASPIRATION
- Asthma exacerbations from inhaled aerosolized acid
- Frequent upper respiratory, sinus, or ear infections
- Aspiration pneumonia

Barrett's epithelium (premalignant) and esophageal adenocarcinoma

CAUSE: Reflux of gastric fluids leads to esophagitis. In chronic esophagitis, the body continuously heals inflamed tissue, eventually replacing healthy esophageal epithelium with premalignant tissue (Barrett's epithelium) or malignant adenocarcinoma.

NURSING ACTIONS: Determine the cause of GERD with the client and review lifestyle changes that can decrease gastric reflux. Monitor nutritional status. Qᴘᴄᴄ

Hiatal hernia

Hiatal hernia (diaphragmatic hernia) is a protrusion of the stomach (in part or in total) above the diaphragm into the thoracic cavity through the hiatus (the opening in the diaphragm). There are two types of hiatal hernia.

Sliding (more common): A portion of the stomach and gastroesophageal junction move above the diaphragm. This generally occurs with increases in intra-abdominal pressure or while the client is in a supine position.

Paraesophageal (rolling): Part of the fundus of the stomach moves above the diaphragm although the gastroesophageal junction remains below the diaphragm.

HEALTH PROMOTION AND DISEASE PREVENTION

- Avoid eating immediately prior to going to bed.
- Avoid foods and beverages that decrease LES pressure (fatty and fried foods, chocolate, coffee, peppermint, spicy foods, tomatoes, citrus fruits, and alcohol).
- Exercise regularly.
- Maintain a healthy weight.
- Elevate the head of the bed on 6-inch blocks.
- Avoid straining or excessive vigorous exercise.
- Avoid wearing clothing that is tight around the abdomen.

DATA COLLECTION

EXPECTED FINDINGS

Presenting manifestations depend on the type of hiatal hernia and are typically worse following a meal.

Sliding: heartburn, reflux, chest pain, dysphagia, belching

Paraesophageal: fullness after eating, sense of breathlessness/suffocation, chest pain, worsening of manifestations when reclining

PHYSICAL FINDINGS
- Pharyngitis
- Inspiratory/expiratory wheeze

DIAGNOSTIC PROCEDURES

Barium swallow with fluoroscopy

Allows visualization of the esophagus.

CLIENT EDUCATION: Use cathartics and increase fluids to evacuate the barium from the GI tract following the procedure. Failure to eliminate the barium places the client at risk for fecal impaction.

Esophagogastroduodenoscopy

Allows visualization of the esophagus and the gastric lining.

NURSING ACTIONS: Verify gag response has returned prior to providing oral fluids or food following the procedure Qs

CT scan of the chest with contrast

Allows visualization of the esophagus and stomach.

NURSING ACTIONS: Check for iodine allergies if IV contrast is to be used. Encourage fluids following procedure to promote dye excretion and minimize risk of acute kidney injury. Monitor BUN/creatinine

PATIENT-CENTERED CARE

MEDICATIONS

Proton pump inhibitors

- Pantoprazole, omeprazole, esomeprazole, rabeprazole, and lansoprazole reduce gastric acid by inhibiting the cellular pump of the gastric parietal cells necessary for gastric acid secretion.
- Long-term use has been related to the development of community-acquired pneumonia and *Clostridium difficile* infections.

NURSING ACTIONS: Monitor for electrolyte imbalances and hypoglycemia in clients who have diabetes mellitus.

CLIENT EDUCATION: Long-term use of PPIs places clients at risk for fractures, especially in older adults. Ⓒ

Antacids

Aluminum hydroxide, magnesium hydroxide, calcium carbonate, and sodium bicarbonate neutralize excess acid and increase LES pressure.

NURSING ACTIONS: Ensure there are no contraindications with other prescribed medications (levothyroxine). Evaluate kidney function in clients taking magnesium hydroxide.

CLIENT EDUCATION: Take antacids when acid secretion is the highest (1 to 3 hr after eating and at bedtime), and separate from other medications by at least 1 hr.

THERAPEUTIC PROCEDURES

Fundoplication: reinforcement of the LES by wrapping a portion of the fundus of the stomach around the distal esophagus

Laparoscopic Nissen fundoplication: minimally invasive with fewer complications

NURSING ACTIONS: Elevate the head of the bed to promote lung expansion.

CLIENT EDUCATION
- Support the incision during movement and coughing to minimize strain on the suture lines.
- Consume a soft diet for the first week postoperatively. Avoid carbonated beverages.
- Ambulate, but avoid heavy lifting.

COMPLICATIONS: Temporary dysphagia, gas bloat syndrome (difficulty burping and distention), atelectasis/pneumonia

COMPLICATIONS

Volvulus: twisting of the esophagus and/or stomach

Obstruction (paraesophageal hernia): blockage of food in the herniated portion of the stomach

Strangulation (paraesophageal hernia): compression of the blood vessels to the herniated portion of the stomach

Iron-deficiency anemia (paraesophageal hernia): results from bleeding into the gastric mucosa due to obstruction

Esophageal varices

Esophageal varices are swollen, fragile blood vessels that are generally found in the submucosa of the lower esophagus, but varices can develop higher in the esophagus or extend into the stomach. **(41.2)**

- Esophageal varices occur as a result of portal hypertension, usually due to cirrhosis of the liver.
- When esophageal varices hemorrhage, it is a medical emergency associated with a high mortality rate. Reoccurrence of esophageal bleeding is common.

HEALTH PROMOTION AND DISEASE PREVENTION

- Avoid alcohol consumption.
- Avoid heavy lifting.
- Avoid straining with bowel movements.
- Chew food completely, as poorly chewed foods can irritate the area.
- Avoid salicylates and other medications that can irritate the esophagus.

DATA COLLECTION

RISK FACTORS

- Portal hypertension (elevated blood pressure in veins that carry blood from the intestines to the liver)
  - Caused by impaired circulation of blood through the liver. Collateral circulation subsequently develops, creating varices in the upper stomach and esophagus. Varices are fragile and can bleed easily.
  - Primary risk factor for esophageal varices
- Alcoholic cirrhosis
- Viral hepatitis
- **OLDER ADULT CLIENTS** frequently have depressed immune function, decreased liver function, and cardiac disorders that make them especially vulnerable to bleeding. Ⓒ

EXPECTED FINDINGS

- The client might not experience manifestations until the varices begin to bleed.
- Hematemesis, melena, and a general deterioration of the client's physical and mental status.
- Activities that precipitate bleeding are the Valsalva maneuver, lifting heavy objects, coughing, sneezing, and alcohol consumption.

PHYSICAL FINDINGS (BLEEDING ESOPHAGEAL VARICES)
- Shock
- Hypotension
- Tachycardia
- Cool, clammy skin

LABORATORY TESTS

Liver function tests indicate a liver disorder.

Hemoglobin and hematocrit tests can indicate anemia secondary to occult bleeding or overt bleeding.

Elevated serum ammonia level indicates an increased nitrogen load from the bleeding varices.

DIAGNOSTIC PROCEDURES

Endoscopy

Therapeutic interventions can be performed during the endoscopy.

NURSING ACTIONS: After the procedure, monitor vital signs and take measures to prevent aspiration.

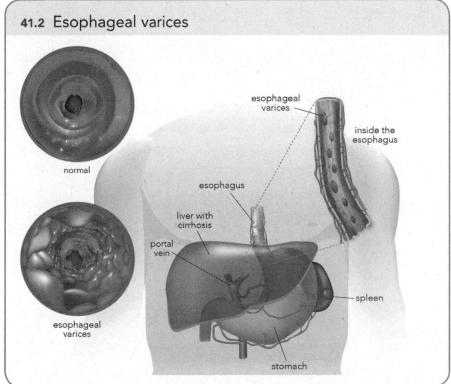

41.2 **Esophageal varices**

normal

esophageal varices

esophageal varices

inside the esophagus

esophagus

liver with cirrhosis

portal vein

spleen

stomach

PATIENT-CENTERED CARE

NURSING CARE Qs

- If bleeding is suspected, ensure the client has IV access with a large-bore needle, monitor vital signs and hematocrit, and monitor for overt and occult bleeding.
- Assist with monitoring if a blood transfusion is prescribed.

MEDICATIONS

Nonselective beta-blockers

- Propranolol is prescribed to decrease heart rate and consequently reduce hepatic venous pressure.
- Used prophylactically (not for emergency hemorrhage).

Vasoconstrictors

- Octreotide is a synthetic form of the hormone somatostatin and decreases the bleeding from the esophageal varices but does not affect the blood pressure.
- Vasopressin causes constriction of the esophageal and proximal gastric veins and reduces portal pressure.

NURSING ACTIONS: Monitor for fluid retention and hyponatremia, as vasopressin has an antidiuretic effect.

THERAPEUTIC PROCEDURES

Endoscopic variceal ligation (EVL)

- EVL (esophageal banding therapy) can be used for acute bleeding.
- During endoscopy, the varices are rubber banded to cut off the circulation to the varices.

NURSING ACTIONS: After the procedure, monitor vital signs and take measures to prevent aspiration.

Endoscopic sclerotherapy

During endoscopy, a sclerosing agent is injected into the varices, resulting in thrombosis of the varicosity.

NURSING ACTIONS
- After the procedure, monitor vital signs and take measures to prevent aspiration.
- Antacids, H_2-receptor blockers, or PPIs can be administered after the procedure to protect the esophagus and prevent acid reflux, which is often caused by sclerotherapy.

Transjugular intrahepatic portal-systemic shunt (TIPS)

- TIPS is used to treat an acute episode of bleeding when EVL and pharmacological measures are not controlling the variceal bleeding. It rapidly lowers the portal pressure. The procedure is costly, and therefore is only used when other measures do not work.
- While the client is under sedation or general anesthesia, a catheter is passed into the liver via the jugular vein in the neck. A stent is then placed between the portal and hepatic veins bypassing the liver. Portal hypertension is subsequently relieved.

NURSING ACTIONS
- Monitor vital signs.
- Keep the head of the bed elevated.

Surgical interventions

- Considered as a last resort. TIPS has replaced many surgical measures. Surgical interventions involve high morbidity and mortality rates.
- Bypass procedures establish a venous shunt that bypasses the liver, decreasing portal hypertension.
  - Common shunts include **splenorenal** (splenic, left renal veins), **mesocaval** (mesenteric vein, vena cava), and **portacaval** (portal vein, inferior vena cava).
  - Clients commonly have a nasogastric tube inserted during surgery to monitor for hemorrhage.

NURSING ACTIONS
- Monitor for an increase in liver dysfunction or encephalopathy.
- Monitor nasogastric tube secretions for bleeding.
- Monitor PT, aPTT, platelets, and INR.

INTERPROFESSIONAL CARE

Alcohol recovery program (varices secondary to alcohol use disorder)

COMPLICATIONS

Hypovolemic shock

Due to hemorrhage from varices

NURSING ACTIONS
- Observe for manifestations of hemorrhage and shock (tachycardia, hypotension).
- Monitor vital signs, Hgb, Hct, and coagulation studies.
- Support therapeutic procedures to stop and control bleeding and to replace fluid loss.

Application Exercises

1. A nurse is caring for a client who has a new diagnosis of gastroesophageal reflux disease (GERD). The nurse should anticipate prescriptions for which of the following medications? (Select all that apply.)

   A. Antacids

   B. Histamine$_2$ receptor antagonists

   C. Opioid analgesics

   D. Fiber laxatives

   E. Proton pump inhibitors

2. A nurse is caring for a client newly admitted with bleeding esophageal varices. The nurse should anticipate a prescription for which of the following medications?

   A. Propranolol

   B. Metoclopramide

   C. Ranitidine

   D. Vasopressin

3. A nurse is collecting data from a client who has GERD. Which of the following findings should the nurse expect?

   A. Absence of saliva

   B. Loss of tooth enamel

   C. Sweet taste in mouth

   D. Absence of eructation

4. A nurse is reinforcing teaching with a client who has a hiatal hernia. Which of the following client statements indicates understanding?

   A. "I can take my medications with soda."

   B. "Peppermint tea will increase my indigestion."

   C. "Wearing an abdominal binder will limit my symptoms."

   D. "I will drink hot chocolate at bedtime to help me sleep."

5. A nurse is reinforcing discharge teaching with a client who is postoperative following fundoplication. Which of the following statements by the client indicates understanding?

   A. "When sitting in my lounge chair after a meal, I will lower the back of it."

   B. "I will try to eat three large meals a day."

   C. "I will elevate the head of my bed on blocks."

   D. "When sleeping, I will lay on my left side."

PRACTICE Active Learning Scenario

A nurse is helping prepare a poster on GERD to be displayed at a community health fair. What should the nurse include in the poster? Use the ATI Active Learning Template: System Disorder to complete this item.

ALTERATION IN HEALTH (DIAGNOSIS)

RISK FACTORS: Describe at least eight.

EXPECTED FINDINGS: Describe at least eight.

Application Exercises Key

1. A. **CORRECT:** Antacids neutralize gastric acid, which irritates the esophagus during reflux.

   B. **CORRECT:** Histamine₂ receptor antagonists decrease acid secretion, which contributes to reflux.

   C. Opioid analgesics are not effective in treating GERD.

   D. Fiber laxatives are not effective in treating GERD.

   E. **CORRECT:** Proton pump inhibitors decrease gastric acid production, which contributes to reflex.

   Ⓝ *NCLEX® Connection: Pharmacological Therapies, Expected Actions/Outcomes*

2. A. Propranolol is not used for clients who are actively bleeding. It can be given prophylactically to decrease portal hypertension.

   B. Metoclopramide decreases motility of the esophagus and stomach.

   C. Following surgical procedures for bleeding esophageal varices, histamine₂ receptor antagonists help protect the esophagus from damage.

   D. **CORRECT:** Vasopressin constricts blood vessels and is used to treat bleeding esophageal varices.

   Ⓝ *NCLEX® Connection: Pharmacological Therapies, Expected Actions/Outcomes*

3. A. Hypersalivation is an expected finding in a client who has GERD.

   B. **CORRECT:** Tooth erosion is an expected finding in a client who has GERD.

   C. A client who has GERD would report a bitter taste in the mouth.

   D. Increased burping is an expected finding in a client who has GERD.

   Ⓝ *NCLEX® Connection: Physiological Adaptation, Basic Pathophysiology*

4. A. The client should avoid carbonated beverages because they affect LES pressure and can exacerbate the effects of a hiatal hernia.

   B. **CORRECT:** Peppermint decreases LES pressure and should be avoided by the client who has a hiatal hernia

   C. The client should avoid tight, restrictive clothing or abdominal binders, which increase intra-abdominal pressure and cause the protrusion of the stomach into the thoracic cavity.

   D. The client should avoid consuming anything immediately prior to bedtime. Additionally, chocolate relaxes the lower esophageal sphincter and should be avoided by a client who has a hiatal hernia.

   Ⓝ *NCLEX® Connection: Physiological Adaptation, Alterations in Body Systems*

5. A. The client should remain upright after eating following a fundoplication.

   B. The client should avoid consuming large meals after a fundoplication.

   C. **CORRECT:** After a fundoplication, the client is instructed to elevate the head of the bed to limit reflux.

   D After a fundoplication, the client should sleep on the right side.

   Ⓝ *NCLEX® Connection: Reduction of Risk Potential, Potential for Complications from Surgical Procedures and Health Alterations*

PRACTICE Answer

Using the ATI Active Learning Template: System Disorder

ALTERATION IN HEALTH (DIAGNOSIS): Gastroesophageal reflux disease (GERD) is a common condition characterized by gastric content and enzyme backflow into the esophagus. These fluids are corrosive to esophageal tissue, causing a delay in their clearance. This further exposes esophageal tissue to the acidic fluids, increasing tissue irritation.

RISK FACTORS
- Obesity
- Older age
- Sleep apnea
- Excessive ingestion of foods that relax the lower esophageal sphincter (fatty and fried foods, chocolate, caffeinated beverages, peppermint, spicy foods, tomatoes, citrus fruits, and alcohol)
- Pregnancy
- Bending at the waist, wearing tight clothing at the waist
- Medications (theophylline, nitrates, calcium channel blockers, anticholinergics, NSAIDs)
- Stress
- Hiatal hernia
- Lying flat

EXPECTED FINDINGS
- Classic report of dyspepsia after eating an offending food or fluid, and regurgitation
- Radiating pain (neck, jaw, or back)
- Report of a feeling of having a heart attack.
- Pyrosis (burning sensation in the esophagus)
- Dyspepsia (indigestion)
- Dysphagia or odynophagia (pain on swallowing)
- Pain that worsens with position (bending, straining, laying down)
- Pain that occurs after eating and lasts 20 min to 2 hr
- Throat irritation (chronic cough, laryngitis), hypersalivation, bitter taste in mouth (caused by regurgitation). Chronic GERD can lead to dysphagia.
- Increased flatus and eructation (burping)
- Tooth erosion
- Pain is relieved (almost immediately) by drinking water, sitting upright, or taking antacids.
- Manifestations occurring four to five times per week on a consistent basis are diagnostic.

Ⓝ *NCLEX® Connection: Physiological Adaptation, Basic Pathophysiology*

CHAPTER 42 *Peptic Ulcer Disease*

A peptic ulcer is an erosion of the mucosal lining of the stomach, esophagus, or duodenum. The most common area for a peptic ulcer is the duodenum. The mucous membranes can become eroded to the point that the epithelium is exposed to gastric acid and pepsin, which can precipitate bleeding and perforation. Perforation that extends through all the layers of the stomach or duodenum can cause peritonitis.

Most peptic ulcers are caused by an infection from gram-negative bacteria *Helicobacter pylori* (*H. pylori*). Contact with the bacteria occurs from food, water, or exposure to body fluids such as saliva. Continued use of NSAIDs and smoking contribute to *H. pylori*. Some people infected with the *H. pylori* bacteria do not develop ulcers.

Stress ulcers occur from an acute period of physiological stressful events (burns, shock, severe sepsis, multiple organ trauma). These ulcers are different clinically from a peptic ulcer and can be present in a ventilated client in the intensive care unit. Curling's ulcer is seen in clients who have burns. Cushing's ulcer can be seen in clients who have head/brain trauma. Bleeding is the primary manifestation of the stress ulcer. Clients experiencing trauma often receive proton-pump inhibitor prophylaxis to prevent the development of stress ulcers.

HEALTH PROMOTION AND DISEASE PREVENTION

- Avoid excessive consumption of alcohol.
- Stop smoking and use of tobacco products.
- Use stress management techniques.
- Avoid NSAIDs as indicated.
- Limit caffeine-containing beverages.
- Consume a balanced diet.
- Engage regularly in exercise.

DATA COLLECTION

RISK FACTORS

Causes of peptic ulcers
- *H. pylori* infection
- NSAID and corticosteroid use
- Smoking
- Severe stress
- Familial tendency
- Hypersecretory states with an increased amount of acidic gastric juices
- Gastrin-secreting benign or malignant tumors of the pancreas
- Type O blood
- Excess alcohol consumption
- Chronic pulmonary or kidney disease
- Zollinger-Ellison syndrome (combination of peptic ulcers, hypersecretion of gastric acid, and gastrin-secreting tumors)
- Pernicious anemia

EXPECTED FINDINGS

- Dyspepsia: heartburn, bloating, nausea, vomiting
  - Vomiting is rare but can be caused by a gastric outlet obstruction.
  - Can be perceived as uncomfortable fullness or hunger
- Dull, gnawing pain or burning sensation at the midepigastrium or the back

42.1 Ulcer pain

GASTRIC ULCER	DUODENAL ULCER
- Pain most commonly occurs before meals and at bedtime.	- Pain that occurs 1.5 to 3 hr after a meal
- Pain is exacerbated by ingestion of food.	- Awakening with pain during the night
- Pain is present for several days or weeks. Pain will then subside and reappear weeks or months later.	- Pain relieved by ingestion of food (food acts as a buffer) or antacid
- Malnourishment	- Well-nourished
- Hematemesis	- Melena
	- Spontaneous vomiting

PHYSICAL FINDINGS
- Pain or epigastric tenderness or abdominal distension (feeling of bloating)
- Bloody emesis (hematemesis)
  - Bright red indicates an active bleed.
  - Coffee-ground appearance indicates it has been sitting in gastric juices.
- Blood in stools (melena)
- Weight loss
- **If GI bleeding is present:** decreased blood pressure, tachycardia, possible diarrhea (blood is a cathartic)

LABORATORY TESTS

***H. pylori* testing:** Gastric samples are collected via endoscopy to test for *H. pylori*.

Urea breath testing: The client exhales into a collection container (baseline), drinks carbon-enriched urea solution, and is asked to exhale into a collection container. The client should take nothing by mouth (NPO) prior to the test. If *H. pylori* is present, the solution will break down and carbon dioxide will be released. Serologic testing documents the presence of *H. pylori* based on antibody assays.

Stool sample tests for the presence of the *H. pylori* antigen

Hemoglobin and hematocrit (unexpected findings secondary to bleeding)

Stool sample for occult blood

White blood count can be elevated if GI bleeding is significant.

Elevated BUN due to digestion of blood in the GI system

DIAGNOSTIC PROCEDURES

Esophagogastroduodenoscopy (EGD)

An EGD provides a definitive diagnosis of peptic ulcers and can be repeated to evaluate the effectiveness of treatment. Gastric samples are obtained to test for *H. pylori*. Refer to **CHAPTER 39: GASTROINTESTINAL DIAGNOSTIC PROCEDURES.**

NURSING ACTIONS
- Monitor vital signs until sedation wears off.
- Keep client NPO until return of gag reflex.
- Monitor for manifestations of perforation (pain, bleeding, fever).

CLIENT EDUCATION: NPO for 6 to 8 hr prior to the exam.

PATIENT-CENTERED CARE

NURSING CARE

- Instruct clients to avoid foods that cause distress (coffee, tea, carbonated beverages).
- Monitor for orthostatic changes in vital signs and tachycardia, as these findings suggest GI bleeding or perforation.
- Administer saline lavage via nasogastric (NG) tube to decrease vomiting.
- Administer medication.
- Decrease environmental stress.
- Encourage rest periods.
- Encourage smoking cessation and avoiding alcohol consumption.
- Monitor laboratory results (hemoglobin, hematocrit, coagulation studies).

MEDICATIONS

Antibiotics

Metronidazole, amoxicillin, clarithromycin, and tetracycline eliminate *H. pylori* infection.

NURSING ACTIONS: A combination of two or three antibiotics can be administered.

CLIENT EDUCATION: Complete a full course of medication.

Histamine₂ receptor antagonists

Ranitidine, famotidine, cimetidine, and nizatidine suppress the secretion of gastric acid by selectively blocking H_2 receptors in parietal cells lining the stomach.
- Used in conjunction with antibiotics to treat ulcers caused by *H. pylori*
- Used to prevent stress ulcers in clients who are NPO after major surgery, have large areas of burns, are septic, or have increased intracranial pressure
- Ranitidine and famotidine can be administered IV in acute situations.
- Ranitidine can be taken with or without food.
- Treatment of peptic ulcer disease is usually started as an oral dose twice a day until the ulcer is healed, followed by a maintenance dose usually taken once a day at bedtime.

CLIENT EDUCATION
- Notify the provider of obvious or occult GI bleeding (coffee-ground emesis).
- Complete the prescribed regimen, even when manifestations subside.

Proton-pump inhibitors

Pantoprazole, esomeprazole, omeprazole, lansoprazole, and rabeprazole suppress gastric acid secretion by irreversibly inhibiting the enzyme that produces gastric acid, and inhibit basal and stimulated acid production.
- Insignificant adverse effects with short-term treatment.
- Long-term use can increase the risk of fractures, pneumonia, acid rebound, and the possibility of developing *Clostridium difficile*.
- Rabeprazole and pantoprazole are enteric-coated tablets and should not be crushed.

CLIENT EDUCATION
- Do not to crush, chew, or break sustained-release capsules.
- Take omeprazole and lansoprazole once per day prior to eating the main meal of the day.
- Take rabeprazole after the morning meal.
- Take esomeprazole 1 hr before meals.
- Avoid alcohol and irritating medications (NSAIDs).
- Complete the prescribed regimen, even when manifestations subside.

Antacids

- Aluminum hydroxide and magnesium hydroxide neutralize acid in the gut. The medication provides relief of manifestations but generally does not accelerate healing.
- Antacids can be given seven times per day, 1 to 2 hr after meals and at bedtime, to neutralize gastric acid, which occurs with food ingestion.

NURSING ACTIONS
- Give 1 to 2 hr apart from other medications to avoid reducing the absorption of other medications.
- Monitor kidney function of clients taking aluminum hydroxide and magnesium hydroxide.

CLIENT EDUCATION
- The intended effect of the antacid is relief of pain and to promote healing of ulcers.
- Take other medications at least 1 to 2 hr before or after taking an antacid.
- Avoid the use of flavored antacids, which delay emptying of the stomach.

Mucosal protectants

- Sucralfate coats the ulcer and protects it from the actions of pepsin and acid.
- Bismuth subsalicylate prevents *H. pylori* from binding to the mucosal wall.
- Oral suspension is easier for the older adult clients to ingest because the tablet form is large and difficult to swallow.

NURSING ACTIONS
- Administer on an empty stomach 1 hr before meals and at bedtime.
- Monitor for adverse effect of constipation.

CLIENT EDUCATION
- If taking bismuth subsalicylate, avoid aspirin products to avoid salicylate overdose.
- Clients taking bismuth subsalicylate can have black stools. This is temporary and harmless.

THERAPEUTIC PROCEDURES

Esophagogastroduodenoscopy

Areas of bleeding can be treated with epinephrine or laser coagulation.

PREPROCEDURE NURSING ACTIONS: Ensure two large-bore IV catheters are initiated.

POSTPROCEDURE NURSING ACTIONS: Monitor vital signs. Keep client NPO until gag reflex returns.

Surgical interventions

Can be used in clients when ulcers do not heal following 12 to 16 weeks of medical treatment, hemorrhage, perforation, or obstruction

Gastrectomy: All or part of the stomach is removed with laparoscopic or open approach.
- **Antrectomy:** The antrum portion (lower portion of stomach) of the stomach is removed.
- **Gastrojejunostomy (Billroth II procedure):** The lower portion of the stomach is excised, the remaining stomach is anastomosed to the jejunum, and the remaining duodenum is surgically closed.

Vagotomy: The vagus nerve is cut to decrease gastric acid production in the stomach. Often done laparoscopically to reduce postoperative complications.

Pyloroplasty: The opening between the stomach and small intestine is enlarged to increase the rate of gastric emptying.

NURSING ACTIONS
- Monitor the incision for evidence of infection.
- Place the client in a semi-Fowler's position to facilitate lung expansion.
- Monitor NG tube drainage. Scant blood can be seen in the first 12 to 24 hr.
- Notify the provider before repositioning or irrigating the NG tube (disruption of sutures). Qs
- Monitor bowel sounds.
- Advance diet as tolerated to avoid undesired effects (abdominal distention, diarrhea).
- Administer medication (analgesics, stool softeners).

CLIENT EDUCATION
- Take vitamin and mineral supplements (vitamin B_{12}, vitamin D, calcium, iron, folate) due to decreased absorption after gastrectomy.
- Consume small, frequent meals while avoiding large quantities of carbohydrates as directed.

INTERPROFESSIONAL CARE

Nutrition consult: Diet that restricts acid-producing foods: milk products, caffeine, decaffeinated coffee, spicy foods, medications (NSAIDs)

COMPLICATIONS

Perforation/hemorrhage

When peptic ulcers perforate or bleed, it is an emergency situation.

- Perforation presents as severe epigastric pain spreading across the abdomen. The pain can radiate into the shoulders, especially the right shoulder due to irritation of the phrenic nerve. The abdomen can become tender and rigid (boardlike). Hyperactive to diminished bowel sounds can be auscultated, and there is rebound tenderness. The client will display manifestations of shock, hypotension, and tachycardia. Perforation is a surgical emergency.
- Gastrointestinal bleeding in the form of hematemesis or melena can cause manifestations of shock (hypotension, tachycardia, dizziness, confusion) and decreased hemoglobin.

NURSING ACTIONS

- Perform frequent data collection of pain and vital signs to detect subtle changes that can indicate perforation or bleeding. Qs
- Provide oxygen and ventilator support as needed.
- Ensure two large-bore IV lines for replacement of blood and fluids are initiated.
- Report findings, prepare the client for endoscopic or surgical intervention, assist with replacement of fluid and blood losses to maintain blood pressure, insert NG tube, and provide saline lavages.

Pernicious anemia

- Occurs due to a deficiency of the intrinsic factor normally secreted by the gastric mucosa.
- Manifestations include pallor, glossitis, fatigue, and paresthesias.

CLIENT EDUCATION: Lifelong monthly vitamin B_{12} injections will be necessary.

Dumping syndrome

This can occur following gastrectomy surgery and is a group of manifestations that occur following eating. A shift of fluid to the abdomen is triggered by rapid gastric emptying or high-carbohydrate ingestion. The rapid release of metabolic peptides following ingestion of a food bolus causes dumping syndrome.

- The client can report a full sensation, weakness, diaphoresis, palpitations, dizziness, and diarrhea. Vasomotor manifestations that can occur 10 to 90 min following a meal are pallor, perspiration, palpitations, headache, feeling of warmth, dizziness, and drowsiness.
- Late manifestations of dumping syndrome can be related to the rapid release of blood glucose, followed by an increase in insulin production resulting in hypoglycemia.

NURSING ACTIONS

- Monitor for vasomotor manifestations.
- Assist/instruct the client to lie down when vasomotor manifestations occur.
- Administer medications.
  - Octreotide subcutaneously can be prescribed if manifestations are severe and not effectively controlled with dietary measures. Octreotide blocks gastric and pancreatic hormones, which can lead to findings of dumping syndrome.
  - Acarbose slows the absorption of carbohydrates.
- Malnutrition and fluid electrolyte imbalances can occur due to altered absorption. Monitor I&O, laboratory values, and weight.

42.2 Vasomotor manifestations

	EARLY MANIFESTATIONS	LATE MANIFESTATIONS
ONSET	Within 30 min after eating	1.5 to 3 hr after eating
CAUSE	Rapid emptying	Excessive insulin release
MANIFESTATIONS	Nausea, vomiting, sweating, and dizziness Tachycardia Palpitations	Dizziness and sweating Tachycardia and palpitations Shakiness and feelings of anxiety Confusion

CLIENT EDUCATION

- Lying down after a meal slows the movement of food within the intestines.
- Limit the amount of fluid ingested at one time.
- Eliminate liquids with meals and for 1 hr prior to and following a meal.
- Consume a high-protein, high-fat, low-fiber, and low- to moderate-carbohydrate diet.
- Avoid milk and sugars (sweets, fruit juice, sweetened fruit, milkshakes, honey, syrup, jelly).
- Consume small, frequent meals rather than large meals.

Pyloric obstruction

- Pyloric obstruction occurs due to scarring, edema, or spasm of the area distal to the pyloric sphincter and prevents emptying of the stomach.
- Manifestations include feeling of fullness, distention, nausea after eating, and emesis consisting of undigested food.

NURSING ACTIONS

- Insert an NG tube for gastric decompression.
- Monitor fluid and electrolyte status.

Application Exercises

1. A nurse is collecting data from a client who has suspected stomach perforation due to a peptic ulcer. Which of the following findings should the nurse expect? (Select all that apply.)

   A. Rigid abdomen

   B. Tachycardia

   C. Elevated blood pressure

   D. Circumoral cyanosis

   E. Rebound tenderness

2. A nurse is reinforcing teaching with a client who has a new diagnosis of dumping syndrome following gastric surgery. Which of the following information should the nurse include?

   A. Eat three moderate-sized meals a day.

   B. Drink at least one glass of water with each meal.

   C. Eat a bedtime snack that contains a milk product.

   D. Increase protein in the diet.

3. A nurse is reinforcing discharge teaching with a client who has an infection due to *Helicobacter pylori (H. pylori)*. Which of the following statements by the client indicates understanding?

   A. "I will continue my prescription for corticosteroids."

   B. "I will schedule a CT scan to monitor improvement."

   C. "I will take a combination of medications for treatment."

   D. "I will have my throat swabbed to recheck for this bacteria."

4. A nurse is collecting data from a client who has a gastric ulcer. Which of the following findings should the nurse expect? (Select all that apply.)

   A. Client reports weight gain.

   B. Client states being awakened by pain during night.

   C. Client reports a sensation of bloating.

   D. Client states that pain occurs before meals.

   E. Client experiences pain upon palpation of the epigastric region.

5. A nurse is reinforcing teaching with a client who has a duodenal ulcer and a new prescription for esomeprazole. Which of the following information should the nurse include? (Select all that apply.)

   A. Take the medication 1 hr before a meal.

   B. Limit NSAIDs when taking this medication.

   C. Expect skin flushing when taking this medication.

   D. Increase fiber intake when taking this medication.

   E. Chew the medication thoroughly before swallowing.

PRACTICE Active Learning Scenario

A nurse is preparing a poster about peptic ulcer disease to be displayed at a community health fair. What information should the nurse include in the poster? Use the ATI Active Learning Template: System Disorder to complete this item.

ALTERATION IN HEALTH (DIAGNOSIS):
Include the types of ulcers.

HEALTH PROMOTION AND DISEASE PREVENTION:
Describe at least three prevention activities.

RISK FACTORS: Describe four risk factors for peptic ulcers.

Application Exercises Key

1. A. **CORRECT:** Manifestations of perforation include a rigid, board-like abdomen.

   B. **CORRECT:** Tachycardia occurs due to gastrointestinal bleeding that accompanies a perforation.

   C. Hypotension is an expected finding in a client who has a perforation and bleeding.

   D. Circumoral cyanosis is not a manifestation of perforation.

   E. **CORRECT:** Rebound tenderness is an expected finding in a client who has a perforation.

   (N) *NCLEX® Connection: Physiological Adaptation, Basic Pathophysiology*

2. A. The client should consume small, frequent meals.

   B. The client should eliminate liquids with meals and for 1 hr prior to and following meals.

   C. The client should avoid milk products.

   D. **CORRECT:** The client should eat a high-protein, high-fat, low-fiber, and moderate- to low-carbohydrate diet.

   (N) *NCLEX® Connection: Reduction of Risk Potential, Potential for Complications from Surgical Procedures and Health Alterations*

3. A. Corticosteroid use is a contributing factor to an infection caused by *H. pylori*.

   B. An esophagogastroduodenoscopy is done to evaluate for the presence of *H. pylori* and to evaluate effectiveness of treatment.

   C. **CORRECT:** A combination of antibiotics and a histamine₂ receptor antagonist is used to treat an infection caused by *H. pylori*.

   D. *H. pylori* is evaluated by obtaining gastric samples, not a throat swab.

   (N) *NCLEX® Connection: Pharmacological Therapies, Medication Administration*

4. A. A client who has a gastric ulcer is expected to report weight loss.

   B. Pain that awakens the client during the night is an expected finding of a duodenal ulcer.

   C. **CORRECT:** A client report of a bloating sensation is an expected finding.

   D. **CORRECT:** A client who has a gastric ulcer will often report pain before meals and at bedtime.

   E. **CORRECT:** Pain in the epigastric region upon palpation is an expected finding.

   (N) *NCLEX® Connection: Physiological Adaptation, Basic Pathophysiology*

5. A. **CORRECT:** The client is instructed to take the medication 1 hr before meals.

   B. **CORRECT:** The client is instructed to limit NSAIDs when on this medication.

   C. Skin flushing is not an adverse effect of this medication.

   D. Fiber intake does not need to be increased when taking this medication.

   E. The client is instructed to swallow the capsule whole. It should not be crushed or chewed.

   (N) *NCLEX® Connection: Pharmacological Therapies, Medication Administration*

PRACTICE Answer

Using the ATI Active Learning Template: System Disorder

ALTERATION IN HEALTH (DIAGNOSIS):
An erosion of the mucosal lining of the stomach or duodenum. Mucous membranes can become eroded to the point that the epithelium is exposed to gastric acid and pepsin, which can precipitate bleeding and perforation. Types of ulcers include gastric, duodenal, and stress ulcers.

HEALTH PROMOTION AND DISEASE PREVENTION
• Avoid excessive intake of alcohol.
• Stop smoking and use of tobacco products.
• Use stress management strategies.
• Avoid NSAIDs.
• Limit caffeine-containing beverages.
• Engage regularly in exercise

RISK FACTORS
• *Helicobacter pylori (H. pylori)*
• NSAID and corticosteroid use
• Smoking
• Severe stress
• Hypersecretory conditions
• Blood type O
• Excess alcohol ingestion
• Chronic pulmonary or kidney disease
• Zollinger-Ellison syndrome

(N) *NCLEX® Connection: Physiological Adaptation, Basic Pathophysiology*

CHAPTER 43 *Acute and Chronic Gastritis*

Cyclooxygenase (COX) is an enzyme that produces mucosal prostaglandins, decreases gastric acid, increases secretion of bicarbonate and cytoprotective mucus, and provides maintenance of submucosal blood flow to protect the gastric mucosa.

Gastritis is not a disease; it is an inflammation in the lining of the stomach, either erosive or nonerosive, and can be acute or chronic.

TYPES OF GASTRITIS

Nonerosive gastritis (acute or chronic) is most often caused by an infection, *Helicobacter pylori.* **(43.1)**

Erosive gastritis is likely caused by NSAIDs, alcohol use disorder, or recent radiation treatment.

Acute gastritis has sudden onset, is of short duration, and can result in gastric bleeding if severe. A severe form of acute gastritis is caused by the ingestion of an irritant (such as a strong acid or alkali) and can result in the development of gangrenous tissue or perforation. Scarring can result, leading to pyloric stenosis.

Chronic gastritis has a slow onset and can be related to autoimmune disease, such as pernicious anemia, and *H. pylori.*

Extensive gastric mucosal wall damage can cause **erosive gastritis (ulcers)** and increase the risk of stomach cancer.

HEALTH PROMOTION AND DISEASE PREVENTION

- Reduce anxiety related to gastritis.
- Follow a prescribed diet.
- Decrease or eliminate alcohol use.
- The client who has pernicious anemia will need vitamin B_{12} injections due to a decrease of the intrinsic factor by the stomach parietal cells.

- Watch for indications of GI bleeding.
- Follow the prescribed medication regimen.
- Eat small, frequent meals, avoiding foods and beverages that cause irritation.
- Report constipation, nausea, vomiting, or bloody stools.
- Stop smoking.
- Do not use cocaine.
- Receive education regarding corticosteroids and NSAIDs.

DATA COLLECTION

RISK FACTORS

- Family member who has *H. pylori* infection
- Family history of gastritis
- Prolonged use of NSAIDs, corticosteroids (stops prostaglandin synthesis)
- Excessive alcohol use
- Bile reflux disease
- Advanced age
- Radiation therapy
- Smoking
- Caffeine
- Cocaine use
- Excessive stress
- Exposure to contaminated food or water
- Chronic kidney disease, which causes an excessive buildup of urea leading to gastric irritation

BACTERIAL INFECTION: *Helicobacter pylori*, Salmonella, Streptococci, Staphylococci, or *Escherichia coli*

AUTOIMMUNE DISEASES: Systemic lupus, rheumatoid arthritis, pernicious anemia

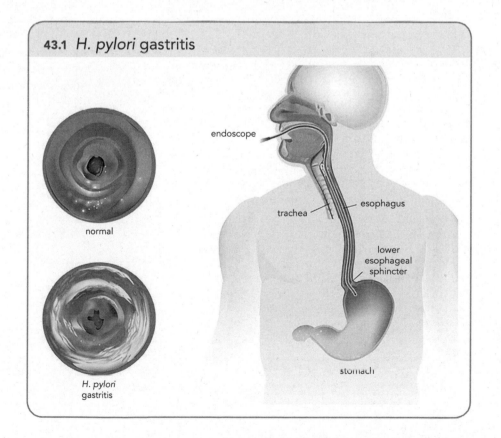

43.1 *H. pylori* gastritis

normal

H. pylori gastritis

endoscope

trachea

esophagus

lower esophageal sphincter

stomach

EXPECTED FINDINGS

PHYSICAL FINDINGS

- Dyspepsia, general abdominal discomfort, indigestion
- Diarrhea
- Headache
- Hiccups that can last for a few hours to several days
- Upper abdominal pain or burning can increase or decrease after eating
- Nausea and vomiting
- Reduced appetite and weight loss
- Abdominal bloating or distention
- Hematemesis (bloody emesis) and stools that test positive for occult blood

> Manifestations can have rapid onset with acute gastritis.
>
> Chronic gastritis can have a sudden massive hemorrhage from the stomach without other manifestations.

Erosive gastritis

- Black, tarry stools; coffee-ground emesis
- Acute abdominal pain

LABORATORY TESTS

Noninvasive tests

CBC to check for anemia

- Female clients: Hgb less than 12 g/dL and RBC less than 4.2 cells/mcL
- Male clients: Hgb less than 14 g/dL and RBC less than 4.7 cells/mcL

Serum and stool antibody/antigen test for presence of *H. pylori*

C13 urea breath test to measure *H. pylori*

DIAGNOSTIC PROCEDURES

Upper endoscopy

A small flexible scope is inserted through the mouth into the esophagus, stomach, and duodenum to visualize the upper digestive tract. This procedure allows for a biopsy, cauterization, removal of polyps, dilation, or diagnosis. (See **CHAPTER 39: GASTROINTESTINAL DIAGNOSTIC PROCEDURES**.)

CLIENT EDUCATION

- Maintain NPO status 6 to 8 hr prior to procedure.
- Have a ride home available after the procedure.
- A local anesthetic will be sprayed onto the back of the throat, but the throat can be sore following the procedure. **Qs**
- Monitor for indications of perforation (chest or abdominal pain, fever, nausea, vomiting, abdominal distention) and have emergency contact numbers available.

PATIENT-CENTERED CARE

NURSING CARE

- Monitor fluid intake and urine output.
- Ensure administration of IV fluids.
- Monitor electrolytes. (Diarrhea and vomiting can deplete electrolytes and cause dehydration.)
- Assist the client in identifying foods that are triggers.
- Provide small, frequent meals and encourage the client to eat slowly.
- Advise the client to avoid alcohol, caffeine, and foods that can cause gastric irritation.
- Assist the client in identifying ways to reduce stress.
- Monitor for indications of gastric bleeding (coffee-ground emesis; black, tarry stools).
- Monitor for findings of anemia (tachycardia, hypotension, fatigue, shortness of breath, pallor, lightheadedness, dizziness, chest pain).

MEDICATIONS

Histamine₂ antagonists

ACTION: Decreases gastric acid output by blocking gastric histamine₂ receptors

MEDICATIONS

- Nizatidine
- Famotidine
- Ranitidine
- Cimetidine

NURSING ACTIONS

- Wait 1 hr before or after to administer antacid. Antacids can decrease the effectiveness of H_2 receptor antagonists.
- Monitor for neutropenia and hypotension.

CLIENT EDUCATION

- Do not smoke or drink alcohol.
- Take oral dose with meals. Take famotidine 1 hr before meals to decrease heartburn, acid indigestion, and sour stomach.
- Wait 1 hr prior to or following H_2 receptor antagonist to take an antacid.
- Monitor for indications of GI bleeding (black stools, coffee-ground emesis).

Antacids

ACTION
- Increases gastric pH and neutralizes pepsin
- Improves mucosal protection

MEDICATIONS
- Aluminum hydroxide
- Magnesium hydroxide with aluminum hydroxide

NURSING ACTIONS
- Do not give to clients who have acute kidney injury or chronic kidney disease.
- Monitor aluminum antacids for aluminum toxicity and constipation. Monitor magnesium antacids for diarrhea or hypermagnesemia.

CLIENT EDUCATION
- Take antacids on an empty stomach.
- Wait 1 hr to take other medications.

Proton pump inhibitors

ACTION: Reduces gastric acid by stopping the hydrogen/potassium ATPase enzyme system in parietal cells, blocking acid production

MEDICATIONS
- Omeprazole
- Lansoprazole
- Rabeprazole sodium
- Pantoprazole
- Esomeprazole

CLIENT EDUCATION
- These medications can cause nausea, vomiting, and abdominal pain.
- Allow 60 min before eating when taking esomeprazole.
- Do not to crush or chew if any of the medications are enteric-coated or sustained-release.
- It can take up to 4 days to see the effects.
- Take medication with or without food according to instructions.

Prostaglandins

ACTION: Replacement for endogenous prostaglandins that stimulates mucosal protection. Reduces gastric acid secretion.

MEDICATIONS: Misoprostol

NURSING ACTIONS
- Can be given with NSAIDs to prevent gastric mucosal damage.
- Can cause abdominal pain and diarrhea.

CLIENT EDUCATION
- Use contraceptives.
- Do not take if there is a chance of becoming pregnant. Qs
- Take with food to reduce gastric effects.

Anti-ulcer/mucosal barriers

ACTION: Inhibits acid and forms a protective coating over mucosa

MEDICATIONS: Sucralfate

NURSING ACTIONS: Wait 30 min before or after to give antacid.

CLIENT EDUCATION
- Take on an empty stomach.
- Do not smoke or drink alcohol.
- Continue to take medication even if manifestations subside.

Antibiotics

ACTION: Eliminates *H. pylori* infection

MEDICATIONS
- Clarithromycin
- Amoxicillin
- Tetracycline
- Metronidazole

NURSING ACTIONS
- Monitor for increased abdominal pain and diarrhea.
- Monitor electrolytes and hydration if fluid is depleted.
- Administer with meals to decrease GI upset.
- Use cautiously in clients who have kidney or hepatic impairment.

CLIENT EDUCATION
- Complete the prescribed dosage.
- Notify the provider of persistent diarrhea, which can indicate superinfection of the bowel.

THERAPEUTIC PROCEDURES

Upper endoscopy: Surgery is prescribed for clients who have ulcerations or significant bleeding, or when nonsurgical interventions are ineffective. (See **CHAPTER 42: PEPTIC ULCER DISEASE.**)

Vagotomy or highly selective vagotomy: A highly selective vagotomy severs only the nerve fibers that control gastric acid secretion, and often is done laparoscopically to reduce postoperative complications. Pyloroplasty is usually done at the same time as the vagotomy.

Partial gastrectomy: Removal of the involved portion of the stomach.

INTERPROFESSIONAL CARE

- A nutritionist can assist in alterations to diet.
- Supportive care might be needed to reduce stress, increase exercise, and stop smoking. Qtc

COMPLICATIONS

Gastric bleeding

CAUSES
- Severe acute gastritis with deep tissue inflammation extending into the stomach muscle.
- In chronic erosive gastritis, bleeding can be slow or profuse as in a perforation of the stomach wall.

NURSING ACTIONS
- Monitor vital signs and airway.
- Care for the client receiving fluid replacement and blood products.
- Monitor CBC and clotting factors.
- Insert a nasogastric (NG) tube for gastric lavage as indicated. Irrigate with normal saline or water to stop active gastric bleed. Obtain an x-ray to confirm placement of NG tube prior to fluid instillation to prevent aspiration. Q_{EBP}
- Monitor NG tube for absence or presence of blood, monitor the amount of bleeding, and prevent gastric dilation.

CLIENT EDUCATION
- Monitor for indications of slow gastric bleeding (coffee-ground emesis; black, tarry stools).
- Seek immediate medical attention with severe abdominal pain or vomiting blood.
- Take medications as directed.

Gastric outlet obstruction

CAUSE: Severe acute gastritis with deep tissue inflammation extending into the stomach muscle

NURSING ACTIONS
- Monitor fluids and electrolytes because continuous vomiting results in loss of chloride (metabolic alkalosis) and severe fluid and electrolyte depletion.
- Provide care for clients receiving fluid and electrolyte replacement. Monitor I&O.
- Prepare to insert a NG tube to empty stomach contents.
- Prepare for a diagnostic endoscopy (NPO status for 6 hr, bowel prep or enema).

CLIENT EDUCATION: Seek medical attention for continuous vomiting, bloating, and nausea.

Dehydration

CAUSE: Loss of fluid due to vomiting or diarrhea

NURSING ACTIONS
- Monitor fluid intake and urine output.
- Ensure the administration of IV fluids if needed.
- Monitor electrolytes.

CLIENT EDUCATION: Contact a provider for vomiting and diarrhea.

Pernicious anemia

CAUSES
- Chronic gastritis can damage the parietal cells. This can lead to reduced production of intrinsic factor, which is necessary for the absorption of vitamin B_{12}.
- Insufficient vitamin B_{12} can lead to pernicious anemia.

NURSING ACTIONS: Monthly vitamin B_{12} injections are needed.

Dumping syndrome

CAUSES: The rapid release of metabolic peptides following the ingestion of a food bolus.

MANIFESTATIONS
- Early manifestations include feeling of fullness, weakness, dizziness, palpitations, sweating, abdominal cramping, and diarrhea.
- Manifestations resolve after having a bowel movement. However, late or residual vasomotor manifestations can occur 10 min to 3 hr after eating.

CLIENT EDUCATION
- Lay down following meals to slow movement of food through intestine and prevent injury. Q_s
- Eat a high-protein, high-fat, low- to moderate-carbohydrate diet
- Eat small meals and limit taking liquids with meals.
- Self-administer octreotide by subcutaneous injection two to three times daily before meals.

Application Exercises

1. A nurse is reinforcing teaching about pernicious anemia with a client who has chronic gastritis. Which of the following information should the nurse include in the teaching?

   A. Pernicious anemia is caused when the cells producing gastric acid are damaged.

   B. Expect a monthly injection of vitamin B_{12}.

   C. Plan to take vitamin K supplements.

   D. Pernicious anemia is caused by an increased production of intrinsic factor.

2. A nurse is reinforcing discharge teaching with a client who has a new prescription for aluminum hydroxide. Which of the following information should the nurse include?

   A. Take the medication with food.

   B. Monitor for diarrhea.

   C. Wait 1 hr before taking other oral medications.

   D. Maintain a low-fiber diet.

3. A nurse is assisting with the plan care for a client who has acute gastritis. Which of the following nursing actions should the nurse recommend for the plan of care? (Select all that apply.)

   A. Evaluate I&O.

   B. Monitor electrolytes.

   C. Provide three large meals per day.

   D. Administer ibuprofen for pain.

   E. Observe stool characteristics.

4. A nurse is reinforcing teaching with a client who has a new prescription for famotidine. Which of the following statements by the client indicates understanding?

   A. "The medicine coats the lining of my stomach."

   B. "The medication should stop the pain right away."

   C. "I will take my pill 1 hr before meals."

   D. "I will monitor for bleeding from my nose."

5. A nurse is reinforcing teaching with a client who has chronic gastritis and is scheduled for a selective vagotomy. Which of the following statements should the nurse include about the purpose of the procedure?

   A. "You will have increased duodenal gastric emptying."

   B. "You will have a reduction of gastric acid secretions."

   C. "You will have an increase of gastric mucus secretion."

   D. "You will have an increased secretion of hydrogen/potassium ATPase enzymes."

PRACTICE Active Learning Scenario

A nurse is reinforcing teaching about acute and chronic gastritis with a client. Which of the following information should the nurse include? Use the ATI Active Learning Template: System Disorder to complete this item.

ALTERATION IN HEALTH (DIAGNOSIS)
- Describe gastritis.
- Compare and contrast acute vs. chronic gastritis.

PATHOPHYSIOLOGY RELATED TO CLIENT PROBLEM:
Describe as related to the client problem.

RISK FACTORS: Describe six.

1. A. Chronic gastritis damages parietal cells, resulting in decreased production of intrinsic factor rather than gastric acid.

    B. **CORRECT:** The client will receive a monthly injection of vitamin B$_{12}$ to treat pernicious anemia due to a decrease of the intrinsic factor by the stomach parietal cells.

    C. Vitamin K supplements are given to clients who have a bleeding disorder.

    D. Parietal cell damage results in insufficient production of intrinsic factor by the stomach parietal cells.

    Ⓝ *NCLEX® Connection: Physiological Adaptation, Alterations in Body Systems*

2. A. The nurse should advise the client to take aluminum hydroxide on an empty stomach.

    B. Aluminum hydroxide can cause constipation.

    C. **CORRECT:** The nurse should advise the client not to take oral medications within 1 hr of an antacid.

    D. The client should increase dietary fiber due to the constipating effect of the medication.

    Ⓝ *NCLEX® Connection: Pharmacological Therapies, Medication Administration*

3. A. **CORRECT:** The nurse should evaluate the client's I&O to prevent electrolyte loss and dehydration.

    B. **CORRECT:** The nurse should monitor the client's electrolyte laboratory values to prevent fluid loss and dehydration.

    C. The nurse should instruct the client to eat small, frequent meals.

    D. The nurse should instruct the client to avoid taking ibuprofen, an NSAID, because of its erosive capabilities.

    E. **CORRECT:** The nurse should instruct the client to report to the provider any indication of the presence of blood in the stools, which can indicate gastrointestinal bleeding.

    Ⓝ *NCLEX® Connection: Physiological Adaptation, Alterations in Body Systems*

4. A. Famotidine decreases gastric acid output. It does not have a protective coating action.

    B. The client might need to take famotidine for several days before pain relief occurs when starting this therapy.

    C. **CORRECT:** The client should take famotidine 1 hr before meals to decrease heartburn, acid indigestion, and sour stomach.

    D. The nurse should instruct the client to monitor for GI bleeding when taking famotidine.

    Ⓝ *NCLEX® Connection: Pharmacological Therapies, Medication Administration*

5. A. Pyloroplasty increases gastric emptying and is performed to widen the opening from the stomach to the duodenum.

    B. **CORRECT:** Selective vagotomy will reduce gastric acid secretions.

    C. Prostaglandin analog medication will stimulate mucosal protection and decrease gastric acid secretions.

    D. A histamine$_2$ antagonist medication will inhibit gastric secretion by inhibiting hydrogen/potassium ATPase enzyme system in the gastric parietal cells.

    Ⓝ *NCLEX® Connection: Reduction of Risk Potential, Diagnostic Tests*

PRACTICE Answer

Using the ATI Active Learning Template: System Disorder

ALTERATION IN HEALTH (DIAGNOSIS): Gastritis is an inflammation of the lining of the stomach as a result of irritation to the mucosa.

- Acute: Sudden onset, short duration, can result in gastric bleeding if severe
- Chronic: Slow onset; when profuse, can damage parietal cells, resulting in pernicious anemia

PATHOPHYSIOLOGY RELATED TO CLIENT PROBLEM: Gastric acid overwhelms the production of COX11 enzymes, which provide mucosal prostaglandins that line the stomach. This results in an erosion of the mucosa and increases the risk for ulcers and stomach cancer.

RISK FACTORS

- Bacterial infection (*H. pylori*, Salmonella, Streptococci, Staphylococci, *E. coli*)
- Family history of *H. pylori* or gastritis
- Prolonged use of NSAIDs or corticosteroids
- Excessive alcohol use
- Bile reflux disease
- Autoimmune diseases
- Advanced age
- Radiation therapy
- Smoking
- Caffeine
- Cocaine use
- Excessive stress
- Exposure to contaminated food or water
- Chronic kidney disease causing gastric irritation from buildup of urea

Ⓝ *NCLEX® Connection: Physiological Adaptation, Alterations in Body Systems*

CHAPTER 44 *Noninflammatory Bowel Disorders*

Noninflammatory bowel disorders can cause pain, changes in bowel pattern, bleeding, and malabsorption. This group of disorders includes hemorrhoids, cancer, hernia, irritable bowel syndrome (IBS), and intestinal obstruction.

Hemorrhoids are distended or edematous intestinal veins resulting from increased intra-abdominal pressure (straining, obesity, prolonged sitting or standing, constipation, weight lifting). Pregnancy increases the risk of hemorrhoids.

Cancer of the small or large intestine can be caused by age-related changes (older than 50 is a greater risk), genetic influence, or chronic bowel disease (Crohn's disease, ulcerative colitis).

Hernia

Bowel herniation is the displacement of the bowel through a weakness of the abdominal muscle into other areas of the abdominal cavity. (44.1)

Incisional hernias can occur as a postsurgical complication due to inadequate healing of the incisional site from malnutrition, infection, or obesity.

A hernia that cannot be moved back into place with gentle palpation is considered irreducible and requires immediate surgical evaluation.

In a hernia that is strangulated, blood supply is cut off to a portion of the bowel, increasing the risk for obstruction, necrosis, and perforation. Findings include abdominal distention, tachycardia, vomiting, and abdominal pain. Surgical intervention is necessary.

DATA COLLECTION

RISK FACTORS

- Male clients (indirect inguinal hernia can be large and descend into the scrotum)
- Older adults (direct hernia) ©
- Increased intra-abdominal pressure due to pregnancy or obesity (femoral, adult-acquired umbilical hernia)
- Genetics (congenital umbilical hernia)

EXPECTED FINDINGS

- Protrusion or lump at involved site (groin area, umbilicus, healed incision)
- Pain if peritoneum becomes irritated

44.1 Hernia

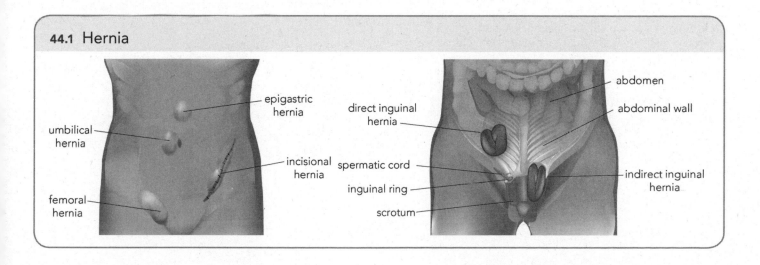

umbilical hernia
epigastric hernia
incisional hernia
femoral hernia

direct inguinal hernia
spermatic cord
inguinal ring
scrotum
abdomen
abdominal wall
indirect inguinal hernia

PATIENT-CENTERED CARE

CLIENT EDUCATION: If the hernia does not require surgery, wear a truss pad with hernia belt during waking hours to prevent the abdominal contents from bulging into the hernia sac. Inspect skin under the pad daily.

POSTOPERATIVE CLIENT EDUCATION
(HERNIORRHAPHY OR HERNIOPLASTY)

- Avoid increased intra-abdominal pressure for 2 to 3 weeks (avoid coughing, straining, and lifting objects greater than 10 lb).
- Apply ice as prescribed and inspect and report redness or swelling at the incisional site.
- Prevent constipation by increasing dietary fiber and fluids.
- Rest for several days and return to work when recommended by the surgeon, usually 1 to 2 weeks postoperatively.

Irritable bowel syndrome

IBS is a disorder of the gastrointestinal system that causes changes in bowel function (chronic diarrhea, constipation, bloating, abdominal pain). IBS can occur after a bowel infection related to changes in the cells and normal flora in the GI tract.

- The etiology of IBS is uncertain, but it is thought that environmental, immunological, genetic, hormonal, and stress influence the development and course of the disease. Food intolerances worsen the manifestations.
- **Environmental factors:** Dairy products, caffeinated beverages, infectious agents
- **Immunological factors:** Cytokine genes (pro-inflammatory interleukins), tumor necrosis factor alpha
- **Stress-related factors:** Anxiety, depression

HEALTH PROMOTION AND DISEASE PREVENTION

- Avoid foods that trigger exacerbation (dairy, wheat, corn, fried foods, alcohol, spicy foods, aspartame).
- Avoid beverages that contain caffeine, alcohol, fructose, or sorbitol.
- Consume 2 to 3 L fluid per day from food and fluid sources.
- Increase fiber intake (approximately 30 to 40 g/day).
- Decrease stress.

DATA COLLECTION

RISK FACTORS

- Female clients
- Stress
- Eating large meals containing a large amount of fat
- Caffeine intake
- Alcohol intake

EXPECTED FINDINGS

- Cramping pain in abdomen
- Abdominal pain (left lower quadrant) due to changes in bowel pattern and consistency
- Flatus
- Nausea with meals or passing stool
- Anorexia
- Abdominal bloating
- Belching
- Diarrhea (diarrhea-predominant IBS)
- Constipation (constipation-predominant IBS)
- Hyperactive or hypoactive bowel sounds

LABORATORY TESTS

CBC, serum albumin, erythrocyte sedimentation rate, and occult stools are typically within the expected reference range.

DIAGNOSTIC TESTS

- IBS is difficult to diagnose with specific tests and is usually based on the presence of specific characteristics, including abdominal pain accompanied by changes in bowel patterns, abdominal distention, feeling that defecation is not complete, and mucus with stools.
- Other criteria can include recurrent abdominal pain for 3 days during a month in the past 3 months, and two or more of the following.
  - Improvement when the client moves bowels
  - Onset when there is a change in frequency of stools
  - Onset when there is a change in appearance of stools

Hydrogen breath test

The client is asked to exhale into a hydrogen analyzer before and after ingesting test sugar. Positive test results indicate excess hydrogen in the bloodstream from bacterial overgrowth or malabsorption.

CLIENT EDUCATION: Remain NPO at least 12 hr prior to test, except for sips of water.

PATIENT-CENTERED CARE

NURSING CARE

- Review strategies to reduce stress.
- Instruct the client to limit the intake of irritating agents (gas-forming foods, caffeine, alcohol).
- Encourage a diet high in fiber and fluids.
- Instruct clients to keep a food diary to record intake and bowel patterns (to adjust diet to prevent exacerbations).

MEDICATIONS

Diarrhea-predominant IBS (IBS-D)

Loperamide
- Decreases peristalsis and increases bulk.
- Can cause drowsiness.
- Discontinue if no response after 48 hr.

Psyllium
- Bulk-forming laxative.
- Discontinue for abdominal cramping, rectal bleeding, and vomiting.
- Monitor for electrolyte imbalance.

Alosetron
- An IBS-specific medication that selectively blocks 5-HT3 receptors that innervate the viscera. The expected result is increased firmness in stools, and decreased urgency and frequency of defecation.
- Indicated for IBS-D in female clients that has lasted more than 6 months and is resistant to conventional management. Use with caution in female clients and only as a last resort.
- Contraindicated for clients who have a history of bowel obstruction, Crohn's disease, ulcerative colitis, impaired intestinal circulation, or thrombophlebitis.

CLIENT EDUCATION
- Manifestations should resolve within 1 to 4 weeks. Discontinue medication after 4 weeks if manifestations persist.
- Avoid concurrent use of psychoactive drugs and antihistamines.
- Report constipation, fever, increasing abdominal pain, fatigue, dark urine, bloody urine, or rectal bleeding immediately because alosetron can cause ischemic colitis. Discontinue medication if these manifestations occur. Qs

Constipation-predominant IBS (IBS-C)

Lubiprostone: An IBS-specific medication that increases fluid secretion in the intestine to promote intestinal motility. This is indicated for IBS-C in female clients.
- Contraindicated for clients who have known or possible bowel obstruction.
- Not effective for treatment of men who have IBS.
- CLIENT EDUCATION: Take with food and water.

Linaclotide
- Increases fluid and motility in the intestine
- Can relieve pain and cramps
- CLIENT EDUCATION: Take daily about 30 min before breakfast.

Intestinal obstruction

Intestinal obstruction can have mechanical or nonmechanical causes. Manifestations vary by type.
- Mechanical obstruction occurs when the bowel is blocked by something outside or inside the intestines (adhesions, tumors, hernias, fecal impactions, strictures due to Crohn's disease, diverticulitis). Complete mechanical obstructions should be addressed surgically.
- Nonmechanical obstructions are caused by diminished peristalsis within the bowel (paralytic ileus). This can occur postoperatively due to the handling of the intestines during surgery.
- Treatment focuses on fluid and electrolyte balance, decompressing the bowel, and relief/removal of the obstruction.

DATA COLLECTION

RISK FACTORS

Mechanical obstructions

- Encirclement or compression of intestine by adhesions, tumors, fibrosis (endometriosis), or strictures (Crohn's disease, radiation)
  - Postsurgical adhesions are often the cause of small bowel obstructions.
  - Carcinomas are often the cause of large intestine obstructions.
  - OLDER ADULT CLIENTS: Diverticulitis, fecal impaction, and tumors are common causes of obstruction. Bowel regimens can be effective in preventing impactions. Ⓖ
- Hernia (bowel becomes trapped in weakened area of abdominal wall)
- Volvulus (twisting) or intussusception (telescoping) of bowel segments **(44.2, 44.3)**

Nonmechanical obstructions

- Nonmechanical obstructions (paralytic ileus) result from decreased or absence of peristalsis secondary to the following.
  - Neurogenic disorders (manipulation of the bowel during major surgery and spinal fracture)
  - Vascular disorders (vascular insufficiency and mesenteric emboli)
  - Electrolyte imbalances (hypokalemia)
  - Inflammatory responses (peritonitis or sepsis)
- Manifestations of nonmechanical obstructions include diffuse, constant pain; significant abdominal distention; and frequent vomiting.

44.2 Bowel intussusception

colon

intussusceptum

ileum

cecum

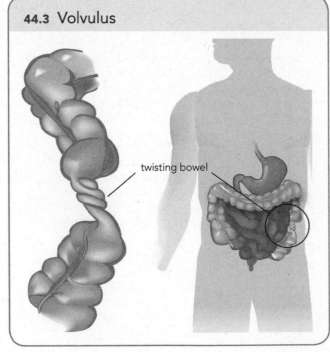

44.3 Volvulus

twisting bowel

EXPECTED FINDINGS

Manifestations vary depending on the location of the obstruction.

Small bowel and large intestine obstructions

- Obstipation: the inability to pass a stool or flatus for more than 8 hr despite feeling the urge to defecate
- Abdominal distention
- High-pitched bowel sounds above site of obstruction (borborygmi) with hypoactive bowel sounds below, or overall hypoactive; absent bowel sounds later in process

Small bowel obstructions

- Severe fluid and electrolyte imbalance
- Metabolic alkalosis
- Visible peristaltic waves (possible)
- Epigastric or upper abdominal distention
- Abdominal pain, discomfort
- Profuse, sudden projectile vomiting with fecal odor
- Rapid dehydration
- High-pitched bowel sounds above the point of obstruction
- No bowel sounds heard below the obstruction

Large intestine obstructions

- Minor fluid and electrolyte imbalance
- Gradual onset
- Metabolic acidosis (possible)
- Significant lower abdominal distention
- Intermittent abdominal cramping with peristaltic waves
- Infrequent vomiting (fecal odor to emesis can indicate a complete intestinal obstruction).
- Diarrhea or ribbon-like stools around an impaction

LABORATORY TESTS

- Increased hemoglobin, BUN, creatinine, and hematocrit can indicate dehydration.
- Increased serum amylase and WBC count can occur with strangulating obstructions.
- Arterial blood gases (ABGs) indicate metabolic imbalance, depending on obstruction type.
- Chemistry profiles reveal decreased sodium, chloride, and potassium.

DIAGNOSTIC PROCEDURES

X-ray: Flat plate and upright abdominal x-rays evaluate the presence of free air and gas patterns. **(44.4)**

Endoscopy determines the cause of obstruction.

CT scan determines the cause and exact location of the obstruction.

PATIENT-CENTERED CARE

NURSING CARE

Nonmechanical cause of obstruction

- NPO with bowel rest.
- Check bowel sounds.
- Provide oral hygiene.
- Care for the client receiving IV fluid and electrolyte replacement (particularly potassium).
- Manage pain (once diagnosis is identified).
- Encourage ambulation.
- Place in semi–Fowler's position.

Mechanical cause of obstruction

- Prepare for surgery and provide preoperative nursing care.
- Withhold intake until peristalsis resumes.

MEDICATIONS

Prokinetics to promote gastric motility (octreotide) in paralytic ileus or partial obstruction.

Broad-spectrum antibiotics, especially with suspected bowel strangulation.

THERAPEUTIC PROCEDURES

Nasogastric (NG) tube with a vent (to prevent damage to the stomach mucosa during continuous suctioning) is inserted to decompress the bowel. Qᴇʙᴘ

NURSING ACTIONS
- Maintain intermittent suction.
- Monitor NG tube patency and placement. Irrigate every 4 hr, or as prescribed.
- Monitor and measure gastric output.
- Monitor nasal area for skin breakdown.
- Provide oral hygiene every 2 hr.
- Monitor vital signs, skin integrity, weight, and I&O.

Surgical interventions

Procedure varies based on cause of obstruction. Can include lysis of adhesions, colon resection, colostomy creation (temporary or permanent), embolectomy, thrombectomy, resection of gangrenous intestinal tissue, or complete colectomy.

Exploratory laparotomy to determine the cause of obstruction and rectify if possible

NURSING ACTIONS
- Ensure the client understands the type of procedure (open or laparoscopic).
- Monitor for hemodynamic instability.
- Ensure the administration of IV fluid replacement and maintenance.

- Monitor bowel sounds.
- Maintain NG tube patency and measure output.
- Clamp NG tube to check the client's tolerance prior to removal.
- Advance diet as tolerated when prescribed, beginning with clear liquids. Clamp tube after eating for 1 to 2 hr.

CLIENT EDUCATION: Report intolerance of intake following NG tube removal (nausea, vomiting, increasing distention).

COMPLICATIONS

Dehydration (small bowel obstruction)

CAUSE: Persistent vomiting

NURSING ACTIONS
- Monitor hydration through evaluation of hematocrit, BUN, orthostatic vital signs, skin turgor/mucous membranes, urine output, and specific gravity. Notify the provider of a fluid imbalance.
- Care for the client receiving IV fluids.

Electrolyte imbalance (small bowel obstruction)

CAUSE: Persistent vomiting

NURSING ACTIONS
- Monitor electrolytes, especially potassium levels. Qs
- Notify the provider of an electrolyte imbalance.
- Care for the client receiving IV fluids to replace electrolytes.

44.4 Radiograph of abdominal obstruction

Metabolic alkalosis (small intestinal obstruction)

CAUSE: Persistent vomiting, leading to a loss of gastric hydrochloride

NURSING ACTIONS
- Monitor for hypoventilation (confusion, hypercarbia), which is a compensatory action by the lungs.
- Review arterial blood gas findings and notify the provider of unexpected laboratory findings.
- Monitor the client receiving fluid and electrolytes.
- Provide oral hygiene to alleviate increased thirst response. Thirst response is decreased in older adults. Provide oral hygiene routinely to ensure maintenance of moist mucous membranes. Ⓒ

Metabolic acidosis (large bowel obstructions)

CAUSE: A lower level obstruction

NURSING ACTIONS
- Monitor for deep, rapid respirations (compensatory action by the lungs), confusion, hypotension, and flushed skin.
- Review arterial blood gas findings and notify the provider of unexpected laboratory findings.

Application Exercises

1. A nurse is reviewing the medical record of a client who has a small bowel obstruction. Which of the following findings should the nurse report to the provider? (Select all that apply.)

   A. Emesis prior to insertion of the nasogastric tube

   B. Urine specific gravity 1.040

   C. Hematocrit 60%

   D. Serum potassium 3.0 mEq/L

   E. WBC 10,000/uL

2. A nurse is contributing to the plan of care for a client who has a small bowel instruction and a nasogastric (NG) tube in place. Which of the following interventions should the nurse recommend for the plan of care? (Select all that apply.)

   A. Document the NG drainage with the client's output.

   B. Irrigate the NG tube every 8 hr.

   C. Check bowel sounds.

   D. Provide oral hygiene every 2 hr.

   E. Monitor NG tube for placement.

3. A nurse is caring for a client who has a small bowel obstruction from adhesions. Which of the following findings should the nurse expect? (Select all that apply.)

   A. Emesis greater than 500 mL with a fecal odor

   B. Report of spasmodic abdominal pain

   C. High-pitched bowel sounds

   D. Abdomen flat with rebound tenderness to palpation

   E. Laboratory findings indicating metabolic acidosis

4. A nurse is collecting data from an older adult client. The nurse should identify which of the following findings as a manifestation of an obstruction of the large intestine due to a fecal impaction?

   A. The client reports he had a bowel movement yesterday.

   B. The client is having small, frequent liquid stools.

   C. The client is flatulent.

   D. The client indicates he vomited once this morning.

5. A nurse is reinforcing discharge teaching with a client who has irritable bowel syndrome (IBS). Which of the following instructions should the nurse include?

   A. Avoid foods that trigger exacerbation.

   B. Consume 15 to 20 g of fiber daily.

   C. Plan three moderate to large meals per day.

   D. Limit fluid intake to 1 L each day.

PRACTICE Active Learning Scenario

A nurse is preparing a poster on caring for clients who have a bowel obstruction. What information should the nurse include on the poster? Use the ATI Active Learning Template: System Disorder to complete this item.

RISK FACTORS: Identify at least two for each form of obstruction.

EXPECTED FINDINGS: Compare and contrast the types of obstructions.

DIAGNOSTIC PROCEDURES: Identify at least two.

Application Exercises Key

1. A. Profuse emesis is an expected finding for a client who has a small bowel obstruction.

   B. **CORRECT:** This urine specific gravity is greater than the expected reference range. An increased urine specific gravity is an indication of dehydration.

   C. **CORRECT:** The Hct is greater than the expected reference range. An elevated Hct indicates hemoconcentration, which is due to dehydration.

   D. **CORRECT:** This serum potassium is less than the expected reference range caused by potassium loss from vomiting. Hypokalemia can cause dysrhythmias, muscle weakness, and lethargy, and requires potassium replacement.

   E. This WBC is within the expected reference range.

   Ⓝ *NCLEX® Connection: Physiological Adaptation, Alterations in Body Systems*

2. A. **CORRECT:** The nurse should document the NG drainage as output. This helps determine the amount of fluid replacement needed.

   B. The NG tube is irrigated every 4 hr to maintain patency.

   C. **CORRECT:** Bowel sounds should be checked to evaluate treatment and resolution of the obstruction.

   D. **CORRECT:** An NG tube promotes mouth breathing. The nurse should provide frequent oral hygiene to provide comfort.

   E. **CORRECT:** The nurse should check the placement of the NG tube prior to irrigation to prevent aspiration and periodically to prevent an increase in abdominal distention.

   Ⓝ *NCLEX® Connection: Reduction of Risk Potential, Potential for Complications of Diagnostic Tests/Treatments/Procedures*

3. A. **CORRECT:** Large amount of emesis with a fecal odor is an expected finding in a client who has a small bowel obstruction.

   B. **CORRECT:** Report of abdominal pain is an expected finding in a client who has a small bowel obstruction.

   C. **CORRECT:** High-pitched bowel sounds are an expected finding of a small or large bowel obstruction.

   D. Abdominal distention is an expected finding in a client who has a small bowel obstruction.

   E. Metabolic alkalosis due to the loss of gastric acid is an expected finding in a client who has a small bowel obstruction.

   Ⓝ *NCLEX® Connection: Physiological Adaptation, Basic Pathophysiology*

4. A. A report of a bowel movement yesterday does not indicate a mechanical obstruction of the large intestine due to a fecal impaction.

   B. **CORRECT:** Small, frequent liquid stools can be passed around a fecal impaction. Other manifestations include constipation and rectal pain.

   C. The presence of flatus does not indicate a mechanical obstruction of the large intestine due to a fecal impaction.

   D. A report of a single episode of vomiting does not indicate a mechanical obstruction of the large intestine due to a fecal impaction. Frequent vomiting is a manifestation of a small-bowel obstruction.

   Ⓝ *NCLEX® Connection: Physiological Adaptation, Basic Pathophysiology*

5. A. **CORRECT:** The client should eliminate foods that trigger exacerbation.

   B. A client who has IBS should increase daily fiber intake to 30 to 40 g.

   C. A client who has IBS should eat small frequent meals.

   D. A client who has IBS should drink 2 to 3 L of fluids per day to promote a consistent bowel pattern.

   Ⓝ *NCLEX® Connection: Physiological Adaptation, Alterations in Body Systems*

PRACTICE Answer

Using the ATI Active Learning Template: System Disorder

RISK FACTORS
- Mechanical
  - Encirclement or compression of intestines by adhesions, tumors, fibrosis, or strictures
  - Volvulus, intussusception
  - Hernia, fecal impaction
  - Small bowel: postsurgical adhesions
  - Large bowel: carcinoma
- Nonmechanical: decreased or absence of peristalsis due to the following
  - Neurogenic (manipulation of the bowel during major surgery) or vascular (mesenteric emboli) disorders
  - Electrolyte imbalances (hypokalemia) and inflammatory responses (peritonitis or sepsis)

EXPECTED FINDINGS
- Mechanical: mild, colicky, intermittent pain
- Nonmechanical: vague, diffuse, constant pain; significant abdominal distention
  - Small bowel obstruction
    - Visible peristaltic waves possible
    - Profuse, sudden projectile vomiting with fecal odor, which relieves pain
    - Severe fluid and electrolyte imbalance, metabolic alkalosis
  - Large bowel obstruction
    - Significant abdominal distention, infrequent vomiting, diarrhea or "ribbon-like" stools around an impaction, minor fluid and electrolyte imbalance, metabolic acidosis (possible)
    - Bowel sounds: hyperactive above and hypoactive below the obstruction, inability to pass a stool, or flatus for more than 8 hr despite urge to defecate

DIAGNOSTIC PROCEDURES
- X-rays (flat plate, upright abdominal)
- Endoscopy
- CT scan

Ⓝ *NCLEX® Connection: Physiological Adaptation, Basic Pathophysiology*

CHAPTER 45 Inflammatory Bowel Disease

Inflammatory bowel disease (IBD) can affect structures or segments along the gastrointestinal (GI) tract. IBD includes both acute and chronic disorders.

Acute and chronic IBD can result in nutritional deficits, altered bowel elimination, infection, pain, and fluid or electrolyte imbalances. The nurse needs to be knowledgeable about acute and chronic IBD to collaborate with the client and interprofessional team in treating and managing these disorders.

ACUTE INFLAMMATORY BOWEL DISEASE

Appendicitis

Inflammation of the appendix. Refer to the **NURSING CARE OF CHILDREN REVIEW MODULE, CHAPTER 22: GASTROINTESTINAL STRUCTURAL AND INFLAMMATORY DISORDERS**.
- Caused by an obstruction of the lumen or opening of the appendix.
- Fecaliths (hard pieces of stool) can be the initial cause of the obstruction.
- Adolescents and young adults are at increased risk.

Peritonitis

Inflammation of the peritoneum
- Results from infection of the peritoneum due to puncture (surgery or trauma), septicemia, or rupture of part of the gastrointestinal tract.
- This can lead to septicemia and is a life-threatening event.

Gastroenteritis

Inflammation of the stomach and small intestine
- Triggered by infection (bacterial, parasitic, viral)
- Vomiting and frequent, watery stools place the client at increased risk for fluid and electrolyte imbalance and impaired nutrition.

CHRONIC INFLAMMATORY BOWEL DISEASE

Ulcerative colitis and Crohn's disease are characterized by frequent stools, crampy abdominal pain, exacerbations, and remissions.

Ulcerative colitis

Edema and inflammation primarily in the rectum and rectosigmoid colon.
- In severe cases, it can involve the entire length of the colon. Mucosa and submucosa become hyperemic (increase in blood flow), and the colon becomes edematous and reddened. It can lead to abscess formation.
- Edema and thickened bowel mucosa can cause partial bowel obstruction. Intestinal mucosal cell changes can lead to colon cancer or insufficient production of intrinsic factor, resulting in insufficient absorption of vitamin B_{12} (pernicious anemia).
- Classified as mild, moderate, severe, or fulminant.

Crohn's disease

Inflammation and ulceration of the GI tract, often at the distal ileum.
- All bowel layers can become involved. Lesions are sporadic. Fistulas are common.
- Can involve the entire GI tract from the mouth to the anus.
- Malabsorption and malnutrition can develop when the jejunum and ileum become involved. Requires supplemental vitamins and minerals, possibly including vitamin B_{12} injections.

Diverticulitis

Inflammation and infection of the bowel mucosa caused by bacteria, food, or fecal matter trapped in one or more diverticula (pouch-like herniations in the intestinal wall)
- Not to be confused with diverticulosis, which is the presence of many small diverticula in the colon without inflammation.
- Not all clients who have diverticulosis develop diverticulitis.
- Diverticula can perforate and cause peritonitis, and or severe bleeding.

DATA COLLECTION

Etiology of ulcerative colitis and Crohn's disease is unknown but possibly due to a combination of genetic, environmental, and immunological causes.

RISK FACTORS

More prevalent in Caucasian (ulcerative colitis), Jewish (ulcerative colitis, Crohn's disease), and African American populations (diverticular disease)

Genetics: Ulcerative colitis and Crohn's disease

Sex and age: The incidence of ulcerative colitis peaks at adolescence to young adulthood (more often in females) and older adulthood (more often in males). Crohn's disease usually develops in adolescents and young adults, but can occur at any age. Diverticulitis occurs more often in older adults and affects males more frequently than females. ©

Tobacco use: Crohn's disease

EXPECTED FINDINGS

Ulcerative colitis

- Abdominal pain/cramping: often left-lower quadrant pain
- Anorexia and weight loss

PHYSICAL FINDINGS
- Fever
- Diarrhea: up to 20 liquid stools per day
- Stools can contain mucus, blood, or pus.
- Abdominal distention, tenderness, or firmness upon palpation
- High-pitched bowel sounds
- Rectal bleeding

Crohn's disease

- Abdominal pain/cramping: often right-lower quadrant pain
- Anorexia and weight loss

PHYSICAL FINDINGS
- Fever
- Diarrhea: five loose stools per day with mucus or pus
- Abdominal distention, tenderness, or firmness upon palpation
- High-pitched bowel sounds
- Steatorrhea

Diverticulitis

- Acute onset of abdominal pain often in left-lower quadrant
- Nausea and vomiting

PHYSICAL FINDINGS
- Fever
- Chills
- Tachycardia

LABORATORY TESTS

Ulcerative colitis

Hematocrit and hemoglobin: Decreased

Erythrocyte sedimentation rate (ESR): Increased

WBC: Increased

C-reactive protein: Increased

Serum albumin: Decreased

Stool for occult blood: Can be positive

K+, Mg, and Ca: Decreased

Crohn's disease

Hematocrit and hemoglobin: Decreased

ESR: Increased

WBC: Increased

C-reactive protein: Increased

Serum albumin: Decreased

Folic acid and B$_{12}$: Decreased

Anti-glycan antibodies: Increased

Stool for occult blood: Can be positive

Urinalysis: WBC

K+, Mg, and Ca: Decreased

Diverticulitis

Hematocrit and hemoglobin: Decreased

ESR: Increased

WBC: Increased

Stool for occult blood: Can be positive

DIAGNOSTIC PROCEDURES

Magnetic resonance enterography: Used with all IBD

CLIENT EDUCATION: Remain NPO for 4 to 6 hr prior to the exam. A contrast medium is used.

Ulcerative colitis

Sigmoidoscopy or colonoscopy: Can diagnose ulcerative colitis

Barium enema: Helpful to distinguish ulcerative colitis from other disease processes

CT scan or MRI: Can identify the presence of abscesses

Stool examination: For the presence of parasites or microbes

Crohn's disease

Endoscopy
- Diagnostic tools such as video capsule endoscopy are being used.
- **Proctosigmoidoscopy**: Performed to identify inflamed tissue.
- **Colonoscopy and sigmoidoscopy**: A lighted, flexible scope is inserted into the rectum to visualize the rectum and large intestine.

Abdominal ultrasound, x-ray, and CT scan: CT scans can show bowel thickening.

Barium enema: Barium is inserted into the rectum as a contrast medium for x-rays. This allows for the rectum and large intestine to be visualized, and is used to diagnose ulcerative colitis. A barium enema can show the presence of diverticulosis and is contraindicated in the presence of diverticulitis due to the risk of perforation.

NURSING ACTIONS
- Monitor postprocedure for manifestations of bowel perforations (rectal bleeding, firm abdomen, tachycardia, hypotension). Qs
- Provide bowel preparation instructions.

FINDINGS
- Small intestine ulcerations and narrowing is consistent with Crohn's disease.
- Ulcerations and inflammation of the sigmoid colon and rectum is significant for ulcerative colitis.

CLIENT EDUCATION
- Remain NPO as required.
- Abdominal discomfort and cramping are possible during the barium enema.

PATIENT-CENTERED CARE

NURSING CARE

Ulcerative colitis and Crohn's disease

- The client should receive instructions regarding the usual course of the disease process.
- The client should receive instructions regarding medication therapy and vitamin supplements.
- The client will need monitoring by colonoscopy due to the increased risk of colon cancer.
- Instruct clients who have extreme or long exacerbations that NPO status and administration of total parenteral nutrition promotes bowel rest while providing adequate nutrition.
- Assist the client in identifying foods that trigger manifestations.
- Monitor for electrolyte imbalance, especially potassium. Diarrhea can cause a loss of fluids and electrolytes.
- Monitor I&O and for dehydration.
- Instruct the client regarding the use of vitamin supplements and B_{12} injections, if needed.

CLIENT EDUCATION
- Seek emergency care for indications of bowel obstruction or perforation (fever, severe abdominal pain, vomiting). Qs
- Eat high-protein, high-calorie, low-fiber foods.
- Avoid caffeine and alcohol.
- Take a multivitamin that contains iron.
- Small frequent meals can reduce the occurrence of manifestations.
- Dietary supplements that are high in protein and low in fiber (elemental and semi-elemental products, canned nutrition beverages) can be used.

Diverticulitis

- For severe manifestations (severe pain, high fever), the client is hospitalized, NPO, and receives nasogastric suctioning, IV fluids, IV antibiotics, and opioid analgesics for pain.
- Instruct the client who has mild diverticulitis about self-care at home.
- Provide the client with instructions to promote normal bowel function and consistency. (Can take bulk-forming laxatives. Drink adequate fluids. Avoid use of enemas.)

CLIENT EDUCATION
- Take medications as prescribed (antibiotics, analgesics, antispasmodics) and get adequate rest.
- Consume a clear liquid diet until manifestations subside. Progress to a low-fiber diet as tolerated.
- Add fiber to the diet once solid foods are tolerated without other manifestations. Slowly advance to a high-fiber diet as tolerated when inflammation resolves.
- Avoid seeds or indigestible material, which can block diverticulum (nuts, popcorn, seeds).
- Avoid foods or drinks that can irritate the bowel. (Avoid alcohol. Limit fat to 30% of daily calorie intake.)

MEDICATIONS FOR ULCERATIVE COLITIS, CROHN'S DISEASE

5-aminosalicylic acid: Anti-inflammatory

Reduces inflammation of the intestinal mucosa and inhibits prostaglandins

Sulfonamides: Sulfasalazine
- These medications are contraindicated if the client has a sulfa allergy.
- Sulfasalazine is given orally.
- Adverse effects include nausea, fever, and rash.
- NURSING ACTIONS
  - Monitor CBC, and kidney and hepatic function.
  - Monitor for the development of agranulocytosis, hemolytic anemia, and macrocytic anemia.

- CLIENT EDUCATION
  - Take the medication with a full glass of water after meals.
  - Avoid sun exposure.
  - Increase fluid intake to 2 L/day.
  - This medication can cause urine, skin, and contact lenses to have a yellow-orange color.
  - Notify the provider if nausea, vomiting, anorexia, sore throat, rash, bruising, or fever occur.
  - Take medication as directed. The usual maintenance dose of sulfasalazine is 2 to 4 g/day.

Nonsulfonamides
- The adverse effects are not as serious as sulfasalazine.
- These medications can be contraindicated if the client has a salicylate or sulfa allergy.
- MEDICATIONS
  - Mesalamine
  - Balsalazide
  - Olsalazine (for clients intolerant to sulfasalazine, rarely used)
- NURSING ACTIONS: Monitor for kidney toxicity.
- CLIENT EDUCATION: Report headache or GI problems (abdominal discomfort, diarrhea).

Corticosteroids

Reduces inflammation and pain
- Used to induce remission
- Not for long-term use due to adverse effects
- Can slow healing

MEDICATIONS
- Prednisone
- Prednisolone
- Hydrocortisone
- Budesonide

NURSING ACTIONS
- For rectal inflammation, topical steroids can be administered by a retention enema.
- Prolonged use can lead to adrenal suppression, osteoporosis, risk of infection, and cushingoid syndrome. Use corticosteroids in low doses to minimize adverse effects.
- Monitor blood pressure.
- Reduce systemic dose slowly.
- Monitor electrolytes and glucose.

CLIENT EDUCATION
- Take the oral dose with food.
- Avoid discontinuing dose suddenly.
- Report unexpected increase in weight or other indications of fluid retention.
- Avoid crowds and other exposures to infectious diseases.
- Report evidence of infection (clients who have Crohn's disease; can mask infection).

Immunosuppressants

Mechanism of action in treatment of IBD is unknown.
- Can take up to 6 months to see therapeutic effects
- Not used as monotherapy
- Reserved for refractory disease due to toxicity

MEDICATIONS
- Cyclosporine
- Methotrexate
- Azathioprine
- Mercaptopurine

NURSING ACTIONS: Monitor for pancreatitis and neutropenia.

CLIENT EDUCATION
- Avoid crowds and other chances of exposures to infectious diseases and report evidence of infection.
- Monitor for indications of bleeding, bruising, or infection.

Immunomodulators

- Suppresses the immune response
- Inhibits tumor necrosis factor, an antibody found in Crohn's disease
- Many adverse effects are possible, including chills, fever, hypotension/hypertension, dysrhythmias, and blood dyscrasias.

MEDICATIONS
- Infliximab
- Adalimumab (self-administered by subcutaneous injection)
- Natalizumab (can cause progressive multi-focal leukoencephalopathy a deadly brain infection)
- Certolizumab

NURSING ACTIONS
- Ensure directions are followed for IV use with care and in accordance with facility policy; can require pretreatment to reduce infusion reactions. Q EBP
- Monitor liver enzymes, coagulation studies, and CBC.

CLIENT EDUCATION
- Avoid crowds and other chances of exposures to infectious diseases and report evidence of infection. The client is at risk for development or reactivation of tuberculosis.
- Monitor and report evidence of bleeding, bruising, or infection, and transfusion or allergic reaction.

Antidiarrheals

- Suppress the number of stools
- Decrease risk of fluid volume deficit and electrolyte imbalance
- Reduce discomfort

MEDICATIONS
- Diphenoxylate and atropine
- Loperamide

NURSING ACTIONS
- Use of antidiarrheals can lead to toxic megacolon (massive dilation of the colon with a risk of the development of gangrene and peritonitis). Use cautiously. Qs
  - Observe for manifestations of toxic megacolon that can result in gangrene and peritonitis (hypotension, fever, abdominal distention, decrease or absence of bowel sounds).
- Observe for indications of respiratory depression, especially in older adult clients.

CLIENT EDUCATION: Due to the central nervous system effects, avoid hazardous activities until the response to the medication is established.

MEDICATION FOR DIVERTICULITIS

Antimicrobials

Treat infection (decrease inflammation in Crohn's disease, ineffective for ulcerative colitis)

MEDICATIONS
- Ciprofloxacin
- Metronidazole
- Sulfamethoxazole-trimethoprim

NURSING ACTIONS
- Discontinue ciprofloxacin for tendon pain (can cause tendon rupture).
- Decreased dose should be used for clients who have impaired kidney function.
- Monitor kidney and hepatic studies.

CLIENT EDUCATION
- Antimicrobials can cause a superinfection. Observe for manifestations of thrush or vaginal yeast infection.
- Urine can darken (expected, harmless effect).
- Monitor for manifestations of CNS effects (numbness of extremities, ataxia, and seizures) and notify the provider immediately.

THERAPEUTIC PROCEDURES

Clients who do not have success with medical treatment or who have complications (bowel perforation, colon cancer) are candidates for surgery.

Ulcerative colitis: Colectomy with or without ileostomy

Crohn's disease
- Laparoscopic strictureplasty to increase the diameter of the bowel for bowel strictures
- Surgical repair of fistulas or in response to other complications related to the disease (perforation)

Diverticulitis (dependent on problem)
- Required for rupture of the diverticulum that results in peritonitis, bowel obstruction, uncontrolled bleeding, or abscess
- Colon resection with or without colostomy

PREOPERATIVE CARE
- Preoperative care is similar to care for clients who have other abdominal surgeries.
- Reinforce preoperative teaching.
- If the creation of a stoma is planned, collaborate with an enterostomal therapy nurse regarding care related to the stoma. Qtc
- Administer antibiotic bowel prep (neomycin).
- Administer cleansing enema or laxative.

POSTOPERATIVE CARE
- Postoperative care is similar to care for clients who have other types of abdominal surgery.
- The client should be NPO and have a nasogastric tube to suction, unless the surgery was performed laparoscopically.
- An ileostomy can drain as much as 1,000 mL/day. Prevent fluid volume deficit. Care for the client receiving IV fluids to replace fluid loss if the client is NPO. Oral hydration is slowly introduced in 1 to 2 days. Qs

CARE AFTER DISCHARGE: Refer the client who has an ostomy to an enterostomal therapist and an ostomy support group.

INTERPROFESSIONAL CARE

- Refer the client for nutritional counseling.
- The client might benefit from complementary therapy (biofeedback, massage, yoga).
- Recommend community support groups or a mental health referral for assistance with coping. Qpcc

COMPLICATIONS

Complications of ulcerative colitis, Crohn's disease, and diverticulitis include bleeding and fluid and electrolyte imbalance. Peritonitis can occur due to perforation of the bowel. Abscess formation can occur as a complication of diverticular disease and Crohn's disease.

Peritonitis

- A life-threatening inflammation of the peritoneum and lining of the abdominal cavity.
- It is often caused by bacteria in the peritoneal cavity.

PHYSICAL FINDINGS
- Rigid, board-like abdomen (hallmark indication)
- Abdominal distention
- Nausea, vomiting
- Rebound tenderness
- Tachycardia
- Fever

NURSING ACTIONS
- Place the client in Fowler's or semi-Fowler's position to promote drainage of peritoneal fluid and improve lung expansion. Q_EBP
- Monitor respiratory status and administer oxygen. Turn, cough, and deep breathe. Provide mechanical ventilation if needed.
- Maintain and monitor nasogastric suction.
- Keep the client NPO.
- Monitor fluid and electrolyte status.
- Monitor for hypovolemia.
- Ensure the administration of IV antibiotics.
- Collaborate with case management to determine home care and wound management needs. Q_TC
- If surgery is performed:
  - Closely monitor postoperative vital signs.
  - Monitor I&O every hour immediately after surgery.
  - Monitor surgical dressing for bleeding.
  - If the client requires wound irrigation postoperatively, use sterile technique, and monitor irrigation intake and output to prevent fluid retention.

CLIENT EDUCATION
- Maintain adequate rest and resume home activity slowly, as tolerated. No heavy lifting for at least 6 weeks.
- Monitor for evidence of return infection. Notify the provider immediately.

Bleeding due to deterioration of the bowel

NURSING ACTIONS
- Observe for indications of rectal bleeding.
- Monitor vital signs.
- Check laboratory values, especially hematocrit, hemoglobin, and coagulation factors.
- Explain to the client the importance of bed rest.

CLIENT EDUCATION: Report rectal bleeding.

Fluid and electrolyte imbalance

Occurs due to loss of fluid through diarrhea, vomiting, and nasogastric suctioning.

NURSING ACTIONS
- Monitor laboratory values, and provide replacement therapy.
- Monitor weight.
- Monitor for indications of fluid volume deficit (loss or absence of skin turgor).

CLIENT EDUCATION
- Record and report the number of loose stools.
- Maintain adequate fluid intake.
- Follow the prescribed diet.

Abscess and fistula formation

Occurs due to the destruction of the bowel wall, leading to an infection

NURSING ACTIONS
- Monitor fluid and electrolytes.
- Observe for manifestations of dehydration.
- Provide a diet high in protein and calories (at least 3,000 calories/day), and low in fiber.
- Administer a vitamin supplement.
- An enterostomal therapist can develop a plan to prevent skin breakdown and promote wound healing. Q_TC
- Monitor for evidence of infection, which can indicate abdominal abscesses or sepsis.
- Ensure the function of drainage devices if used.

Toxic megacolon

Occurs due to inactivity of the colon. Massive dilation of the colon occurs, and the client is at risk for perforation.

NURSING ACTIONS
- Maintain nasogastric suction.
- Care for the client receiving IV fluids and electrolytes.
- Administer medications (antibiotics, corticosteroids).
- Prepare the client for surgery (usually an ileostomy) if the client does not begin to show improvement within 72 hr.

Application Exercises

1. A nurse is reviewing the serum laboratory data of a client who has an acute exacerbation of Crohn's disease. Which of the following laboratory tests should the nurse expect to be elevated? (Select all that apply.)

   A. Hematocrit

   B. Erythrocyte sedimentation rate

   C. WBC

   D. Folic acid

   E. Albumin

2. A nurse is collecting data from a client who has been taking prednisone following an exacerbation of inflammatory bowel disease. The nurse should identify which of the following findings as the priority?

   A. Client reports difficulty sleeping.

   B. The client's urine is positive for glucose.

   C. Client reports having an elevated body temperature.

   D. Client reports gaining 4 lb in the last 6 months.

3. A nurse is reinforcing teaching with a client who has a new prescription for sulfasalazine. Which of the following instructions should the nurse include in the teaching?

   A. "Take the medication 2 hr after eating."

   B. "Discontinue this medication if your skin turns yellow-orange."

   C. "Notify the provider if you experience a sore throat."

   D. "Expect your stools to turn black."

4. A nurse is reinforcing discharge teaching with a client who has Crohn's disease. Which of the following instructions should the nurse include in the teaching?

   A. Decrease intake of calorie-dense foods.

   B. Drink canned protein supplements.

   C. Increase intake of high fiber foods.

   D. Take a bulk-forming laxative daily.

5. A nurse in a clinic is reinforcing teaching with a client who has ulcerative colitis. Which of the following statements by the client indicates understanding of the teaching?

   A. "I will plan to limit fiber in my diet."

   B. "I will restrict fluid intake during meals."

   C. "I will switch to black tea instead of drinking coffee."

   D. "I will try to eat three moderate to large meals a day."

PRACTICE Active Learning Scenario

A nurse is reinforcing teaching with a client who has diverticulitis. What should the nurse include in the teaching? Use the ATI Active Learning Template: System Disorder to complete this item.

PATHOPHYSIOLOGY RELATED TO CLIENT PROBLEM

RISK FACTORS: Identify two.

EXPECTED FINDINGS: Identify two expected findings.

DIAGNOSTIC PROCEDURES: Identify three.

CLIENT EDUCATION: Describe dietary teaching.

Application Exercises Key

1. A. Hematocrit is decreased as a result of chronic blood loss.

   B. **CORRECT:** Increased erythrocyte sedimentation rate is a finding in a client who has Crohn's disease as a result of inflammation.

   C. **CORRECT:** Increased WBC is a finding in a client who has Crohn's disease.

   D. A decrease in folic acid level is indicative of malabsorption due to Crohn's disease.

   E. A decrease in serum albumin is indicative of malabsorption due to Crohn's disease.

   (N) *NCLEX® Connection: Reduction of Risk Potential, Laboratory Values*

2. A. The client is at risk for sleep deprivation because prednisone can cause anxiety and insomnia. However, another finding is the priority.

   B. The client is at risk for hyperglycemia because prednisone can cause glucose intolerance. However, another finding is the priority.

   C. **CORRECT:** The greatest risk to the client is infection because prednisone can cause immunosuppression. Therefore, indications of an infection, such as an elevated body temperature, are the priority finding.

   D. The client is at risk for weight gain because prednisone can cause fluid retention. However, another finding is the priority.

   (N) *NCLEX® Connection: Pharmacological Therapies, Adverse Effects/ Contraindications/Side Effects/Interactions*

3. A. Sulfasalazine should be taken right after meals and with a full glass of water to reduce gastric upset and prevent crystalluria.

   B. Yellow-orange coloring of the skin and urine is a harmless effect of sulfasalazine.

   C. **CORRECT:** Sulfasalazine can cause blood dyscrasias. The client should monitor and report any manifestations of infection, such as a sore throat.

   D. Sulfasalazine can cause thrombocytopenia and bleeding. Black stools are a manifestation of gastrointestinal bleeding, and the client should report this to the provider.

   (N) *NCLEX® Connection: Pharmacological Therapies, Medication Administration*

4. A. A high-protein diet is recommended for the client who has Crohn's disease.

   B. **CORRECT:** A high-protein diet is recommended for the client who has Crohn's disease. Canned protein supplements are encouraged.

   C. A low-fiber diet is recommended for the client who has Crohn's disease to reduce inflammation.

   D. Bulk-forming laxatives are recommended for the client who has diverticulitis.

   (N) *NCLEX® Connection: Physiological Adaptation, Alterations in Body Systems*

5. A. **CORRECT:** A low-fiber diet is recommended for the client who has ulcerative colitis to reduce inflammation.

   B. A client who has dumping syndrome should avoid fluids with meals.

   C. Caffeine can increase diarrhea and cramping. The client should avoid caffeinated beverages, such as black tea.

   D. Small, frequent meals are recommended for the client who has ulcerative colitis.

   (N) *NCLEX® Connection: Physiological Adaptation, Alterations in Body Systems*

PRACTICE Answer

Using the ATI Active Learning Template: System Disorder

PATHOPHYSIOLOGY RELATED TO CLIENT PROBLEM: Inflammation and infection of the bowel mucosa caused by bacteria or fecal matter trapped in one or more diverticula (pouches in the intestine)

RISK FACTORS
• Older adult clients
• Male clients

EXPECTED FINDINGS
• Decreased hemoglobin and hematocrit
• Stool can be positive for occult blood.

DIAGNOSTIC PROCEDURES
• Abdominal x-ray
• CT scan
• Colonoscopy
• Sigmoidoscopy

CLIENT EDUCATION
• Consume clear liquid until manifestations subside. Progress to a low fiber diet as tolerated. Add fiber once solid foods are tolerated. Slowly advance to a high-fiber diet.
• Avoid seeds or indigestible material (nuts, popcorn, seeds).
• Avoid alcohol. Limit fat to 30% of daily caloric intake.

(N) *NCLEX® Connection: Physiological Adaptation, Alterations in Body Systems*

CHAPTER 46
Cholecystitis and Cholelithiasis

Cholecystitis is an inflammation of the gallbladder wall. Gallstones (cholelithiasis) obstructing the cystic or common bile ducts is the most common cause of cholecystitis. Obstruction slows the flow of bile from the gallbladder to the duodenum causing bile to back up and the gallbladder to become inflamed.

Cholelithiasis is the presence of stones in the gallbladder related to the precipitation of bile or cholesterol into stones. Bile aids in the digestion of fats. It is produced in the liver and stored in the gall bladder. Cholecystitis can be acute or chronic, and can obstruct the pancreatic duct, causing pancreatitis. It can also cause the gallbladder to rupture, resulting in secondary peritonitis.

HEALTH PROMOTION AND DISEASE PREVENTION

- Consume a low-fat diet rich in HDL sources (seafood, nuts, olive oil).
- Participate in a regular exercise program.
- Do not smoke.

DATA COLLECTION

RISK FACTORS

- More common in females (hormone therapy and use of some oral contraceptives)
- High-fat diet
- Obesity (impaired fat metabolism, high cholesterol)
- Genetic predisposition
- Older adults (decreased contractility, more likely to develop gallstones) ©
- Type 2 diabetes mellitus (high triglycerides) or Crohn's disease
- Low-calorie, liquid protein diets
- Rapid weight loss (increases cholesterol)
- Native American or Hispanic American ethnicity

EXPECTED FINDINGS

- Sharp pain in the right upper quadrant, often radiating to the right shoulder
- Pain with deep inspiration during right subcostal palpation (Murphy's sign)
- Intense pain (increased heart rate, pallor, diaphoresis) with nausea and vomiting after ingestion of high-fat food caused by biliary colic
- Rebound tenderness (Blumberg's sign performed by the provider or advanced practice nurse)
- Dyspepsia, eructation (belching), flatulence
- Fever

PHYSICAL FINDINGS

- Jaundice, clay-colored stools, steatorrhea (fatty stools), dark urine, and pruritus (accumulation of bile salts in the skin) in clients who have chronic cholecystitis (due to biliary obstruction).
- OLDER ADULT CLIENTS who have diabetes mellitus can have atypical presentation of cholecystitis (absence of pain or fever). ©

LABORATORY TESTS

- Increased WBC and erythrocyte sedimentation rate indicates inflammation.
- Direct, indirect, and total serum bilirubin increased if bile duct obstructed.
- Amylase and lipase increased with pancreatic involvement.
- Aspartate aminotransferase (AST), lactate dehydrogenase (LDH), gamma-glutamyl transpeptidase (GGT), and alkaline phosphatase (ALP) (increased with liver dysfunction) can indicate the common bile duct is obstructed.

DIAGNOSTIC PROCEDURES

Ultrasound visualizes gallstones and a dilated common bile duct.

Abdominal x-ray or CT scan can visualize calcified gallstones and an enlarged gallbladder.

Hepatobiliary scan (HIDA) assesses the patency of the biliary duct system after an IV injection of contrast.

Endoscopic retrograde cholangiopancreatography (ERCP) allows for direct visualization using an endoscope that is inserted through the esophagus and into the common bile duct via the duodenum. A sphincterotomy with gallstone removal can be done during this procedure. (Refer to **CHAPTER 39: GASTROINTESTINAL DIAGNOSTIC PROCEDURES.**)

Magnetic resonance cholangiopancreatography combines the use of oral/IV contrast with an MRI. This test assists the provider in determining the cause of cholecystitis or cholelithiasis.

PATIENT-CENTERED CARE

NURSING CARE

Administer analgesics as needed.

MEDICATIONS

Analgesics

- Opioid analgesics (morphine sulfate, hydromorphone) are preferred for acute biliary pain.
- An NSAID, such as ketorolac, is used for mild to moderate pain. Monitor for GI bleeding.

Bile acid

Bile acid (chenodiol, ursodiol) gradually dissolves cholesterol-based gallstones.

NURSING ACTIONS: Use caution in clients who have liver conditions or disorders with varices.

CLIENT EDUCATION
- Report abdominal pain, diarrhea, or vomiting.
- The medication is limited to 2 years of administration and requires a gallbladder ultrasound every 6 months during the first year to determine effectiveness.

COMPLEMENTARY THERAPIES

Goldenseal

An herb that promotes bilirubin and bile secretion and blocks bacterial growth.

NURSING ACTIONS: Warn the client that goldenseal stimulates uterine contractions, and not to take it when pregnant or lactating.

THERAPEUTIC PROCEDURES

Extracorporeal shock wave lithotripsy

Shock waves are used to break up stones. This is best for nonsurgical candidates of normal weight who have small, cholesterol-based stones.

NURSING ACTIONS
- Instruct and assist client to lay on fluid-filled pad for delivery of shock waves.
- Administer analgesia.

CLIENT EDUCATION
- Several procedures can be required to break up all stones.
- The client might have pain intraprocedure due to gallbladder spasms or movement of the stones.

Cholecystectomy

- Removal of the gallbladder with a laparoscopic, minimally invasive, or open approach
- The client usually goes home within 24 hr if a laparoscopic approach is used. An open approach can require hospitalization for 1 to 2 days.

NURSING ACTIONS
- **Laparoscopic approach:** Provide immediate postoperative care. Instruct the client regarding pain control.
- **Minimally invasive approach:** Natural orifice transluminal endoscopic surgery (NOTES). Explain to the client that this surgical procedure is performed through entry of the mouth, vagina, or rectum. This approach eliminates visible incisions and decreases the risk of complications for the client. Instruct the client regarding pain control.
- **Open approach:** The provider may place a Jackson-Pratt drain in the gallbladder bed or a T-tube in the common bile duct.
- The provider less commonly places a T-tube in the common bile duct to drain bile if there were intraoperative complications involving the bile duct.
- **Care of the drainage tube**
  - Clients can have a Jackson-Pratt drain or other drainage tube placed intraoperatively to prevent accumulation of fluid in the gallbladder bed.
  - Monitor and record drainage (initially serosanguineous stained with green-brown bile).
  - Administer antibiotics to decrease the risk for infection.
- **Care of the T-tube**
  - Instruct client to report an absence of drainage with manifestations of nausea and pain (can indicate obstruction in the T-tube).
  - Inspect the surrounding skin for evidence of infection or bile leakage.
  - If prescribed, elevate the T-tube above the level of the abdomen to prevent the total loss of bile.
  - Monitor and record the color and amount of drainage.
  - Clamp the tube 1 hr before and after meals to provide the bile necessary for food digestion.
  - Monitor stools for color (stools clay-colored until biliary flow is reestablished).
  - Monitor for bile peritonitis (pain, fever, jaundice).
  - Monitor and document response to food.
  - Expect removal of the tube in 1 to 3 weeks.

CLIENT EDUCATION
- **Laparoscopic or NOTES approach**
  - Ambulate frequently to minimize free air pain, common following laparoscopic surgery (under the right clavicle, shoulder, scapula).
  - Monitor the incision for evidence of infection or wound dehiscence (laparoscopic approach).
  - Report indications of bile leak (pain, vomiting, abdominal distention) to the provider.
  - Resume activity gradually and as tolerated, and to resume the preoperative diet.

- **Open approach**
  - Resume activity gradually. Avoid heavy lifting for 4 to 6 weeks.
  - Begin with clear liquids and advance to solid foods as peristalsis returns.
  - Report sudden increase in drainage, foul odor, pain, fever, or jaundice. Qs
  - Take showers instead of baths while the drainage tube is in place.
  - The color of stools should return to brown in about a week, and diarrhea is common.
- **Dietary counseling**
  - Consume a low-fat diet (reduce dairy products and avoid fried foods, chocolate, nuts, gravies). The client can have increased tolerance of small, frequent meals.
  - Avoid gas-forming foods (beans, cabbage, cauliflower, broccoli).
  - Reduce weight.
  - Take fat-soluble vitamins or bile salts to enhance absorption and aid with digestion.

COMPLICATIONS

Obstruction of the bile duct

This can cause ischemia, gangrene, and a rupture of the gallbladder wall. A rupture of the gallbladder wall can cause a local abscess or peritonitis (rigid, board-like abdomen, guarding), which requires a surgical intervention and administration of broad spectrum antibiotics.

Bile peritonitis

This can occur if adequate amounts of bile are not drained from the surgical site. This is a rare but potentially fatal complication

NURSING ACTIONS
- Monitor for pain, fever, and jaundice.
- Report findings to the provider immediately.

Postcholecystectomy syndrome

Manifestations of gallbladder disease can continue after surgery. The client will report findings similar to those experienced prior to surgery related to pain and nausea. Manifestations can recur immediately or months later.

NURSING ACTIONS
- Monitor pain characteristics and other reported findings.
- Instruct client on the need for possible further diagnostic evaluation.

Application Exercises

1. A nurse is reviewing discharge instructions with a client who is postoperative following open cholecystectomy with T-tube placement. Which of the following instructions should the nurse include in the teaching? (Select all that apply.)

   A. Take baths rather than showers.

   B. Clamp T-tube for 1 hr before and after meals.

   C. Replace the drainage system daily.

   D. Expect to have the T-tube removed 3 days postoperatively.

   E. Expect brown-green drainage from the tube.

2. A nurse is reviewing nutrition teaching for a client who has cholecystitis. The nurse should identify that which of the following food choices is most likely to trigger cholecystitis?

   A. Brownie with nuts

   B. Bowl of mixed fruit

   C. Grilled turkey

   D. Baked potato

3. A nurse is reviewing preoperative teaching with a client scheduled for a laparoscopic cholecystectomy. Which of the following should the nurse include?

   A. "The scope will be passed through your rectum."

   B. "You might have shoulder pain after surgery."

   C. "You will have a Jackson-Pratt drain in place after surgery."

   D. "You should limit how often you walk for 1 to 2 weeks."

4. A nurse is reviewing a new prescription for ursodiol with a client who has cholelithiasis. Which of the following information should the nurse include?

   A. This medication is used to decrease acute biliary pain.

   B. This medication requires thyroid function monitoring every 6 months.

   C. This medication is not recommended for clients who have diabetes mellitus.

   D. This medication dissolves gallstones gradually over a period of up to 2 years.

5. A nurse in a clinic is reviewing the laboratory reports of a client who has suspected cholelithiasis. Which of the following is an expected finding?

   A. Serum amylase 80 units/L

   B. WBC 9,000/mm³

   C. Direct bilirubin 2.1 mg/dL

   D. Alkaline phosphatase (ALP) 25 units/L

Application Exercises Key

1. A. The client should not soak in bath water while the T-tube is in place due to the increased risk for introduction of organisms and infection.

   B. **CORRECT:** Clamping the T-tube 1 hr before and after meals allows bile needed for digestion of food to remain in the body.

   C. The nurse should inform the client that drainage can be emptied from the T-tube system and the client will not have to change it.

   D. The T-tube usually remains in place for 1 to 3 weeks postoperatively.

   E. **CORRECT:** The purpose of the T-tube is to drain bile from the common bile duct. The client should expect to see brown-green drainage.

   ⓝ *NCLEX® Connection: Reduction of Risk Potential, Therapeutic Procedures*

2. A. **CORRECT:** Foods that are high in fat, such as a brownie with nuts, can cause cholecystitis.

   B. Fruits are low in fat and not associated with cholecystitis. A low-calorie diet can trigger cholecystitis.

   C. Turkey is low in fat and not associated with cholecystitis. A liquid protein diet can trigger cholecystitis.

   D. Baked potatoes are low in fat and not associated with cholecystitis. Rapid weight loss can trigger cholecystitis.

   ⓝ *NCLEX® Connection: Basic Care and Comfort, Nutrition and Oral Hydration*

3. A. The natural orifice transluminal endoscopic surgery (NOTES) approach might require entry through the rectum.

   B. **CORRECT:** Shoulder pain is an expected finding postoperatively due to free air that is introduced into the abdomen during laparoscopic surgery.

   C. An open cholecystectomy can require drain placement, such as a JP or T-tube.

   D. The client should ambulate frequently following a laparoscopic surgical approach to minimize the free air that has been introduced.

   ⓝ *NCLEX® Connection: Reduction of Risk Potential, Potential for Complications of Diagnostic Tests/Treatments/Procedures*

4. A. Opioid analgesics are preferred for the treatment of acute biliary pain.

   B. The client should have an ultrasound of the gallbladder every 6 months during the first year of treatment to determine effectiveness of the medication.

   C. Clients who have liver conditions or disorders with varices should use ursodiol cautiously.

   D. **CORRECT:** Ursodiol is a bile acid that gradually dissolves cholesterol-based gallstones. The client can take this medication for up to 2 years.

   ⓝ *NCLEX® Connection: Pharmacological Therapies, Medication Administration*

5. A. The nurse should expect the client who has cholelithiasis to have an elevated serum amylase level if pancreatic involvement is present. A serum amylase of 80 units/L is within the expected reference range.

   B. The nurse should expect the client who has cholelithiasis to have an elevated WBC level due to inflammation. WBC 9,000/mm³ is within the expected reference range.

   C. **CORRECT:** The nurse should expect the client who has cholelithiasis to have an elevated direct bilirubin level if the bile duct is obstructed. A direct bilirubin level of 2.1 mg/dL is greater than the expected reference range.

   D. The nurse should expect the client who has cholelithiasis to have an elevated ALP level if the common bile duct is obstructed. An ALP of 25 units/L is less than the expected reference range.

   ⓝ *NCLEX® Connection: Reduction of Risk Potential, Laboratory Values*

PRACTICE Active Learning Scenario

A nurse is assisting with a program on gallbladder disease with a group of clients at a health fair. What information should the nurse expect to include? Use the ATI Active Learning Template: System Disorder to complete this item.

RISK FACTORS: Describe at least four.

EXPECTED FINDINGS: Describe at least eight findings.

CLIENT EDUCATION: Describe three preventative activities.

PRACTICE Answer

Using the ATI Active Learning Template: System Disorder

RISK FACTORS
- Female sex (hormone therapy, and some oral contraceptives)
- High-fat or low-calorie, liquid protein diets
- Obesity
- Genetic predisposition
- Age older than 60 years
- Type 2 diabetes mellitus
- Rapid weight loss
- Native American or Hispanic American ethnicity

EXPECTED FINDINGS
- Sharp pain in the right upper quadrant that often radiates to the right shoulder
- Pain upon deep inspiration during right subcostal palpation
- Intense pain with nausea and vomiting after ingestion of high-fat food
- Dyspepsia
- Eructation (belching)
- Flatulence
- Fever
- Jaundice
- Clay-colored stools
- Steatorrhea (fatty stools)
- Dark urine
- Pruritus

CLIENT EDUCATION
- Get regular exercise.
- Stop smoking.
- Consume a low-fat diet rich in HDL sources (seafood, nuts, olive oil).

ⓝ *NCLEX® Connection: Physiological Adaptation, Basic Pathophysiology*

CHAPTER 47 *Pancreatitis*

The pancreas secretes insulin, glucagon, and digestive enzymes that break down carbohydrates, proteins, and fats.

Pancreatitis is an autodigestion of the pancreas by pancreatic digestive enzymes that activate prematurely before reaching the intestines. Pancreatitis can result in pancreatic inflammation, necrosis, and hemorrhage. Manifestations of an acute attack include severe, constant, knifelike pain (left upper quadrant, midepigastric, radiating to the back).

Acute pancreatitis is an inflammatory process due to activated pancreatic enzymes autodigesting the pancreas.

Chronic pancreatitis is a progressive, destructive disease of inflammation and fibrosis of the pancreas. Chronic pancreatitis includes chronic calcifying pancreatitis (often associated with alcohol use disorder), chronic obstructive pancreatitis (often associated with cholelithiasis), autoimmune pancreatitis, and idiopathic and hereditary pancreatitis.

HEALTH PROMOTION AND DISEASE PREVENTION

- Avoid excessive alcohol consumption.
- Eat a low-fat diet.

DATA COLLECTION

RISK FACTORS

- Biliary tract disease: Gallstones can cause a blockage where the common bile duct and pancreatic duct meet.
- Alcohol use: The primary cause of chronic pancreatitis is alcohol use disorder. Times of increased alcohol consumption, such as vacations or holidays, are associated with acute pancreatitis.
- Increased age: Pancreatitis is more common in older adults. Ⓖ
- Endoscopic retrograde cholangiopancreatography (ERCP) (postprocedure complication)
- Gastrointestinal surgery
- Metabolic disturbances (hyperlipidemia, hyperparathyroidism, hypercalcemia)
- Kidney disease or transplant
- Genetic predisposition
- Trauma
- Penetrating ulcer (gastric or duodenal)
- Medication toxicity
- Viral infections: coxsackievirus B and human immunodeficiency virus
- Cigarette smoking

EXPECTED FINDINGS

- Sudden onset of severe, boring pain (goes through the body)
  - Epigastric, radiating to back, left flank, or left shoulder
  - Worse when lying down
- Pain relieved somewhat by fetal position or sitting upright, bending forward
- Pain that occurs or worsens after food or alcohol consumption
- Nausea and vomiting
- Weight loss

PHYSICAL FINDINGS
- Seepage of blood-stained exudates into tissue as a result of pancreatic enzyme actions
  - Ecchymoses on the flanks: Turner's sign (47.1)
  - Bluish-gray periumbilical discoloration: Cullen's sign (47.2)
- Generalized jaundice
- Absent or decreased bowel sounds (possible paralytic ileus)
- Warm, moist skin
- Fruity breath (evidence of hyperglycemia)
- Ascites
- Tetany due to hypocalcemia
  - Trousseau's sign: hand spasm when blood pressure cuff is inflated
  - Chvostek's sign: facial twitching when facial nerve is tapped

LABORATORY TESTS

- **Serum amylase** increases within 12 to 24 hr, and remains increased for 2 to 3 days (continued elevation can indicate pancreatic abscess or pseudocyst).
- **Serum lipase** increases slowly but remains increased for up to 2 weeks.
  - Urine amylase remains increased for up to 2 weeks.
  - Increases in enzymes indicate pancreatic cell injury.

  > MEMORY AID: In pancreatitis, the "ases" (aces) are high.

- **WBC count:** Increased due to infection and inflammation
- **Platelets:** Decreased
- **Serum calcium and magnesium:** Decreased due to fat necrosis with pancreatitis
- **Serum liver enzymes and bilirubin:** Increased with associated biliary dysfunction
- **Serum glucose:** Increased due to a decrease in insulin production by the pancreas
- **Erythrocyte sedimentation rate:** Elevated

DIAGNOSTIC PROCEDURES

CT scan with contrast reliably diagnoses acute pancreatitis.

PATIENT-CENTERED CARE

NURSING CARE

- Rest the pancreas.
  - NPO: No food until pain-free
  - For severe pancreatitis: Total parenteral nutrition or jejunal feedings (contraindicated if paralytic ileus develops, less risk of hyperglycemia)
  - When diet is resumed: Bland, high protein, low-fat diet with no stimulants (caffeine); small, frequent meals QEBP
  - Administer antiemetic as needed
  - Nasogastric tube: Gastric decompression (for severe vomiting or paralytic ileus)
  - No alcohol consumption
  - No smoking
  - Limit stress
  - Pain management
- Position the client for comfort (fetal, side-lying, head of the bed elevated, sitting up or leaning forward).
- Administer analgesics and other medications.
- Monitor blood glucose, and provide insulin as needed (potential for hyperglycemia).
- Monitor hydration status (orthostatic blood pressure, I&O, laboratory values).
- Monitor IV fluids and electrolyte replacement.

47.1 Turner's sign

47.2 Cullen's sign

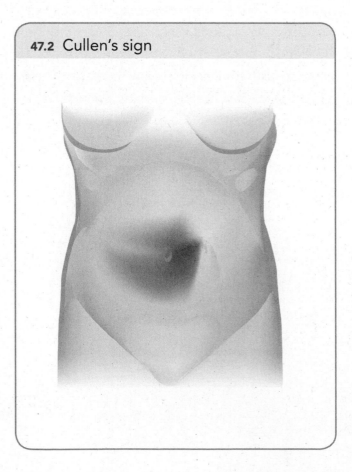

MEDICATIONS

Opioid analgesics

Morphine or hydromorphone for acute pain

Meperidine is discouraged due to the risk of seizures, especially in older adult clients. Ⓢ

Antibiotics: Imipenem

Antibiotics are generally indicated for clients who have acute necrotizing pancreatitis.

NURSING ACTIONS
- Monitor for evidence of infection.
- Monitor for seizures.

Histamine receptor antagonists: Ranitidine

Decreases gastric acid secretion.

CLIENT EDUCATION: Take 1 hr before or 1 hr after antacid.

Proton pump inhibitors: Omeprazole

Decreases gastric acid secretion.

NURSING ACTIONS: Monitor for hypomagnesemia.

Pancreatic enzymes: Pancrelipase

Aid with digestion of fats and proteins when taken with meals and snacks.

CLIENT EDUCATION
- Contents of capsules can be sprinkled on nonprotein foods.
- Drink 8 oz water following pancrelipase.
- Wipe lips and rinse mouth after taking (to prevent skin breakdown or irritation).
- Take pancrelipase after antacid or histamine receptor antagonists.
- Take pancrelipase with every meal and snack.

THERAPEUTIC PROCEDURES

- ERCP to create an opening in the sphincter of Oddi if pancreatitis is caused by gallstones
- Cholecystectomy if pancreatitis is a result of cholecystitis and gallstones
- Sphincterotomy to enlarge the pancreatic duct sphincter
- Endoscopic pancreatic necrosectomy and natural orifice transluminal endoscopic surgery (NOTES) to remove necrotic tissue
- Pancreaticojejunostomy (Roux-en-Y) to reroute drainage of pancreatic secretions into jejunum

INTERPROFESSIONAL CARE

- Recommend a dietary referral for postpancreatitis diet and nutritional supplements when oral intake is resumed.
- Recommend home health services for clients regarding nutritional needs, possible wound care, and assistance with ADLs, if indicated. Ⓠᴛᴄ
- Clients or family members who have alcohol use disorder can benefit from Alcoholics Anonymous (AA).

CLIENT EDUCATION

Chronic pancreatitis due to alcohol use: Avoid alcohol intake and caffeinated beverages, and participate in support groups for individuals who have alcohol use disorder. Ⓠᴘᴄᴄ

COMPLICATIONS

Hypovolemia

Up to 6 L of fluid can be third-spaced; caused by retroperitoneal loss of protein-rich fluid from proteolytic digestion. The client can develop hypovolemic shock.

NURSING ACTIONS: Monitor vital signs, electrolytes, and for hypotension and tachycardia. Monitor IV fluid and electrolyte replacement.

Pancreatic infection

Pseudocyst (outside pancreas); abscess (inside pancreas)

CAUSE: Leakage of fluid out of damaged pancreatic duct

MANIFESTATIONS: Fever, epigastric mass, nausea, vomiting, jaundice

NURSING ACTIONS
- Monitor for rupture and hemorrhage.
- Maintain sump tube if placed for drainage of cyst.
- Monitor skin around tube for breakdown secondary to corrosive enzymes.

Type 1 diabetes mellitus

CAUSE: Lack or absence of insulin (due to destruction of pancreatic beta cells)

NURSING ACTIONS
- Monitor blood glucose.
- Administer insulin.
- Inform the client about long-term diabetes management.

Left lung effusion and atelectasis

- More common complication in older adult clients Ⓖ
- Can precipitate pneumonia

CAUSES
- Splinting of chest due to pain upon coughing and deep breathing
- Pancreatic ascites

NURSING ACTIONS: Monitor for hypoxia, and provide ventilatory support.

Coagulation defects

Disseminated intravascular coagulopathy

CAUSES: Release of thromboplastic endotoxins secondary to necrotizing hemorrhagic pancreatitis

NURSING ACTIONS: Monitor coagulation studies and for bleeding.

Multi-system organ failure

Inflammation of pancreas appears to trigger systemic inflammation.

CAUSE: Necrotizing hemorrhagic pancreatitis

NURSING ACTIONS
- Administer treatments.
- Monitor for evidence of organ failure (respiratory distress, jaundice, oliguria). Ⓠs
- Report unexpected findings to provider.

Application Exercises

1. A nurse is collecting data from a client who has acute pancreatitis. Which of the following findings is the priority to report?

   A. History of cholelithiasis

   B. Elevated serum amylase level

   C. Decrease in bowel sounds upon auscultation

   D. Hand spasms when blood pressure is checked

2. A nurse is preparing to administer pancrelipase to a client who has pancreatitis. Which of the following actions should the nurse take?

   A. Instruct the client to chew the medication before swallowing.

   B. Offer 8 oz water following medication administration.

   C. Administer the medication 30 min before meals.

   D. Sprinkle the contents on peanut butter.

3. A nurse is collecting data from a newly admitted client who has pancreatitis. Which of the following findings should the nurse expect?

   A. Pain in right upper quadrant radiating to right shoulder

   B. Pain that is worse when sitting upright

   C. Pain that is worse when in a fetal position

   D. Epigastric pain radiating to the left shoulder

4. A nurse is collecting data from a client who has pancreatitis. Which of the following actions should the nurse take to check for the presence of Cullen's sign?

   A. Tap lightly at the costovertebral margin on the client's back.

   B. Palpate the right lower quadrant.

   C. Inspect the skin around the umbilicus.

   D. Auscultate the area below the scapula.

5. A nurse is reinforcing nutrition teaching with a client who has pancreatitis. Which of the following statements by the client indicates understanding? (Select all that apply.)

   A. "I plan to eat small, frequent meals."

   B. "I will eat easy-to-digest foods with limited spice."

   C. "I will use skim milk when cooking."

   D. "I plan to drink regular cola."

   E. "I will limit alcohol intake to two drinks per day."

PRACTICE Active Learning Scenario

A nurse is reviewing the plan of care for a client who has pancreatitis. What interventions should the nurse expect to find in the plan? Use the ATI Active Learning Template: System Disorder to complete this item.

ALTERATION IN HEALTH (DIAGNOSIS): Describe the classic presentation of pancreatitis.

LABORATORY TESTS: Describe four tests and expected findings.

NURSING CARE: Describe at least six nursing actions.

Application Exercises Key

1. A. A history of cholelithiasis indicates the client is at risk for chronic obstructive pancreatitis. However, another finding is the priority to report.

   B. A continuous elevation of amylase can indicate the client is at risk for pancreatic abscess or pseudocyst. However, another finding is the priority to report. Increased serum amylase is an expected finding for 2 to 3 days with acute pancreatitis.

   C. Decreased bowel sounds indicate the client is at risk for paralytic ileus from acute pancreatitis. However, another finding is the priority to report.

   D. **CORRECT:** The greatest risk to this client is injury from ECG changes and hypotension induced by hypocalcemia. Hand spasms when taking blood pressure is an indication of hypocalcemia.

   Ⓝ NCLEX® Connection: Physiological Adaptation, Alterations in Body Systems

2. A. The client should swallow pancrelipase without chewing it to reduce irritation and slow the release of the medication.

   B. **CORRECT:** The client should drink an 8 oz glass of water following administration of pancrelipase.

   C. The client should take pancrelipase with every meal and snack.

   D. The client can sprinkle the contents of the pancrelipase capsule on nonprotein foods.

   Ⓝ NCLEX® Connection: Pharmacological Therapies, Expected Actions/Outcomes

3. A. A client who has cholecystitis will report pain in the right upper quadrant radiating to the right shoulder.

   B. A client who has pancreatitis will report pain being worse when lying down and relieved by sitting up.

   C. A client who has pancreatitis will report pain relieved by assuming the fetal position.

   D. **CORRECT:** A client who has pancreatitis will report severe, boring epigastric pain that radiates to the back, left flank, or left shoulder.

   Ⓝ NCLEX® Connection: Physiological Adaptation, Basic Pathophysiology

4. A. This action checks for tenderness at McBurney's point which can indicate pyelonephritis.

   B. This action checks for the presence of rebound tenderness, which can indicate appendicitis.

   C. **CORRECT:** Cullen's sign is indicated by a bluish-gray discoloration in the periumbilical area.

   D. This action is part of focused data collection of the lung fields.

   Ⓝ NCLEX® Connection: Reduction of Risk Potential, Diagnostic Tests

5. A. **CORRECT:** A client who has pancreatitis should consume small, frequent meals to reduce gastrointestinal stimulation.

   B. **CORRECT:** A client who has pancreatitis should consume bland, easy-to-digest foods to reduce gastrointestinal stimulation.

   C. **CORRECT:** A client who has pancreatitis should choose low-fat foods to reduce gastrointestinal stimulation.

   D. The client should choose caffeine-free beverages to reduce gastrointestinal stimulation. Regular cola contains caffeine.

   E. The client who has pancreatitis should avoid any alcohol intake.

   Ⓝ NCLEX® Connection: Basic Care and Comfort, Nutrition and Oral Hydration

PRACTICE Answer

Using the ATI Active Learning Template: System Disorder

ALTERATION IN HEALTH (DIAGNOSIS): Severe, constant, knifelike pain (left upper quadrant, midepigastric, radiating to the back)

LABORATORY TESTS
- Serum amylase (increases within 12 to 24 hr, remains increased for 2 to 3 days)
- Serum lipase value (increases slowly and remains increased for up to 2 weeks)
- Urine amylase remains increased for up to 2 weeks
- Increased WBC count due to inflammation/infection
- Decreased serum calcium and magnesium
- Serum liver enzymes and bilirubin increased with associated biliary dysfunction
- Serum glucose increased

Ⓝ NCLEX® Connection: Physiological Adaptation, Basic Pathophysiology

NURSING CARE
- Maintain NPO status until the client is pain-free.
- Reinforce teaching about total parenteral nutrition or jejunal feedings (contraindicated if paralytic ileus develops).
- Maintain nasogastric tube (for severe vomiting or paralytic ileus).
- Resume diet beginning with bland, high protein, low-fat foods and no caffeine.
- Provide small, frequent meals.
- Administer antiemetics as needed.
- Limit stress.
- Provide analgesia for pain.
- Remind the client to not consume alcohol or smoke.

CHAPTER 48 *Hepatitis and Cirrhosis*

Hepatitis is an inflammation of liver cells. Hepatitis can be caused by a viral or toxic agent, or as a secondary infection in conjunction with another virus. It is classified as acute or chronic.

Cirrhosis is permanent scarring of the liver that is usually caused by chronic inflammation.

Hepatitis

- Viral hepatitis is the most common type of hepatitis.
- Toxic and drug-induced hepatitis occurs secondary to an exposure to a chemical or medication agent such as alcohol, industrial toxins, ephedra, or acetaminophen.
- Hepatitis can occur in conjunction with other viruses such as varicella-zoster, cytomegalovirus, or herpes simplex.
- After exposure to a virus or toxin, the liver becomes enlarged from the inflammatory process. As the disease progresses, there is an increase in inflammation and necrosis, interfering with blood flow to the liver.
- Individuals infected with hepatitis can remain free of manifestations during the incubation period, and further transmit the disease unknowingly

Major categories of viral hepatitis
- Hepatitis A virus (HAV)
- Hepatitis B virus (HBV)
- Hepatitis C virus (HCV)
- Hepatitis D virus (HDV)
- Hepatitis E virus (HEV)

HEALTH PROMOTION AND DISEASE PREVENTION

- Provide community health education interventions on transmission and exposure.
- Follow CDC immunization recommendations.
- Follow CDC isolation precautions.
- Use safe injection practices. Qᵉⁱ
  - Aseptic technique for preparation and administration of parenteral medications
  - Sterile, single-use, disposable needle and syringe for each injection
  - Single-dose vials whenever possible
  - Needleless systems or safety caps

- Use personal protective equipment (gown, gloves, goggles) appropriate to the type of exposure.
  - Hepatitis A: Clients who are incontinent of stool
  - Hepatitis B or C: Exposure to blood
- Use proper hand hygiene (before preparing and eating food, after using the toilet or changing a diaper).
- When traveling to underdeveloped countries, drink purified water, and avoid sharing eating utensils and bed linens.

DATA COLLECTION

RISK FACTORS

Hepatitis A

ROUTE OF TRANSMISSION: Fecal-oral

RISK FACTORS
- Ingestion of contaminated food or water, especially shellfish
- Close personal contact with an infected individual

Hepatitis B

ROUTE OF TRANSMISSION: Blood

RISK FACTORS
- Unprotected sex with infected individual
- Infants born to infected mothers
- Contact with infected blood
- Substance use disorder (injectable substances)

Hepatitis C

ROUTE OF TRANSMISSION: Blood

RISK FACTORS
- Substance use disorder (injectable substances)
- Blood, blood products, or organ transplants
- Contaminated needle sticks
- Unsanitary tattoo equipment
- Sexual contact

Hepatitis D

ROUTE OF TRANSMISSION: Coinfection with HBV

RISK FACTORS
- Substance use disorder (injectable substances)
- Unprotected sex with infected individual

Hepatitis E

ROUTE OF TRANSMISSION: Fecal-oral

RISK FACTORS: Ingestion of food or water contaminated with fecal waste

Additional risk factors

- Unscreened blood transfusions (prior to 1992)
- Hemodialysis
- Percutaneous exposure (dirty needles, sharp instruments, body piercing, tattooing, use of another person's substance use paraphernalia or personal hygiene tools)
- Unprotected sexual intercourse with a hepatitis-infected person, sex with multiple partners, anal sex
- Ingestion of food prepared by a hepatitis-infected person who does not practice proper sanitation precautions
- Travel/residence in underdeveloped country (using tap water to clean food products, drinking contaminated water)
- Eating or living in crowded environments (correctional facilities, dormitories, universities, long-term care facilities, military base housing)

EXPECTED FINDINGS

- Failure to take personal precautions with blood and body fluid
- Influenza-like manifestations
  - Fatigue
  - Decreased appetite with nausea
  - Abdominal pain
  - Joint pain

PHYSICAL FINDINGS

- Fever
- Vomiting
- Dark-colored urine
- Clay-colored stool
- Jaundice

LABORATORY TESTS Qebp

Prothrombin time (PT) and INR: possibly elevated due to decreased liver production of clotting factors.

Positive viral antibody testing indicates presence of infection.

Positive immunoglobulin testing can indicate liver inflammation, or the body's attempt to provide immunity against the virus.

Hepatitis A

Alanine aminotransferase (ALT): Elevated (expected reference range 4 to 36 units/L)

Aspartate aminotransferase (AST): Elevated (expected reference range 0 to 35 units/L)

Alkaline phosphatase (ALP): Normal or elevated (expected reference range 30 to 120 units/L)

Total bilirubin level: Elevated (expected reference range 0.3 to 1.0 mg/dL)

Hepatitis A virus antibodies (anti-HAV): Presence indicates hepatitis A.

Hepatitis B

ALT: Elevated

AST: Elevated

ALP: Normal or elevated

Total bilirubin level: Elevated

Hepatitis C

ALT: Elevated

AST: Elevated

ALP: Normal or elevated

Total bilirubin level: Elevated

Enzyme immunoassay (EIA) and other assay testing: Presence detects hepatitis C infection.

DIAGNOSTIC PROCEDURES

Liver biopsy

This is the most definitive diagnostic approach, and it is used to identify the intensity of the infection, and the degree of liver damage.

PREPROCEDURE NURSING ACTIONS

- Explain the procedure.
- Witness informed consent.
- Ensure the client fasts starting at midnight on the day of the procedure in case surgery is needed due to a complication. Qci
- Administer medications.

INTRAPROCEDURE NURSING ACTIONS

- Assist the client into the supine position with the upper right quadrant of the abdomen exposed.
- Assist the client with relaxation techniques.
- Instruct the client to exhale and hold for at least 10 seconds while the needle is inserted. Qci
- Instruct the client to resume breathing once the needle is withdrawn.
- Apply pressure to the puncture site.

POSTPROCEDURE NURSING ACTIONS

- Assist the client to a right side–lying position and maintain for several hours.
- Monitor vital signs and for abdominal pain.
- Check for bleeding from the puncture site.
- Observe for manifestations of pneumothorax (dyspnea, cyanosis, restlessness) due to accidental puncture of the pleura or lung.

PATIENT-CENTERED CARE

NURSING CARE

- Most clients will be cared for in the home unless they are acutely ill.
- Enforce contact precautions if indicated.
- Provide a high-carbohydrate, high-calorie, low- to moderate-fat, and low- to moderate-protein diet, and small, frequent meals to promote nutrition and healing.
- Promote hepatic rest and the regeneration of tissue.
  - Administer only necessary medications.
  - Avoid over-the-counter medications or herbal supplements.
  - Avoid alcohol.
  - Limit physical activity.
- Instruct the client and family regarding measures to prevent the transmission of the disease to others at home. Qpcc
  - Avoid sexual intercourse until hepatitis antibody testing is negative.
  - Use proper hand hygiene.
- Provide culturally sensitive care.

MEDICATIONS

Hepatitis A

- Hepatitis A immunization is recommended for postexposure protection.
- Immunoglobulin is recommended for postexposure protection for clients older than 40 years, younger than 12 months, who have chronic liver disease, who are immunosuppressed, or who are allergic to the vaccine.

Hepatitis B, D

Acute infection: No medications; supportive care

Chronic infection: Antiviral medications (adefovir dipivoxil, interferon alfa-2b, peginterferon alfa-2a, lamivudine, entecavir, telbivudine)

Hepatitis C

Combination therapy with peginterferon alfa-2a and ribavirin is the preferred treatment.

Hepatitis E

No medications; supportive care

INTERPROFESSIONAL CARE

Possible consults with infection control, social worker, primary care provider, or community resources

COMPLICATIONS

Chronic hepatitis
- Ongoing inflammation of the liver cells
- Results from hepatitis B, C, or D
- Increases the client's risk for liver cancer

Fulminating hepatitis
- Extremely severe and potentially fatal form of viral hepatitis.
- Clients develop manifestations of viral hepatitis, then within hours or days develop severe liver failure.
- No medications, supportive care.

Cirrhosis of the liver: Permanent scarring of the liver that is usually caused by chronic inflammation

Liver cancer

Liver failure: Irreversible damage to liver cells, with decreased ability to function adequately to meet the body's needs

Cirrhosis

- Cirrhosis is extensive scarring of the liver caused by necrotic injury or a reaction to inflammation over a prolonged period of time. Normal liver tissue is replaced with fibrotic tissue that lacks function.
- Portal and periportal areas of the liver are primarily involved, affecting the liver's ability to handle the flow of bile. Nodules block the bile ducts and normal blood flow throughout the liver. The development of new bile channels causes an overgrowth of tissue and liver scarring/enlargement.

HEALTH PROMOTION AND DISEASE PREVENTION

- Stay current on immunizations.
- Avoid drinking alcohol, and engage in an alcohol recovery program if needed. Qpcc

Types of cirrhosis

Postnecrotic: Caused by viral hepatitis, or some medications or toxins

Laennec's: Caused by chronic alcohol use disorder

Biliary: Caused by chronic biliary obstruction or autoimmune disease

Cardiac: Caused by cor pulmonale from chronic right-sided heart failure

DATA COLLECTION

RISK FACTORS

- Alcohol use disorder
- Chronic viral hepatitis (hepatitis B, C, or D)
- Autoimmune hepatitis (destruction of the liver cells by the immune system)
- Steatohepatitis (fatty liver disease causing chronic inflammation)
- Damage to the liver caused by medications, substances, toxins, and infections
- Chronic biliary cirrhosis (bile duct obstruction, bile stasis, hepatic fibrosis)
- Cardiac cirrhosis resulting from severe right heart failure inducing necrosis and fibrosis due to lack of blood flow

EXPECTED FINDINGS

- Fatigue
- Weight loss, abdominal pain, distention
- Pruritus (severe itching of skin)
- Confusion or difficulty thinking (due to the buildup of waste products in the blood and brain that the liver is unable to get rid of)
- Personality and mentation changes, emotional lability, euphoria, depression

PHYSICAL FINDINGS
- Cognitive changes
- Altered sleep/wake pattern
- Gastroesophageal bleeding (enlarged esophageal veins [varices] develop and burst, causing vomiting and passing of blood in bowel movements) or portal hypertensive gastropathy, which is bleeding of gastric mucosa
- Splenomegaly caused from backup of blood into the spleen, which can cause thrombocytopenia and platelet destruction
- Ascites (bloating or swelling due to fluid buildup in abdomen and legs)
- Jaundice (yellowing of skin) and icterus (yellowing of the eyes) from decreased excretion of bilirubin, resulting in an increase of circulating bilirubin levels
- Petechiae (round, pinpoint, red-purple lesions), ecchymoses (large yellow and purple-blue bruises), nosebleeds, hematemesis, melena (decreased synthesis of prothrombin, deteriorating hepatic function)
- Palmar erythema (redness, warmth of the palms of the hands)
- Spider angiomas (red lesions, vascular in nature with branches radiating on the nose, cheeks, upper thorax, shoulders)
- Dependent peripheral edema of extremities and sacrum
- Asterixis (liver flapping tremor): coarse tremor characterized by rapid, nonrhythmic extension and flexion of the wrists and fingers
- Fetor hepaticus (liver breath): fruity or musty odor

LABORATORY TESTS Q EBP

Serum liver enzymes: Elevated initially

Lactate dehydrogenase (LDH), ALT, and AST are elevated due to hepatic inflammation. ALT and AST return to normal when liver cells are no longer able to create an inflammatory response. ALP increases in cirrhosis due to intrahepatic biliary obstruction.

ALT: Expected reference range 4 to 36 units/L

AST: Expected reference range 0 to 35 units/L

ALP: Expected reference range 30 to 120 units/L

Serum bilirubin: Elevated

Bilirubin levels are elevated in cirrhosis due to the inability of the liver to excrete bilirubin.

Bilirubin, indirect (unconjugated): Elevated (expected reference range 0.2 to 0.8 mg/dL)

Bilirubin, total: Elevated (expected reference range 0.3 to 1.0 mg/dL)

Serum protein

- Decreased due to the lack of hepatic synthesis
- Expected reference range 6.4 to 8.3 g/dL

Serum albumin

- Decreased due to the lack of hepatic synthesis
- Expected reference range 3.5 to 5 g/dL

Hematological tests

RBC: Decreased
- Expected reference range, females 4.2 to 5.4 million/uL
- Expected reference range, males 4.7 to 6.1 million/uL

Hemoglobin: Decreased
- Expected reference range, females 12 to 16 g/dL
- Expected reference range, males 14 to 18 g/dL

Hematocrit: Decreased
- Expected reference range, females 37% to 47%
- Expected reference range, males 42% to 52%

Platelet count: Decreased (expected reference range 150,000 to 400,000/mm³)

PT/INR

- Prolonged due to decreased synthesis of prothrombin
- PT expected reference range 11 to 12.5 sec
- INR expected reference range 0.8 to 1.1

Ammonia levels

- Increase when hepatocellular injury (cirrhosis) prevents the conversion of ammonia to urea for excretion.
- Expected reference range 10 to 80 mcg/dL

Serum creatinine levels

- Can increase due to deteriorating kidney function, which can occur as a result of advanced liver disease
- Expected reference range, females 0.5 to 1.1 mg/dL
- Expected reference range, males 0.6 to 1.3 mg/dL

DIAGNOSTIC PROCEDURES

Ultrasound: Used to detect ascites, hepatomegaly, splenomegaly, biliary stones, biliary obstruction

Abdominal x-rays and CT scan: Used to visualize possible hepatomegaly, ascites, splenomegaly

MRI: Used to visualize mass lesions and determine whether the liver is malignant or benign

Liver biopsy (most definitive)

- A liver biopsy identifies the progression and extent of the cirrhosis.
- To minimize the risk of hemorrhage, a radiologist may perform the biopsy through the jugular vein and down into the hepatic vein to obtain tissue for a microscopic evaluation.
- Fluoroscopy can increase safety for cirrhosis clients due to an increased risk for bleeding complications. Qᴏɪ

Esophagogastroduodenoscopy: Detects the presence of esophageal varices, ulcerations in the stomach, or duodenal ulcers and bleeding. The client undergoes moderate (conscious) sedation.

Endoscopic retrograde cholangiopancreatography: Provides visualization of the biliary tract to assist in removing stones, to collect specimens for biopsy, and for stent placement

PATIENT-CENTERED CARE

NURSING CARE Qᴘᴄᴄ

Respiratory status: Monitor oxygen saturation levels and distress. Provide comfort measures by positioning the client to ease respiratory effort (can be compromised by plasma volume excess and ascites). Have the client sit in a chair or elevate the head of the bed to 30° with feet elevated.

Skin integrity: Monitor closely for skin breakdown. Implement measures to prevent pressure ulcers. Pruritus, which is associated with jaundice, will cause the client to scratch. Encourage washing with cold water and applying lotion to decrease the itching.

Fluid balance: Monitor for indications of fluid volume excess. Keep strict I&O, obtain daily weights, and monitor ascites and peripheral edema. Restrict fluids and sodium if prescribed.

Vital signs: Monitor vital signs and pain level.

Neurological status: Monitor for deteriorating mental status and dementia consistent with hepatic encephalopathy. Monitor for asterixis (coarse tremor of wrists and fingers) and fetor hepaticus (fruity breath odor). Lactulose can be given to aid in excretion of ammonia.

Nutritional status: High-carbohydrate, high-protein, moderate-fat, and low-sodium diet with vitamin supplements such as thiamine, folate, and multivitamins

Gastrointestinal status: In the presence of ascites, measure abdominal girth daily over the largest part of the abdomen. Mark the location of tape for consistency. Observe for potential bleeding complications.

Pain status: Monitor pain. Administer analgesics and gastrointestinal antispasmodics as needed.

MEDICATIONS Qᴇʙᴘ

Because the metabolism of most medications is dependent upon a functioning liver, general medications are administered sparingly (especially opioids, sedatives, barbiturates).

Diuretics: Decrease excessive fluid in the body.

Beta-blocking agent: Used for clients who have varices to prevent bleeding.

Lactulose: Used to promote excretion of ammonia from the body through the stool.

Nonabsorbable antibiotic: An alternative to lactulose.

THERAPEUTIC PROCEDURES

Paracentesis

Used to relieve ascites.

PREPROCEDURE NURSING CARE
- Explain the procedure.
- Witness informed consent.
- Measure vital signs and weight.
- Assist the client to void to reduce the risk of injury to the bladder. Qᴏɪ
- Weigh client.

INTRAPROCEDURE NURSING CARE
- Position the client supine with head of bed elevated.
- Assist the client with relaxation techniques.
- Apply dressing over puncture site.

POSTPROCEDURE NURSING CARE
- Monitor vital signs.
- Maintain bed rest.
- Measure the fluid, and document amount and color.
- Send specimen to the laboratory.
- Check puncture site dressing for drainage.
- Weigh client.

Endoscopic variceal ligation/ endoscopic sclerotherapy

- Varices are either sclerosed or banded endoscopically.
- There is a decreased risk of hemorrhage with banding.

Transjugular intrahepatic portosystemic shunt

Performed in interventional radiology for clients who require further intervention with ascites or hemorrhage.

Surgical bypass shunting procedures

This is a last resort for clients who have portal hypertension and esophageal varices. Ascites is shunted from the abdominal cavity to the superior vena cava.

Liver transplantation

- Portions of healthy livers from deceased donors (most commonly trauma victims) or living donors can be used for transplant.
- The transplanted liver portion will regenerate and grow in size based on the needs of the body.
- The client must meet the transplant criteria to be eligible.
- Clients who have severe cardiac and respiratory disease, metastatic malignant liver cancer, or alcohol/substance use disorder are not candidates for liver transplantation.

PREPROCEDURE NURSING ACTIONS
- Use an interprofessional approach.
- Witness informed consent.

POSTPROCEDURE NURSING ACTIONS Qpcc
- Closely monitor during the immediate postoperative period in an intensive care unit.
- Monitor vital signs frequently.
- Monitor neurological status.
- Monitor for acute graft rejection (tachycardia, fever, right upper quadrant pain, change in bile color or increased jaundice, increased ALT and AST levels).
- Monitor for infection (fever; excessive, foul-smelling drainage).
- Monitor for clotting problems (blood in drainage tubes, petechiae).
- Monitor for hepatic complications (decreased bile drainage, increased right upper quadrant pain with distention, nausea, vomiting, increased jaundice).
- Monitor for acute kidney injury (change in urine output, increased BUN and creatinine levels, electrolyte imbalance).
- Administer immunosuppressant agents.
- Administer antibiotic prophylaxis.
- Obtain blood cultures.
- Keep T-tube in dependent position. Empty frequently, documenting amount and description.

INTERPROFESSIONAL CARE

- A dietitian can assist with specific diet needs.
- Recommend appropriate referrals (social services, Alcoholics Anonymous, Al-Anon).

CLIENT EDUCATION Qpcc

- Abstain from alcohol and engage in an alcohol recovery program if needed.
  - Helps prevent further scarring and fibrosis of liver
  - Allows healing and regeneration of liver tissue
  - Prevents irritation of the stomach and esophagus lining
  - Helps decrease the risk of bleeding
  - Helps prevent other life-threatening complications
- Consult with the provider prior to taking any over-the-counter medications or herbal supplements. Qqi
- Follow diet guidelines.
  - High-calorie, moderate-fat diet
  - Low-sodium diet (if the client has excessive fluid in the peritoneal cavity)
  - Low-protein (if encephalopathy, elevated ammonia)
  - Small, frequent, well-balanced nutritional meals
  - Supplemental vitamin-enriched liquids
  - Replacement and administration of vitamins due to the inability of the liver to store them
  - Fluid intake restrictions if serum sodium is low

COMPLICATIONS

Portal systemic encephalopathy

Clients who have a poorly functioning liver are unable to convert ammonia and other waste products to a less toxic form. These products are carried to the brain and cause neurological manifestations. Clients take medications such as lactulose to reduce the ammonia levels in the body via intestinal excretion. Ammonia is formed when dietary protein is broken down by intestinal flora.

NURSING ACTIONS
- Administer lactulose.
- Monitor laboratory findings, including potassium, because clients can become hypokalemic with increased stools from the lactulose therapy.
- Monitor for changes in the level of consciousness and orientation.
- Report asterixis (flapping of the hands) and fetor hepaticus (liver breath) immediately to the provider. These indicate that encephalopathy is worsening.

CLIENT EDUCATION: Adhere to the prescribed diet.

Esophageal varices

Impaired circulation of blood through the liver causes portal hypertension (elevated blood pressure in veins that carry blood from the intestines to the liver). The body develops collateral circulation, creating varices in the upper stomach and esophagus. Varices are fragile and can bleed easily.

NURSING ACTIONS
- Assist with saline lavage (vasoconstriction), esophagogastric balloon tamponade, blood transfusions, ligation and sclerotherapy, and shunts to stop bleeding and reduce the risk for hypovolemic shock.
- Monitor hemoglobin level and vital signs.
- Monitor for any bleeding.

Acute graft rejection post liver transplantation

Typically occurs between 4 and 10 days after surgery

MANIFESTATIONS OF REJECTION
- Tachycardia
- Upper right flank pain
- Jaundice
- Laboratory findings indicative of liver failure

CAUSES: Graft vs. host disease (recipient's bone marrow creates T-cells to attack the new organ)

NURSING ACTIONS
- Early diagnosis of graft rejection is necessary to successfully prevent total rejection of the liver.
- Administer immunosuppressants.
- Monitor laboratory findings.

CLIENT EDUCATION
- Take immunosuppressants and monitor white blood cell count.
- Report indications of rejection to the provider immediately.

PRACTICE Active Learning Scenario

A nurse is caring for a client who has hepatitis C and will undergo liver biopsy. Use the ATI Active Learning Template: Diagnostic Procedure to complete the following.

DESCRIPTION OF PROCEDURE

NURSING INTERVENTIONS (PRE, INTRA, POST): One each preprocedure, intraprocedure, and postprocedure.

POTENTIAL COMPLICATIONS: Identify one potential complication of the procedure.

Application Exercises

1. A nurse is contributing to the plan of care for a client who has hepatitis B with ascites. Which of the following interventions should the nurse recommend?
   - A. Initiate contact precautions.
   - B. Weigh the client weekly.
   - C. Measure abdominal girth every 48 hr.
   - D. Provide a high-calorie, high-carbohydrate diet.

2. A nurse is reviewing the medical record of a client who has a new diagnosis of hepatitis C. Which of the following laboratory findings should the nurse expect?
   - A. Prothrombin time 8 sec
   - B. Total bilirubin 4.5 mg/dL
   - C. Aspartate aminotransferase (AST) 35 units/L
   - D. Alanine aminotransferase (ALT) 15 IU/L

3. A nurse is collecting data from a client who has advanced cirrhosis. Which of the following findings indicates the client is experiencing hepatic encephalopathy? (Select all that apply.)
   - A. Anorexia
   - B. Change in orientation
   - C. Asterixis
   - D. Ascites
   - E. Fetor hepaticus

4. A nurse is caring for a client who has cirrhosis. Which of the following medications should the nurse expect to administer to this client? (Select all that apply.)
   - A. Diuretic
   - B. Beta-blocking agent
   - C. Opioid analgesic
   - D. Lactulose
   - E. Sedative

5. A nurse is reinforcing teaching with a client who has hepatitis B about home care. Which of the following instructions should the nurse include? (Select all that apply.)
   - A. Limit physical activity.
   - B. Avoid alcohol.
   - C. Take acetaminophen for comfort.
   - D. Wear a mask when in public places.
   - E. Eat small frequent meals.

Application Exercises Key

1. A. Hepatitis B is transmitted via blood. Standard precautions are adequate.

   B. The nurse should plan to obtain daily weights to monitor fluid status.

   C. The nurse should track the client's abdominal girth daily by measuring over the largest part of the abdomen, which will vary by client.

   D. **CORRECT:** The client who has hepatitis B should have a diet high in calories and carbohydrates to promote healing of the liver tissue.

   (N) *NCLEX® Connection: Physiological Adaptation, Basic Pathophysiology*

2. A. The nurse should expect a client who has hepatitis to have a prothrombin time that is within or above the expected reference range due to reduced clotting factor production.

   B. **CORRECT:** The nurse should expect a client who has a new diagnosis of hepatitis C to have an increased total bilirubin; a finding of 4.5 mg/dL is above the expected reference range.

   C. AST is elevated in clients who have hepatitis C infection; 35 units/L is within the expected reference range.

   D. ALT is elevated in clients who have hepatitis C infection; 15 units/L is within the expected reference range.

   (N) *NCLEX® Connection: Reduction of Risk Potential, Laboratory Values*

3. A. Anorexia is present in clients who have liver dysfunction, but is not an indication of hepatic encephalopathy.

   B. **CORRECT:** A change in orientation indicates hepatic encephalopathy due to the effect of toxins on the brain in a client who has advanced cirrhosis.

   C. **CORRECT:** Asterixis, a coarse tremor of the wrists and fingers, is observed as a late complication in a client who has cirrhosis and hepatic encephalopathy. The nurse should report asterixis immediately.

   D. Ascites can be present in a client who has liver dysfunction, but it is not an indication of hepatic encephalopathy.

   E. **CORRECT:** Fetor hepaticus, a fruity breath odor, is a finding of hepatic encephalopathy due to buildup of toxic wastes in the client who has advanced cirrhosis. The nurse should report fetor hepaticus immediately.

   (N) *NCLEX® Connection: Reduction of Risk Potential, Potential for Alterations in Body Systems*

4. A. **CORRECT:** Diuretics facilitate excretion of excess fluid from the body in clients who have cirrhosis.

   B. **CORRECT:** Beta-blocking agents are prescribed for clients who have cirrhosis to prevent bleeding from varices.

   C. The liver metabolizes opioid analgesics. The nurse should not expect to administer this type of medication to a client who has cirrhosis.

   D. **CORRECT:** Lactulose is prescribed for a client who has cirrhosis to aid in the elimination of ammonia in the stool.

   E. The liver metabolizes most sedatives. The nurse should not expect to administer this type of medication to a client who has cirrhosis.

   (N) *NCLEX® Connection: Pharmacological Therapies, Expected Actions/Outcomes*

5. A. **CORRECT:** Limiting physical activity and taking frequent rest breaks conserves energy and assists in the recovery process for a client who has hepatitis B.

   B. **CORRECT:** A client who has hepatitis B should avoid alcohol consumption because it is metabolized in the liver.

   C. A client who has hepatitis B should avoid taking acetaminophen because it is metabolized in the liver and could worsen the client's condition.

   D. Hepatitis B is a blood-borne disease. Wearing a mask is not necessary to prevent transmission to others.

   E. **CORRECT:** The client who has hepatitis B should eat small, frequent meals to promote improved nutrition due to anorexia.

   (N) *NCLEX® Connection: Physiological Adaptation, Alterations in Body Systems*

PRACTICE Answer

Using the ATI Active Learning Template: Diagnostic Procedure

DESCRIPTION OF PROCEDURE: A liver biopsy is a procedure to collect a sample of liver tissue for diagnostic testing. A needle is inserted in the intercostal space between the two right lower ribs and into the liver. An aspirate of liver tissue is then collected.

NURSING ACTIONS (PRE, INTRA, POST)

- Preprocedure
  - Explain the procedure to the client/family.
  - Witness informed consent.
  - Ensure the client has been fasting since midnight.
  - Administer medication.

- Intraprocedure
  - Assist the client into the supine position with the upper right quadrant of the abdomen exposed.
  - Assist the client with relaxation techniques.
  - Instruct the client to exhale and hold for at least 10 seconds while the needle is inserted.
  - Instruct the client to resume breathing once the needle is withdrawn.
  - Apply pressure to the puncture site.

- Postprocedure
  - Assist the client to a right side-lying position and maintain for several hours.
  - Monitor vital signs.
  - Monitor for abdominal pain.
  - Check for bleeding from puncture site.

POTENTIAL COMPLICATIONS

- Bleeding
- Bile peritonitis
- Pneumothorax

(N) *NCLEX® Connection: Reduction of Risk Potential, Potential for Complications of Diagnostic Tests/Treatments/Procedures*

When reviewing the following chapters, keep in mind the relevant topics and tasks of the NCLEX outline, in particular:

Basic Care and Comfort

ELIMINATION: Identify the client at risk for impaired elimination (medication, hydration status).

NONPHARMACOLOGICAL COMFORT INTERVENTIONS
Assist in planning comfort interventions for the client with impaired comfort.

Monitor the client's response to nonpharmacological interventions.

NUTRITION AND ORAL HYDRATION
Monitor the client's intake and output.

Reinforce client teaching on special diets based on the client's diagnosis/nutritional needs and cultural considerations (high protein, kosher diet, calorie restriction).

Reduction of Risk Potential

LABORATORY VALUES: Reinforce client teaching on the purposes of laboratory tests.

POTENTIAL FOR COMPLICATIONS OF DIAGNOSTIC TESTS/TREATMENTS/PROCEDURES
Identify the client's response to diagnostic tests/treatments/procedures.

Identify the client's risk and implement interventions.

Physiological Adaptation

ALTERATIONS IN BODY SYSTEMS: Provide care to the client undergoing peritoneal dialysis.

FLUID AND ELECTROLYTE IMBALANCES
Identify signs and symptoms of fluid and/or electrolyte imbalances.

Provide interventions to restore the client's fluid and/or electrolyte balance.

Monitor the client's response to interventions to correct fluid and/or electrolyte imbalance.

UNEXPECTED RESPONSE TO THERAPIES: Promote recovery of the client from unexpected negative responses to therapy (such as urinary tract infection).

CHAPTER 49 *Renal Diagnostic Procedures*

Renal diagnostic procedures and laboratory assessments evaluate kidney function. By testing kidney function, providers can diagnose diseases and evaluate the efficacy of treatment.

LABORATORY TESTS

Serum creatinine

Results from protein and muscle breakdown
- Increases in creatinine can be the result of kidney disease, urinary obstruction, decreased renal blood flow, or nephrotoxic medications.
- Increases in creatinine reflect a decrease in the ability of the kidney to filter the blood (glomerular filtration rate [GFR]).
- Creatinine levels are dependent upon age and sex.
- Serum creatinine values remain constant in older adults unless they have kidney disease. Ⓖ

Blood urea nitrogen (BUN)

Results from the breakdown of protein in the liver, creating the byproduct urea nitrogen, which is then excreted by the kidneys
- Factors affecting BUN that can be related to liver or kidney function are dehydration, infection, chemotherapy, steroid therapy, and gastrointestinal bleeding.
- The expected reference range for BUN is 10 to 20 mg/dL in adults, with a slightly higher expected value for older adult clients.

Cystatin C

- A protein resulting from cellular metabolism that is used to evaluate GFR.
- Levels are not affected by factors affecting BUN and creatinine levels.
- The expected reference range for females is 0.52 to 0.9 mg/L and males is 0.56 to 0.98 mg/L

Urinalysis

Evaluates waste products from the kidney and detects urologic disorders
- Collection of an early-morning specimen provides a more concentrated sample.
- If urinary tract infection is suspected, a midstream, clean-catch sample should be obtained.
- Urinalysis identifies color; clarity; specific gravity; acidity or alkalinity; and presence of medication and substance metabolites, glucose, ketone bodies, WBCs, RBCs, and protein.
- Glucose, ketone bodies, and protein (including leukocyte esterase and nitrites) are not usually present in urine and can indicate diabetes mellitus; fat metabolism; infection; or, after a cytology analysis, cancer.
- Urine for culture and sensitivity identifies bacteria and determines the type of antibiotic to treat the infection.
- A 24-hr urine collection measures creatinine, urea nitrogen, sodium, chloride, calcium, catecholamines, and proteins.
  - **Guidelines for collecting a 24-hr urine specimen**
    - Reinforce client teaching regarding the testing procedure.
      - Void prior to defecating.
      - Avoid placing toilet paper into urine collection container.
    - To begin the test, have the client void. The test begins at the time of first void. This first void is discarded. However, all subsequent urine is collected for the next 24 hr.
    - Post notices on the client's medical record and over the toilet alerting all personnel of the ongoing test.
    - Collect all urine voided over the next 24 hr in an approved container that is kept on ice or refrigerated.
    - Collect the last urine sample as close to the end of the 24 hr as possible.
    - Take laboratory requisition and container with the urine to the laboratory.
    - The test must be restarted if any urine is missed.
- A 24-hr collection for creatinine clearance measures the GFR for clients who have impaired kidney function.

RENAL DIAGNOSTIC PROCEDURES

Radiography (x-ray)

- An x-ray of the kidneys, ureters, and bladder (KUB or a "flat plate")
- Allows for visualization of structures and to detect renal calculi, strictures, calcium deposits, or obstructions

NURSING ACTIONS
- Ask female clients if they are pregnant.
- Tell clients to remove clothes over the area and all jewelry and metal objects.

COMPLICATIONS: No known complications

CT scan

- Provides cross sectional imaging of the renal system to check for kidney size, obstruction or structural abnormalities, cysts, or masses.
- IV contrast dye (iodine-based) enhances images.

NURSING ACTIONS
- Evaluate for client iodine allergy if contrast is to be used.
- Determine if client is claustrophobic.
- Encourage fluid intake following procedure to increase renal elimination of dye.
- Monitor for allergic reaction to dye (dyspnea, tachycardia, rash, pruritus). Qs
- Monitor urinary output following the procedure.

COMPLICATIONS: Dye can cause acute kidney injury.

MRI

- Provides three-dimensional images of renal system.
- Useful for staging cancer and determining the presence of trauma. Similar to a CT.
- Clients lie down and have to remain still for the test.

CONTRAINDICATIONS: Implanted metal objects (pacemakers, surgical clips, inner ear implants, metal fragments in eyes, implanted ports)

COMPLICATIONS: Poor imaging if a client is unable to lie still

Ultrasound

- Determines the size of kidneys; images the ureters, bladder, masses, cysts, calculi, and obstructions of the lower urinary tract.
- Measures urine content in the bladder.
- Good alternative to excretory urography.

NURSING ACTIONS: Provide skin care by removing gel after the procedure.

COMPLICATIONS: Minimal risk for the client

Cystography, cystourethrography, voiding cystourethrogram (VCUG)

- Detects urethral or bladder injury after instillation of contrast dye through a urinary catheter to provide an image of the bladder (cystography) and the ureters (cystourethrography).
- VCUG detects via an x-ray during urination whether urine refluxes into the ureters.

NURSING ACTIONS
- Determine the presence of client allergy to iodine contrast media. Qs
- Ask female clients if they are pregnant.
- Monitor for infection for the first 72 hr after the procedure.
- Encourage increased fluid intake to dilute urine and minimize burning on urination.
- Monitor urine output (less than 30 mL/hr) if suspected pelvic or urethral trauma.
- Contrast dye does not reach the bloodstream or the kidneys and is not nephrotoxic.

COMPLICATIONS: Urinary tract infection due to catheter placement
- Cloudy, foul-smelling urine
- Urgency
- Urine positive for leukocyte esterase and nitrites, sediment, and RBCs

Kidney biopsy

Removal of a sample of tissue by excision or needle aspiration for cytological (histological) examination
- Clients receive sedation and ongoing monitoring.

PREPROCEDURE NURSING ACTIONS
- Ensure informed consent is obtained.
- Review coagulation studies.
- Nothing by mouth for 4 to 6 hr.

POSTPROCEDURE NURSING ACTIONS
- Ensure client remains on bed rest for 6 to 24 hr following procedure
- Monitor vital signs following sedation.
- Monitor dressings and urinary output (hematuria). Hematuria should decrease with time and no longer be present 24 hr following procedure
- Review Hgb and Hct values.
- Administer PRN pain medication.
- Encourage fluid intake (unless contraindicated)
- Monitor for indications of hemorrhage (hypotension; tachycardia; back, flank, or shoulder pain; dizziness).
- Monitor for indications of liver or bowel perforation (decreased bowel sounds, pain, rigidity, and guarding of abdomen).

COMPLICATIONS
- Hemorrhage
- Infection
  - Cloudy, foul-smelling urine
  - Urgency
  - Urine positive for leukocyte esterase and nitrites, sediment, and RBCs

CLIENT EDUCATION Qpcc
- Avoid strenuous activities for 2 weeks.
- Report increased temperature, bleeding, or burning with urination to the provider.

Cystoscopy, cystourethroscopy

Used to discover abnormalities of bladder wall (cystoscopy) or occlusions of ureter or urethra (cystourethroscopy) by direct visualization
- Clients receive anesthesia for the procedure.

NURSING ACTIONS
- Check for indications of bleeding and infection. Monitor for infection for the first 72 hr after the procedure.
- PREPROCEDURE
  - Ensure informed consent is obtained
  - NPO after midnight.
  - Administer laxative or enemas for bowel preparation the night before the procedure.

- **INTRAPROCEDURE**
  - Monitor vital signs.
  - General and local anesthesia are options.
  - Place the client in lithotomy position.
- **POSTPROCEDURE**
  - Monitor vital signs and urine output.
  - Document the amount and color of urine (can be pink-tinged).
  - Irrigate urinary catheter with a solution of mannitol or sorbitol irrigation if blood clots are present or the urine output is decreased or absent.
  - Encourage oral fluids to increase urine output and reduce any burning sensation with urination.
  - Instruct client to call for assistance prior to standing or walking.
  - Monitor for manifestations of infection or sepsis (hyperpyrexia, flushing, chills, hypotension, tachycardia).

COMPLICATIONS
- Possible urinary tract infection/sepsis from instrumentation
  - Cloudy, foul-smelling urine
  - Urgency
  - Urine positive for leukocyte esterase, nitrites, sediment, and RBCs
- Urinary retention
- Perforation of bladder or ureters

CLIENT EDUCATION Qpcc
- Monitor and report urinary retention, red-tinged urine, and increasing pain in lower abdomen.
- Increase oral fluid intake to decrease dysuria and reduce the risk of infection.
- Report fever, shaking chills, or prolonged dysuria.
- Discomfort can be managed with the use of warm sitz baths or warm moist compresses to the lower abdomen.

Retrograde pyelogram, cystogram, urethrogram

- Identifies obstruction or structural disorders of the ureters and renal pelvis of the kidneys (pyelogram) by instilling contrast dye during a cystoscopy
- Identifies fistulas, diverticula, stones and tumors in the bladder (cystogram) and urethra (urethrogram) by instilling contrast dye during a cystoscopy

PREPROCEDURE NURSING ACTIONS
- Ensure informed consent is obtained.
- NPO after midnight. (Older adult clients can have reduced fasting times.)
- Administer laxative or enemas for bowel preparation the night before the procedure.
- Check for iodine allergy.
- Review kidney function studies.
- Ask female clients if they are pregnant.

POSTPROCEDURE NURSING ACTIONS
- Monitor vital signs and urine output.
- Document the amount and color of urine (can be pink-tinged).
- Encourage oral fluids to increase urine output.
- Monitor the administration of intravenous fluids.
- Instruct clients to call for assistance prior to standing or walking.

- Monitor for manifestations of infection or sepsis (fever, flushing, chills, hypotension, tachycardia).
- Clients who take metformin are at increased risk for hypoglycemia and acidosis. Metformin should be held for 24 hr prior to and following the procedure pending kidney function studies.
- Older adult clients are at increased risk of acute kidney injury and weakness. Ⓖ

COMPLICATIONS
- Possible urinary tract infection/sepsis from instrumentation
  - Cloudy, foul-smelling urine
  - Urgency
  - Urine positive for leukocyte esterase, nitrites, sediment, and RBCs
- Urinary retention
- Perforation of bladder or ureters

Renal scan

- Checks renal blood flow and estimates GFR after IV injection of radioactive material to produce a scanned image of the kidneys
- Determines the presence of renovascular hypertension

PREPROCEDURE NURSING ACTIONS
- Ask female clients if they are pregnant.
- Encourage the client to drink fluids prior to the scan.

POSTPROCEDURE NURSING ACTIONS
- Check blood pressure frequently during and after the procedure if the client receives captopril during the procedure to change the blood flow to the kidneys.
- Alert clients about possible orthostatic hypotension following the procedure if they received captopril.
- Increase fluid intake if hypotension occurs and also to promote excretion of the radioisotope.

COMPLICATIONS
- Radioactive material does not cause nephrotoxicity.
- Clients are not at risk from radioactive material they excrete in the urine.

Excretory urography

Detects obstruction and parenchymal masses, and determines the size of the kidneys. IV contrast dye (iodine-based) enhances the images.

NURSING ACTIONS: Same as KUB
- **PREPROCEDURE**
  - Encourage increased fluids the day before procedure.
  - Bowel cleansing with a laxative or an enema to remove fecal contents, fluid, and gas from the colon for a clearer visualization.
  - NPO after midnight.
  - Determine allergies to iodine, seafood, eggs, milk, or chocolate, or if the client has asthma.
  - Check creatinine and BUN levels.
  - Withhold metformin for 24 hr before the procedure (risk for lactic acidosis from contrast dye with iodine).

- **POSTPROCEDURE**
  - Monitor parenteral fluid administration and encourage oral fluids to flush dye through the renal system and prevent complications.
  - Diuretics can increase dye excretion.
  - Check creatinine and BUN serum levels before resuming metformin.

COMPLICATIONS

- Dye can cause acute kidney injury.
- Possible urinary tract infection/sepsis from instrumentation
  - Cloudy, foul-smelling urine
  - Urgency
  - Urine positive for leukocyte esterase, nitrites, sediment, and RBCs

CONSIDERATIONS FOR OLDER ADULT CLIENTS

- Kidney size and function decrease with aging. ©
- Blood flow adaptability decreases, especially during a hypotensive or hypertensive crisis.
- GFR decreases by half the rate of a young adult.
- Diabetes mellitus, hypertension, and heart failure can affect GFR.
- Kidney injury can occur more easily from contrast dyes and medication due to decreased kidney size, blood flow, and GFR.
- Tubular changes can cause urgency and nocturnal polyuria.
- A weak urinary sphincter muscle in females, tissue atrophy related to menopause, and a shorter urethra can cause incontinence and urinary tract infections.
- An enlarged prostate can cause urinary retention and infection.
- Bladder muscle weakening can cause incomplete emptying of the bladder.
- More frequent urination is the result of decreased bladder capacity and decreased ability of the kidneys to concentrate urine.

Application Exercises

1. A nurse is reinforcing teaching with a client who will have an x-ray of the kidneys, ureters, and bladder. Which of the following statements should the nurse include?

   A. "You will receive contrast dye during the procedure."

   B. "An enema is necessary before the procedure."

   C. "You will need to lie in a prone position during the procedure."

   D. "The procedure determines whether you have a kidney stone."

2. A nurse is monitoring a client who had a kidney biopsy for postoperative complications. Which of the following complications should the nurse identify as causing the greatest risk to the client?

   A. Infection

   B. Hemorrhage

   C. Hematuria

   D. Pain

3. A nurse is caring for a client who has type 2 diabetes mellitus and will have excretory urography. Prior to the procedure, which of the following actions should the nurse take? (Select all that apply.)

   A. Identify an allergy to seafood.

   B. Withhold metformin for 24 hr.

   C. Administer an enema.

   D. Obtain a serum coagulation profile.

   E. Check for asthma.

4. A nurse is preparing to begin a 24-hr urine collection for a client. Which of the following actions should the nurse take?

   A. Store collected urine in a designated container at room temperature.

   B. Discard the first voiding when beginning the test.

   C. Post a notice on the client's door regarding the testing.

   D. Document any urine collection that was missed during the 24 hr of the testing.

5. A nurse is collecting data from a client who has returned to the medical-surgical unit following a CT scan of the kidneys with IV contrast. Which of the following findings should the nurse identify as an indication the client is experiencing an allergic reaction to the contrast material?

   A. Bradycardia

   B. Pink-tinged urine

   C. Hyperpyrexia

   D. Pruritus

PRACTICE Active Learning Scenario

A nurse is contributing to the plan of care for a client who will undergo a cystoscopy with retrograde pyelogram. What information should the nurse recommend for the plan of care? Use the ATI Active Learning Template: Diagnostic Procedure to complete this item.

DESCRIPTION OF PROCEDURE: Define the procedure.

INDICATIONS: Identify one indication for cystoscopy and two for retrograde pyelogram.

NURSING INTERVENTIONS (PRE, INTRA, POST): Describe two nursing actions for preprocedure and two for postprocedure.

Application Exercises Key

1. A. Clients do not receive any contrast dye for this procedure as they would for excretory urography.

   B. Clients do not receive an enema before this procedure because it does not affect the gastrointestinal system.

   C. The client will lie supine, not prone.

   D. **CORRECT:** The nurse should explain to the client that a KUB can identify renal calculi, strictures, calcium deposits, and obstructions of the urinary system.

   Ⓝ *NCLEX® Connection: Reduction of Risk Potential, Potential for Complications of Diagnostic Tests/Treatments/Procedures*

2. A. The client is at risk for infection of the kidney because a biopsy is an invasive procedure. However, another complication is the priority.

   B. **CORRECT:** The greatest risk to the client following a kidney biopsy is hemorrhage due to a lack of clotting at the puncture site. The nurse should report this finding to the provider immediately.

   C. The client is at risk for hematuria, which is a common complication during the first 48 to 72 hr after the biopsy. However, another complication is the priority.

   D. The client is at risk for pain after a kidney biopsy because blood in and around the kidney causes pressure on the nerves in the area. However, another complication is the priority.

   Ⓝ *NCLEX® Connection: Reduction of Risk Potential, Potential for Complications from Surgical Procedures and Health Alterations*

3. A. **CORRECT:** Clients who have an allergy to seafood are at higher risk for an allergic reaction to the contrast dye they will receive during the procedure.

   B. **CORRECT:** Clients who take metformin are at risk for lactic acidosis from the contrast dye with iodine they will receive during the procedure.

   C. **CORRECT:** Clients should receive an enema to remove fecal contents, fluid, and gas from the colon for a more clear visualization.

   D. A serum coagulation profile is essential for a client prior to a kidney biopsy because of the risk of hemorrhage from the procedure.

   E. **CORRECT:** Clients who have asthma have a higher risk of an exacerbation as an allergic response to the contrast dye they will receive during the procedure.

   Ⓝ *NCLEX® Connection: Reduction of Risk Potential, Potential for Complications of Diagnostic Tests/Treatments/Procedures*

4. A. The nurse should store collected urine in an approved container that is kept on ice or refrigerated.

   B. **CORRECT:** The nurse should begin the testing period after discarding the first voiding.

   C. The nurse should post notices on the client's medical record and over the toilet alerting all personnel of the ongoing test. However, placing a notice on the client's door is a violation of privacy laws.

   D. In the event the client urinates without collecting it in the approved container, the test must be started again. A full 24 hr of urine collection is needed for accurate testing.

   Ⓝ *NCLEX® Connection: Pharmacological Therapies, Expected Actions/Outcomes*

5. A. A client who has an allergic reaction to contrast media can experience tachycardia rather than bradycardia.

   B. A client who undergoes cystoscopic examination can have pink-tinged urine. However, this is not an indication of an allergic reaction to contrast media.

   C. A client who develops a urinary tract infection following an invasive renal diagnostic test (cystogram, pyelogram) can develop a fever. However, hyperpyrexia is not an indication of an allergic response to contrast media.

   D. **CORRECT:** A client who develops an allergic reaction to contrast media used during a CT of the renal pelvis can experience manifestations such as tachycardia, dyspnea, rash, and pruritus.

   Ⓝ *NCLEX® Connection: Reduction of Risk Potential, Potential for Complications of Diagnostic Tests/Treatments/Procedures*

PRACTICE Answer

Using ATI Active Learning Template: Diagnostic Procedure

DESCRIPTION OF PROCEDURE
- Cystoscopy is instrumentation into the urinary tract to inspect the bladder wall.
- Retrograde pyelogram is the injection of dye up the ureters to inspect the ureters and pelvis of the kidney.

INDICATIONS
- Cystoscopy discovers abnormalities of the bladder wall (cysts, tumors, stones).
- Retrograde pyelogram discovers obstructions or structural disorders of the ureters and kidney pelvis (strictures, stones, mass).

NURSING INTERVENTIONS (PRE, INTRA, POST)
- Preprocedure
  - Ensure informed consent is obtained.
  - NPO after midnight.
  - Administer laxative or enemas for bowel preparation the night before the procedure.
  - Check client for iodine allergy.
  - Review kidney function studies.
  - Ask female clients if they are pregnant.

- Postprocedure
  - Monitor vital signs and urine output.
  - Document the amount and color of urine (can be pink-tinged).
  - Irrigate urinary catheter with a solution of mannitol or sorbitol irrigation if blood clots are present or the urine output is decreased or absent.
  - Encourage oral fluids to increase urine output.
  - Monitor the administration of IV fluids.
  - Instruct the client to call for assistance prior to standing or walking.
  - Monitor for manifestations of infection or sepsis.
  - Clients who take metformin are at increased risk for hypoglycemia and acidosis. Metformin should be held for 24 hr prior to and following the procedure pending kidney function studies.

Ⓝ *NCLEX® Connection: Reduction of Risk Potential, Potential for Complications from Surgical Procedures and Health Alterations*

UNIT 8   NURSING CARE OF CLIENTS WHO
HAVE RENAL DISORDERS
SECTION: DIAGNOSTIC AND THERAPEUTIC PROCEDURES

CHAPTER 50 *Hemodialysis and Peritoneal Dialysis*

Dialysis can sustain life for clients who have acute kidney injury or chronic kidney disease. Dialysis does not replace the hormonal functions of the kidneys. Two types of dialysis are hemodialysis and peritoneal dialysis.

FUNCTIONS OF DIALYSIS

- Rids the body of excess fluid and electrolytes
- Achieves acid-base balance
- Eliminates waste products
- Restores internal homeostasis by osmosis, diffusion, and ultrafiltration

Hemodialysis

Hemodialysis shunts blood from the body through a dialyzer and back into circulation. Hemodialysis requires vascular access.

INDICATIONS

POTENTIAL DIAGNOSES

- Acute kidney injury
- Chronic kidney disease
- Substance overdose
- Persistent hyperkalemia
- Hypervolemia that does not respond to diuretics

CLIENT PRESENTATION

- Fluid volume changes, electrolyte and pH imbalances, and nitrogenous wastes.
- Hemodialysis is based on manifestations, not the glomerular filtration rate.
- Manifestations include fluid overload, neurological changes, bleeding, and uremia (cognitive impairment, pruritus, nausea, vomiting).

CONSIDERATIONS

PREPROCEDURE

NURSING ACTIONS

- Check for informed consent.
- The client will have a temporary hemodialysis dual-lumen catheter or subcutaneous device until the provider inserts a long-term device and it is available for access. Specifically trained staff will access and maintain these accesses.
- Monitor the patency of a long-term device: arteriovenous (AV) fistula or AV graft (presence of bruit, palpable thrill, adequate distal pulses, and evidence of peripheral perfusion).
- Communicate with the health care team the need to avoid measuring blood pressure, administering injections, performing venipunctures, or inserting IV catheters on or into the client's arm that has an access site. Elevate the extremity following surgical creation of an AV fistula to reduce swelling.
- Obtain vital signs, laboratory values (BUN, serum creatinine, electrolytes, Hct), and weight.
- Discuss medications to withhold until after dialysis with the provider. Withhold any dialyzable medications and medications that lower blood pressure.

CLIENT EDUCATION: Clients will need hemodialysis three times per week, for 3- to 5-hr sessions. The provider will insert two needles, one into an artery and the other into a vein.

POSTPROCEDURE

NURSING ACTIONS

- Monitor vital signs and laboratory values (BUN, serum creatinine, electrolytes, Hct). Decreases in blood pressure and changes in laboratory values are common following dialysis.
- Compare the client's preprocedure weight with the postprocedure weight as a way to estimate the amount of fluid the procedure removed.

  1 L fluid equals 1 kg (2.2 lb).

- Monitor for the following.
  ○ Complications (hypotension, clotting of vascular access, headache, muscle cramps, bleeding, cardiac dysrhythmias)
  ○ Indications of bleeding or infection at the access site
  ○ Manifestations of disequilibrium syndrome (mental status changes, seizures, headache, vomiting)
  ○ Manifestations of hypovolemia (hypotension, dizziness, tachycardia)
- Avoid invasive procedures for 4 to 6 hr after dialysis due to the risk of bleeding as a result of anticoagulation.

CLIENT EDUCATION

- AV fistula or AV graft precautions. **Qs**
- Alert the nurse of early indications of disequilibrium syndrome, such as nausea and headache.
- Check the access site at intervals following dialysis. Apply light pressure if bleeding.

- Check the graft for patency by checking for a thrill or bruit.
- Monitor the access site for manifestations of infection, such as fever, redness, drainage, or swelling.
- Contact the provider if bleeding from the insertion site lasts longer than 30 min following dialysis, for no thrill/bruit, or manifestations of infection.
- Take medications and supplements to replace folate loss.
- Eat well-balanced meals to include foods high in folate (beans, green vegetables), and take supplements. Each exchange during dialysis depletes protein, requiring the client to increase protein intake over predialysis limitations, but it still might require some restriction.
- Avoid lifting heavy objects with the access-site arm.
- Avoid carrying objects that compress or constrict the extremity.
- Avoid sleeping on top of the extremity with the access device.
- Perform hand exercises that promote fistula maturation.

COMPLICATIONS

Clotting/infection of the access site

- Anticoagulants prevent blood clots from forming.
- Cannulation can introduce infections at the access site.
- Immunosuppressive disorders increase the risk for infection.
- Advanced age is a risk factor for dialysis-induced hypotension and access site complications due to chronic illnesses or fragile veins. Ⓖ

NURSING ACTIONS
- Monitor for hemorrhage at the insertion site.
- Ensure aseptic technique for device cannulation.
- Avoid compression of the access site.
- Avoid venipuncture or blood pressure measurements on the extremity with the access site.
- Check the graft site for a palpable thrill or audible bruit indicating vascular flow.
- Monitor the access site for redness, swelling, and drainage.
- Monitor for fever.

Disequilibrium syndrome

Disequilibrium syndrome results from too rapid a decrease of BUN and circulating fluid volume. It can result in cerebral edema and increased intracranial pressure.
- Early recognition of disequilibrium syndrome is essential. Manifestations include nausea, vomiting, changes in level of consciousness, seizures, and agitation.
- Advanced age is a risk factor for dialysis disequilibrium and hypotension due to rapid changes in fluid and electrolyte status. Ⓖ

NURSING ACTIONS
- Implement seizure precautions.
- Monitor for and report manifestations of disequilibrium syndrome.

Hypotension

Antihypertensive therapy and rapid fluid depletion during dialysis can cause hypotension.

NURSING ACTIONS
- Monitor for indications of hypotension.
- Lower the head of the bed.

Anemia

Blood loss and removal of folate during dialysis can contribute to the anemia that often accompanies chronic kidney disease (from decreased RBC production due to decreased erythropoietin secretion).

NURSING ACTIONS
- Administer erythropoietin to stimulate the production of RBC.
- Monitor Hgb and RBC level.
- Monitor for hypotension and tachycardia.
- Assist with blood product replacement therapy.

Infectious diseases

Blood transfusions and frequent blood access due to hemodialysis pose a risk for transmission of bloodborne infections such as HIV and hepatitis B and C.

NURSING ACTIONS
- Use sterile equipment and skin antisepsis.
- Use standard precautions.

Peritoneal dialysis

- Peritoneal dialysis involves instillation of hypertonic dialysate solution into the peritoneal cavity and subsequent dwell times followed by drainage of the dialysate solution that includes the waste products. The peritoneum serves as the filtration membrane.
- The client should have an intact peritoneal membrane, without adhesions from infection or multiple surgeries.

INDICATIONS

- Peritoneal dialysis is the treatment of choice for the older adults who require dialysis.
- Peritoneal dialysis treats clients requiring dialysis who:
  - Are unable to tolerate anticoagulation.
  - Have difficulty with vascular access.
  - Have a chronic infection or are unstable.
  - Have a chronic disease, such as diabetes mellitus, heart failure, or severe hypertension.

CONSIDERATIONS

PREPROCEDURE

NURSING ACTIONS
- Determine dry weight (without dialysate instillation), vital signs, serum electrolytes, creatinine, BUN, and blood glucose.
- Determine the client's ability to self-perform peritoneal dialysis and follow sterile technique.
  - Level of alertness
  - Past experience with dialysis
  - Understanding of procedure
- Instruct the client about the procedure.

CLIENT EDUCATION
- The client can feel a sensation of fullness when the dialysate is dwelling. There can be discomfort initially with dialysate infusion.
- Continuous ambulatory peritoneal dialysis (CAPD) requires 7 days/week for 4 to 8 hr. Clients can continue normal activities during CAPD.
- Continuous-cycle peritoneal dialysis (CCPD) is a 24-hr dialysis. The exchange occurs at night while the client is sleeping. The final exchange is left in to dwell during the day.
- Automated peritoneal dialysis (APD) is a 30-min exchange repeated over 8 to 10 hr while the client is sleeping.

INTRAPROCEDURE

NURSING ACTIONS
- Monitor vital signs frequently during initial dialysis of clients in an acute setting
- Monitor serum glucose level (dialysate contains glucose, a hypertonic solution).
- Record the amount of inflow compared to outflow of dialysate.
- Monitor the color (should be clear, light yellow) and amount (should equal or exceed the amount of dialysate inflow) of outflow.
- Monitor for manifestations of infection (fever; bloody, cloudy, or frothy dialysate return; drainage at access site) and for complications (respiratory distress, abdominal pain, insufficient outflow, discolored outflow).
- Check the access site dressing for wetness (risk of dialysate leakage) and exit-site infections.
- Warm the dialysate prior to instilling. Avoid the use of microwave ovens, which cause uneven heating.
- Adhere to the times for infusion, dwell, and outflow.
- Maintain surgical asepsis of the catheter insertion site and when accessing the catheter.
- Keep the outflow bag lower than the client's abdomen (drain by gravity, prevent reflux).
- Reposition the client if inflow or outflow is inadequate.
- Carefully milk the peritoneal dialysis catheter if a fibrin clot has formed.
- Provide emotional support to the client and family.

POSTPROCEDURE

NURSING ACTIONS: Monitor weight, serum electrolytes, creatinine, BUN, and blood glucose.

CLIENT EDUCATION
- Home care of the access site.
- How to perform peritoneal dialysis exchanges at home. Provide support for home peritoneal dialysis with home visits. Q℗cc
- Seek additional information from the National Kidney Foundation for local support groups.
- Follow instructions carefully and take all medications.
- Take essential minerals and vitamins with supplements of phosphorus, calcium, sodium, and potassium.
- Older adult clients might be unable to care for a peritoneal access site due to cognitive or physical deficits. ©
- Body image changes from bloating can be a concern.

COMPLICATIONS

Peritonitis

Peritoneal dialysis can allow micro-organisms into the peritoneum and cause peritonitis.

NURSING ACTIONS
- Maintain surgical asepsis during the procedure.
- Monitor for infection, such as fever, purulent drainage, redness, swelling, and cloudy or discolored drained dialysate.

CLIENT EDUCATION
- Use strict sterile technique during exchanges.
- Notify the provider about any indications of infection.

Infection at the access site

- Infection at the access site can result from leakage of dialysate. Access-site infections can cause peritonitis.
- Older adults are at increased risk for access site complications due to chronic illnesses and fragile veins. ©

NURSING ACTIONS
- Maintain surgical asepsis at the access site.
- Observe the site for wetness from a leaking catheter.
- Monitor for infection (fever, purulent drainage, redness, swelling).

CLIENT EDUCATION
- Use strict sterile technique during exchanges.
- Notify the provider of any indications of infection. Qs
- Watch the site for leakage, and prevent tugging or twisting of the tubing.

Protein loss

Peritoneal dialysis can remove protein from the blood as well as excess fluid, wastes, and electrolytes.

NURSING ACTIONS
- Increase the client's dietary intake of protein over predialysis restrictions.
- Monitor serum albumin levels.

CLIENT EDUCATION: Follow the renal diet with an increase in dietary protein.

Hyperglycemia and hyperlipidemia

- Hyperglycemia can result from the hyperosmolarity of the dialysate.
- The blood can absorb glucose from the dialysate.
- Hyperlipidemia can also occur from long-term therapy and lead to hypertension.

NURSING ACTIONS
- Monitor serum glucose.
- Administer insulin for glycemic control.
- Administer antilipemic medication for triglyceride control.

CLIENT EDUCATION
- Check serum glucose.
- Follow the diet the provider recommends.
- Take antihypertensive medications for elevated blood pressure.

Poor dialysate inflow or outflow

- Obstruction or twisting of the tubing can decrease the flow.
- Constipation is a common cause of poor inflow or outflow.

NURSING ACTIONS
- Reposition the client if inflow or outflow is inadequate.
- Milk the tubing to break up fibrin clots.
- Check the tubing for kinks or closed clamps.

CLIENT EDUCATION
- Avoid constipation by using stool softeners and consuming a diet high in fiber.
- Check the tubing for kinks. The client should know how to remove a fibrin clot.
- Monitor the inflow and outflow, and change position or lower or raise the dialysate bag to improve flow.
- Prevent constipation with diet and stool softeners.
- Lie supine with head slightly elevated during CCPD and APD treatment.

Application Exercises

1. A nurse is reinforcing teaching with a client who has chronic kidney disease and is to begin hemodialysis. Which of the following information should the nurse include?

   A. Hemodialysis restores kidney function.

   B. Hemodialysis replaces hormonal function of the renal system.

   C. Hemodialysis allows an unrestricted diet.

   D. Hemodialysis returns a balance to serum electrolytes.

2. A nurse is caring for a client who has acute kidney injury and is scheduled for hemodialysis. Which of the following actions should the nurse take? (Select all that apply.)

   A. Review the medications the client currently takes.

   B. Check the AV fistula for a bruit.

   C. Calculate the client's hourly urine output.

   D. Measure the client's weight.

   E. Check serum electrolytes.

   F. Use the access site area for venipuncture.

3. A nurse is contributing to the plan of care for a client who received hemodialysis. Which of the following interventions should the nurse recommend? (Select all that apply.)

   A. Check BUN and serum creatinine.

   B. Administer medications the nurse withheld prior to dialysis.

   C. Observe for manifestations of hypovolemia.

   D. Monitor the access site for bleeding.

   E. Measure blood pressure on the extremity with AV access.

4. A nurse is caring for a client who develops disequilibrium syndrome after receiving hemodialysis. Which of the following actions should the nurse take?

   A. Administer an opioid medication.

   B. Monitor for hypertension.

   C. Check level of consciousness.

   D. Recommend an increase in the dialysis exchange rate.

5. A nurse is caring for a client who will undergo peritoneal dialysis. Which of the following actions should the nurse plan to take? (Select all that apply.)

   A. Monitor serum glucose levels.

   B. Report cloudy dialysate return.

   C. Warm the dialysate in a microwave oven.

   D. Monitor for shortness of breath.

   E. Check the access site dressing for wetness.

   F. Maintain medical asepsis when accessing the catheter insertion site.

PRACTICE Active Learning Scenario

A nurse is reviewing complications that a client can develop from peritoneal dialysis. What complications and nursing actions should the nurse include in the review? Use the ATI Active Learning Template: Diagnostic Procedure to complete this item.

DESCRIPTION OF PROCEDURE: Write out the name, and define the diagnostic test.

POTENTIAL COMPLICATIONS: List three.

NURSING INTERVENTIONS: List two nursing actions for each of the three complications.

Application Exercises Key

1. A. Hemodialysis does not restore kidney function, but it sustains the life of a client who has chronic kidney disease.

   B. Hemodialysis does not replace hormonal function of the renal system due to tissue damage causing dysfunction of the renin-angiotensin-aldosterone system.

   C. Hemodialysis does not allow an unrestricted diet. It requires a diet high in folate and more protein than predialysis restrictions allowed, and low in sodium, potassium, and phosphorus.

   D. **CORRECT:** The nurse should explain to the client that hemodialysis restores electrolyte balance by removing excess sodium, potassium, fluids, and waste products, and also restores acid-base balance.

   Ⓝ *NCLEX® Connection: Reduction of Risk Potential, Therapeutic Procedures*

2. A. **CORRECT:** By reviewing the medications the client currently takes, the nurse can determine which medications to withhold until after dialysis.

   B. **CORRECT:** Checking the AV fistula for a bruit determines the patency of the fistula for dialysis.

   C. The client's hourly urine output can vary with the remaining kidney function and does not determine the need for dialysis.

   D. **CORRECT:** Measuring the client's weight before dialysis is essential for comparing it with the client's weight after dialysis.

   E. **CORRECT:** Checking the serum electrolytes determines the need for dialysis and can help with evaluating effectiveness of the dialysis.

   F. The nurse should never use the access site area for venipuncture because compression from the tourniquet can cause loss of the vascular access.

   Ⓝ *NCLEX® Connection: Reduction of Risk Potential, Potential for Complications of Diagnostic Tests/Treatments/Procedures*

3. A. **CORRECT:** The nurse should check the BUN and serum creatinine to determine the presence and degree of uremia or waste products that remain following dialysis.

   B. **CORRECT:** Prior to dialysis, the nurse should withhold medications the treatment can partially dialyze. After the treatment, the nurse should administer the previously held medications.

   C. **CORRECT:** A client who is postdialysis is at risk for hypovolemia due to a rapid decease in fluid volume.

   D. **CORRECT:** The nurse should monitor the access site for bleeding because the client receives heparin during the procedure to prevent clotting of blood.

   E. The nurse should never measure blood pressure on the extremity that has the AV access site because it can cause collapse of the AV fistula or graft.

   Ⓝ *NCLEX® Connection: Reduction of Risk Potential, Therapeutic Procedures*

4. A. The nurse should not administer an opioid medication because it can make it difficult to monitor the client's condition. The provider can prescribe medication to decrease seizure activity.

   B. The nurse should monitor for hypotension due to rapid change in fluids and electrolytes causing disequilibrium syndrome.

   C. **CORRECT:** The nurse should check the client's level of consciousness. A rapid change in urea levels following hemodialysis can cause increased intracranial pressure and decrease the client's level of consciousness.

   D. The nurse should recommend a decrease the dialysis exchange rate, as disequilibrium syndrome is caused by rapid changes in fluid and electrolyte status.

   Ⓝ *NCLEX® Connection: Reduction of Risk Potential, Potential for Complications of Diagnostic Tests/Treatments/Procedures*

5. A. **CORRECT:** The nurse should monitor serum glucose levels because the dialysate solution contains glucose.

   B. **CORRECT:** The nurse should monitor for and report cloudy dialysate return, which indicates infection. Expected dialysate outflow is a clear, light-yellow solution.

   C. The nurse should avoid warming the dialysate in a microwave oven, which causes uneven heating of the solution.

   D. **CORRECT:** The nurse should monitor for shortness of breath, which can indicate inability to tolerate a large volume of dialysate.

   E. **CORRECT:** The nurse should check the access site dressing for wetness and look for kinking, pulling, clamping, or twisting of the tubing, which can increase the risk for exit-site infections.

   F. The nurse should maintain surgical asepsis when accessing the catheter insertion site to prevent infection from contamination.

   Ⓝ *NCLEX® Connection: Reduction of Risk Potential, Potential for Complications of Diagnostic Tests/Treatments/Procedures*

PRACTICE Answer

Using ATI Active Learning Template: Diagnostic Procedure

DESCRIPTION OF PROCEDURE: Peritoneal dialysis to instill a hypertonic dialysate solution into the peritoneal cavity, allow the solution to dwell for prescribed amount of time, and drain the solution that includes the waste products.

POTENTIAL COMPLICATIONS/NURSING INTERVENTIONS

Peritonitis
- Maintain surgical asepsis.
- Monitor color of outflow solution.
- Monitor for pain and fever.

Protein loss
- Increase dietary intake of protein.
- Monitor albumin level.

Hyperglycemia
- Monitor serum glucose level.
- Administer insulin.

Poor dialysate inflow or outflow
- Reposition the client.
- Milk the tubing to break up fibrin clots.
- Check the tubing for kinks or closed clamps.
- Encourage stool softeners and high-fiber diet to prevent constipation.

Ⓝ *NCLEX® Connection: Reduction of Risk Potential, Potential for Complications of Diagnostic Tests/Treatments/Procedures*

CHAPTER 51   *Polycystic Kidney Disease, Acute Kidney Injury, and Chronic Kidney Disease*

The kidneys regulate fluid, acid-base and electrolyte balance, and eliminate wastes from the body. Several disorders affect the renal system and its ability to function, including acute kidney injury, chronic kidney disease, and polycystic kidney disease.

Kidney failure is diagnosed as acute kidney injury or chronic kidney disease. Without aggressive treatment, or when complicating pre-existing conditions exist, acute kidney injury can result in chronic kidney disease.

Acute kidney injury

Acute kidney injury (AKI) also called acute renal failure (ARF) is the sudden cessation of kidney function that occurs when blood flow to the kidneys is significantly compromised. Manifestations occur abruptly.

PHASES

Onset: Begins with the onset of the event, ends when oliguria develops, and lasts for hours to days.

Oliguria: Begins with the kidney insult; urine output is 100 to 400 mL/24 hr with or without diuretics; and lasts for 1 to 3 weeks. Fluid volume overload can lead to heart failure, electrolyte imbalance, and metabolic acidosis.

Diuresis: Begins when the kidneys start to recover; diuresis of a large amount of fluid occurs, 1000 mL to 2000 mL per day; and can last for 2 to 6 weeks. Death can result from dehydration and imbalances in serum sodium or potassium levels.

Recovery: Continues until kidney function is fully restored and can take up to 12 months. Urine is more concentrated, and electrolytes return to expected reference range.

TYPES

Prerenal: Occurs as a result of volume depletion and prolonged reduction of blood flow to the kidneys, which leads to ischemia of the nephrons. Occurs before damage to the kidney. Early intervention to restore fluid volume deficit can reverse AKI and prevent chronic kidney disease (CKD).

Intrarenal: Occurs as a result of direct damage to the kidney from lack of oxygen (acute tubular necrosis), toxins, or vascular disease to the kidney vascular system.

Postrenal: Occurs as a result of bilateral obstruction of the ureters, bladder, or urethra that can cause a back-up of urine into the kidneys.

HEALTH PROMOTION AND DISEASE PREVENTION

- Drink at least 2 L of fluid daily. Consult with the provider about prescribing fluid restrictions.
- Stop smoking.
- Maintain a healthy weight.
- Use NSAIDs and other medications cautiously.
- Control diabetes and hypertension to prevent complications.
- Take all antibiotics prescribed for infections.

DATA COLLECTION

RISK FACTORS

Prerenal acute kidney injury

- Renal vascular obstruction
- Shock
- Decrease in cardiac output can cause a decrease in renal profusion
- Sepsis
- Hypovolemia
- Peripheral vascular resistance
- Use of aspirin, ibuprofen, or NSAIDs
- Liver failure

Intrarenal acute kidney injury

- **Physical injury:** trauma
- **Hypoxic injury:** renal artery or vein stenosis or thrombosis
- **Chemical injury:** from nephrotoxic agents (antibiotics, contrast dye, heavy metals, blood transfusion reaction, alcohol, cocaine)
- **Immunologic injury:** infection, vasculitis, acute glomerulonephritis, acute tubular necrosis, hepatorenal syndrome

Postrenal acute kidney injury

- Stone, tumor, bladder atony
- Prostate hyperplasia, urethral stricture
- Spinal cord disease or injury

EXPECTED FINDINGS

In most cases, the findings of AKI are related to waste buildup and a decrease in urine output. However, AKI can affect almost every body system.
- CARDIOVASCULAR: fluid overload (dependent and generalized edema), dysrhythmia (hyperkalemia)
- RESPIRATORY: crackles, decreased oxygenation, shortness of breath
- RENAL: scant to normal or excessive urine output, depending on the phase; possible hematuria
- NEUROLOGICAL: lethargy, muscle twitching, seizures
- INTEGUMENTARY: dry skin and mucous membranes

The nurse should also collect data for findings associated with the underlying cause.

LABORATORY TESTS

- Serum creatinine gradually increases 1 to 2 mg/dL every 24 to 48 hr, or 1 to 6 mg/dL in 1 week or less.
- Blood urea nitrogen (BUN) can increase to 80 to 100 mg/dL within 1 week.
- Urine specific gravity varies in postrenal type; can elevate up to 1.030 in prerenal type or the urine is dilute as low as 1.000 in intrarenal type.
- Serum electrolytes: Sodium decreased (prerenal azotemia) or increased (intrarenal azotemia); hyperkalemia; hyperphosphatemia; hypocalcemia
- Hemoglobin and hematocrit: decreased due to a decrease in erythropoietin secretion
- Urinalysis: presence of sediment (protein, RBC, casts)
- ABG: metabolic acidosis

DIAGNOSTIC PROCEDURES

- X-ray of the pelvis, or kidneys, urethra, and bladder (KUB) to detect calculi, hydronephrosis, and to determine size of kidneys
- Ultrasound to detect an obstruction in the urinary tract
- CT scan without contrast dye or MRI to detect anatomical changes, tumors, or other obstruction; patency of ureters; and renal perfusion.
- Kidney biopsy to detect immunological disease or determine kidney dysfunction reversibility and need for dialysis therapy
- Nuclear medicine tests (cystography, retrograde pyelography)

PATIENT-CENTERED CARE

NURSING CARE

- Identify and assist with correcting the underlying cause.
- Monitor fluid intake and output.
- Review laboratory values (BUN, creatinine, electrolytes, hemoglobin, hematocrit).
- Avoid using nephrotoxic medications. If necessary, give these medications sparingly and decrease the medication dosage.
- Monitor for edema and manifestations of heart failure or pulmonary edema.
- Restrict fluid intake as prescribed.
- Monitor for flank pain, nausea, and vomiting (nephrolithiasis).
- Monitor for cardiac dysrhythmias.
- Monitor daily weights.
- Ask about changes in urination stream or difficulty starting the stream of urine.
- Check the urine for blood or particles.
- Treat fever or infection promptly to prevent increase in the client's metabolic rate.
- Provide skin care to prevent injury (bathe with cool water, reposition frequently, provide adequate moisture).
- Provide psychosocial support to the client and family. Reinforce teaching with the client and family about prescribed treatments.
- Reinforce teaching with the client to perform coughing and deep breathing exercises, if lethargic.

NUTRITION
- Implement potassium, phosphate, sodium, and magnesium restrictions if prescribed (depending on the stage of injury).
- Restrict fluid intake if prescribed.
- High-protein diet replaces the high rate of protein breakdown due to stress from the illness.
- Possible total parenteral nutrition (TPN).

MEDICATIONS

- Ask the charge nurse to administer IV fluid therapy as a fluid challenge to promote kidney perfusion or as fluid replacement if the client is in the diuretic phase.
- Administer oral diuretics (furosemide, ethacrynic acid) to promote an increase in filtration of blood by the kidneys.
- Administer calcium channel blocker to prevent the movement of calcium into the kidney cells, to maintain cell integrity, and increase the glomerular filtration rate (GFR) when the client has AKI from medication nephrotoxicity.
- Administer sodium polystyrene sulfonate to replace sodium with potassium in the intestinal tract to promote potassium excretion.
- Administer sorbitol to induce a bowel movement to promote excretion of excess potassium.
- In an emergency, IV medications (dextrose, insulin, calcium) can reduce potassium levels.
- Severe metabolic acidosis can require administration of sodium bicarbonate.
- For hyperphosphatemia, administer phosphate-binding agents.

THERAPEUTIC PROCEDURES

- Continuous kidney replacement therapy
- Hemodialysis
- Peritoneal dialysis

INTERPROFESSIONAL CARE

- Dietitian to calculate protein, calorie, and fluid needs
- Nephrology services to monitor kidney function

Chronic kidney disease

CKD is a progressive, irreversible kidney disease.

- A client who has CKD doesn't initially have manifestations except during periods of stress (infection, surgery, and trauma). As kidney dysfunction progresses, manifestations become apparent.
- Older adult clients have an increased risk for CKD related to the aging process (decreased number of functioning nephrons, decreased GFR). ⑤
- Older adults clients who are on bed rest, have confusion, have a lack of thirst, and do not have easy access to water are at a higher risk for dehydration leading to CKD.
- End-stage kidney disease (ESKD) is when the kidneys lose the ability to function.

STAGES

CKD is comprised of three stages.

- **Stage 1:** No buildup of metabolic waste in the blood, polyuria, nocturia, and lower specific gravity
- **Stage 2:** Increase in metabolic waste in the blood causing an elevation in BUN and creatinine, glomerular filtration rate decreases, oliguria, and peripheral edema
- **Stage 3:** End-stage kidney disease; rise in metabolic waste in the blood, imbalance in fluid and electrolytes, inability to maintain homeostasis

HEALTH PROMOTION AND DISEASE PREVENTION

- Drink at least 2 L water daily. Consult with the provider regarding any restrictions.
- Stop smoking.
- Limit alcohol intake.
- Use diet and exercise to manage weight and prevent or control diabetes and hypertension.
- Adhere to medication prescription guidelines to prevent kidney damage.
- Test for albumin in the urine yearly (clients who have diabetes or hypertension).
- Take all antibiotics until completed.
- Limit over-the-counter NSAIDs. Qs

DATA COLLECTION

- ESKD exists when 90% of the functioning nephrons are destroyed and are no longer able to maintain fluid, electrolyte, and acid–base homeostasis.
- Dialysis or kidney transplantation can maintain life, but neither is a cure for CKD.

RISK FACTORS

- Acute kidney injury
- Diabetes mellitus
- Chronic glomerulonephritis, nephrotic syndrome, sickle cell disease
- Nephrotoxic medications (gentamicin, NSAIDs) or substances
- Hypertension, especially in African American clients
- Autoimmune disorders (systemic lupus erythematosus)
- Polycystic kidney disease
- Pyelonephrosis
- Renal artery stenosis
- Recurrent severe infections especially streptococcal bacteria
- Cirrhosis of the liver

EXPECTED FINDINGS

- Nausea, fatigue, lethargy, involuntary movement of legs, depression, intractable hiccups
- Manifestations of CKD are related to fluid volume overload in most cases.
  - **Neurologic:** lethargy, decreased attention span, blurred speech, tremors or jerky movements, ataxia, seizures, coma
  - **Cardiovascular:** fluid overload (jugular distention; sacrum, ocular, or peripheral edema), hypertension, dysrhythmias, heart failure, orthostatic hypotension, peaked T wave on ECG (hyperkalemia)
  - **Respiratory:** uremic halitosis with deep sighing, yawning, shortness of breath, tachypnea, hyperpnea, Kussmaul respirations, crackles, pleural friction rub, frothy pink sputum
  - **Hematologic:** anemia (pallor, weakness, dizziness), ecchymosis, petechiae, melena
  - **Gastrointestinal:** ulcers in mouth and throat, foul breath, blood in stools, vomiting
  - **Musculoskeletal:** osteodystrophy (thin fragile bones)
  - **Renal:** urine contains protein, blood, particles; change in amount, color, concentration
  - **Skin:** decreased skin turgor, yellow cast, dryness, pruritus, urea crystals on skin (uremic frost)
  - **Reproductive:** erectile dysfunction

LABORATORY TESTS

Urinalysis: Hematuria, proteinuria, and decrease in specific gravity.

Serum creatinine: Gradual increase over months to years for CKD exceeding 4 mg/dL. Levels can increase to 15 to 30 mg/dL.

BUN: Gradual increase with elevated serum creatinine over months to years for CKD. Levels can increase 10 to 20 times the creatinine finding.

Serum electrolytes: Decreased sodium (dilutional) and calcium; increased potassium greater than 5 mEq/L, phosphorus, and magnesium.

CBC: Decreased hemoglobin and hematocrit causing anemia secondary to the loss of erythropoietin secretions in CKD.

DIAGNOSTIC PROCEDURES

Radiologic procedures to detect disease processes, obstruction, and arterial defects
- Ultrasound
- Kidneys, ureter, and bladder (KUB)
- Computerized tomography (CT)
- Magnetic resonance imaging (MRI) without contrast dye
- Aortorenal angiography
- Cystoscopy
- Retrograde pyelography
- Kidney biopsy

PATIENT-CENTERED CARE

NURSING CARE

- Report and monitor irregular findings
  - URINARY ELIMINATION PATTERNS: amount, color, odor, and consistency
  - VITAL SIGNS: blood pressure can be increased or decreased
  - WEIGHT: 1 kg (2.2 lb) daily weight increase is approximately 1 L fluid retained.
- Check and monitor vascular access or peritoneal dialysis insertion site.
- Obtain a detailed medication, herb, and supplement history to determine the client's risk for continued kidney injury.
- Control protein intake based on the client's stage of CKD and type of dialysis prescribed.
- Restrict dietary sodium, potassium, phosphorous, and magnesium.
- Provide a diet that is high in carbohydrates and moderate in fat.
- Restrict intake of fluids (based on urinary output).
- Monitor for weight gain trends.
- Adhere to meticulous cleaning of areas on skin not intact and access sites to control infections.
- Balance the client's activity and rest.

- Prepare the client for hemodialysis, peritoneal dialysis, and hemofiltration if indicated.
- Provide skin care in order to increase comfort and prevent breakdown.
- Protect the client from injury. Qs
- Provide emotional support to the client and family.
- Encourage the client to ask questions and discuss fears.
- Administer medications.
- Auscultate lungs for pulmonary edema.
- Provide frequent mouth rinses due to uremic halitosis caused by urea waste in the blood.

MEDICATIONS

See the **PN PHARMACOLOGY REVIEW MODULE** for detailed information on these medications.

> ! Avoid administering antimicrobial medications (aminoglycosides and amphotericin B, vancomycin), NSAIDs, and IV contrast dye, which are nephrotoxic.

Angiotensin-converting enzymes (ACE) inhibitors and angiotensin receptor blockers (ARBs) decrease proteinuria and can decrease the progression of CKD by lowering the client's blood pressure.

Digoxin: a cardiac glycoside that increases contractility of the myocardium and promotes cardiac output for acute cases of heart failure during stage 2 of CKD
- Monitor digoxin laboratory levels and expect dosages to be reduced due to slow excretion of the medication with CKD.
- Monitor carefully for manifestations of digoxin toxicity (nausea, vomiting, anorexia, vision changes).
- Monitor potassium level. Qs
- Administer digoxin after dialysis.

Sodium polystyrene increases elimination of serum potassium.
- Restrict sodium intake. Sodium polystyrene contains sodium and can cause fluid retention and hypertension, a complication of CKD.

Epoetin alfa stimulates production of red blood cells; given for anemia

Ferrous sulfate an iron supplement to prevent severe iron deficiency anemia

Calcium carbonate
- Taken with meals to bind phosphate in food and stop phosphate absorption.
- Administer 2 hr before or after other medications
- Can cause constipation, so clients can require a stool softener.

Furosemide: a loop-diuretic administered to excrete excess fluids, reduce blood pressure and decrease potassium levels.
- Avoid administering to a client who has ESKD.
- Clients can also receive thiazide diuretics, potassium-sparing diuretics, and osmotic diuretics.

THERAPEUTIC PROCEDURES

- Peritoneal dialysis
- Hemodialysis
- Kidney transplantation

INTERPROFESSIONAL CARE

- Nephrology services to manage dialysis or kidney failure
- Nutritional services to manage nutritional needs

CLIENT EDUCATION Q$_{EBP}$

- Monitor the daily intake of carbohydrates, proteins, sodium, and potassium.
- Monitor fluid intake according to prescribed fluid restriction.
- Avoid antacids containing magnesium.
- Take rest periods from activity.
- Educate the client who is receiving hemodialysis or peritoneal dialysis on an outpatient basis.
- Measure blood pressure and weight at home.
- Ask questions and discuss fears.
- Follow prescribed diet, exercise, and take prescription medication.
- Notify the provider if skin breakdown occurs.

CARE AFTER DISCHARGE

- Contact nephrology services if the client is to receive outpatient dialysis.
- Refer the client to a community support group relating to the disease.
- Consult nutritional services for dietary needs.
- Refer the client to a smoking-cessation support group and counseling if needed.

COMPLICATIONS

Potential complications include electrolyte imbalance, dysrhythmias, fluid overload, hypertension, metabolic acidosis, secondary infection, and uremia.

Polycystic kidney disease

- Polycystic kidney disease (PKD) is a congenital disorder where clusters of fluid-filled cysts develop in the nephrons. Healthy kidney tissue is replaced by multiple non-functioning cysts. For additional information, refer to the PKD Foundation (https://pkdcure.org).
- PKD is hereditary and the cause is from a genetic mutation.
- PKD is more common in white clients.

FORMS: There are two forms of PKD.
- **Autosomal dominant trait:** Most common form. Cysts begin to multiply when the client reaches age 30.
- **Autosomal recessive trait:** Multiple cysts are present at birth.

DATA COLLECTION

EXPECTED FINDINGS

- Familial history of PKD
- Anxiety, guilt
- Abdominal and flank pain
  - Dull pain indicates increased kidney size or possible cyst infection.
  - Sharp pain indicates ruptured cyst or possible renal lithiasis (kidney stone).
- Headaches
- Hypertension caused by kidney ischemia from the enlarging cysts
- Enlarged abdominal girth
- Constipation
- Bloody or cloudy urine
- Renal lithiasis
- Hyponatremia
- Nocturia (excessive urination at night)
- Progressive kidney failure

LABORATORY TESTS

- Urinalysis
- Hematuria, proteinuria, and bacteria indicating infection
- Gradual increase of serum creatinine, BUN, creatinine clearance

DIAGNOSTIC PROCEDURES

Radiologic procedures detect disease processes and cysts.
- Ultrasound
- CT
- MRI

PATIENT-CENTERED CARE

NURSING CARE

HYPERTENSION CONTROL
- Controlling blood pressure is the highest nursing priority for clients who have PKD.
- Manage hypertension with medication.
- Reinforce teaching with the client and family how to measure and record blood pressure readings and daily weights.

PAIN MANAGEMENT
- Encourage the client to take prescribed pain medications and implement nonpharmacological pain methods, such as relaxation, deep breathing, guided imagery, and distraction. Use NSAIDs cautiously in clients who have kidney disease.
- Apply dry heat to abdomen or flank areas to reduce discomfort.

INFECTION PREVENTION
- Administer antibiotics (ciprofloxacin, trimethoprim/sulfamethoxazole). Monitor for antibiotic-induced nephrotoxicity by evaluating serum creatinine levels and urinary output.
- Monitor urine specific gravity to determine kidney function and hydration status.

CONSTIPATION PREVENTION
- Provide adequate oral fluid intake (as allowed per prescribed fluid restrictions), increase dietary fiber, and encourage client to ambulate.
- Auscultate bowel sounds and ask about frequency of bowel movements.
- Administer stool softeners.

THERAPEUTIC PROCEDURE

Needle aspiration and drainage of cysts

CLIENT EDUCATION

- Monitor blood pressure and weight daily.
- Notify the provider if experiencing an elevated temperature.
- Maintain a low-sodium diet.
- Inform the provider if there are any changes in urine or bowel movements.
- Take all medications as prescribed.

CARE AFTER DISCHARGE
- Assist with a referral to a community support group related to the disease.
- Collaborate with nutritional services for dietary needs.

Application Exercises

1. A nurse is contributing to the plan of care for a client who has prerenal acute kidney injury (AKI) following abdominal aortic aneurysm repair. Urinary output is 60 mL in the past 2 hr, and blood pressure is 92/58 mm Hg. The nurse should anticipate which of the following interventions?

    A. Prepare the client for a CT scan with contrast dye.

    B. Administer ketorolac for pain.

    C. Administer a fluid challenge.

    D. Position the client in reverse Trendelenburg.

2. A nurse is contributing to the plan of care for a client who has postrenal AKI due to metastatic cancer. The client has a serum creatinine of 5 mg/dL. Which of the following interventions should the nurse recommend? (Select all that apply.)

    A. Provide a high-protein diet.

    B. Check the urine for blood.

    C. Monitor for intermittent anuria.

    D. Weigh the client once per week.

    E. Provide NSAIDs for pain.

3. A nurse is assisting in the planning of care for a client who has chronic kidney disease. Which of the following actions should the nurse include in the plan of care? (Select all that apply.)

    A. Auscultate lungs for pulmonary edema.

    B. Provide frequent mouth rinses.

    C. Restrict fluids based on urinary output.

    D. Provide a high-sodium diet.

    E. Monitor for weight gain trends.

4. A nurse is checking a client's laboratory findings. Which of the following findings is expected for a client who has stage 3 chronic kidney disease?

    A. Blood urea nitrogen (BUN) 15 mg/dL

    B. Hemoglobin 14.4 g/dL

    C. Serum creatinine 1.1 mg/dL

    D. Serum potassium 6.0 mEq/L

5. A nurse is reviewing the medical record of a client who has intrarenal acute kidney injury (AKI). Which of the following factors should the nurse identify as the cause of this form of AKI?

    A. Shock

    B. Prostate hyperplasia

    C. Cocaine use disorder

    D. Liver failure

PRACTICE Active Learning Scenario

A nurse is preparing to administer medication to a client who has chronic kidney disease (CKD). What information should the nurse consider when administering medication? Use the ATI Active Learning Template: Medication to complete this item.

MEDICATION: Identify three medications the nurse should expect to administer.

THERAPEUTIC USES: Describe how the medication is used to treat CKD.

NURSING INTERVENTIONS: Describe two for each medication.

Application Exercises Key

1. A. CT scan using contrast dye can cause further injury to the kidney nephrons when a client has acute kidney injury.

    B. Ketorolac is an NSAID that can cause further injury to the kidney nephrons and is contraindicated for a client who has acute kidney injury.

    C. **CORRECT:** The nurse should ask the charge nurse to administer a fluid challenge for hypovolemia. Hypovolemia can reduce blood flow to the kidneys causing low urinary output and blood pressure.

    D. The nurse should position the client in a modified Trendelenburg position with the head flat and feet elevated, to treat hypotension.

    Ⓝ *NCLEX® Connection: Physiological Adaptation, Alterations in Body Systems*

2. A. **CORRECT:** The nurse should provide a high-protein diet to replace the high rate of protein breakdown and loss that occurs with acute kidney injury.

    B. **CORRECT:** The nurse should check the urine for blood, stones, and particles indicating an obstruction of the renal system.

    C. **CORRECT:** The nurse should check for intermittent anuria due to obstruction or damage to kidneys or urinary structures.

    D. The nurse should weigh the client daily to monitor for fluid retention due to acute kidney injury.

    E. The nurse should not administer NSAIDs, which are toxic to the nephrons in the kidney.

    Ⓝ *NCLEX® Connection: Physiological Adaptation, Alterations in Body Systems*

3. A. **CORRECT:** The nurse should auscultate the client's lungs for pulmonary edema, which can indicate fluid overload and heart failure.

    B. **CORRECT:** The nurse should provide frequent mouth rinses due to uremic halitosis caused by urea waste in the blood.

    C. **CORRECT:** The nurse should restrict fluids based on urinary output to prevent fluid volume overload.

    D. The nurse should monitor serum sodium and reduce the client's dietary sodium intake.

    E. **CORRECT:** The nurse should monitor for weight gain trends that can indicate fluid volume overload.

    Ⓝ *NCLEX® Connection: Physiological Adaptation, Alterations in Body Systems*

4. A. The nurse should expect a client who has stage 3 CKD to have an elevated BUN. A BUN of 15 mg/dL is within the expected reference range.

    B. The nurse should expect a client who has stage 3 CKD to have a decreased hemoglobin. A hemoglobin of 14.4 g/dL is within the expected reference range.

    C. The nurse should expect a client who has stage 3 CKD to have a creatinine level as high as 30 mg/dL. A creatinine level of 1.1 mg/dL is within the expected reference range.

    D. **CORRECT:** The client in stage 3 chronic kidney disease can have a potassium level greater than 5.0 mEq/L.

    Ⓝ *NCLEX® Connection: Reduction of Risk Potential, Laboratory Values*

5. A. Shock is a causative factor of prerenal AKI

    B. Prostate hyperplasia is a causative factor of postrenal AKI.

    C. **CORRECT:** The nurse should identify nephrotoxic agents, such as cocaine, as a causative factor of intrarenal AKI.

    D. Liver failure is a causative factor of prerenal AKI.

    Ⓝ *NCLEX® Connection: Physiological Adaptation, Basic Pathophysiology*

PRACTICE Answer

Using the ATI Active Learning Template: Medication

MEDICATION
- Digoxin
- Sodium polystyrene
- Calcium carbonate
- Furosemide

THERAPEUTIC USES
- Digoxin: A cardiac glycoside, increases contractility of the myocardium and promotes cardiac output.
- Sodium polystyrene: Increases elimination of potassium.
- Calcium carbonate: Binds to phosphate in food and stops phosphate absorption.
- Furosemide: A loop diuretic that causes diuresis of excess fluids and can lower potassium levels.

NURSING INTERVENTIONS
- Digoxin
  - Monitor serum digoxin and potassium levels.
  - Monitor for manifestations of toxicity (nausea, vomiting, anorexia, visual changes).
- Sodium polystyrene
  - Monitor for hypokalemia.
  - Restrict sodium intake.

- Calcium carbonate
  - Administer this medication with meals, 2 hr before or after other medications.
  - Administer a stool softener with this medication.
- Furosemide
  - Monitor intake and output and blood pressure.
  - Avoid administering to a client who has end-stage kidney disease.

Ⓝ *NCLEX® Connection: Pharmacological Therapies, Expected Actions/Outcomes*

CHAPTER 52 *Infections of the Renal and Urinary System*

The renal system includes the kidneys and the urinary system. The function of the renal system includes maintaining fluid volume, removing waste, regulating blood pressure, maintaining acid-base balance, producing erythropoietin, and activating vitamin D.

There are three components to the urinary system: the ureter, bladder, and urethra. The function of the urinary system is to store and remove urine.

Urinary tract infections are infections of the urinary system, and pyelonephritis is an infection of the kidney and renal pelvis. Acute and chronic glomerulonephritis can develop from a systemic infection and involves the glomeruli of the kidney or the area responsible for filtering particles from the blood to make urine.

Urinary tract infection

- A urinary tract infection (UTI) refers to any portion of the lower urinary tract (ureters, bladder, urethra, prostate). UTIs include the following.
  - Cystitis
  - Urethritis
  - Prostatitis
- An upper UTI refers to conditions such as pyelonephritis (inflammation of the kidney pelvis).
- *Escherichia coli* often causes UTIs. Other organisms include enterobacteriaceae micro-organisms (klebsiella, proteus), pseudomonas, and *Staphylococcus saprophyticus*.
- Untreated UTIs can lead to pyelonephritis and urosepsis, which can result in septic shock and death.

DATA COLLECTION

RISK FACTORS

- FEMALE CLIENTS
  - Short urethra predisposes females to UTIs
  - Close proximity of the urethra to the rectum
  - Decrease in estrogen levels in aging clients promotes atrophy of the urethral opening toward the rectum (increases the risk of urosepsis) Ⓖ
  - Sexual intercourse
  - Frequent use of feminine hygiene sprays, tampons, sanitary napkins, spermicidal jellies
  - Pregnancy
  - Poorly fitted diaphragm
  - Hormonal influences within the vaginal flora
  - Synthetic underwear and pantyhose
  - Wet bathing suits
  - Frequent submersion into baths or hot tubs
- Alkaline urine, which promotes bacterial growth
- Indwelling urinary catheters (significant source of infection in clients who are hospitalized)
- Stool incontinence
- Bladder distention
- Urinary conditions (anomalies, stasis, calculi, residual urine)
- Possible genetic links
- Disease (diabetes mellitus)
- OLDER ADULT CLIENTS Ⓖ
  - Increase in the risk of bacteremia, sepsis, and shock
  - Incomplete bladder emptying from an enlarged prostate or prostatitis in males
  - Bladder prolapse in females
  - Inability to empty bladder (neurogenic bladder) as a result of a stroke or Parkinson's disease
  - Fecal incontinence with poor perineal hygiene
  - Hypoestrogen in females affecting the mucosa of the vagina and urethra, causing bacteria to adhere to the mucosal surface
  - Renal complications increase due to a decrease in the number of functioning nephrons and fluid intake

EXPECTED FINDINGS

- Lower back or lower abdominal discomfort and tenderness over the bladder area
- Nausea
- Urinary frequency and urgency
- Dysuria, bladder cramping, spasms
- Feeling of incomplete bladder emptying or retention of urine
- Perineal itching
- Hematuria (red-tinged, smoky, coffee-colored urine)
- Pyuria (WBCs in the urine sample)
- Fever
- Vomiting
- Voiding in small amounts
- Nocturia
- Urethral discharge
- Cloudy or foul-smelling urine

OLDER ADULT MANIFESTATIONS ⓖ
- Confusion
- Incontinence
- Loss of appetite
- Nocturia and dysuria
- Hypotension, tachycardia, tachypnea, and fever (indications of urosepsis)

LABORATORY TESTS

Urinalysis and urine culture and sensitivity

NURSING ACTIONS
- Reinforce teaching with the client regarding proper technique for the collection of a clean-catch urine specimen.
- Collect catheterized urine specimens using sterile technique.

EXPECTED FINDINGS
- Bacteria, sediment, positive for white blood cells (WBCs) and red blood cells (RBCs)
- Positive leukocyte esterase and nitrates indicates UTI

WBC count and differential

- If urosepsis is suspected
- White blood cell count equal to or greater than 10,000/mm³ with a shift to the left, indicating an increase in the number of immature cells (neutrophils) in response to infection

Rule out sexually transmitted infections

- STIs can cause manifestations of a UTI.
- *Chlamydia trachomatis*, *Neisseria gonorrhoeae*, and herpes simplex can cause acute urethritis.
- Trichomonas or candida can cause acute vaginal infections.

DIAGNOSTIC PROCEDURES

- Cystoscopy to help determine the cause of complicated UTIs.
- Cystourethroscopy to detect strictures, calculi, tumors, and cystitis.
- Computed tomography (CT) scan to detect pyelonephritis.
- Ultrasonography to detect cysts, tumors, calculi, and abscesses.
- Transrectal ultrasonography to detect prostate and bladder conditions in males.

PATIENT-CENTERED CARE

NURSING CARE

- Promote fluid intake up to 3 L daily. Consult with the provider if the client needs fluid restrictions.
- Administer antibiotic medications.
- Encourage clients to urinate every 2 to 4 hr instead of waiting until the bladder is completely full.
- Recommend warm sitz bath two or three times a day to provide comfort.
- Encourage clients to shower daily to promote good body hygiene.
- Avoid the use of indwelling catheters if possible. This reduces the risk for infection.
- Pregnant clients require immediate and effective treatment to prevent pyelonephritis that can result in preterm labor. Qₛ

MEDICATIONS

See the **PN PHARMACOLOGY REVIEW MODULE** for more detailed information.

Fluoroquinolones, nitrofurantoin, trimethoprim, sulfonamides

Antibiotics treat urinary infections by directly killing bacteria and inhibiting bacterial reproduction. Qᴇʙᴘ
- Penicillins and cephalosporins are administered less frequently because the medication is less effective and tolerated.
- Nitrofurantoin is an antibacterial medication used for the treatment of UTIs caused by susceptible micro-organisms.

NURSING ACTIONS: Before administering sulfonamide antibiotics, ask the client about an allergy to sulfa.

CLIENT EDUCATION
- Take all of the prescribed antibiotics even if manifestations subside.
- Take the medication with food.
- Avoid direct exposure to sunlight because fluoroquinolones or sulfonamides can cause sun-sensitivity and increase the risk for a sunburn, even for dark-skinned individuals.
- Take fluoroquinolones or sulfonamides with a full glass of water and increase total daily fluid intake because the medication can precipitate in the renal tubules.
- Monitor and report watery diarrhea that can indicate pseudomembranous colitis.

Phenazopyridine

- Bladder analgesic to treat manifestations of a UTI
- The medication will not treat the infection, but it will help relieve bladder discomfort; pain, burning, itching, urgency, and frequency.

CLIENT EDUCATION

- Medication will turn urine orange and can stain skin and clothing.
- Take the medication with food to decrease gastrointestinal irritation.

INTERPROFESSIONAL CARE

Consult with urology services for managing UTIs.

CLIENT EDUCATION

- Drink at least 3 L fluid daily.
- Bathe daily to promote good body hygiene.
- Empty bladder every 2 to 4 hr instead of waiting until the bladder is completely full.
- Urinate before and after intercourse.
- Drink cranberry juice to decrease the risk of infection. QEBP
  - The compound in cranberries might stop certain bacteria from adhering to the mucosa of the urinary tract.
  - Clients who have chronic cystitis should avoid cranberry juice, which irritates the bladder.
- Empty the bladder as soon as there is an urgency to void.
- For female clients
  - Wipe the perineal area from front to back.
  - Avoid using bubble baths, and feminine products and toilet paper containing perfumes.
  - Avoid sitting in wet bathing suits.
  - Avoid wearing pantyhose with slacks or tight clothing.

CARE AFTER DISCHARGE: Urology services can be consulted for management of long-term antibiotic therapy for chronic UTIs.

COMPLICATIONS

Urethral obstruction, pyelonephritis, chronic kidney disease, urosepsis, septic shock, and death

Pyelonephritis

- Pyelonephritis is an infection and inflammation of the kidney pelvis, calyces, and medulla. The infection usually begins in the lower urinary tract with organisms ascending into the kidney pelvis.
- *Escherichia coli* organisms are frequently the cause of acute pyelonephritis.
- Repeated infections can create scarring that changes the blood flow to the kidney, glomerulus, and tubular structure.
- Filtration, reabsorption, and secretion are impaired, which results in a decrease in kidney function.
- **Acute pyelonephritis** is an active bacterial infection that can cause the following.
  - Interstitial inflammation
  - Tubular cell necrosis
  - Abscess formation in the capsule, cortex, or medulla
  - Temporarily altered kidney function (this rarely progresses to chronic kidney disease)
- **Chronic pyelonephritis** is the result of repeated infections that cause progressive inflammation and scarring.
  - This can result in the thickening of the calyces and postinflammatory fibrosis with permanent renal tissue scarring.
  - It is more common with obstructions, urinary anomaly, and vesicoureteral urine reflux.
  - Reflux of urine occurs at the junction where the ureter connects to the bladder.

DATA COLLECTION

RISK FACTORS

- Males older than 65 who have prostatitis and hypertrophy of the prostate (stasis of urine) Ⓖ
- Chronic urinary stone disorders (stones harbor bacteria)
- Spinal cord injury (clients have a higher incidence of reflux from neurogenic bladder)
- Pregnancy causing increase in pressure on the urinary system that can cause reflux or retention of urine
- Congenital malformations
- Bladder tumors
- Chronic illness (diabetes mellitus, hypertension, chronic cystitis)
- Alkaline urine promotes bacterial growth.
- Incomplete bladder emptying is more common among older adult clients. Ⓖ
- Older adult clients can exhibit gastrointestinal or pulmonary manifestations instead of febrile responses because their temperature can vary at a lower-than-normal state. Causes are inadequate diet, loss of adipose tissue, lack of exercise, and reduction in the client's thermoregulator. Ⓖ

EXPECTED FINDINGS

- Chills
- Colicky-type abdominal pain
- Nausea, vomiting
- Malaise, fatigue
- Burning, urgency, and frequency with urination
- Costovertebral tenderness
- Flank and back pain
- Nocturia
- Fever
- Tachycardia
- Tachypnea
- Hypertension
- Inability to concentrate urine or conserve sodium (chronic pyelonephritis)
- Asymptomatic bacteremia

LABORATORY TESTS

- Urinalysis and urine culture and sensitivity: same as for a UTI (positive leukocyte esterase and nitrites, WBCs, and bacteria).
- WBC count and differential: same as for a UTI.
- Positive blood cultures indicates the presence of bacteria if a systemic infection is present.
- Serum creatinine and blood urea nitrogen (BUN) are elevated during acute episodes and consistently elevated with chronic infection.
- C-reactive protein is elevated during exacerbating inflammatory processes of the kidneys. Erythrocyte sedimentation rate (ESR) is elevated during acute or chronic inflammation.

DIAGNOSTIC PROCEDURES

- An x-ray of the kidneys, ureters, and bladder (KUB) can demonstrate calculi or structural abnormalities.
- Ultrasonography to detect cysts, tumors, calculi, and abscesses.
- Gallium scan: a nuclear medicine test that uses injectable radioactive dye to visualize organs, glands, bones, and blood vessels that have infection and inflammation.
- Intravenous pyelogram can demonstrate calculi, structural, or vascular abnormalities.
- Renal computed tomography (CT) or magnetic resonance imaging (MRI) to determine the location of an obstruction causing pyelonephritis.

PATIENT-CENTERED CARE

NURSING CARE

- Monitor the following.
  - Nutritional status
  - Intake and output
  - Fluid and electrolyte balance
  - Temperature
  - Onset, quality, duration, and severity of pain
- Increase fluid intake to 2 L/day unless contraindicated.
- Administer antipyretic, such as acetaminophen, as needed for fever and opioid analgesics for pain associated with pyelonephritis.
- Provide emotional support.
- Assist with personal hygiene.

MEDICATIONS

See the **PN PHARMACOLOGY REVIEW MODULE** for more detailed information.

Opioid analgesics (opioid agonists), morphine sulfate, and morphine: For moderate to severe pain

Antibiotics Q̇EBP
- Mild to moderate pyelonephritis treated at home for 14 days with the following.
  - Anti-infective: trimethoprim, sulfamethoxazole/trimethoprim
  - Quinolone antibiotic: ciprofloxacin levofloxacin
- Severe pyelonephritis treated in the hospital for 24 to 48 hr with IV medication.

THERAPEUTIC PROCEDURES

Reinforce preoperative teaching.
- Check with the client on understanding of the purpose of the surgery and expected outcomes.
- Plan to receive intravenous antibiotics and analgesics.

Pyelolithotomy: The removal of a large stone from the kidney that causes infections and blocks the flow of urine from the kidney

Nephrectomy: The removal of the kidney when all procedures to clear the client of infection were unsuccessful

Ureteroplasty: Done to repair or revise the ureter and can involve reimplantation of the ureter in the bladder wall to preserve the function of the kidney and eliminate infection

Provide postoperative care
- Check the dressings and incision.
- Balance rest and activities.
- Reinforce with the client about monitoring for indications of infection.
- Reinforce with the client about the role of nutritious meals and adequate fluid intake.

INTERPROFESSIONAL CARE

- Urology services to manage pyelonephritis
- Nutritional services to promote adequate calories

CLIENT EDUCATION

- Consume adequate nutrition and calories that the nutritional services recommend.
- Drink at least 2 L fluids daily unless otherwise indicated by the provider.
- Take medications as prescribed.
- Notify the provider if acute onset of pain occurs or a fever is present.
- Express fears and anxiety related to the disease.
- Take rest periods from activity as needed.

CARE AFTER DISCHARGE: Home care services if the client needs assistance with medications or nutritional therapy.

COMPLICATIONS

- **Septic shock** (hypotension, tachycardia, fever) due to bacterial organism entering the blood stream
- **Chronic kidney disease** (elevated BUN, creatinine, electrolytes) from inflammation and infection that causes fibrosis of the kidney pelvis and calyx, scarring, and changes in the blood vessels and the glomerular and tubular filtration system
- **Hypertension** (related to fluid and sodium retention) indicating chronic kidney disease that causes destruction of the filtration system of the kidney due to infection

Glomerulonephritis

Immunologic kidney disorder that can start in the kidneys (genetic basis and immune-inducing inflammation) or occurs as a result of other health disorders (lupus erythematosus, diabetic nephropathy) and results in glomerular injury

- Can lead to end-stage kidney disease (ESKD), often referred to as end-stage renal disease.
- Acute glomerulonephritis often occurs following an infection.
- Chronic glomerulonephritis develops over a period of 20 to 30 years.

DATA COLLECTION

RISK FACTORS

- Recent infection, particularly of the skin or upper respiratory tract
- Recent travel or other possible exposure to bacteria, viruses, fungi, or parasites
- Presence of systemic diseases (systemic lupus erythematosus, Goodpasture syndrome)
- Recent surgery or illness

EXPECTED FINDINGS

- Anorexia
- Nausea and vomiting
- Dysuria
- Oliguria
- Fatigue
- Hypertension
- Headache
- Difficulty breathing
- Crackles
- S_3 heart sound
- Weight gain
- Periorbital edema, facial edema, and upper extremity edema
- Reddish-brown or cola-colored urine
- Older adult clients are likely to have the less common manifestations of circulatory overload, which can be confused with heart failure. Ⓖ

LABORATORY TESTS

- Urinalysis shows red blood cells and protein.
- Glomerular filtration rate is decreased.
- Blood, skin, or throat cultures can be indicated.
- 24-hr urine collection for protein assay (increased in acute glomerulonephritis and decreased in chronic glomerulonephritis).
- Serum blood urea nitrogen and creatinine are increased.
- Antistreptolysin-O titers are increased after group A beta hemolytic streptococcus infection.
- Anti-nuclear antibody (ANA) presence.
- Altered electrolytes; hyperkalemia, hyperphosphatemia, hypocalcemia.

DIAGNOSTIC PROCEDURES

- Kidney biopsy to diagnose the condition, determine prognosis, and treatment.
- Ultrasound to determine kidney size.

PATIENT-CENTERED CARE

NURSING CARE

- Coordinate care to conserve client energy.
- Consult with provider to determine if fluid restriction is needed.
- Administer antibiotics.
- Reinforce the teaching of relaxation exercises to decrease stress.
- Monitor blood pressure.
- Monitor respiratory status.
- Monitor fluid and electrolytes.

MEDICATIONS

See the **PN PHARMACOLOGY REVIEW MODULE** for more detailed information.

Antibiotics: Penicillin, erythromycin, or azithromycin is prescribed for glomerulonephritis infection due to streptococcal infection. Q<small>EBP</small>

Antihypertensives: To control hypertension, recommend angiotensin-converting enzyme (ACE) or angiotensin-receptor blockers (ARBs)

Glucocorticoids: To decrease the risk of kidney failure

INTERPROFESSIONAL CARE

- Collaborate with provider and nutritional support regarding any potassium or protein restriction in diet.
- Dialysis or plasmapheresis can be necessary.

CLIENT EDUCATION

- Complete full course of antibiotics.
- Monitor weight daily and report increases to provider.
- Maintain dietary and fluid restrictions.
- Follow basic infection control practices, such as hand hygiene.

CARE AFTER DISCHARGE

- Refer to home care services for dialysis or plasmapheresis if needed.
- Follow up as the provider directs.

Application Exercises

1. A nurse is contributing to the plan of care for a client who has chronic pyelonephritis. Which of the following actions should the nurse recommend? (Select all that apply.)

   A. Assist with a referral for nutrition counseling.

   B. Encourage daily fluid intake of 1 L.

   C. Palpate the costovertebral angle.

   D. Monitor urinary output.

   E. Administer antibiotics.

2. A nurse is caring for a client who has a urinary tract infection (UTI). Which of the following is the priority intervention by the nurse?

   A. Offer a warm sitz bath.

   B. Recommend drinking cranberry juice.

   C. Encourage increased fluids.

   D. Administer an antibiotic.

3. A nurse is reviewing information with a female client who has frequent urinary tract infections. Which of the following information should the nurse include? (Select all that apply.)

   A. Avoid sitting in a wet bathing suit.

   B. Wipe the perineal area back to front following elimination.

   C. Empty the bladder when there is an urge to void.

   D. Wear synthetic fabric underwear.

   E. Take a shower daily.

4. A nurse is caring for several clients. Which of the following clients are at risk for developing pyelonephritis? (Select all that apply.)

   A. A client who is at 32 weeks of gestation

   B. A client who has kidney calculi

   C. A client who has a urine pH of 4.2

   D. A client who has a neurogenic bladder

   E. A client who has diabetes mellitus

5. A nurse is checking urinalysis results for four clients. Which of the following urinalysis results indicates a urinary tract infection?

   A. Positive for hyaline casts

   B. Positive for leukocyte esterase

   C. Positive for ketones

   D. Positive for crystals

PRACTICE Active Learning Scenario

A nurse is reinforcing teaching with a client who has chronic pyelonephritis. What information should the nurse include? Use the ATI Active Learning Template: System Disorder to complete this item.

ALTERATION IN HEALTH (DIAGNOSIS)

COMPLICATIONS: List three, and explain why these occur.

CLIENT EDUCATION: Include three education points.

Application Exercises Key

1. A. **CORRECT:** The client requires adequate nutrition to promote healing.

   B. The nurse should encourage fluid intake of 2 L daily to maintain dilute urine.

   C. **CORRECT:** The nurse should gently palpate the costovertebral angle for flank tenderness, which can indicate inflammation and infection.

   D. **CORRECT:** The nurse should monitor urinary output to ensure that 1 to 3 L of urine is excreted daily.

   E. **CORRECT:** The nurse should administer antibiotics to treat the bacteriuria and decrease progressive damage to the kidney.

   Ⓝ *NCLEX® Connection: Physiological Adaptation, Alterations in Body Systems*

2. A. The nurse should offer a warm sitz bath to provide temporary relief of the manifestations of the UTI. However, another action is the priority.

   B. The nurse should recommend that the client drink cranberry juice to prevent a UTI in the future. However, another action is the priority.

   C. The nurse should encourage the client to increase fluid intake to dilute the urine, and flush the kidneys to relieve the manifestations of the UTI. However, another action is the priority.

   D. **CORRECT:** The greatest risk to the client is injury to the renal system and sepsis from the UTI. The priority intervention is to administer antibiotics.

   Ⓝ *NCLEX® Connection: Pharmacological Therapies, Medication Administration*

3. A. **CORRECT:** The client should avoid sitting in a wet bathing suit, which can increase the risk for a UTI by colonization of bacteria in a moist, warm environment.

   B. The client should wipe the perineal area from front to back after elimination to prevent contaminating the urethra with bacteria.

   C. **CORRECT:** The client should empty the bladder when there is an urge to void. Retaining urine for an extended period of time increases the risk for a UTI.

   D. The client should wear cotton underwear that absorbs moisture and keeps the perineal area drier, thus decreasing colonization of bacteria that can cause a UTI.

   E. **CORRECT:** The client should take a shower daily to promote good body hygiene and decrease colonization of bacteria in the perineal area that can cause a UTI.

   Ⓝ *NCLEX® Connection: Physiological Adaptation, Alterations in Body Systems*

4. A. **CORRECT:** A client who is at 32 weeks of gestation is at risk for developing pyelonephritis because increased pressure on the urinary system during pregnancy causes reflux or retention of urine.

   B. **CORRECT:** A client who has kidney calculi is at risk for pyelonephritis because stones harbor bacteria.

   C. The expected reference range for urine pH is 4.6 to 8.0. Alkaline urine promotes bacteria growth. The client who has a urine pH of 4.2 has acidic urine.

   D. **CORRECT:** The client who has a neurogenic bladder can retain urine, promoting bacterial growth and causing pyelonephritis.

   E. **CORRECT:** The client who has diabetes mellitus is at risk of pyelonephritis because glucose in the urine promotes bacterial growth.

   Ⓝ *NCLEX® Connection: Physiological Adaptation, Basic Pathophysiology*

5. A. Hyaline casts in the urine can indicate proteinuria and can occur following exercise.

   B. **CORRECT:** A positive leukocyte esterase indicates a urinary tract infection.

   C. Ketones in the urine is a manifestation of poorly controlled diabetes mellitus or starvation.

   D. Crystals in the urine can indicate a potential for kidney stone formation.

   Ⓝ *NCLEX® Connection: Reduction of Risk Potential, Laboratory Values*

PRACTICE Answer

Using the ATI Active Learning Template: System Disorder

ALTERATION IN HEALTH (DIAGNOSIS):
Chronic pyelonephritis is a repetitive infection and inflammation of the kidney pelvis, calyces, and medulla that generally begins from bacteria that ascends from a lower urinary tract infection.

COMPLICATIONS
- Septic shock caused by micro-organisms entering the bloodstream from the infected kidney
- Chronic kidney disease caused by inflammation, fibrosis, and scarring of the kidney filtration structure
- Hypertension (related to fluid and sodium retention) indicating chronic kidney disease caused by destruction of the filtration system of the kidney from infection

CLIENT EDUCATION
- Consume at least 2 L of fluids daily.
- Take all medications as prescribed.
- Notify the provider of acute, rapid onset of pain.
- Verbalize fears and anxiety.
- Balance rest and activity.

Ⓝ *NCLEX® Connection: Physiological Adaptation, Alterations in Body Systems*

UNIT 8 NURSING CARE OF CLIENTS WHO HAVE RENAL DISORDERS
SECTION: RENAL SYSTEM DISORDERS

CHAPTER 53 *Renal Calculi*

Urolithiasis is the presence of calculi (stones) in the urinary tract. The majority of calculi contain calcium phosphate or calcium oxalate, but other substances (uric acid, struvite, cystine) can compose a renal calculus.

A diet high in calcium is not believed to increase the risk of calculi formation unless there is a pre-existing metabolic disorder or renal tubular defect. Reoccurrence increases in clients who have a family history.

Most clients can expel calculi without invasive procedures. Factors that influence the spontaneous passing of a renal calculus include composition, size, and location of the calculus.

DATA COLLECTION

RISK FACTORS

- Cause is unknown
- Higher incidence in males
- Recurrent urinary tract infection
- Urinary tract lining that is damaged
- Urine flow that is decreased, concentrated, and contains particles (calcium)
- Metabolic defects
  - Increased intestinal absorption or decreased kidney excretion of calcium
  - Increased oxalate production (genetic) or inability to metabolize oxalate from foods (black tea, spinach, beets, Swiss chard, chocolate, peanuts)
  - Increased production or decreased clearance of purines (contributing to increased uric-acid levels)
- High alkalinity or acidity of urine
- Urinary stasis, urinary retention, immobilization, dehydration
- History of intestinal bypass surgery (increased absorption of oxalate)
- Decrease in fluid intake or increase in the incidence of dehydration among older adult clients Ⓖ

EXPECTED FINDINGS

- Severe pain (renal colic)
  - Pain intensifies as the calculus moves through the ureter.
  - Flank pain suggests calculi are located in the kidney or ureter.
  - Flank pain that radiates to the abdomen, scrotum, testes, or vulva suggests calculi in the ureter or bladder.
- Urinary frequency or dysuria (calculi in the bladder)
- Fever
- Diaphoresis
- Pallor
- Nausea/vomiting due to the severity of the pain
- Tachycardia, tachypnea, increased blood pressure (pain), or decreased blood pressure (shock)
- Oliguria/anuria occurs with calculi that obstruct urinary flow. Urinary tract obstruction is a medical emergency and immediate treatment is necessary to preserve kidney function.
- Hematuria (dark brown or smoky-looking urine) ⓠEBP

LABORATORY TESTS

Urinalysis

- Infection manifests with an alteration in the odor of the urine and an increase in urine turbidity.
- RBCs, WBCs, and bacteria (presence of infection) increase.
- Crystals noted on microscopic exam
- Abnormal serum calcium, phosphate, and uric-acid levels in the presence of metabolic disorders/defects

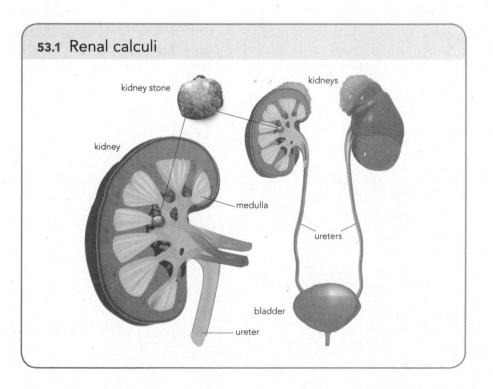

53.1 Renal calculi

kidney stone

kidneys

kidney

medulla

ureters

bladder

ureter

DIAGNOSTIC PROCEDURES

Radiology examination

X-ray of kidney, ureters, bladder (KUB), or intravenous pyelogram (IVP) is used to confirm the presence and location of calculi. IVP is contraindicated if there is a urinary obstruction.

CT or MRI

A CT (noncontrast helical scan) or MRI identifies cystine or uric-acid calculi, which is not detectable on standard x-rays.

Renal ultrasound or cystoscopy

These can confirm the diagnosis.

PATIENT-CENTERED CARE

NURSING CARE

- Report laboratory and diagnostic findings to the provider.
- Provide preoperative and postoperative care as indicated.
- Administer medications.
- Strain all urine to check for passage of the calculus, and save the calculus for laboratory analysis.
- Encourage an increase of oral intake to 3 L/day unless contraindicated.
- Assist with administration of IV fluids.
- Encourage ambulation to promote passage of the calculus.
- Monitor pain status, I&O, and urinary pH.

MEDICATIONS

Analgesics

Opioids
- Administer morphine sulfate when pain is 3 or greater on a pain scale of 0 to 10 during the acute onset of calculi pain.
- Treat moderate to severe pain with opioid medication. These medications act on the mu and kappa receptors that help alleviate pain. Activation of these receptors produces analgesia (pain relief), respiratory depression, euphoria, sedation, and a decrease in GI motility.
- Use cautiously with clients who have asthma or emphysema due to the risk of respiratory depression.
- NURSING ACTIONS
  ○ Check the client frequently.
  ○ Watch for evidence of respiratory depression, especially in older adult clients. If respirations are 12/min or less, stop the medication and notify the provider immediately. ⓖ
  ○ Monitor vital signs for hypotension and decreased respirations.
  ○ Determine level of sedation (drowsiness, level of consciousness).
- CLIENT EDUCATION: Drink plenty of fluids to prevent constipation.

NSAIDs
- Ketorolac treats mild to moderate pain, fever, and inflammation.
- NURSING ACTIONS: Observe for indications of bleeding.
- CLIENT EDUCATION
  ○ Watch for bleeding (dark stools, blood in stools).
  ○ Notify the provider if abdominal pain occurs, which can be due to gastric ulceration.

Spasmolytic medications

Oxybutynin alleviates pain by decreasing bladder spasms that can result from the renal calculi moving down the ureter into the bladder.

NURSING ACTIONS
- Collect data for history of glaucoma, as this medication increases intraocular pressure. Qᴘᴄᴄ
- Monitor for dizziness and tachycardia.
- Monitor for urinary retention.

CLIENT EDUCATION
- Report palpitations and problems with voiding or constipation.
- Dizziness and dry mouth are common. Suck on hard candies to alleviate dry mouth.

Antibiotics

Administer gentamicin and cephalexin to treat UTI that can cause renal calculi.

NURSING ACTIONS
- Monitor laboratory results for culture and sensitivity of infective organism.
- Administer medication with food to decrease GI distress.
- Monitor for nephrotoxicity and ototoxicity for clients taking gentamicin.

CLIENT EDUCATION
- Urine can have foul odor related to the antibiotic.
- Report loose stools related to the medication.

INTERPROFESSIONAL CARE

Urology services consult for management of urolithiasis.

Nutritional services consult for dietary modifications concerning foods related to calculi formation.

THERAPEUTIC PROCEDURES

Extracorporeal shock wave lithotripsy (ESWL)

- Uses shock-wave energies that pass through water, bounce off a reflector, move through the soft flank tissue, and break the calculi into fragments
- Requires moderate sedation or general anesthesia to prevent the client from moving during the procedure
- ECG monitoring during the procedure

NURSING ACTIONS
- Monitor for gross hematuria. Strain urine following the procedure and send stone fragments to the laboratory for analysis.
- Administer analgesics.

CLIENT EDUCATION

- The procedure uses moderate sedation or general anesthesia.
- Increase fluid to 4000 mL/day to flush calculi fragments through the urinary tract.
- Expect bruising at the location where the shock waves are generated, generally through the soft tissue of the flank area.
- Hematuria can occur postprocedure.

Surgical interventions

Stenting is the placement of a small tube in the ureter during a ureteroscopy to dilate the ureter and allow passage of a calculus.

Retrograde ureteroscopy uses a basket, forceps, or loop on the end of the ureteroscope to grasp and remove the calculus.

Percutaneous ureterolithotomy/nephrolithotomy is the insertion of an ultrasonic or laser lithotripter into the ureter or kidney to grasp and extract the calculus.

Open surgery uses a surgical incision to remove large or impacted calculi (staghorn calculi) or for calculi when other approaches are unsuccessful.

- **Ureterolithotomy:** into the ureter
- **Pyelolithotomy:** into the kidney pelvis
- **Nephrolithotomy:** into the kidney

CARE AFTER DISCHARGE: Recommend a nutritionist consult for dietary modifications concerning foods related to calculi formation. Qᴛᴄ

CLIENT EDUCATION: The role of diet and medications in the treatment and prevention of renal calculi.

- **Calcium phosphate**
  - Limit intake of food high in animal protein (reduction of protein intake decreases calcium precipitation).
  - Limit sodium intake.
  - Reduced calcium intake (dairy products) is individualized.
  - Treat underlying conditions that cause hypercalcemia (hyperparathyroidism)
  - Increase daily fluid intake to 2 to 3 liters.
  - Report any manifestations of urinary tract infection
- **Calcium oxalate**
  - Avoid oxalate sources (spinach, black tea, rhubarb, cocoa, beets, pecans, peanuts, okra, chocolate, wheat germ, lime peel, Swiss chard). Qᴘᴄᴄ
  - Limit sodium intake.
  - MEDICATIONS
    - Thiazide diuretics (hydrochlorothiazide) increase calcium reabsorption and increases urinary output.
    - Sodium cellulose phosphate reduces the intestinal absorption of calcium.
- **Struvite** (magnesium ammonium phosphate): Manifests from an increase in urinary tract infections. Administer antibiotics and acetohydroxamic acid to inhibit bacteria growth that contributes to this type of stone formation.

- **Uric acid** (urate)
  - Decrease intake of purine sources: organ meats, poultry, fish, gravies, red wine, sardines.
  - MEDICATIONS
    - Allopurinol prevents the formation of uric acid.
    - Potassium or sodium citrate or sodium bicarbonate alkalinizes the urine.
- **Cystine**
  - Alkalinize the urine by consuming potassium citrate or lemonade.
  - Consume fluids up to 3 L/day.
  - MEDICATIONS
    - Tiopronin prevents crystallization of cystine.

COMPLICATIONS

Urosepsis

Occurs when a urinary tract infection spreads to the client's bloodstream. This complication is potentially life-threatening due to organ failure and shock, and the nurse should report manifestations immediately. Qs

NURSING ACTIONS
- Monitor for indications of a urinary tract infection (fever, tachycardia, increased urine turbidity, urine odor, elevated serum WBC count, client report of pain with urination).
- Obtain urine culture and sensitivity and monitor for the results.
- Review the plan of care for antibiotic therapy.
- Monitor urinary output and report if less than 30 mL/hr.
- Monitor vital signs, neurological status, color, and appearance of the client's skin every 2 hr.
- Increase fluid intake.
- Provide adequate nutrition.

Obstruction

A calculus can block the passage of urine into the kidney, ureter, or bladder. Urinary output can be diminished or absent.

NURSING ACTIONS
- Notify the provider immediately.
- Assist with preparing the client for removal of the calculus.

Hydronephrosis

Occurs when a calculus blocks a portion of the urinary tract. The urine backs up and causes distention of the kidney.

NURSING ACTIONS
- Notify the provider immediately.
- Assist with preparing the client for removal of the calculus.

Application Exercises

1. A nurse is assisting with the admission assessment of a client who has renal calculi. Which of the following findings should the nurse expect?

   A. Bradycardia

   B. Diaphoresis

   C. Nocturia

   D. Bradypnea

2. A nurse is reinforcing discharge instructions with a client who had spontaneous passage of a calcium phosphate renal calculus. Which of the following instructions should the nurse include in the teaching? (Select all that apply.)

   A. Limit intake of food high in animal protein.

   B. Reduce sodium intake.

   C. Strain urine for 48 hr.

   D. Report burning with urination to the provider.

   E. Increase fluid intake to 3 L/day.

3. A nurse is reinforcing teaching with a client who is scheduled for extracorporeal shock wave lithotripsy (ESWL). Which of the following statements by the client indicates understanding of the teaching?

   A. "I will be fully awake during the procedure."

   B. "Lithotripsy will reduce my chances of having stones in the future."

   C. "I will report any bruising that occurs to my doctor."

   D. "Straining my urine following the procedure is important."

4. A nurse is caring for a client who has a left renal calculus and an indwelling urinary catheter. Which of the following findings is the priority for the nurse to report to the provider?

   A. Flank pain that radiates to the lower abdomen

   B. Client report of nausea

   C. Absent urine output for 1 hr

   D. Serum WBC count 15,000/mm^3

5. A nurse reinforcing discharge teaching with a client who has spontaneously passed a calcium oxalate calculus. To decrease the chance of recurrence, the client should avoid which of the following foods? (Select all that apply.)

   A. Red meat

   B. Black tea

   C. Cheese

   D. Peanuts

   E. Spinach

PRACTICE Active Learning Scenario

A nurse is contributing to the plan of care for a client who has renal calculi and prescriptions for morphine and oxybutynin for pain control. What should the nurse take into consideration when administering these medications? Use the ATI Active Learning Template: Medication to complete this item.

THERAPEUTIC USES: Identify the rationale for administering morphine and oxybutynin.

COMPLICATIONS: Identify adverse effects the nurse should monitor for when administering each of these medications.

NURSING INTERVENTIONS: Identify nursing considerations and client education the nurse should reinforce when administering each of these medications.

Application Exercises Key

1. A. Tachycardia is associated with renal calculi.

   B. **CORRECT:** Diaphoresis is associated with renal calculi.

   C. Oliguria associated with renal calculi.

   D. Tachypnea is associated with renal calculi.

   Ⓝ *NCLEX® Connection: Physiological Adaptation, Basic Pathophysiology*

2. A. **CORRECT:** The client should limit the intake of food high in animal protein, which contains calcium phosphate.

   B. **CORRECT:** The client should limit intake of sodium, which affects the precipitation of calcium phosphate in the urine.

   C. The client does not need to continue straining urine once the calculus has passed.

   D. **CORRECT:** The client should report burning with urination to the provider because this can indicate a urinary tract infection.

   E. **CORRECT:** The client should increase fluid intake to 2 to 3 L/day. A decrease in fluid intake can cause dehydration, which increases the risk of calculi formation.

   Ⓝ *NCLEX® Connection: Physiological Adaptation, Alterations in Body Systems*

3. A. The client can receive moderate sedation or general anesthesia to prevent movement during the procedure.

   B. Lithotripsy does not decrease the rate of recurrence of renal calculi. Lithotripsy breaks the calculi into fragments, which then pass into urine.

   C. The client can have bruising in the flank area following the procedure and does not need to notify the provider of this expected finding.

   D. **CORRECT:** The nurse should tell the client to strain urine following the lithotripsy procedure to collect the stone fragments for laboratory analysis.

   Ⓝ *NCLEX® Connection: Reduction of Risk Potential, Diagnostic Tests*

4. A. Flank pain radiating to the lower abdomen is expected as a renal calculus moves down the ureter. The nurse should provide the client with analgesia. However, another finding is the priority.

   B. Nausea is an expected finding related to severe pain as the calculi moves down the ureter. The nurse should administer an antiemetic to the client. However, another finding is the priority

   C. **CORRECT:** The greatest risk to the client is obstruction of urine flow by the renal calculus resulting in damage to the kidney. Therefore, absence of urine output is the priority finding for the nurse to report to the provider.

   D. An elevated serum WBC is a common finding associated with a renal calculus and can indicate a urinary tract infection. The nurse should determine whether the client requires an antibiotic. However, another finding is a priority.

   Ⓝ *NCLEX® Connection: Reduction of Risk Potential, Potential for Complications of Diagnostic Tests/Treatments/Procedures*

5. A. Consuming animal protein increases the risk of formation of calcium phosphate or uric acid stones.

   B. **CORRECT:** The client who has renal calculi composed of calcium oxalate should avoid intake of black tea because it is a source of oxalate.

   C. Consuming dairy products increases the risk of formation of calcium phosphate stones.

   D. **CORRECT:** The client who has renal calculi composed of calcium oxalate should avoid intake of peanuts because it is a source of oxalate.

   E. **CORRECT:** The client who has renal calculi composed of calcium oxalate should avoid intake of spinach because it is a source of oxalate.

   Ⓝ *NCLEX® Connection: Basic Care and Comfort, Nutrition and Oral Hydration*

PRACTICE Answer

Using the ATI Active Learning Template: Medication

THERAPEUTIC USES
- Morphine sulfate, an opioid, is administered during the first 24 hr to treat moderate to severe pain associated with acute renal calculi.
- Oxybutynin, a spasmolytic, is administered to provide pain relief by decreasing bladder spasms resulting from renal calculi.

COMPLICATIONS
- Morphine sulfate: respiratory depression, euphoria, sedation, decreased GI motility
- Oxybutynin: dizziness, tachycardia, urinary retention, dry mouth, constipation

NURSING INTERVENTIONS
- Morphine sulfate
  - Administer cautiously for clients who have asthma or emphysema due to the risk of respiratory depression.
  - Monitor frequently for respiratory depression, especially in older adults. If respirations are 12/min or less, stop the medication and notify the provider immediately.
  - Monitor vital signs frequently for hypotension.
  - Encourage the client to drink plenty of fluids to prevent constipation.

- Oxybutynin
  - Determine prior to administration if the client has a history of glaucoma, as this medication increases intraocular pressure.
  - Monitor for dizziness and tachycardia.
  - Monitor for urinary retention.
  - Instruct the client to report palpitations and problems with voiding or constipation.
  - Inform the client that dizziness and dry mouth are common with the medication.
  - Encourage the client to suck on hard candies to alleviate dry mouth.

Ⓝ *NCLEX® Connection: Physiological Adaptation, Alterations in Body Systems*

When reviewing the following chapters, keep in mind the relevant topics and tasks of the NCLEX outline, in particular:

Basic Care and Comfort

ELIMINATION: Perform an irrigation of the client's urinary catheter, bladder, wound, ear, nose, or eye.

NUTRITION AND ORAL HYDRATION: Monitor the client's intake and output.

Reduction of Risk Potential

DIAGNOSTIC TESTS: Perform diagnostic testing (blood glucose, oxygen saturation, testing for occult blood).

LABORATORY VALUES
Compare the client's laboratory values to normal laboratory values.

Monitor diagnostic or laboratory test results.

POTENTIAL FOR ALTERATIONS IN BODY SYSTEMS: Monitor the client's output for changes from baseline (nasogastric emesis, stool, urine).

Physiological Adaptation

ALTERATIONS IN BODY SYSTEMS
Provide care to correct the client's alteration in body systems.

Reinforce education to the client regarding care and condition.

Notify the primary health care provider of a change in the client's status.

BASIC PATHOPHYSIOLOGY: Apply knowledge of pathophysiology to monitoring the client for alterations in body systems.

CHAPTER 54 *Diagnostic and Therapeutic Procedures for Female Reproductive Disorders*

Diagnostic procedures are used to evaluate the structure, condition, and function of a female client's reproductive tissues and organs. Biopsies serve a therapeutic purpose in removing abnormal tissue. Nurses should be knowledgeable about the therapeutic intent and nursing care for a hysterectomy.

Pelvic exam with Papanicolaou and human papilloma virus tests

The provider performs bimanual examination of the cervix, uterus, fallopian tubes, and ovaries. The provider inserts two gloved fingers into the vagina and traps the reproductive structures between the fingers of the one hand and the fingers of the opposite hand that is on the abdomen. Palpation of the structures is done during this time.

Two tests are used for cervical cancer screening, the Papanicolaou (Pap) test and the test for human papilloma virus (HPV). Both can be performed prior to the pelvic examination. **(54.1)**
- **Pap test** is used to identify precancerous and cancerous cells of the cervix.
- **HPV test** is used to identify HPV infections that can lead to cervical cancer.

CONSIDERATIONS

PREPROCEDURE Qpcc

NURSING ACTIONS
- Have the client empty bladder.
- Place the client in the lithotomy position and drape appropriately.
- Explain to the client how the procedure will be carried out.
- Have all necessary equipment available (gloves, vaginal speculum, lubricant, cervical scraping tools, glass slides, fixative, tissues, perineal pad).

CLIENT EDUCATION
- Schedule the test when not menstruating.
- Use of vaginal medications, douching, or sexual intercourse within the past 24 hr can alter test results.

INTRAPROCEDURE

NURSING ACTIONS
- Remain with the client and provide support.
- Have ready the necessary equipment for the provider during procedure.
- Transfer specimens to slides and apply fixative to slides.

POSTPROCEDURE

NURSING ACTIONS
- Provide the client with perineal pad and tissues.
- Inform the client of the time frame for results to be available.

CLIENT EDUCATION
- Minimal bleeding can occur from the cervix.
- Follow up with provider if results are abnormal.

54.1 Pap and HPV screening guidelines

The American Cancer Society provides guidelines for the prevention and early detection of cervical cancer. See www.cancer.org. QEBP

Testing recommendations by age

Age	Recommendation
21	All women begin screening for cervical cancer.
21 TO 29	Pap test every 3 years. HPV unnecessary unless needed following an abnormal Pap test.
30 TO 65	Pap and HPV every 5 years.
OLDER THAN 65	May discontinue testing if regular screenings have been negative. If diagnosed with cervical precancer, continue to screen.

Screening is unnecessary for females who have had a hysterectomy with removal of the cervix and have a negative history of cervical cancer.

Females who are at high risk for cervical cancer need to be screened more frequently based on the advice of the provider.

Colposcopy and cervical biopsy

A colposcopy is the examination of the tissues of the vagina and cervix using an electric microscope. Typically, the provider also performs a biopsy. Several options are available.

- The provider may perform an endocervical curettage if a lesion is visible.
- A cone biopsy is an extensive surgical biopsy. The provider excises a cone-shaped sample of tissue to remove potentially harmful cells. In some cases, anesthesia is used for the procedure. Margins of the excised tissue are examined to ensure removal of all harmful cells. The surgeon may destroy the cells using a scalpel, cryosurgery (extreme cold, which freezes the tissue), lasers, or loop electrosurgical excision (LEEP). LEEP uses an electric current, and the laser procedure uses a laser beam that vaporizes the abnormal tissue.
- The best time to perform the procedure is in the early phase of the menstrual cycle because the cervix is less vascular.

INDICATIONS

Pap tests that demonstrate atypical or abnormal cells must be followed up with a colposcopy and cervical biopsy.

CONSIDERATIONS

PREPROCEDURE

NURSING ACTIONS
- Provide psychological support.
- Explain the procedure to the client.
- Preprocedure care is the same as that for a Pap test, except a sterile biopsy cup will be needed instead of the other equipment.

CLIENT EDUCATION: When the specimen is obtained, expect to experience temporary discomfort and cramping.

POSTPROCEDURE

NURSING ACTIONS
- Postprocedure care is the same as for a Pap test.
- Provide client with perineal pad and tissues.

CLIENT EDUCATION Qᴘᴄᴄ
- Rest for the first 24 hr after the procedure.
- Abstain from sexual intercourse and avoid using a douche, vaginal creams, or tampons until all discharge has stopped (usually about 2 weeks).
- Avoid lifting heavy objects for approximately 2 weeks to allow time for the cervix to heal.
- Use analgesics as directed, but avoid the use of aspirin because it can cause bleeding. Qˢ
- Report excessive bleeding, fever, or foul-smelling drainage to the provider.

COMPLICATIONS

Bleeding

Heavy bleeding can result from the excision of tissue.

NURSING ACTIONS: Monitor for heavy bleeding.

CLIENT EDUCATION: Notify the provider of heavy vaginal bleeding.

Infection

Infection can result from this invasive procedure.

NURSING ACTIONS: Observe for fever, chills, severe pain, foul odor, or purulent vaginal discharge.

CLIENT EDUCATION: Notify the provider regarding manifestations of infection.

Endometrial biopsy

A thin, hollow tube is inserted through the cervix, and a curette or suction equipment is used to obtain the endometrial tissue sample.

INDICATIONS

POTENTIAL DIAGNOSES: Endometrial biopsies are done to check for uterine cancer as well as evaluate for menstrual irregularities and potential causes of infertility.

CLIENT PRESENTATION: Abnormal or postmenopausal bleeding

CONSIDERATIONS

PREPROCEDURE

NURSING ACTIONS
- Obtain the client's menstrual history.
- Administer an analgesic prior to the procedure.
- Prepare the client using same procedure as pelvic examination.
- Witness consent.
- Have the client empty her bladder.

CLIENT EDUCATION Qᴘᴄᴄ
- Biopsies are done without sedation.
- Expect to feel some discomfort and cramping.
- Use relaxation techniques.

POSTPROCEDURE

NURSING ACTIONS: Postprocedure care is the same as that for a Pap test.

CLIENT EDUCATION

- Rest on the examination table until cramping has diminished.
- Spotting can be present for 1 to 2 days.
- Results will be available in approximately 72 hr.
- Abstain from sexual intercourse and avoid using a douche, vaginal creams, or tampons until all discharge has stopped (usually about 1 to 2 days).
- Notify the provider of heavy vaginal bleeding, fever, severe pain, or foul discharge.

COMPLICATIONS

Bleeding

Heavy vaginal bleeding is a potential complication of an endometrial biopsy.

NURSING ACTIONS: Monitor for heavy bleeding.

CLIENT EDUCATION: Notify the provider of heavy vaginal bleeding.

Infection

Infection can result from this invasive procedure.

NURSING ACTIONS: Observe for fever, chills, severe pain, foul odor, and purulent vaginal discharge.

CLIENT EDUCATION: Notify the provider regarding manifestations of infection.

Screening for reproductive disorders (sexually transmitted infections)

Syphilis

There are two serologic (blood) studies used to screen for syphilis. QEBP

- Venereal disease research laboratory (VDRL): the oldest test for syphilis that is still performed
- Rapid plasma reagin (RPR): a newer test for syphilis and has replaced the VDRL test in many institutions

INTERPRETATION OF FINDINGS

- Both tests are done using a sample of blood and reported as nonreactive (negative for syphilis) or reactive (positive for syphilis).
- False positives can occur secondary to infection, pregnancy, malignancies, and autoimmune disorders.
- If either test is reactive, diagnosis should be confirmed using one of the following tests.
  - Fluorescent treponemal antibody absorbed (FTA–ABS)
  - Microhemagglutination assays for antibody to *T. pallidum*

Human immune deficiency virus (HIV)

The enzyme immunoassay (EIA) test and Western blot assay are used to detect the presence of HIV.

INTERPRETATION OF FINDINGS

- The EIA test, formerly the enzyme-linked immunosorbent assay (ELISA), is an antibody test used to measure response to HIV. The test is typically positive 3 weeks to 3 months after the infection occurs, but it can be delayed for as long as 36 months. False positive results can occur, so further testing is needed.
- If the EIA is positive, the Western blot assay is used to confirm the diagnosis of HIV.

Genital herpes

Although a diagnosis of genital herpes can be based on the client's history and physical, it can be confirmed with laboratory testing, which include the following.

- **Herpes viral culture:** Fluid from a lesion is obtained using a swab and placed in a cup for culture.
- **Polymerase chain reaction (PRC) test:** Identifies genetic material of the virus. Cells from a lesion, blood, or other body fluids can be tested. Identifies type of virus (herpes simplex 1 [HSV 1] or herpes simplex 2 [HSV 2]).
- **Antibody test:** Blood is tested for antibodies to the virus. Some tests can identify the type of virus (HSV 1 and HSV 2).

Mammography

During a mammogram, the x-ray machine mechanically compresses a breast both vertically and horizontally while radiologic pictures are taken of the breast.

INDICATIONS

Screening mammograms detect breast cancer lesions in women who do not have manifestations. Screening mammograms decrease cancer death rates because the treatment options and outcomes are best when the cancer is detected early. Q𝐄𝐁𝐏

> Many organizations provide guidelines for screening mammograms, including the American Cancer Society and the U.S. Preventive Services Task Force. For current guidelines, see www.cancer.org and www.uspreventiveservicestaskforce.org.

Diagnostic mammograms are used when a screening mammogram reveals abnormal findings or when breast cancer manifestations are present. The diagnostic mammogram provides a more detailed picture and is more accurate than the screening mammogram.

There are two types of mammography screening tools. Traditional mammography images are stored on film. Digital mammography takes an electronic image, which can be stored electronically. Both types are effective diagnostic tools. However, the digital mammogram can be more useful in clients who have dense breast tissue. It is also more costly.

A breast ultrasound can be used to determine whether a mass is fluid-filled (cyst) or a solid mass, which could be a cancerous lesion. A wire needle biopsy can be used if the abnormal area is too small to be palpated. Ultrasound is used to identify the area of concern. Then a small wire is placed into the area. Subsequently the surgeon performs a biopsy using the wire to locate the area.

CONSIDERATIONS

PREPROCEDURE Q𝐏𝐂𝐂

CLIENT EDUCATION
- Avoid the use of deodorant, lotion, or powders in the axillary region or on the breasts prior to the exam.
- Do not have a mammogram if pregnant.

INTRAPROCEDURE

Radiologic technicians are often the members of the health care team who perform mammograms.

CLIENT EDUCATION: Slight, temporary discomfort is expected when the breast is compressed.

POSTPROCEDURE

CLIENT EDUCATION
- The client will be contacted about results of diagnostic examination.
- Practice self-breast examinations.
- Follow the advice of provider regarding when to return for a follow-up mammogram.

Hysterosalpingography

- Visualization of the cervix, uterus, and fallopian tubes by x-ray with injection of contrast dye
- Performed 2 to 5 days following menstrual period to avoid harm to an existing pregnancy

INDICATIONS

- Evaluation of fibroids, tumors, and fistulas
- Determine fertility

CONSIDERATIONS

PREPROCEDURE

NURSING ACTIONS Q𝐬
- Confirm date of client's last menstrual cycle.
- Monitor for allergy to iodine.
- Witness informed consent.
- Prepare client as for a pelvic exam.

INTRAPROCEDURE

NURSING ACTIONS
- Remain with the client and provide support.
- Have ready the necessary equipment for the provider during the procedure.

POSTPROCEDURE

NURSING ACTIONS
- Provide the client with perineal pad and tissues.
- Inform the client of the time frame for results to be available.

CLIENT EDUCATION Q𝐏𝐂𝐂
- Minimal bleeding can occur from the cervix.
- Take analgesics as prescribed for pelvic cramping and referred pain to the shoulder.
- Notify the provider if bleeding continues for 4 or more days and report any manifestations of infection (fever, severe pain, foul discharge).

Hysterectomy

- A hysterectomy is the removal of the uterus.
- A bilateral salpingo oophorectomy is the removal of the ovaries and fallopian tubes.
- There are three methods of performing a hysterectomy.
  - Abdominal approach, also known as a total abdominal hysterectomy
  - Vaginal approach
  - Laparoscopy-assisted vaginal hysterectomy
- There are a number of options available for a client who requires a hysterectomy or other reproductive procedure. In some cases, the decision regarding which procedure is based on the client's preference in conjunction with the surgeon's recommendation.
  - Total hysterectomy: Uterus and cervix are removed.
  - Subtotal hysterectomy: Uterus is removed; cervix is not.
  - Bilateral salpingo oophorectomy: Ovaries and fallopian tubes are removed.
  - Panhysterectomy: Uterus, cervix, ovaries, and fallopian tubes are removed.
  - Radical hysterectomy: Uterus, cervix, upper part of the vagina, and adjacent tissue (including lymph nodes) are removed.
- To treat leiomyomas (benign fibroid tumors), uterine-sparing procedures are available.

INDICATIONS

POTENTIAL DIAGNOSES
- Uterine cancer
- Noncancerous conditions: fibroids, endometriosis (inflammation of the endometrium), and genital prolapse that cause pain, bleeding, or emotional stress

CLIENT PRESENTATION
- Painful intercourse
- Hypermenorrhea
- Pelvic pressure
- Urinary urgency or frequency
- Constipation

CONSIDERATIONS

PREPROCEDURE

NURSING ACTIONS Qs
- Ensure that clients have discontinued use of anticoagulant medications, aspirin, nonsteroidal anti-inflammatory drugs (NSAIDs), and vitamin E.
- Rule out pregnancy.
- Administer preoperative antibiotics.
- Place antiembolism stockings.
- Measure psychological status.
- Maintain NPO status.
- Ensure that informed consent has been obtained.

CLIENT EDUCATION Qs
- How to turn, cough, and deep breathe, and the importance of early ambulation
- How to use an incentive spirometer
- Information about preoperative and postoperative medications

POSTPROCEDURE Qebp

NURSING ACTIONS
- Monitor for vaginal bleeding. Excess bleeding is more than one saturated pad in 4 hr.
- An indwelling urinary catheter is generally inserted intraoperatively and in place for the first 24 hr postoperatively.

Priority interventions following total abdominal hysterectomy
- Measure vital signs (fever, hypotension).
- Monitor breath sounds (risk of atelectasis; turn, cough, and deep breathe; use of incentive spirometry; ambulation).
- Auscultate bowel sounds (risk of paralytic ileus).
- Monitor urine output. (Call the provider if less than 30 mL/hr.)
- Assist with IV fluid and electrolyte replacement until bowel sounds return.
- Check the incision (infection, integrity, risk of dehiscence).
- Observe for indications of thrombophlebitis (warmth, tenderness, edema).
- Take thromboembolism precautions (sequential compression devices, ambulation).
- Monitor blood loss (Hgb and Hct, vital signs).

CLIENT EDUCATION
- Consume a well-balanced diet that is high in protein and vitamin C for wound healing, and high in iron if anemic.
- If the ovaries have been removed, menopausal manifestations can develop. Discuss issues related to hormone therapy with the client.
- Restrict activity (heavy lifting, strenuous activity, driving, stairs, sexual activity) for as long as 6 weeks depending on the procedure that was performed. Qs
- Avoid the use of tampons.
- Notify the surgeon of temperatures greater than 37.8° C (100° F), foul-smelling drainage from incision, pain, redness, swelling in calf, or burning on urination.

COMPLICATIONS

Complications for clients following a hysterectomy are similar to that of clients who are postoperative following other abdominal surgeries.

Hypovolemic shock

Hypovolemic shock due to blood loss is a potential complication following a hysterectomy.

NURSING ACTIONS
- Monitor vital signs, Hgb, and Hct.
- Check for excessive vaginal bleeding (more than one saturated perineal pad in 4 hr).
- Provide fluid replacement therapy and blood transfusions as indicated.

Infection

Can be indicated by foul-smelling vaginal drainage, temperatures greater than 37.8° C (100° F), and redness, swelling, or drainage at the site of the incision.

Psychological reactions

Psychological reactions can occur months to years after surgery.

NURSING ACTIONS
- Encourage the client to discuss the positive aspects of life.
- Understand that occasional sadness in the client is normal, but persistent sadness or depression indicates a need for counseling assistance.

CLIENT EDUCATION: Attend a support group. Qpcc

Application Exercises

1. A nurse is reviewing the facility's testing process and procedures for human immune deficiency virus (HIV) with a new employee. Which of the following information should the nurse include in the review?

    A. The enzyme immunoassay (EIA) test is typically reactive within 72 hr after the client is infected with HIV.

    B. The Western blot assay is used to confirm diagnosis of HIV.

    C. The polymerase chain reaction (PRC) test is used to confirm diagnosis of HIV.

    D. CD4+ cell counts are elevated in a client who is infected with HIV.

2. A nurse is reinforcing teaching with a client prior to her first mammogram. Which of the following statements should the nurse include in the teaching?

    A. "You should not take any aspirin products prior to the mammogram."

    B. "Do not apply any deodorant the day of the exam."

    C. "You will need to avoid sexual intercourse the day before the mammogram."

    D. "You should avoid exercise prior to the exam."

3. A nurse is preparing a client for her first Papanicolaou (Pap) test. Which of the following statements should the nurse make?

    A. "You should urinate immediately after the procedure is over."

    B. "You will not feel any discomfort."

    C. "You may experience some bleeding after the procedure."

    D. "You will need to hold your breath during the procedure."

4. A nurse in a provider's office is reviewing a client's laboratory results, which shows a positive rapid plasma regain (RPR). The nurse should identify which of the following tests will be administered to the client to confirm the diagnosis of syphilis?

    A. Venereal disease research laboratory (VDRL)

    B. D-dimer

    C. Fluorescent treponemal antibody absorbed (FTA-ABS)

    D. Papanicolaou (Pap) test

5. A nurse is reinforcing teaching with a client who is to undergo a cervical biopsy. Which of the following information should the nurse include in the instructions? (Select all that apply.)

    A. "The procedure is painless."

    B. "Avoid heavy lifting for approximately 2 weeks after the procedure."

    C. "Heavy bleeding is common during the first 12 hours after the procedure."

    D. "Plan to rest for the first 72 hours after the procedure."

    E. "Avoid the use of tampons for 2 weeks after the procedure."

PRACTICE Active Learning Scenario

A nurse is assisting with the plan of care for a client who is to have a total abdominal hysterectomy. Use the ATI Active Learning Template: Therapeutic Procedure to complete this item.

NURSING ACTIONS (PRE, INTRA, POST): List at least two nursing actions the nurse should include preprocedure and at least four actions the nurse should include postprocedure.

Application Exercises Key

1. A. The EIA test is typically reactive 3 weeks to 3 months after the infection occurs, but it can be delayed for as long as 36 months.

   B. **CORRECT:** Confirming HIV is a two-step process. If the EIA is positive, a second test (the Western blot assay) is done.

   C. The PRC test is used to confirm the diagnosis of genital herpes.

   D. The nurse should expect the CD4+ cell counts to be decreased elevated in a client who is infected with HIV.

   Ⓝ *NCLEX® Connection: Reduction of Risk Potential, Laboratory Values*

2. A. Taking aspirin products does not alter the accuracy of a mammogram.

   B. **CORRECT:** Applying deodorant or powder can alter the accuracy of a mammogram by causing a shadow to appear.

   C. Having sexual intercourse does not alter the accuracy of a mammogram.

   D. Exercising does not alter the accuracy of a mammogram.

   Ⓝ *NCLEX® Connection: Reduction of Risk Potential, Diagnostic Tests*

3. A. The client is instructed to urinate immediately before the procedure.

   B. The client can experience discomfort when the provider obtains the cervical sample.

   C. **CORRECT:** The client can experience a small amount of vaginal bleeding due to scraping of the cervix.

   D. The client should use relaxation techniques, such as taking deep breaths during the procedure.

   Ⓝ *NCLEX® Connection: Reduction of Risk Potential, Diagnostic Tests*

4. A. The VDRL is another screening test for syphilis.

   B. The D-dimer is a test used to measure fibrin in the blood and rule out the presence of a clot or help diagnose disseminated intravascular coagulation.

   C. **CORRECT:** The fluorescent treponemal antibody absorbed is used to confirm the diagnosis of syphilis.

   D. The Papanicolaou (Pap) test is used to detect cervical cell changes that can indicate cancer.

   Ⓝ *NCLEX® Connection: Reduction of Risk Potential, Laboratory Values*

5. A. Typically the client will experience temporary discomfort and cramping when the specimen is obtained.

   B. **CORRECT:** The client should avoid heavy lifting until the cervix has healed, which takes approximately 2 weeks.

   C. Some bleeding is common after a cervical biopsy, but excessive bleeding is a complication and should be reported to the provider.

   D. The client should plan to rest for the first 24 hr after the procedure.

   E. **CORRECT:** The client should not use tampons until the cervix has healed, which takes approximately 2 weeks.

   Ⓝ *NCLEX® Connection: Reduction of Risk Potential, Diagnostic Tests*

PRACTICE Answer

Using the ATI Active Learning Template: Therapeutic Procedure

NURSING ACTIONS (PRE, INTRA, POST)

Preprocedure
- Maintain NPO status.
- Ensure that informed consent has been obtained.
- Instruct the client to turn, cough, and deep breathe; to use the incentive spirometer; and regarding the importance of early ambulation
- Instruct the client about preoperative and postoperative medications.
- Rule out pregnancy.
- Ensure that clients who have been taking anticoagulant medications, aspirin, nonsteroidal anti-inflammatory drugs (NSAIDs), or vitamin E have discontinued their use.
- Administer preoperative antibiotics.
- Place antiembolism stockings.
- Measure psychological status.

Postprocedure
- Monitor vaginal bleeding. The client should have no more than one saturated perineal pad in 4 hr.
- Maintain indwelling urinary catheter and monitor urine output. The client should have at least 30 mL/hr.
- Monitor vital signs.
- Monitor breath sounds and use of incentive spirometer.
- Assist with ambulation.
- Auscultate bowel sounds.
- Assist with IV fluid and electrolyte replacement.
- Check the incision.
- Monitor the Hgb and Hct.
- Observe for indications of thrombosis and take thromboembolism precautions.
- Instruct the client about diets that promote wound healing (high protein and vitamin C).
- Instruct the client to restrict activity.
- If ovaries have been removed, discuss issues related to hormone therapy.
- Remind the client to avoid the use of tampons.
- Tell the client to notify the surgeon of temperature greater than 37.8° C (100° F), foul-smelling drainage from incision, pain, redness, swelling in calf, and burning on urination.
- Measure psychological status.

Ⓝ *NCLEX® Connection: Reduction of Risk Potential, Potential for Complications from Surgical Procedures and Health Alterations*

CHAPTER 55 *Menstrual Disorders and Menopause*

The average age of menarche (first menses) is 12.4 years but can occur from 9 to 17 years. Evaluation by a provider is indicated if an adolescent has not begun menstruation by 16.5 years of age.

Menstrual cycles are typically 28 days long, with a range from 23 to 35 days. The first day of menstruation is day 1 of a menstrual cycle. Ovulation typically occurs around day 14. Menstruation begins 14 days after ovulation and typically lasts 4 to 6 days, but it can continue for up to 9 days. Monthly menstruation often causes minor discomfort, such as uterine cramping, a feeling of heaviness in the pelvic area along with backache and breast tenderness.

Menstrual cycles continue until menopause or surgical removal of the uterus. Menopause is when ovulation ceases and menstrual cycles become irregular and eventually stop. The median age of onset of menopause is 51 years.

Menstrual disorders

Painful menstruation (dysmenorrhea) is common in adolescents and young females. In many clients, this pain is significantly decreased after the birth of a child or as the client becomes older.

Dysfunctional uterine bleeding (DUB) is believed to be due to a hormonal imbalance of decreased estrogen and can include menorrhagia and metrorrhagia.
- **Menorrhagia** is excessive menstrual bleeding (in amount and duration), possibly with clots that saturates more than one tampon or pad per hour.
- **Metrorrhagia** is bleeding between menstrual periods. It is more common in clients who are entering menopause and in adolescent clients.

Amenorrhea is the absence of menses. In a client who has had menstrual cycles, this can be an indication of pregnancy, a medical disorder or a hormone imbalance (thyroid disorder, structural disorders of the reproductive system). A common cause is low percentage of body fat in clients who are involved in sports or strenuous physical activity. Anorexia nervosa also can result in amenorrhea due to a decrease in body fat.

Premenstrual syndrome (PMS) is thought to be caused by an imbalance between estrogen and progesterone, and increased prolactin and aldosterone levels during the luteal phase (between ovulation and the start of menstruation) of the menstrual cycle.
- Manifestations can vary among clients and can vary for an individual client from one cycle to the next. Common manifestations include irritability, impaired memory, depression, poor concentration, mood swings, binge eating, breast tenderness, bloating, weight gain, headache, and back pain.
- **Premenstrual dystrophic disorder (PMDD)** is a severe form of PMS seen in only a small number of clients (3% to 8%), and it consists of debilitating premenstrual mood manifestations that interfere with a client's ability to carry out daily activities. With either condition, manifestations begin a few days before the menstrual period and end a few days after the onset of the menstrual period.

Endometriosis is characterized by an overgrowth of endometrial tissue that extends outside the uterus into the fallopian tubes, onto the ovaries, and into the pelvis. Blockage of the fallopian tubes by endometrial tissue is a common cause of infertility.

DATA COLLECTION

When collecting data on a client who has a menstrual disorder the nurse should determine the following.
- Menstrual history (age of first menses, monthly cycle)
- Timing and regularity of the menstrual cycle, and duration along with the amount of the menstrual flow.
- Sexual history
- Nutritional history

EXPECTED FINDINGS

- Report of premenstrual depression, irritability, changes in appetite, abdominal bloating, fatigue, emotional lability, or fluid retention
- Characteristics of flow
- Characteristics and location of pain during menstrual cycle
- Pelvic tenderness during palpation of the lower abdomen and the pelvic examination
- Metabolic disorders (thyroid disorders)

LABORATORY TESTS

Hemoglobin and hematocrit can be below the expected reference range due to excessive blood loss.

CA-125 is an immunodiagnostic test in which findings are elevated in ovarian cancer. Endometriosis and other conditions can also cause CA-125 to be elevated above the expected reference range.

DIAGNOSTIC PROCEDURES

Endometrial biopsy determines the relationship between menstrual flow and the hormone cycle, as well as possible pathologic reasons for bleeding, such as uterine cancer.

Transvaginal ultrasound can identify the presence of uterine fibroids, endometrial abnormalities, or leiomyomas.

Laparoscopy can identify inflammation, edema, and possible abscess of pelvic structures.

PATIENT-CENTERED CARE

MEDICATIONS

Hormonal contraceptives

- Can be used to decrease manifestations of PMS, PMDD, dysmenorrhea, endometriosis, and DUB
- Can be the initial treatment for endometriosis

Diuretic

An aldosterone antagonist (spironolactone) can be used to treat bloating and weight gain associated with PMS and PMDD.

Leuprolide: synthetic luteinizing hormone

- Reduces the follicle-stimulating and luteinizing hormone levels in DUB
- Suppresses estrogen and testosterone production in the body, making it an effective treatment for endometriosis (promotes atrophy of ectopic tissue)
- Can cause birth defects, so the client should use a reliable form of contraception **Qs**
- Can cause decreased libido and increased risk of osteoporosis

NSAIDs: ibuprofen

- Prescribed for endometriosis to inhibit production of prostaglandins and relieve pain.
- Aids in treatment of pain and discomfort related to PMS and PMDD

Oral iron supplements

Used to treat anemia associated with DUB

SSRIs: fluoxetine, sertraline

Used to treat the emotional and physical manifestations of PMS and PMDD

THERAPEUTIC PROCEDURES

Dysfunctional uterine bleeding

Dilatation and curettage: Used to diagnose and treat DUB. The cervix is dilated, and the wall of the uterus is scraped with a curette. Endometrium scraped from the uterine wall is sent to the laboratory for examination.

Endometrial ablation: Used to remove endometrial tissue in the uterus. The tissue may be removed by laser, heat, electricity, or cryotherapy.

Hysterectomy: If other treatments are unsuccessful

Endometriosis

Laparoscopic removal of ectopic tissue and adhesions: A laser may be used to remove tissue.

Menopause

- Menopause is the period during which there is a permanent cessation of menses. Menses will appear on an infrequent cycle for a period of time, which can be 4 to 5 years. Menopause is considered complete when no menses have occurred for 12 months.
- The client can have natural or surgically induced menopause when the ovaries are removed in premenopausal clients.

DATA COLLECTION

EXPECTED FINDINGS

Vasomotor manifestations: Hot flashes, palpitations, night sweats, headaches, and irregular menses

Genitourinary: Atrophic vaginitis, shrinking of labia, decreased vaginal secretions, dyspareunia, increased vaginal pH, vaginal dryness and atrophy, and incontinence.

Psychological: Mood swings, changes in sleep patterns, decreased REM sleep

Skeletal: Decreased bone density

Cardiovascular: Decreased HDL, increased LDL

Dermatological: Decreased skin elasticity, loss of hair on the head and pubic area

Reproductive: Breast tissue changes

LABORATORY TESTS

Follicle-stimulating hormone (FSH): Increased during menopause

Blood, urine, and saliva hormone levels: Estrogens, progesterone, testosterone

DIAGNOSTIC PROCEDURES

Pelvic examination with Papanicolaou (Pap) test to rule out cancer in cases of abnormal bleeding

Breast examination with mammogram to rule out cancer in cases of a palpable change from predominantly glandular tissue to fatty tissue

Biopsy of uterine lining in cases of undiagnosed abnormal uterine bleeding in a client older than 40 years of age, or in a client whose menses has stopped for 1 year and bleeding has begun again

Bone mineral density measurement using dual-energy x-ray absorptiometry (DXA) to determine the client's risk for osteoporosis

PATIENT-CENTERED CARE

MEDICATIONS

Menopausal hormone replacement therapy (HRT)

- Estrogen deficiency manifestations occur naturally as part of the aging process during menopause. HRT is prescribed to suppress hot flashes associated with menopause, to prevent atrophy of vaginal tissue, and to reduce the risk of fractures due to osteoporosis. For a client who has a uterus, HRT includes estrogen and progestin. For a client who no longer has a uterus (following a hysterectomy), estrogen alone is prescribed.
- Many preparations of HRT are available (oral, transdermal, intravaginal, intramuscular). The provider may prescribe HRT as a continuous, combined estrogen-progesterone therapy or a variety of cyclic patterns.
- Based on their individual risk factors and health care needs, clients should discuss the risks and benefits of using HRT with their providers.
  - The risk associated with the use of HRT depends on many factors (the age of the client, personal/family history, regimen prescribed).
  - HRT places clients at risk for a number of adverse conditions (coronary heart disease; myocardial infarction [MI]; deep-vein thrombosis; stroke; endometrial, ovarian, and breast cancer).
- If HRT is required for management of menopausal manifestations, the recommendation is to use HRT on a short-term basis.

CLIENT EDUCATION

- Advantages and disadvantages of HRT; HRT can be beneficial in the prevention of age-related problems (osteoporosis, fractures).
- Atrophic vaginitis, which is characterized by vaginal burning and bleeding, pruritus, and painful intercourse, can improve with HRT. Vaginal instillations of estrogen can be the best option because systemic absorption is reduced.
- Self-administration of HRT.
- Quit smoking immediately, if applicable.

- How to prevent and monitor the development of venous thrombosis Qs
  - Avoid wearing knee-high stockings, and restrictive clothing or socks.
  - Note and report manifestations of unilateral leg pain, edema, warmth, and redness.
  - Avoid sitting for long periods of time.
  - Take short walks throughout the day to promote circulation.
  - Perform frequent ankle pumps, and move and stretch legs.
- Female clients often experience manifestations of MI different from the classic chest pain often reported by male clients. Seek assistance immediately if manifestations of an MI (dyspnea, jaw discomfort, indigestion, pain between the shoulders) develop.
- If oral therapy causes nausea, taking medication with food can help.
- If the client is using vaginal creams or suppositories of estrogen compounds, be sure to refrain from inserting them prior to intercourse, or the client's partner can absorb some of the product.

Alternative therapies

- Ask the client about use of complementary and alternative therapies (black cohosh, chasteberry, St. John's wort, ginseng, red clover) to relieve the effects of menopause. Research regarding their usefulness is inconsistent.
- Phytoestrogens interact with estrogen receptors in the body, which can result in a decrease in the manifestations of menopause. Vegetables such as dandelion greens, alfalfa sprouts, black beans, and soy beans contain phytoestrogens. QEBP
- Vitamins E and B_6 are reported to decrease hot flashes in some clients.

CLIENT EDUCATION: Older adult clients can decrease the risk of osteoporosis by performing regular weight-bearing exercises; increasing intake of high-protein and high-calcium foods; avoiding alcohol, caffeine, and tobacco; and taking calcium with vitamin D supplements. Ⓒ

COMPLICATIONS

Embolic complications

Risks increased by concurrent smoking
- Myocardial infarction, especially during the first year of therapy
- Stroke
- Venous thrombosis: thrombophlebitis, especially during the first year of therapy

Cancer

- In some studies, long-term use of HRT has been found to increase the risk for breast cancer.
- Studies indicate lowering the risk of colon cancer.
- Some studies indicate that long-term use of estrogen-only HRT increases the risk for ovarian and endometrial cancer.

Application Exercises

1. A nurse is reinforcing teaching about menstruation with an adolescent female client. Which of the following statements should the nurse include? (Select all that apply.)

   A. "The average age of onset of menstruation is 10."

   B. "The range for a typical menstrual cycle is between 23 and 35 days."

   C. "The first day of the menstrual cycle begins with the last day of the menstrual period."

   D. "Ovulation typically occurs around the 14th day of the menstrual cycle."

   E. "A menstrual period can last as long as 9 days."

2. A nurse is reviewing the medical record of a client who has premenstrual syndrome (PMS). The nurse should identify that which of the following medications are used to treat PMS? (Select all that apply.)

   A. Fluoxetine

   B. Spironolactone

   C. Ethinyl estradiol/drospirenone

   D. Ferrous sulfate

   E. Methylergonovine

3. A nurse in a provider's office is providing information to a client who has dysfunctional uterine bleeding (DUB). Which of the following client statements indicate understanding of the information? (Select all that apply.)

   A. "My heavy bleeding can be due to a hormonal imbalance."

   B. "If I experience menstrual pain, I should take aspirin."

   C. "I can't take oral contraceptives, because I have heavy uterine bleeding."

   D. "My doctor may perform a D&C to find out what's causing my abnormal bleeding."

   E. "My condition is more common in people who are in their 30s."

4. A nurse is providing support to a client who has a new diagnosis of endometriosis. The nurse should inform the client that which of the following conditions is a possible complication of endometriosis?

   A. Insulin resistance

   B. Infertility

   C. Vaginitis

   D. Pelvic inflammatory disease

5. A nurse is reviewing the medical record of a client who is menopausal. Which of the following findings should the nurse expect? (Select all that apply.)

   A. Increased vaginal secretions

   B. Decreased bone density

   C. Increased HDL level

   D. Decreased skin elasticity

   E. Increased pubic hair growth

   F. Decreased follicle-stimulating hormone level

PRACTICE Active Learning Scenario

A nurse is instructing a client who is being evaluated for premenstrual syndrome (PMS) to journal her manifestations to aid in diagnosis. Use the ATI Active Learning Template: System Disorder to complete this item.

EXPECTED FINDINGS: Identify six manifestations of PMS.

Application Exercises Key

1. A. Although some females experience the onset of menstruation as early as age 9, the average age is 12.4 years.

   B. **CORRECT:** Although a typical menstrual cycle is 28 days, a range of 23 to 35 days is considered a regular menstrual cycle.

   C. The first day of the menstrual cycle begins with the first day of the menstrual period.

   D. **CORRECT:** The first half of the menstrual cycle is the follicular phase, and the second half is the luteal phase. Ovulation typically occurs around the middle of the cycle, or day 14 in a 28-day cycle.

   E. **CORRECT:** A menstrual period typically lasts from 4 to 6 days but can continue for up to 9 days.

   Ⓝ *NCLEX® Connection: Physiological Adaptation, Alterations in Body Systems*

2. A. **CORRECT:** Fluoxetine, an SSRI, is used to treat the emotional manifestations of PMS (irritability, mood swings) and has an added effect of treating physical manifestations.

   B. **CORRECT:** Spironolactone is a diuretic and can reduce bloating and weight gain associated with PMS.

   C. **CORRECT:** Oral contraceptives can be prescribed to reduce the manifestations of PMS.

   D. Oral iron supplements, such as ferrous sulfate, are used to treat anemia associated with dysfunctional uterine bleeding.

   E. Methylergonovine is used to treat postpartum hemorrhage.

   Ⓝ *NCLEX® Connection: Pharmacological Therapies, Expected Actions/Outcomes*

3. A. **CORRECT:** DUB can be caused by a progesterone deficiency.

   B. The client should avoid aspirin due to the increased risk for bleeding. NSAIDs can be recommended as needed for menstrual pain or discomfort.

   C. Contraceptives can be prescribed to treat DUB.

   D. **CORRECT:** When the provider performs a dilatation and curettage, endometrium scraped from the uterine wall is sent to the laboratory for evaluation.

   E. DUB is more common in adolescent clients and in clients who are nearing menopause.

   Ⓝ *NCLEX® Connection: Physiological Adaptation, Alterations in Body Systems*

4. A. Insulin resistance is a complication of polycystic ovary syndrome.

   B. **CORRECT:** Infertility is a complication of endometriosis because endometrial tissue overgrowth can block the fallopian tubes.

   C. Vaginitis is typically caused by an infection.

   D. Pelvic inflammatory disease is caused by an infection of the pelvic organs.

   Ⓝ *NCLEX® Connection: Physiological Adaptation, Alterations in Body Systems*

5. A. Clients who are menopausal are expected to have decreased vaginal secretions.

   B. **CORRECT:** Clients who are menopausal are expected to have decreased bone density.

   C. Clients who are menopausal are expected to have a decreased HDL level and increased LDL level.

   D. **CORRECT:** Clients who are menopausal are expected to have decreased skin elasticity.

   E. Clients who are menopausal are expected to have a loss of hair on the head and in the pubic area.

   F. Clients who are menopausal are expected to have an increased follicle-stimulating hormone (FSH) level.

   Ⓝ *NCLEX® Connection: Health Promotion and Maintenance, Aging Process*

PRACTICE Answer

Using the ATI Active Learning Template: System Disorder

EXPECTED FINDINGS
- Irritability
- Impaired memory
- Depression
- Poor concentration
- Mood swings
- Binge eating
- Breast tenderness
- Bloating
- Weight gain
- Headache
- Back pain

Ⓝ *NCLEX® Connection: Physiological Adaptation, Basic Pathophysiology*

CHAPTER 56 Disorders of Female Reproductive Tissue

Pelvic organ prolapse occurs when the client's pelvic floor muscles and ligaments become weakened or damaged, resulting in a cystocele or rectocele. A cystocele is a protrusion of the posterior bladder through the anterior vaginal wall. It is caused by weakened pelvic muscles and structures. A rectocele is a protrusion of the anterior rectal wall through the posterior vaginal wall. It is caused by a defect of the pelvic structures, a difficult delivery, a forceps delivery, or chronic constipation with straining. Uterine prolapse is another form of pelvic organ prolapse caused by stretching of the ligaments that support the uterus within the pelvis.

Medical treatment is possible for clients who have a cystocele or a rectocele causing mild manifestations. If treatment is unsuccessful, the provider may recommend surgical intervention.

Fibrocystic breast change is a noncancerous breast condition. It is most common in younger clients. It occurs less frequently in postmenopausal clients. The changes are thought to occur due to cyclic hormonal changes. Fibrosis (of connective tissue) and cysts (fluid-filled sacs) develop.

Cystocele and rectocele

HEALTH PROMOTION AND DISEASE PREVENTION

- Clients who are at risk should lose weight if obese.
- Eat high-fiber diets and drink adequate fluids to prevent constipation.

DATA COLLECTION

RISK FACTORS

- Cystocele and rectocele can develop in older adult clients, usually following menopause as thinning of the vaginal wall occurs.
- Older adult clients are more susceptible to constipation and chronic bearing down during elimination, which can displace weakened structures. ⓒ

Cystocele

- Obesity
- Postmenopause (loss of estrogen)
- Family history
- Multiparity
- Increased abdominal pressure during pregnancy
- Strain and injury during vaginal childbirth

Rectocele

- Pelvic structure defects
- Obesity
- Aging
- Chronic constipation with straining to defecate
- Family history
- Difficult vaginal childbirth necessitating repair of a tear

EXPECTED FINDINGS

Cystocele

- Urinary frequency and urgency
- Stress incontinence
- History of frequent urinary tract infections
- Sense of vaginal fullness
- Dyspareunia
- Fatigue
- Back and pelvic pain

Rectocele

- Constipation or the need to place fingers in the vagina to elevate the rectocele to complete evacuation of feces
- Sensation of a mass in the vagina
- Pelvic/rectal pressure or pain
- Dyspareunia
- Fecal incontinence
- Uncontrollable flatus
- Hemorrhoids

DIAGNOSTIC PROCEDURES

Cystocele

- A pelvic examination reveals a bulging of the anterior vaginal wall when the client is instructed to bear down.
- Bladder ultrasound measures residual urine.
- Urine culture and sensitivity is used to diagnose urinary tract infection associated with urinary stasis.
- A cystography is performed to identify the degree of bladder protrusion.
- An x-ray can help determine the degree of cystocele.

Rectocele

- A pelvic examination reveals a bulging of the posterior vaginal wall when the client is instructed to bear down.
- A rectal examination reveals the presence of a rectocele.

PATIENT-CENTERED CARE

THERAPEUTIC PROCEDURES

Intravaginal estrogen is used to prevent atrophy of the pelvic muscles in clients who are postmenopausal.

Bladder training contributes to urinary continence.

Vaginal pessary (56.1)
- A removable rubber, plastic, or silicone device inserted into the vagina to provide support and block protrusion of other organs into the vagina.
- The provider selects the type of pessary and ensures that it fits correctly.
- Provides temporary support for the uterus or bladder when surgery is contraindicated or refused.
- NURSING ACTIONS: Ensure that the client does not have a latex allergy if a rubber pessary is prescribed. Qs
- CLIENT EDUCATION
  ○ How to insert, remove, and clean the device.
  ○ Routine checks by the provider are necessary to ensure proper fit, and to monitor for complications.
  ○ Notify the provider of pain, discomfort, or vaginal discharge.

Kegel exercises
- Exercises the client performs to strengthen the pelvic floor muscles, which results in reduction or prevention of pelvic organ prolapse and stress urinary incontinence
- CLIENT EDUCATION: How to perform the exercises
  ○ Contract the circumvaginal and perirectal muscles.
  ○ Tighten pelvic muscles.
  ○ Gradually increase the contraction period to 10 seconds.
  ○ Follow each contraction period with a relaxation period of 10 seconds.
  ○ Perform while lying down, sitting, and standing.
  ○ Perform the exercises 30 to 80 times daily.
  ○ Keep abdominal muscles relaxed during contractions.

Transvaginal repair is performed to treat prolapse of pelvic organs. Vaginal mesh or tape is used to create a sling that re-suspends pelvic organs and supports the pelvic floor.

Anterior-posterior repair: Surgical repair of both a cystocele and a rectocele.

Hysterectomy may be performed at the same time as cystocele or rectocele repair.

Cystocele

Anterior colporrhaphy: Using a vaginal or laparoscopic approach, the pelvic muscles are shortened and tightened, resulting in increased bladder support.

Rectocele

Posterior colporrhaphy: Using a vaginal/perineal approach, the pelvic muscles are shortened and tightened, resulting in a reduction of rectal protrusion into the vaginal canal.

POSTOPERATIVE NURSING ACTIONS
- Provide routine postoperative care to prevent complications.
- Administer analgesics, antimicrobials, and stool softeners/laxatives.
- Apply a warm compress to the abdomen to decrease discomfort.
- Suggest that the client take frequent sitz baths to soothe the perineal area.
- Provide a low-residue diet until normal bowel function returns.

CLIENT EDUCATION Qs

- Notify the provider about indications of infection (elevated temperature, pulse, or respirations; foul-smelling or purulent vaginal discharge; consistent pain).
- Avoid straining at defecation; sneezing; coughing; lifting; and sitting, walking, or standing for prolonged periods following surgery.
- Tighten and support pelvic muscles when coughing or sneezing.
- Postoperative restrictions: avoid strenuous activity, lifting anything weighing greater than 5 lb, and sexual intercourse for 6 weeks.
- The sutures are absorbable and do not require removal.

COMPLICATIONS

Complications are similar to those associated with a vaginal hysterectomy.
- Vaginal erosion and serious infection has led to the recall of some surgical mesh or tape used to repair pelvic organ prolapse. For more information, see www.fda.gov.
- Provide the client with written information from the manufacturer regarding the specific product used. Qs
- Dyspareunia (painful sexual intercourse) is a possible complication due to surgical alteration of the vaginal orifice.

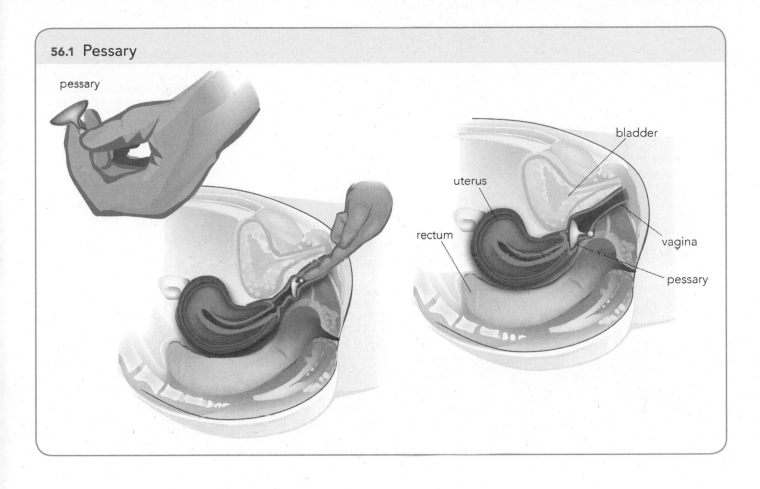

56.1 Pessary

pessary

bladder

uterus

rectum

vagina

pessary

Fibrocystic breast changes

DATA COLLECTION

RISK FACTORS

- Premenopausal status
- Postmenopausal hormone replacement therapy

EXPECTED FINDINGS

- Breast pain
- Tender lumps, commonly in upper outer quadrant
- Nipple discharge

PHYSICAL FINDINGS: Palpable rubberlike lumps, usually in the upper outer quadrant

DIAGNOSTIC PROCEDURES

History, physical exam, and mammography

Breast ultrasound is used to confirm the diagnosis.

Fine-needle aspiration of a large cyst is used to confirm the diagnosis or to reduce pain due to fluid build-up.

PATIENT-CENTERED CARE

NURSING CARE

- Suggest that the client reduce the intake of salt before menses, wear a supportive bra, and apply either local heat or cold to temporarily reduce pain.
- Suggest avoiding caffeine, chocolate, and smoking. These are factors believed to contribute to fibrocystic changes.
- Discuss the risks (liver disease, stroke) of hormonal medication therapy with clients considering this form of treatment.
- Encourage the client to follow the provider's recommendations and to journal the effectiveness of the treatment plan.
- Inform the client that having fibrocystic breast changes does not increase the risk of breast cancer. Qpcc

MEDICATIONS

- Over-the-counter analgesics (acetaminophen, ibuprofen)
- Oral contraceptives or hormonal medication therapy if manifestations are severe to suppress estrogen/progesterone secretion
- Diuretics to decrease breast engorgement

Application Exercises

1. A nurse is reinforcing education with a client about how to perform Kegel exercises. Which of the following instructions should the nurse include? (Select all that apply.)

   A. Perform exercises about 50 times each day.

   B. Contract the circumvaginal and perirectal muscles.

   C. Gradually increase the contraction period to 10 seconds.

   D. Follow each contraction with at least a 10-second relaxation period.

   E. Perform while sitting, lying, and standing.

   F. Tighten abdominal muscles during contractions.

2. A nurse is collecting data from a client who is scheduled for an anterior colporrhaphy. Which of the following client statements should the nurse expect?

   A. "I have to push the feces out of a pouch in my vagina with my fingers."

   B. "I have pain and bleeding when I have a bowel movement."

   C. "I have had frequent urinary tract infections."

   D. "I am embarrassed by uncontrollable flatus."

3. A nurse is reviewing the medical record of a client who has a cystocele. Which of the following findings is a risk factor for the development of this disorder?

   A. BMI 18

   B. Nulliparity

   C. Chronic constipation

   D. Postmenopause

4. A nurse is assisting with the discharge of a client following an anterior and posterior colporrhaphy. Which of the following instructions should the nurse provide?

   A. "Do not bend over for at least 6 weeks."

   B. "You can lift objects as heavy as 10 pounds."

   C. "Do not engage in intercourse for at least 6 weeks."

   D. "You might have foul-smelling drainage for the first week after surgery."

5. A nurse in a provider's office is reviewing the medical record of a client who has fibrocystic breast changes. Which of the following findings should the nurse expect?

   A. Palpable rubberlike lump in the upper outer quadrant

   B. BRCA1 gene mutation

   C. Elevated CA-125

   D. *Peau d'orange* dimpling of the breast

PRACTICE Active Learning Scenario

A nurse is preparing to assist with an educational session for a group of clients on medications used to treat fibrocystic breast changes. Use the ATI Active Learning Template: Medication to complete this item.

THERAPEUTIC USES: Identify three types of medications used to treat the condition, and provide a brief description of the purpose of the medications in treating fibrocystic breast changes.

Application Exercises Key

1. A. **CORRECT:** The client should perform Kegel exercises 30 to 80 times a day.

   B. **CORRECT:** The client should contract the circumvaginal and perirectal muscles as if trying to stop the flow of urine or passing flatus.

   C. **CORRECT:** The client should hold the contraction for 10 seconds. She might need to gradually increase the contraction period to reach this goal.

   D. **CORRECT:** The client should follow each contraction with a relaxation period of 10 seconds.

   E. **CORRECT:** The client can perform the exercises while lying, sitting, or standing.

   F. The client should relax other muscles, such as those in the abdomen and thighs.

   Ⓝ *NCLEX® Connection: Reduction of Risk Potential, Therapeutic Procedures*

2. A. Pouching of feces in an expected finding associated with a rectocele. The surgical procedure for a rectocele is posterior colporrhaphy.

   B. Pain and bleeding with a bowel movement is an expected finding associated with a rectocele.

   C. **CORRECT:** Due to urinary stasis associated with a cystocele, this finding is an expected finding of a cystocele. The surgery for a cystocele is an anterior colporrhaphy.

   D. Uncontrollable flatus is an expected finding associated with a rectocele.

   Ⓝ *NCLEX® Connection: Physiological Adaptation, Basic Pathophysiology*

3. A. Obesity is a risk factor for the development of a cystocele. A BMI of 18 indicates the client is underweight.

   B. Multiparity is a risk factor for the development of a cystocele.

   C. Constipation is a risk factor for the development of a rectocele.

   D. **CORRECT:** Advancing age and loss of estrogen related to postmenopausal status are risk factors for the development of a cystocele.

   Ⓝ *NCLEX® Connection: Health Promotion and Maintenance, Health Promotion/Disease Prevention*

4. A. The client does not have a restriction regarding bending over.

   B. The client should not lift an object that weighs more than 5 lb.

   C. **CORRECT:** The client should refrain from intercourse to allow time for the surgical site to heal, which is typically about 6 weeks.

   D. Foul-smelling drainage is an indication of infection, which should be reported to the provider.

   Ⓝ *NCLEX® Connection: Reduction of Risk Potential, Therapeutic Procedures*

5. A. **CORRECT:** Clients who have fibrocystic breast changes typically have breast pain and rubbery palpable lumps in the upper outer quadrant of the breasts.

   B. BRCA1 gene mutation is a risk factor for breast cancer.

   C. An elevated CA-125 is a finding associated with ovarian cancer.

   D. *Peau d'orange* dimpling of the breast is a finding associated with breast cancer.

   Ⓝ *NCLEX® Connection: Physiological Adaptation, Basic Pathophysiology*

PRACTICE Answer

Using ATI Active Learning Template: Medication

THERAPEUTIC USES

- Analgesics (acetaminophen, ibuprofen) are used to relieve pain.
- Oral contraceptives or hormonal medication therapy suppress estrogen/progesterone secretion.
- Diuretics decrease breast engorgement.

Ⓝ *NCLEX® Connection: Pharmacological Therapies, Expected Actions/Outcomes*

CHAPTER 57 *Diagnostic Procedures for Male Reproductive Disorders*

Changes to the prostate gland are common as clients age, and routine diagnostic procedures are recommended to evaluate these changes. Enlargement of the prostate gland is usually benign and referred to as benign prostatic hyperplasia (BPH). Prostate cancer is one of the most common forms of cancer in males. Q͏ᴇʙᴘ

Diagnostic procedures for male reproductive disorders include prostate-specific antigen (PSA), early prostate cancer antigen (EPCA-2), digital rectal exam (DRE), and transrectal ultrasound (TRUS).

Prostate-specific antigen, early prostate cancer antigen, and digital rectal exam

PSA measures the amount of a protein produced by the prostate gland in the bloodstream. It is performed prior to the DRE because a rise in PSA can occur due to the irritation that occurs upon palpation of the gland. A sample of blood is used to determine the PSA level. Q͏ᴇʙᴘ

EPCA-2 measures the amount of protein in the blood that is only produced by abnormal prostate cells.

DRE is done in an office or clinic.
- The client lies in the lithotomy position, on his side, or standing while leaning over the examination table. The provider places a gloved, lubricated finger in the client's anus and palpates the posterior portion of the prostate gland through the rectal wall. This allows for an estimation of the size, shape, and consistency of the gland. The client also can be placed on his side or in the lithotomy position for the exam. Q͏ᴘᴄᴄ
- If the DRE reveals an abnormality, the location of the potentially cancerous prostate lesion is determined by ultrasonography and confirmed by a biopsy.

INDICATIONS

- Many providers recommend an annual PSA and DRE for male clients older than 50 years to help ensure early detection of prostate cancer. BPH tends to develop earlier in African American clients and clients who have a family history of prostate cancer; therefore they should begin screening at an earlier age.
- Because the EPCA-2 is highly sensitive in detecting prostate cancer, some providers use this test in place of a biopsy. The EPCA-2 is also used to monitor the client's response to treatment for prostate cancer.
- For additional information regarding screening for and treatment of prostate cancer, see www.cdc.gov.

CLIENT PRESENTATION: As the prostate gland enlarges, it encroaches on the urethra and causes diminished flow and retention of urine. Blood can also be found in the urine. These findings can indicate BPH or prostate cancer.

INTERPRETATION OF FINDINGS

PSA: An increase can indicate that a client has prostate cancer.
- PSA levels increase with age. For a client younger than 50 years of age, a PSA level of 2.5 ng/mL is within the expected range.
- The client can have an elevated PSA level for up to 6 weeks following a urinary tract infection.
- A PSA value greater than 4 ng/mL requires further evaluation. An elevated PSA is an indication of a number of conditions (cancer, BPH, acute prostatitis).

EPCA-2: A value of 30 ng/mL or greater is highly suggestive of prostate cancer.

DRE: Abnormal findings during the DRE include an abnormally large and hard prostate with an irregular shape or lumps.

Transrectal ultrasound (TRUS)

- With the client in a left, side-lying position, a probe is inserted into the client's rectum, and sound waves are bounced off the surface of the prostate gland to provide an image.
- The provider may prescribe an enema prior to the procedure.
- The client is instructed to void immediately prior to the procedure.
- The procedure is contraindicated for clients who have a latex allergy. The rectal ultrasound probe is covered by a latex sac. Therefore, it is important to check the client for a latex allergy prior to the procedure. Q͏ꜱ

INDICATIONS

A TRUS is done if a client's PSA is elevated or the DRE reveals a possible abnormality.

INTERPRETATION OF FINDINGS

If an irregularity is found, the image is used to guide a needle biopsy.

Application Exercises

1. A nurse is caring for an older adult client who is having an annual physical exam. Which of the following findings indicates additional follow-up is needed in regard to the prostate gland? (Select all that apply.)

A. Prostate-specific antigen (PSA) is 7.1 ng/mL.

B. A digital rectal exam (DRE) reveals an enlarged and nodular prostate.

C. The client reports a weak urine stream.

D. The client reports urinating once during the night.

E. Smegma is present below the glans of the penis.

2. A nurse is reinforcing teaching with a client who is scheduled for a transrectal ultrasound (TRUS). Which of the following information should the nurse include?

A. "This procedure will determine whether you have prostate cancer."

B. "The procedure is contraindicated if you have an allergy to eggs."

C. "Sound waves will be used to create a picture of your prostate."

D. "You should avoid having a bowel movement for 1 hr prior to the procedure."

PRACTICE Active Learning Scenario

A nurse in a provider's office is reinforcing teaching with an older adult client who is scheduled for a prostate-specific antigen (PSA) test and a digital rectal exam (DRE). Use the ATI Active Learning Template: Diagnostic Procedure to complete this item.

DESCRIPTION OF PROCEDURE: Include the order in which they are performed.

INDICATIONS: Identify two factors that the nurse should discuss with the client that place the client at risk for prostate cancer.

Application Exercises Key

1. A. **CORRECT:** Although the PSA level is typically elevated in older adult clients, PSA greater than 4 ng/mL warrants additional follow-up.

   B. **CORRECT:** An enlarged and nodular prostate is a possible indication of prostate cancer and requires further evaluation.

   C. **CORRECT:** A weak urine stream is a manifestation of benign prostatic hyperplasia and warrants follow-up

   D. Urinating once during the night is an expected finding for an older adult male client.

   E. Smegma is a normal secretion that can accumulate beneath the glans penis.

   Ⓝ *NCLEX® Connection: Health Promotion and Maintenance, Health Promotion/Disease Prevention*

2. A. A biopsy or EPCA-2 is used to make the diagnosis of prostate cancer.

   B. A TRUS is contraindicated if the client has an allergy to latex.

   C. **CORRECT:** A transrectal ultrasound creates an image of the prostate using sound waves.

   D. The provider may prescribe an enema prior to the procedure to decrease the interference of feces with obtaining accurate test results.

   Ⓝ *NCLEX® Connection: Reduction of Risk Potential, Diagnostic Tests*

PRACTICE Answer

Using ATI Active Learning Template: Diagnostic Procedure

DESCRIPTION OF PROCEDURE
- PSA: A blood sample is taken to measure a specific protein produced by the prostate gland that is present in the bloodstream. The PSA is performed first because examination of the prostate irritates the prostate and can cause the PSA to rise.
- DRE: With the client standing and leaning over the exam table, lying on his side, or in the lithotomy position, the examiner uses a gloved, lubricated finger to palpate the prostate through the rectal wall to identify any abnormalities in size, shape, and consistency.

INDICATIONS
- Age greater than 50 years
- Black ancestry
- Family history of prostate cancer

Ⓝ *NCLEX® Connection: Reduction of Risk Potential, Diagnostic Tests*

CHAPTER 58

CHAPTER 58 *Benign Prostatic Hyperplasia*

As an adult male ages, the prostate gland enlarges. When the enlargement of the gland begins to cause urinary dysfunction, it is called benign prostatic hyperplasia (BPH). BPH is a common condition of the older adult male. BPH can significantly impair the outflow of urine from the bladder, making a client susceptible to infection and retention. Excessive amounts of urine retained can cause reflux of urine into the kidney, dilating the ureter, causing kidney infections and affecting kidney function.

DATA COLLECTION

RISK FACTORS

- Increased age (older than 50 years)
- Western diet (high fat, protein, carbohydrate; low fiber)
- Diabetes mellitus, heart disease
- African American race
- Family history of BPH

EXPECTED FINDINGS

- The International Prostate Symptom Score (I-PSS) is a data collection tool used to determine the severity of manifestations and their effect on the client's quality of life. The client rates the severity of lower urinary tract manifestations using a 0-to-5 scale and also rates his quality of life as affected by urinary tract manifestations.
- Clients who have BPH typically report urinary frequency, urgency, hesitancy (difficulty initiating urine flow), or incontinence; incomplete emptying of the bladder; dribbling post-voiding; nocturia; diminished force of urinary stream; straining with urination; and hematuria.
- Urinary stasis and persistent urinary retention lead to frequent urinary tract infections.
- If BPH persists, back flow of urine into the ureters and kidney can lead to kidney damage.

LABORATORY TESTS

Urinalysis and culture: WBCs elevated and bacteria present with urinary tract infection

CBC: WBCs elevated if systemic infection present, RBCs possibly decreased due to hematuria

BUN and creatinine: Elevated, indicating kidney damage

Prostate-specific antigen (PSA): To rule out prostate cancer

Culture and sensitivity of prostatic fluid: Can be performed if fluid is expressed during digital rectal examination

DIAGNOSTIC PROCEDURES

Digital rectal exam will reveal an enlarged, hardened, and smooth prostate.

Transrectal ultrasound with needle aspiration biopsy is performed to rule out prostate cancer in the presence of an enlarged prostate.

Early prostate cancer antigen serum blood test may be prescribed instead of a biopsy to rule out prostate cancer.

PATIENT-CENTERED CARE

NURSING CARE

CLIENT EDUCATION

- Frequent ejaculation releases retained prostatic fluids, thereby decreasing the size of the prostate.
- Drink at least 3 L of fluids daily (unless contraindicated) to reduce dysuria and prevent urinary tract infections.
- Urinate when the urge is initially felt.
- Avoid bladder stimulants, such as alcohol and caffeine.
- Avoid medications that cause decreased bladder tone (anticholinergics, decongestants, antihistamines).
- Medication is used for conservative treatment of BPH.

MEDICATIONS

The goal of medication for BPH is to re-establish uninhibited urine flow out of the bladder.

Dihydrotestosterone (DHT)-lowering medications

5-alpha reductase inhibitor (5-ARI), such as finasteride
- DHT-lowering medications reduce the conversion of testosterone to DHT.
- Decreasing DHT often causes a decrease in the size of the prostate.

CLIENT EDUCATION

- It can take 6 months to 1 year before effects of the medication are evident.
- Impotence and a decrease in libido are possible adverse effects.
- Report breast enlargement to the provider.
- Finasteride is teratogenic to a male fetus. The medication is potentially absorbed through the skin. Clients who are pregnant or who could become pregnant should avoid contact with tablets that are crushed or broken and with the semen of a client currently taking this medication. **Qs**

Alpha-blocking agents: tamsulosin

- Alpha adrenergic receptor antagonists cause relaxation of the smooth muscle in the bladder outlet and prostate gland.
- These agents decrease pressure on the urethra, thereby re-establishing a stronger urine flow and decreasing the manifestations of BPH.

CLIENT EDUCATION
- Orthostatic hypotension can occur. Slowly change position.
- Concurrent use with cimetidine can potentiate the hypotensive effect.

THERAPEUTIC PROCEDURES

Transurethral needle ablation (TUNA)

Low-level radiation is used to shrink the prostate.

Transurethral microwave therapy (TUMT)

Heat is applied to the prostate to decease its size.

Prostatic stent

Placed to keep the urethra patent, especially if client is a poor candidate for surgery

Interstitial laser coagulation

- Also called contact laser prostatectomy
- Laser energy is used to coagulate excess prostatic tissue.

Electrovaporization of the prostate

High-frequency electrical current is used to cut and vaporize excess tissue.

Surgical resection

An option for clients who do not receive adequate relief from conservative measures

Transurethral incision of the prostate (TUIP)

Involves incisions into the prostate and bladder neck to widen the urethra and relieve constriction
- Tissue is not removed with this procedure.
- It is minimally invasive and typically performed in an outpatient setting.

Holmium laser enucleation of the prostate (HoLEP)

Uses a laser to remove excess prostatic tissue that is obstructing the client's urethra
- The tissue is then moved to the bladder, where the client eliminates it in the urine.
- The client often has an indwelling urinary catheter that is left in place overnight.

Transurethral resection of the prostate (TURP)

The most common surgical procedure for BPH
- TURP is performed using a resectoscope (similar to a cystoscope) that is inserted through the urethra and trims away excess prostatic tissue, enlarging the passageway of the urethra through the prostate gland.
- Irrigating fluid carries resected tissue into the bladder to be flushed out.
- Typically, epidural and spinal anesthesia are used.

PREOPERATIVE NURSING ACTIONS
- Carefully collect data from cardiovascular, respiratory, and renal systems.
- Ensure that the client fully understands the procedure and what to expect postoperatively.

POSTOPERATIVE NURSING ACTIONS
- Postoperative treatment for a TURP usually includes placement of an indwelling three-way catheter.
  - The urinary catheter drains urine and allows for instillation of a continuous bladder irrigation (CBI) of normal saline (isotonic) or another prescribed irrigating solution to keep the catheter free from obstruction.
  - The rate of the CBI is adjusted to keep the irrigation return pink or lighter. For example, if bright-red or ketchup-appearing (arterial) bleeding with clots is observed, the nurse should increase the CBI rate.
  - If the catheter becomes obstructed (bladder spasms, reduced irrigation outflow), turn off the CBI and irrigate with 50 mL irrigation solution using a large piston syringe or per facility or surgeon protocol. Contact the surgeon if unable to dislodge the clot.
  - Record the amount of irrigating solution instilled (generally very large volumes) and the amount of return. The difference equals urine output.
  - The catheter has a large balloon (30 to 45 mL). The catheter is taped tightly to the leg, creating traction so that the balloon will apply firm pressure to the prostatic fossa to prevent bleeding. This makes the client feel a continuous need to urinate. Instruct the client to not void around the catheter as this causes bladder spasms. Avoid kinks in the tubing.
- Monitor vital signs and urinary output (amount, color, clarity, odor).
- Monitor ability to control urine flow without incontinence or dribbling.
- Administer/provide increased fluids.
- Monitor for bleeding (persistent bright-red bleeding unresponsive to increase in CBI and traction on the catheter or reduced Hgb levels) and report to the provider.
- Assist the client to ambulate as soon as possible to reduce the risk of deep-vein thrombosis and other complications that occur due to immobility.

- Administer medications.
  - Analgesics discomfort from (surgical manipulation or incision)
  - Antispasmodics (bladder spasms)
  - Antibiotics (prophylaxis)
  - Stool softeners (prevent straining)
- When the catheter is removed, monitor urinary output. The initial voiding following removal can be uncomfortable, red in color, and contain clots. The color of the urine should progress toward amber in 2 to 3 days. Instruct the client that expected output is 150 to 200 mL every 3 to 4 hr. The client should contact the provider if unable to void. Q𝖤𝖡𝖯
- Obtain a bladder scan as indicated to monitor urinary retention after catheter removal.

CLIENT EDUCATION
- Avoid heavy lifting, strenuous exercise, straining, and sexual intercourse for the prescribed length of time (usually 2 to 6 weeks).
- Drink 12 or more 8-oz glasses of water each day unless contraindicated.
- Avoid nonsteroidal anti-inflammatory medications due to increased risk for bleeding.
- Avoid bladder stimulants (caffeine, alcohol).
- If urine becomes bloody, stop activity, rest, and increase fluid intake.
- Contact the surgeon for persistent bleeding or obstruction (less than expected output or distention).

COMPLICATIONS

Complications of procedures to treat BPH include regrowth of prostate tissue and reoccurrence of bladder neck obstruction.

TURP complications

- Urethral trauma, urinary retention, bleeding, and infection
- Fluid volume excess with hyponatremia, also known as "transurethral syndrome"

NURSING ACTIONS
- Monitor the client and intervene for bleeding.
- Provide antibiotic prophylaxis to the client.
- Monitor for manifestations of fluid volume excess and hyponatremia.

PRACTICE Active Learning Scenario

A nurse is reinforcing teaching with a client who has a new prescription for finasteride about the medication. Use the ATI Active Learning Template: Medication to complete this item.

THERAPEUTIC USES: Identify the therapeutic use of this medication for this client.

CLIENT EDUCATION: Identify four instructions the nurse should include.

Application Exercises

1. A nurse in a provider's office is collecting history data from a client who is undergoing an evaluation for benign prostatic hyperplasia (BPH). The nurse should identify that which of the following findings are indicative of this condition? (Select all that apply.)
   - A. Backache
   - B. Frequent urinary tract infections
   - C. Weight loss
   - D. Hematuria
   - E. Urinary incontinence

2. A nurse is caring for a client who has a new diagnosis of benign prostatic hyperplasia (BPH). The nurse should anticipate a prescription for which of the following medications?
   - A. Oxybutynin
   - B. Diphenhydramine
   - C. Ipratropium
   - D. Tamsulosin

3. A nurse is reinforcing instructions with a client who is scheduled for a transurethral resection of the prostate (TURP) about his postoperative care. Which of the following information should the nurse include in the teaching?
   - A. "You may have a continuous sensation of needing to void even though you have a catheter."
   - B. "You will be on bed rest for the first 2 days after the procedure."
   - C. "You will be instructed to limit your fluid intake after the procedure."
   - D. "Your urine should be clear yellow the evening after the surgery."

4. A nurse is reinforcing discharge instructions with a client who is postoperative following a TURP. Which of the following instructions should the nurse include? (Select all that apply.)
   - A. Avoid sexual intercourse for 3 months after the surgery.
   - B. If urine appears bloody, stop activity and rest.
   - C. Avoid drinking caffeinated beverages.
   - D. Take a stool softener once a day.
   - E. Treat pain with ibuprofen.

Application Exercises Key

1. A. Backache occurs in the presence of prostate cancer that has spread to other areas of the body.

   B. **CORRECT:** In the presence of BPH, pressure on urinary structures leads to urinary stasis, which in turn promotes the occurrence of urinary tract infections.

   C. Weight loss occurs in the presence of prostate cancer.

   D. **CORRECT:** Hematuria occurs in the presence of BPH.

   E. **CORRECT:** Overflow incontinence occurs in the presence of BPH due to an increased volume of residual urine.

   Ⓝ *NCLEX® Connection: Physiological Adaptation, Basic Pathophysiology*

2. A. Oxybutynin is an anticholinergic medication that is used to treat overactive bladder. Anticholinergic medications are contraindicated for a client who has BPH. Oxybutynin causes urinary retention.

   B. Diphenhydramine is an antihistamine and is contraindicated for a client who has BPH. Diphenhydramine causes urinary retention.

   C. Ipratropium is an anticholinergic medication used to treat asthma and other respiratory conditions. Ipratropium causes urinary retention.

   D. **CORRECT:** Tamsulosin is an alpha adrenergic receptor antagonist that relaxes the bladder outlet and the prostate gland, which improves urinary flow.

   Ⓝ *NCLEX® Connection: Pharmacological Therapies, Expected Actions/Outcomes*

3. A. **CORRECT:** To reduce the risk of postoperative bleeding, the client will have a catheter with a large balloon that places pressure on the internal sphincter of the bladder. Pressure on the sphincter causes a continuous sensation of needing to void.

   B. The client is ambulated early in the postoperative period to reduce the risk of deep-vein thrombosis and other complications that occur due to immobility.

   C. The client is encouraged to increase his fluid intake unless contraindicated by another condition. A liberal fluid intake reduces the risks of urinary tract infection and dysuria.

   D. The client's urine is expected to be pink the first 24 hr after surgery.

   Ⓝ *NCLEX® Connection: Reduction of Risk Potential, Therapeutic Procedures*

4. A. The client should follow the provider's instructions, which typically includes avoidance of sexual intercourse for 2 to 6 weeks after the surgery.

   B. **CORRECT:** Excessive activity can cause recurrence of bleeding. The client should rest to promote reclotting at the incisional site.

   C. **CORRECT:** The client should avoid caffeine and other bladder stimulants.

   D. **CORRECT:** The client should take a stool softener to keep the stool soft and thus prevent the complication of bleeding at the time of a bowel movement.

   E. The client should avoid taking nonsteroidal anti-inflammatory drugs because they can cause bleeding.

   Ⓝ *NCLEX® Connection: Reduction of Risk Potential, Therapeutic Procedures*

PRACTICE Answer

Using the ATI Active Learning Template: Medication

THERAPEUTIC USES: Finasteride inhibits 5-alpha reductase, an enzyme which converts testosterone to dihydrotestosterone. Production of testosterone in the prostate gland is reduced, which in turn reduces the size of prostate tissue.

CLIENT EDUCATION
- The medication is prescribed on a long-term basis. It can take as long as 1 year before the effects of the medication are evident.
- Impotence and a decreased libido are possible adverse effects.
- Report breast enlargement to the provider.
- Finasteride is teratogenic to the male fetus. The medication can be absorbed through the skin. Clients who are pregnant or who could become pregnant should avoid contact with tablets that are crushed or broken and with the semen of a client currently taking this medication.

Ⓝ *NCLEX® Connection: Pharmacological Therapies, Expected Actions/Outcomes*

ⓝ *NCLEX® Connections*

When reviewing the following chapters, keep in mind the relevant topics and tasks of the NCLEX outline, in particular:

Basic Care and Comfort

ASSISTIVE DEVICES: Contribute to the care of the client using an assistive device (feeding devices, telecommunication devices, touch pad, communication board).

MOBILITY/IMMOBILITY

Check the client for mobility, gait, strength, and motor skills.

Provide for mobility needs (ambulation, range of motion, transfer, repositioning, use of adaptive equipment).

Reinforce client teaching on methods to maintain mobility (active/passive range of motion, strengthening, isometric exercises).

Maintain the client's correct body alignment.

Provide care to an immobilized client (traction, bedridden).

NONPHARMACOLOGICAL COMFORT INTERVENTIONS

Apply therapies for comfort and treatment of inflammation/swelling (apply heat and cold treatments, elevate limb).

Provide nonpharmacological measures for pain relief (imagery, massage, repositioning).

Reduction of Risk Potential

POTENTIAL FOR ALTERATIONS IN BODY SYSTEMS

Identify the client with an increased risk for insufficient blood circulation (immobilized limb, diabetes mellitus).

Perform circulatory checks.

Apply and check proper use of compression stockings/sequential compression devices.

Physiological Adaptation

ALTERATIONS IN BODY SYSTEMS

Perform wound care and/or dressing change.

Perform care for the client after a surgical procedure.

Remove wound sutures or staples.

Reinforce education to the client regarding care and condition.

MEDICAL EMERGENCIES: Notify the primary health care provider about the client's unexpected response/emergency situation.

CHAPTER 59 *Musculoskeletal Diagnostic Procedures*

Imaging studies are the primary diagnostic procedures for musculoskeletal disorders. Muscle weakness is an indication for evaluating the conduction of electrical impulses. Arthroscopy assesses the condition of a joint and allows the repair of tears and other joint defects.

Musculoskeletal diagnostic procedures include arthroscopy, nuclear scans (bone scan, gallium scan, thallium scan), dual-energy x-ray absorptiometry scans (DXA), electromyography (EMG), and nerve conduction studies. Other diagnostic procedures that help detect joint problems and identify musculoskeletal structures are x-ray studies, ultrasound, computed tomography (CT) scans, and magnetic resonance imaging (MRI).

Arthroscopy

- Allows visualization of the internal structures of a joint, most commonly the knee or shoulder joints.
- It is a sterile procedure.
- Uses a flexible fiber-optic endoscope to visualize and repair joints and tissues.
- Number and placement of incisions depend on the area of the joint undergoing visualization and the extent of the repair.
- Infection in the joint and a lack of joint mobility are contraindications for arthroscopy.

INDICATIONS

POTENTIAL DIAGNOSES: A client who has a joint injury can undergo arthroscopy to ascertain the extent of damage, during which the provider can use the arthroscope to repair a torn ligament or meniscus or perform a synovial biopsy.

CLIENT PRESENTATION: Joint swelling, pain, crepitus, and instability

CONSIDERATIONS

PREPROCEDURE

NURSING ACTIONS
- Reinforce teaching with the client about postprocedure exercises (straight-leg raising, quadriceps setting isometrics) or recommend referral to a physical therapist.
- Ensure that the client signed the informed consent form.
- Instruct the client regarding fasting and medication use prior to the procedure.
- Reinforce explanation of the procedure.

CLIENT EDUCATION: Practice postoperative joint exercises.

POSTPROCEDURE

NURSING ACTIONS
- Postprocedure care is on an outpatient basis.
- Monitor for pain, neurovascular status, swelling, and dressings for excessive bleeding on the limb every hour or per the facility's protocol. **Qs**

CLIENT EDUCATION
- Apply ice for the first 24 hr.
- Elevate the extremity for 12 to 24 hr.
- Take an analgesic for pain.
- Apply a splint or sling.
- Maintain activity restrictions.
- Use crutches if the provider allows limited weight bearing.
- Monitor the color and temperature of the extremity, as well as pain and sensation.
- Notify the provider of any changes, such as swelling, increased joint pain, thrombophlebitis, or infection (redness, swelling, purulent drainage).

COMPLICATIONS

Infection

Complications are uncommon after this procedure, but infection can occur as with any procedure that disrupts the integrity of the skin.

CLIENT EDUCATION: Notify the provider immediately of swelling, redness, or fever.

Nuclear scans

Bone scans

Bone scans evaluate the entire skeletal system.
- A radionuclide test involves a radioactive isotope via injection 2 to 3 hr before scanning.
- Bone scans can detect hairline bone fractures, tumors, fractures, and diseases of the bone (osteomyelitis, osteoporosis, vertebral compression fractures).
- Bone scans are becoming less common due to the increased availability of MRI equipment.

Gallium and thallium scans

Gallium and thallium scans are more sensitive for detecting bone problems than a bone scan.
- The radioisotope migrates to tissues of the brain, liver, and breast, and helps detect disease of these organs.
- The client receives the radionuclide injection 4 to 6 hr before scanning.
- The scan takes 30 to 60 min and can require sedation to help the client lie still during that time. Repeat scanning occurs at 24, 48, and 72 hr.

INDICATIONS

Gallium and thallium scans

POTENTIAL DIAGNOSES
- Arthritis
- Osteomyelitis
- Fractures
- Osteoporosis
- Primary or metastatic bone cancer
- Bone pain of unknown origin

CLIENT PRESENTATION: Bone pain

CONSIDERATIONS

PREPROCEDURE

NURSING ACTIONS
- Inform the client about the procedure.
- Check for allergy to radioisotope or conditions that would prevent performing the procedure (pregnancy, kidney disease).

CLIENT EDUCATION
- Lie still during the entire procedure.
- Empty the bladder before the procedure to promote visualization of pelvic bones. Q̲EBP

POSTPROCEDURE

CLIENT EDUCATION
- Following the procedure, no radioactive precautions are needed.
- Drink fluids to increase excretion of radioisotope in the urine and feces.

Dual-energy x-ray absorptiometry

- DXA scans estimate the density of bone mass—usually in the hip or spine—and the presence/extent of osteoporosis.
- Helps to determine fracture risk.
- DXA scans use two beams of radiation. A computer analyzes the findings and a radiologist interprets them. No contrast material is used. Clients receive a score that relates their amount of bone density to that of other people with demographic similarities.
- Clients lie on an x-ray table during scanning of the hip or spine.

Note: These scores are not gender-specific.

INDICATIONS

POTENTIAL DIAGNOSES
- Osteoporosis
- Postmenopausal state (baseline: at age 40)

CLIENT PRESENTATION
- Loss of height
- Bone pain
- Fractures

CONSIDERATIONS

NURSING ACTIONS: Inform the client about the procedure.

CLIENT EDUCATION
- Follow up with the provider to discuss possible supplements and medications if bone loss is present.
- Stay dressed but remove metallic objects.

Electromyography and nerve conduction studies

EMG and nerve conduction studies determine the presence and cause of muscle weakness.

EMG

- Clients undergo EMG at the bedside or in an EMG laboratory.
- The technician places thin needles in the muscle under study. Electrodes attach the needles to an oscilloscope, which records electrical activity at rest and during a muscle contraction.

Nerve conduction study

- The technician attaches surface or needle electrodes to the skin.
- Low electrical currents go through the electrodes, producing a recording of the muscle response to the stimulus.

INDICATIONS

POTENTIAL DIAGNOSES
- Neuromuscular disorders
- Motor neuron disease
- Peripheral nerve disorders (carpal tunnel)

CONSIDERATIONS

PREPROCEDURE

NURSING ACTIONS
- Inform the client about what to expect.
- Determine whether the client takes an anticoagulant, because anticoagulation is a contraindication for this procedure due to the risk for bleeding within the muscle with needle insertion.
- Check for any skin infections in the area to be tested. Infection is a contraindication for this procedure due to the risk for transmission of the infection to the muscle. Qs
- Ask whether the client takes any muscle relaxants. The provider might discontinue these prior to the procedure to ensure accurate test results.
- Make sure the client signed the consent form.

CLIENT EDUCATION
- Avoid the application of cream or lotion to the area on the day of the procedure.
- Do not to drink any fluids containing caffeine and refrain from smoking at least 3 hr before the test.
- Discomfort is possible during needle insertion and when the electrical current goes through the electrodes.
- The client might have to flex her muscle during needle insertion.

POSTPROCEDURE

CLIENT EDUCATION
- Some bruising can occur at needle insertion sites.
- Report swelling or tenderness at any of the sites to the provider.
- Apply ice to prevent hematoma formation at the needle insertion sites and to reduce swelling or warm compresses to relieve residual discomfort.

Application Exercises

1. A nurse is reinforcing preoperative teaching with a client who is to undergo an arthroscopy to repair a shoulder injury. Which of the following statements should the nurse include? (Select all that apply.)
   - A. "Avoid damage or moisture to the cast on your arm."
   - B. "Inspect your incision daily for indications of infection."
   - C. "Apply ice packs to the area for the first 24 hours."
   - D. "Keep your arm in a dependent position."
   - E. "Perform isometric exercises."

2. A nurse is contributing to the plan of care for a client who is postoperative following an arthroscopy of the knee. Which of the following actions should the nurse take? (Select all that apply.)
   - A. Inspect color and temperature of the extremity.
   - B. Apply warm compresses to incision sites.
   - C. Place pillows under the extremity.
   - D. Administer analgesic medication.
   - E. Check pulse and sensation in the foot.

3. A nurse is reinforcing teaching with a client who is to have a bone scan. Which of the following statements should the nurse include?
   - A. "You will receive an injection of a radioactive isotope when the scanning procedure begins."
   - B. "You will be inside a tube-like structure during the procedure."
   - C. "You will need to take radioactive precautions with your urine for 24 hours after the procedure."
   - D. "You will have to urinate just before the procedure."

4. A nurse is reinforcing teaching with clients at a health fair about dual-energy x-ray absorptiometry (DXA) scans. Which of the following information should the nurse include in the teaching? (Select all that apply.)
   - A. "The test requires the use of contrast material."
   - B. "The hip and spine are the usual areas the device scans."
   - C. "The scan detects osteoarthritis."
   - D. "Bone pain can indicate a need for a scan."
   - E. "At age 40, you should have a baseline scan."

5. A nurse is contributing to the plan of care for a client who will undergo an electromyography (EMG). Which of the following actions should the nurse include in the plan of care? (Select all that apply.)
   - A. Check for bruising.
   - B. Apply ice to insertion sites.
   - C. Determine whether the client takes a muscle relaxant.
   - D. Instruct the client to flex her muscles during needle insertion.
   - E. Expect swelling, redness, and tenderness at the insertion sites.

Application Exercises Key

1. A. The client should wear a sling to immobilize the arm of the affected shoulder to limit activity and promote healing.

   B. **CORRECT:** The client should inspect the incision for evidence of infection (redness, swelling, purulent drainage).

   C. **CORRECT:** The client should apply ice packs to the affected area for the first 24 hr to reduce swelling and discomfort.

   D. The client should elevate the affected extremity for 12 to 24 hr to reduce swelling.

   E. **CORRECT:** The client should perform the isometric exercises as prescribed and directed.

   Ⓝ *NCLEX® Connection: Reduction of Risk Potential, Potential for Complications from Surgical Procedures and Health Alterations*

2. A. **CORRECT:** Inspecting color and temperature of the affected extremity helps identify alterations in circulation.

   B. Cold compresses on the incisional site for the first 24 hr help decrease swelling and pain.

   C. **CORRECT:** Elevating the leg helps decrease swelling and pain in the affected extremity.

   D. **CORRECT:** Administering analgesic medication helps relieve joint pain in the affected extremity.

   E. **CORRECT:** Checking pulse and sensation of the affected extremity helps identify alterations in circulation.

   Ⓝ *NCLEX® Connection: Reduction of Risk Potential, Potential for Complications from Surgical Procedures and Health Alterations*

3. A. The radioactive isotope is injected through an IV 2 to 3 hr before the scanning.

   B. The procedure does not use a tube-like structure as for an MRI.

   C. Radioactive precautions for urine are not necessary following the procedure.

   D. **CORRECT:** The client will need to urinate prior to the procedure. An empty bladder promotes visualization of the pelvic bones.

   Ⓝ *NCLEX® Connection: Reduction of Risk Potential, Diagnostic Tests*

4. A. DXA scan does not require contrast material.

   B. **CORRECT:** The most common areas for a DXA scan are the hip and spine for more clear visualization of a large area of bone.

   C. A DXA scan detects osteoporosis, not osteoarthritis.

   D. **CORRECT:** Bone pain, loss of height, and fractures can indicate the need for a DXA scan.

   E. **CORRECT:** A baseline scan at age 40 is helpful for comparison with a scan during the postmenopausal period.

   Ⓝ *NCLEX® Connection: Reduction of Risk Potential, Diagnostic Tests*

5. A. **CORRECT:** Some bruising can occur at the needle insertion sites.

   B. **CORRECT:** The nurse should apply ice to the insertion sites to prevent hematoma development.

   C. **CORRECT:** The nurse should collect data regarding the client's medications to determine whether she takes a muscle relaxant, which can decrease the accuracy of the test results.

   D. **CORRECT:** The nurse should ask the client to flex her muscles for an easier insertion of the needle into the muscle.

   E. The nurse should instruct the client to report swelling, redness, and tenderness at the insertion sites to the provider because this can indicate an infection.

   Ⓝ *NCLEX® Connection: Reduction of Risk Potential, Potential for Complications of Diagnostic Tests/Treatments/Procedures*

PRACTICE Active Learning Scenario

A nurse is reinforcing teaching with a client who is having a gallium scan. Which of the following information should the nurse include in the teaching? Use the ATI Active Learning Template: Diagnostic Procedure to complete this item.

DESCRIPTION OF PROCEDURE

INDICATIONS: List three.

NURSING INTERVENTIONS (PRE, POST): List two preprocedure and one postprocedure.

PRACTICE Answer

Using ATI Active Learning Template: Diagnostic Procedure

DESCRIPTION OF PROCEDURE: A gallium scan involves a radioisotope (radionuclide) that is injected 4 to 6 hr before the scan to view the bones. The radionuclide also migrates to the tissues of the brain, liver, and breast and is used to detect disease of these organs.

INDICATIONS: Detect fractures, osteoporosis, bone lesions, osteomyelitis, and arthritis.

NURSING INTERVENTIONS (PRE, POST)
- Preprocedure
  - Check for allergy to radioisotopes.
  - Check for existing conditions, such as pregnancy or kidney disease, that are contraindications for the procedure.
  - Have the client empty the bladder before the procedure.
- Postprocedure: Inform the client to increase fluid intake to promote the excretion of the radioisotope in the urine and feces.

Ⓝ *NCLEX® Connection: Reduction of Risk Potential, Diagnostic Tests*

UNIT 10   NURSING CARE OF CLIENTS WHO HAVE
MUSCULOSKELETAL DISORDERS
SECTION: DIAGNOSTIC AND THERAPEUTIC PROCEDURES

CHAPTER 60 *Arthroplasty*

Most musculoskeletal surgical procedures are performed to repair damaged joints, particularly the knees and the hips. A noncemented press-fit prosthesis is used for clients who are active, young, or overweight.

Arthroplasty is surgical removal of a diseased joint due to osteoarthritis, osteonecrosis, rheumatoid arthritis, trauma, or congenital anomalies, and replacing it with prosthetics or artificial components made of metal and/or plastic.

Total joint arthroplasty, also called total joint replacement, involves replacement of all components of an articulating joint.

Total knee arthroplasty involves the replacement of the distal femoral component, tibia plate, and patellar button. This is a surgical option when conservative measures fail. (60.1)

Unicondylar knee replacement is done when the joint is diseased in one compartment.

Total hip arthroplasty involves the replacement of the acetabular cup, femoral head, and femoral stem. (60.2)

Hemiarthroplasty refers to half of a joint replacement. Fractures of the femoral neck are treated with replacement of the femoral component.

INDICATIONS

The goal of both hip and knee arthroplasty is to eliminate pain, restore joint motions, and improve functional status and quality of life.

POTENTIAL DIAGNOSES
• Knee and hip arthroplasty treats degenerative disease (osteoarthritis, rheumatoid arthritis).
• Osteonecrosis is a necrosis of the bone secondary to lack of blood flow due to trauma or chronic steroid therapy.

CLIENT PRESENTATION
• Pain when bearing weight on the joint (walking, running)
• Joint crepitus and stiffness
• Joint swelling (primarily in the knees)

60.1 Artificial knee joint

femur
metal surface
plastic surface
tibia

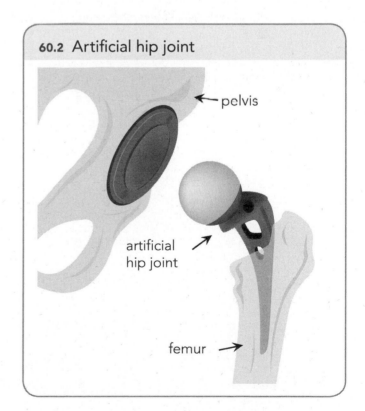

60.2 Artificial hip joint

pelvis
artificial hip joint
femur

CONSIDERATIONS

CONTRAINDICATIONS

- Recent or active infection (urinary tract infection), which can cause micro-organisms to migrate to the surgical area and cause the prosthesis to fail
- Arterial impairment to the affected extremity
- Client inability to follow the postsurgical regimen
- A comorbid condition (uncontrolled diabetes mellitus or hypertension, advanced osteoporosis, progressive inflammatory condition, unstable cardiac or respiratory conditions)

PREPROCEDURE

NURSING ACTIONS: Review diagnostic test results.
- **CBC, urinalysis, electrolytes, BUN, creatinine:** Determine surgical readiness, and rule out anemia, infection, or organ failure. Epoetin alfa is often prescribed several weeks preoperatively to increase Hgb for a client who has mild anemia.
- **Chest x-ray:** Rule out pulmonary surgical contraindications (infection, tumor).
- **ECG:** Gather baseline rhythm to identify cardiovascular surgical contraindications (dysrhythmia).

CLIENT EDUCATION
- Postoperative care includes incentive spirometry, transfusion, surgical drains, dressing, pain control, transfer, exercises, and activity limits.
- An overhead trapeze bar and ambulatory assistive devices (walkers, crutches, canes) can be used.
- Autologous blood donation involves donating blood prior to procedure to transfuse during or after the procedure.
- Scrub the surgical site with a prescribed antiseptic soap the night before and the morning of surgery to decrease bacterial count on skin, which reduces the chance of infection. Q**EBP**
- Wear clean clothes and sleep on clean linens the night before surgery.
- Take antihypertensive and other medications the surgeon allows with a sip of water the morning of surgery.
- Use an abduction pillow and specific turning procedures to prevent dislocation of the prosthesis.
- The provider will prescribe prophylactic antibiotics just prior to surgery to prevent infection.

INTRAPROCEDURE

- General or spinal anesthesia is used.
- Joint components are removed and replaced with artificial components.
- Components are either cemented in place or a press-fit, noncemented prosthesis is used. Components that do not use cement are stabilized when the bone grows into the prosthesis. Weight bearing is delayed several weeks until the femoral shaft has grown into the prosthesis.

POSTPROCEDURE

CLIENT EDUCATION
- Extensive physical therapy is required to regain mobility. The client is discharged home or to an acute rehabilitation facility. If discharged home, outpatient or in-home therapy is provided. Home care is usually available for 4 to 6 weeks. Q**TC**
- Monitor for evidence of incisional infection (fever, increased redness, swelling, purulent drainage).
- Care for the incision (clean daily with soap and water).
- Monitor for deep vein thrombosis (swelling, redness, pain in calf), pulmonary embolism (shortness of breath, chest pain), and bleeding, especially if taking an anticoagulant.
- Perform deep breathing and coughing, and use incentive spirometer to prevent respiratory complications.

Knee arthroplasty

NURSING ACTIONS
- Provide postoperative care to prevent complications (venous thromboembolism developing into deep vein thrombosis [DVT], which can lead to a pulmonary embolism, anemia, infection, neurovascular compromise).
- Older adult clients are at a higher risk for medical complications related to chronic conditions, including hypertension, diabetes mellitus, coronary artery disease, and obstructive pulmonary disease. Ⓖ
- A continuous passive motion (CPM) machine is often prescribed to promote motion in the knee, promote circulation, and prevent scar tissue formation. CPM is usually placed and initiated immediately after surgery. CPM provides passive range of motion from full extension to the prescribed amount of flexion. Follow the prescribed duration of use, but turn it off during meals.
- Positions of flexion of the knee are limited to avoid flexion contractures.
  - Avoid positioning the bed in a way that the knees are flexed or placing pillows behind the knee.
  - Place one pillow under the lower calf and foot to cause a slight extension of the knee joint and to prevent flexion contractures. The knee can also rest flat on the bed.
- To prevent pressure ulcers from developing on the heels, place a small blanket or pillow slightly above the ankle area to keep heels off the bed.
- Provide medications to promote comfort and participation in early ambulation.
  - **Analgesics:** Opioids (epidural, PCA, IV, oral), NSAIDs
  - **Peripheral nerve blockade:** Inject the femoral or sciatic nerve with a local anesthetic, or the client can receive a continuous infusion of local anesthetic directly into sciatic or femoral nerve.
    - A continuous peripheral nerve block provides localized pain relief.
    - Monitor for systemic effects of local anesthetic (metallic taste, tinnitus, slurred speech, decreased respiratory rate, hypotension, bradycardia, restlessness, seizure).

- On postoperative day 1, the client should start quadriceps-strengthening exercises and straight-leg raises by straightening the leg and pushing the back of the knees against the bed. Physical therapy usually continues after discharge.
- Administer antiobiotics postoperatively to prevent infection.
- Administer anticoagulants to prevent thrombus formation (warfarin, fondaparinux, rivaroxaban, or low-molecular-weight heparin, such as enoxaparin). Apply sequential compression devices, foot pumps, and antiembolism stockings to prevent venous thromboembolism formation that can develop into DVT.
- Apply ice or cold therapy to the incisional area to reduce postoperative swelling.
- Monitor neurovascular status of the surgical extremity (movement, sensation, color, pulse, capillary refill) every 2 to 4 hr, and compare with the contralateral extremity.
- Monitor frequently for overt bleeding and manifestations of hypovolemia (hypotension, tachycardia).
- Monitor the compression bandage and wound suction drain for excessive drainage.
- Monitor the autotransfusion drainage system, if used, and assist with blood reinfusion.

CLIENT EDUCATION
- Dislocation is uncommon following total knee arthroplasty.
- Kneeling and deep-knee bends are limited indefinitely.

Hip arthroplasty

NURSING ACTIONS
- Provide postoperative care to prevent complications.
- Check the dressing site frequently, noting any evidence of bleeding. Monitor and record drainage from surgical drains.
- Monitor daily laboratory values, including Hgb and Hct levels. Hgb and Hct can continue to drop for 48 hr after surgery. Assist with the use of autologous blood from presurgery donation, or blood salvaged intraoperatively or postoperatively, using collection devices for postoperative blood replacement as needed. Blood transfusions are often administered for Hgb levels less than 9 g/dL.
- Monitor the neurovascular status of the surgical extremity (movement, sensation, color, pulse, capillary refill, and compare with contralateral extremity) every 2 to 4 hr.
- Encourage deep breathing and coughing, and use of incentive spirometer to prevent respiratory complications.
- The client might have a drain at the surgical site placed to a suction reservoir, and an indwelling urinary catheter.

- Administer prescribed medications.
  - **Analgesics:** Opioids (epidural, PCA, IV, oral), NSAIDs
  - **Antibiotics:** Generally administered 30 min before the surgical incision is made as a prophylaxis, and postoperatively to prevent infection
  - **Anticoagulant:** Warfarin, dalteparin, fondaparinux, rivaroxaban, or low-molecular-weight heparin, such as enoxaparin
- Provide early ambulation.
  - Transfer the client out of bed from his unaffected side into a chair or wheelchair.
  - Weight-bearing status is determined by the orthopedic surgeon and by choice of cemented (usually partial/full weight-bearing as tolerated) vs. noncemented prostheses (usually only partial or minimal weight-bearing [toe touch] until after a few weeks of bone growth).
  - Use assistive (walker) and adaptive (raised toilet seat, grab bars, and shower chairs) devices when caring for the client. Qs
  - Apply ice to the surgical site following ambulation as a nonpharmacological measure to decrease pain and discomfort.
- Use total hip precautions to prevent dislocation of the new joint. Place the client supine with the head slightly elevated and the affected leg in a neutral position. Place a pillow or abduction device between the legs when turning to the unaffected side, or leave in place if the client has altered mental status and cannot follow hip precautions. Qpcc
- Monitor for new joint dislocation: acute onset of pain, reports hearing a pop, internal rotation of the affected extremity, and shortened affected extremity.
- Arrange for and instruct the client about the use of raised toilet seats and care items (long-handled shoehorn, dressing sticks).

CLIENT EDUCATION
- Follow position restrictions to avoid dislocation.
  - Use elevated seating and a raised toilet seat.
  - Use straight chairs with arms.
  - Use an abduction pillow or regular pillow, if prescribed, between the legs while turning, or while in bed, if restless.
  - Externally rotate the toes.
  - Use extended handles on shoehorns and dressing sticks to prevent hip flexion greater than 90°.
  - Avoid hip flexion greater than 90°.
  - Avoid low chairs.
  - Do not cross the legs for at least 3 months.
  - Do not internally rotate the toes.
  - Continue to follow the exercise program at home.

COMPLICATIONS

HIP ARTHROPLASTY

Venous thromboembolism

Can develop into a DVT resulting in a pulmonary embolism, a life-threatening complication after total hip arthroplasty

NURSING ACTIONS
- Monitor for manifestations of pulmonary embolism, including acute dyspnea, tachycardia, and pleuritic chest pain.
- Follow venous thromboembolism prophylaxis (pharmacological management, antiembolic stockings, sequential compression devices or foot pumps while in bed).
- Encourage plantar flexion, dorsiflexion, and circumduction exercises to prevent clot formation.
- Encourage early ambulation with physical and occupational therapy.

Hip dislocation, infection, anemia, neurovascular compromise

- Older adult clients are at an increased risk for medical complications related to chronic conditions, including hypertension, diabetes mellitus, coronary artery disease, and obstructive pulmonary disease. Ⓖ
- Older adult clients are an increased risk for a potentially life-threatening complication (venous thromboembolism formation that develops into DVT, pulmonary emboli) due to age and compromised circulation before surgery.
- Clients who are obese or who have a history of venous thromboembolism formation are also at increased risk for developing DVT or pulmonary emboli.

NURSING ACTIONS: Monitor for bleeding.

Application Exercises

1. A nurse is reviewing the health record of a client who is to undergo total joint arthroplasty. The nurse should recognize which of the following findings as a contraindication to this procedure?

   A. Age 78 years

   B. History of cancer

   C. Previous joint replacement

   D. Bronchitis 2 weeks ago

2. A nurse is admitting a client to the orthopedic unit following a total knee arthroplasty. Which of the following actions should the nurse take? (Select all that apply.)

   A. Check continuous passive motion device settings.

   B. Palpate dorsal pedal pulses.

   C. Place a pillow under the knees.

   D. Elevate heels off the bed.

   E. Apply heat therapy to the incision.

3. A nurse is assisting with planning discharge teaching for a client who had a total hip arthroplasty. Which of the following instructions should the nurse include? (Select all that apply.)

   A. Clean the incision daily with soap and water.

   B. Turn the toes inward when sitting or lying.

   C. Sit in a straight-backed armchair.

   D. Bend at the waist when putting on socks.

   E. Use a raised toilet seat.

4. A nurse is collecting data on a client who is scheduled to undergo a right knee arthroplasty. The nurse should expect which of the following findings? (Select all that apply.)

   A. Skin reddened over the joint

   B. Pain when bearing weight

   C. Joint crepitus

   D. Swelling of the affected joint

   E. Limited joint motion

5. A nurse is assisting with a preoperative teaching plan for a client who is scheduled to have a total hip arthroplasty. Which of the following should the nurse include in the teaching plan? (Select all that apply.)

   A. Complete autologous blood donation.

   B. Sit in a low reclining chair.

   C. Cross legs when in bed.

   D. Use an abductor pillow when turning.

   E. Perform isometric exercises.

PRACTICE Active Learning Scenario

A nurse is preparing to administer enoxaparin to a client who had a total knee arthroplasty. What should the nurse consider before administering the medication? Use the ATI Active Learning Template: Medication and the Pharmacology Review Module to complete this item.

EXPECTED PHARMACOLOGICAL ACTION: Define.

NURSING INTERVENTIONS: List two nursing interventions.

CLIENT EDUCATION: List three client teaching points.

Application Exercises Key

1. A. Age greater than 70 is not a contraindication for a total joint arthroplasty unless there are comorbid factors.

   B. History of cancer is not a contraindication for a total joint arthroplasty unless there are comorbid factors.

   C. Previous joint arthroplasty surgery is not a contraindication for total joint arthroplasty unless there are comorbid factors.

   D. **CORRECT:** Recent bronchitis or infection can cause micro-organisms to migrate to the surgical area and cause the prosthesis to fail. This client is at risk for postoperative pulmonary complications.

   Ⓝ *NCLEX® Connection: Reduction of Risk Potential, Potential for Complications from Surgical Procedures and Health Alterations*

2. A. **CORRECT:** The nurse should check the continuous passive motion device settings to determine if the settings are as prescribed.

   B. **CORRECT:** The nurse should check the strength of the pulses of both lower extremities to help determine adequate circulation.

   C. The nurse should place one pillow under the lower calf and foot to cause a slight extension of the knee joint and to prevent flexion contractures. The knee can also rest flat on the bed.

   D. **CORRECT:** The nurse should prevent pressure ulcers on the client's heels by elevating the heels off the bed with a pillow.

   E. The nurse should apply cold therapy to reduce postoperative swelling.

   Ⓝ *NCLEX® Connection: Reduction of Risk Potential, Potential for Complications from Surgical Procedures and Health Alterations*

3. A. **CORRECT:** The client should wash the surgical incision daily with soap and water to decrease the risk of infection.

   B. The client should externally rotate toes to prevent dislocation of the hip prosthesis.

   C. **CORRECT:** Using a straight-backed armchair decreases the chance of bending at a greater than 90° angle, which can cause dislocation of the hip prosthesis.

   D. Bending at the waist places the hip in a position greater than a 90° angle, which can cause dislocation of the hip prosthesis.

   E. **CORRECT:** Using a toilet riser decreases the chance of bending greater than 90°, which can cause dislocation of the hip prosthesis.

   Ⓝ *NCLEX® Connection: Reduction of Risk Potential, Potential for Complications from Surgical Procedures and Health Alterations*

4. A. Skin over the knee that is red can indicate infection and is not an expected finding.

   B. **CORRECT:** Pain when bearing weight is an expected finding due to degeneration of the joint.

   C. **CORRECT:** Joint crepitus due to degeneration of the joint tissue is an expected finding.

   D. **CORRECT:** Swelling of the affected joint due to degeneration of the joint tissue is an expected finding.

   E. **CORRECT:** Limited joint motion is due to degeneration of the joint tissue and is an expected finding.

   Ⓝ *NCLEX® Connection: Physiological Adaptation, Basic Pathophysiology*

5. A. **CORRECT:** The nurse should encourage the client to donate autologous blood to use postoperatively.

   B. The nurse should have the client sit in a hard-back chair to keep the hip at a 90° angle. This prevents dislocation of the joint.

   C. The nurse should instruct the client to avoid crossing his legs to prevent dislocation of the prosthesis.

   D. **CORRECT:** The nurse should instruct the client to place an abductor device or pillow between the legs when turning to prevent dislocation of the affected hip.

   E. **CORRECT:** The nurse should instruct the client to perform isometric exercises to prevent blood clots and maintain muscle tone.

   Ⓝ *NCLEX® Connection: Reduction of Risk Potential, Potential for Complications of Diagnostic Tests/Treatments/Procedures*

PRACTICE Answer

Using ATI Active Learning Template: Medication

EXPECTED PHARMACOLOGICAL ACTION: Enoxaparin is an anticoagulant. Use low molecular-weight heparin after abdominal and orthopedic surgery to prevent deep vein thrombosis that may lead to pulmonary embolism.

NURSING INTERVENTIONS
- Do not expel the air bubble from the syringe before injection to prevent the loss of medication and allow the client to receive all the medication during the injection.
- Rotate injection sites.
- Monitor for manifestations of unexplained bleeding.

CLIENT EDUCATION
- Use a soft toothbrush and shave with an electric razor to prevent bleeding.
- Avoid over-the-counter medication unless prescribed.
- Do not take enoxaparin with garlic, ginger, ginkgo, or feverfew. These supplements can increase the risk of bleeding.

Ⓝ *NCLEX® Connection: Pharmacological Therapies, Medication Administration*

CHAPTER 61 *Amputations*

Amputation is the removal of a body part, most commonly an extremity. Amputations are elective due to complications of peripheral vascular disease and arteriosclerosis, congenital deformities, chronic osteomyelitis, or malignant tumor; or traumatic due to an accident.

Amputations are described in regard to the extremity and whether they are located above or below the designated joint. Disarticulation describes an amputation performed through a joint.

The higher the level of amputation, the greater the amount of effort required to use a prosthesis. The level of the amputation is determined by the presence of adequate blood flow needed for healing.

Older adult clients are poor candidates for prosthetic training due to the amount of energy required for ambulation. Ⓖ

Significant changes to body image occur after an amputation and should be addressed during the perioperative and rehabilitative phases.

UPPER EXTREMITY AMPUTATIONS

- Upper extremity amputations include above- and below-the-elbow amputations, wrist and shoulder disarticulations, and finger amputations.
- Traumatic amputation caused by accidents, war, or injury is the primary cause of upper extremity amputations.
- Other causes include vasospastic disease, malignancy, and infection of the extremity.

LOWER EXTREMITY AMPUTATIONS

- Lower extremity amputations include above- and below-the-knee amputations, hip and knee disarticulations, Syme's amputation (removal of foot with ankle saved), and mid-foot and toe amputations.
- Lower extremity amputations are usually done due to peripheral vascular disease as a result of arteriosclerosis and diabetes mellitus.
- Every effort is made to save as much of the extremity as possible. Even loss of the big toe can significantly affect balance, gait, and push-off ability during ambulation. Salvage of the knee instead of a below-the-knee amputation increases function.

HEALTH PROMOTION AND DISEASE PREVENTION

- Clients who have diabetes mellitus should monitor blood glucose and maintain it within the expected reference range.
- Use safety measures when working with heavy machinery or in areas where there is a risk of electrocution or burns.
- Quit or do not start smoking, maintain a healthy weight, and exercise regularly.
- Maintain good foot care and seek early medical attention for nonhealing wounds.

DATA COLLECTION

RISK FACTORS

- Traumatic injury (motor vehicle crashes, industrial equipment, war-related injuries)
- Thermal injury (frostbite, electrocution, burns)
- Peripheral vascular disease related to diabetes mellitus
- Malignancy
- Older adult clients have a higher risk of peripheral vascular disease and diabetes mellitus resulting in decreased tissue perfusion and peripheral neuropathy. Both conditions place older adult clients at risk for lower extremity amputation. Ⓖ

CHRONIC DISEASE PROCESSES
- Peripheral vascular disease resulting in ischemia/gangrene
- Diabetes mellitus resulting in peripheral neuropathy and peripheral vascular disease
- Infection (osteomyelitis)
- Congenital defects

EXPECTED FINDINGS

Decreased tissue perfusion

- Client report of pain
- History of injury or disease process precipitating amputation
- Altered peripheral pulses (can use Doppler if needed)
- Differences in temperature of extremities (level of leg at which temperature becomes cool)
- Altered color of extremities (black indicates gangrene; cyanosis indicates vascular compromise)
- Presence of infection and open wounds
- Lack of sensation in the affected extremity

NURSING ACTIONS
Neurological checks

- Monitor capillary refill by comparing extremities. In older adult clients, capillary refill can be difficult to monitor due to thickened and opaque nails.
- Observe for edema, necrosis, and lack of hair distribution of the extremity due to inadequate peripheral circulation.
- Monitor for circulation, movement, and sensation of the extremity.

DIAGNOSTIC PROCEDURES

To determine blood flow at various levels of an extremity

Angiography: Allows visualization of peripheral vasculature and areas of impaired circulation

Doppler laser and ultrasonography studies: Measures speed of blood flow in an extremity

Transcutaneous oxygen pressure (TcPO$_2$): Measures oxygen pressures in an extremity to indicate blood flow in the extremity, which is a reliable indicator for healing

Ankle-brachial index: Measures difference between ankle and brachial systolic pressures

PATIENT-CENTERED CARE

NURSING CARE

Preoperative

- Involve the client in decision to amputate, and explain what to expect postoperatively.
- Expect clients to experience stages of denial and anger.
- Reinforce teaching about phantom limb pain.
- Reinforce teaching about muscle strengthening exercises.

Postoperative

- Prevent postoperative complications (hypovolemia, pain, infection).
- Elevate for the first 24 to 48 hr (lower extremities are usually not elevated longer than 24 hr due to the risk of hip contractures).
- Monitor surgical site for bleeding. Monitor vital signs frequently.

- Monitor tissue perfusion of end of residual limb.
  - Palpate residual limb for warmth. Heat can indicate infection.
  - Compare pulse most proximal to incision with pulse in other extremity.
- Monitor for manifestations of infection and nonhealing of incision. Infection can lead to osteomyelitis.
  - Amputation might not heal if performed below the level of adequate tissue perfusion.
  - Position the affected extremity in dependent position to promote blood flow/oxygenation.
  - Administer antibiotics and change dressings if open amputation was performed.
  - Record characteristics of drainage (amount, color, odor).
  - Keep a tourniquet at the bedside in case of hemorrhage.

Management of traumatic amputation

- Implement a medical emergency system (EMS).
- Apply direct pressure using gauze (if available) or clean cloth to prevent life-threatening hemorrhage.
- Elevate the extremity above the heart to decrease blood loss.
- Wrap the severed extremity in dry sterile gauze (if available) or in a clean cloth, and place in a sealed plastic bag. Submerge the bag in ice water (one part ice and three parts water), and send with the client.

Pain

- Monitor and treat pain.
- Differentiate between phantom limb and incisional pain.
- Incisional pain is treated with analgesics.

Phantom limb pain

- The sensation of pain in the location of the extremity following the amputation
- Related to severed nerve pathways and is a frequent complication in clients who experienced chronic limb pain before the amputation.
- Can be experienced immediately after surgery, up to several weeks, or indefinitely.
- Occurs less frequently following traumatic amputation.
- Often described as deep and burning, cramping, shooting, or aching.
- Treated much differently from incisional pain.
- IV infusion of ketamine can reduce or eliminate phantom pain.
  - Administration of calcitonin during the first week after having an amputation can decrease phantom limb pain.
  - Administering beta blockers, such as propranolol, can relieve the continual dull, burning sensation associated with the amputated limb.
  - Administering antiepileptics (gabapentin, pregabalin) can relieve sharp, stabbing, and burning phantom limb pain.
  - Some clients have relief from antispasmodics, such as baclofen, and antidepressant medications.

- ○ Recognize that pain is real and manage it accordingly.
- ○ Alternative treatment for phantom limb pain can include nonpharmacological methods (massage, heat, transcutaneous electrical nerve stimulation [TENS], ultrasound therapy, biofeedback, relaxation therapy).
- ○ A stump stocking with an electromagnetic shield blocks external electromagnetic impulses from outside sources, which are thought to cause phantom pain.
- ○ Virtual reality goggles help visualize the limb as whole.
- ○ Reinforce teaching with the client how to push the residual limb down toward the bed while supported on a soft pillow. This helps reduce phantom limb pain and prepare the limb for a prosthesis.

Client perception and feelings regarding amputation

- Allow the client and family to grieve for the loss of the body part and change in body image.
- Feelings can include depression, anger, withdrawal, and grief.
- Monitor the psychosocial well-being of the client. Observe for feelings of altered self-concept and self-esteem, and willingness and motivation for rehabilitation.
- Facilitate a supportive environment for the client and family so grief can be processed. Refer the client to religious/spiritual adviser, social worker, or counselor.
- Rehabilitation should include adaptation to a new body image and integration of prosthetic and adaptive devices into self-image.

Residual limb preparation and prosthesis fitting

Residual limb must be shaped and shrunk in preparation for prosthetic training.

SHRINKAGE INTERVENTIONS
- Wrap the stump, using elastic bandages (figure-eight wrap) to prevent restriction of blood flow and decrease edema.
- Use a stump shrinker sock (easier for the client to apply).
- Use an air splint (plastic inflatable device) inflated to protect and shape the residual limb and for easy access to inspect the wound.

NURSING ACTIONS
- Explain how to care for and wrap the residual limb, and how to perform limb-strengthening exercises.
- Reinforce proper application and care of the prosthesis.
- Explain how to safely transfer and use mobility devices and adaptive aids. Qs
- Explain how to manage phantom limb pain.

CLIENT EDUCATION
- Amputation can alter sense of balance due to a disruption in the body's center of gravity
- Use a mirror to monitor the stump daily for redness, or abrasions.
- Wash the stump daily with bacteriostatic soap and completely rinse and dry it.

- Replace the stump sock daily.
- Apply the prosthesis immediately when getting out of bed to reduce swelling.
- Perform exercises to increase strength.
- Replace shoes frequently to prevent falls
- Clean the prosthesis socket daily with a damp cloth. Dry the prosthesis socket thoroughly.
- Consult with the prosthetic orthotist for prosthetic adjustments and yearly checks.

THERAPEUTIC PROCEDURES

Closed amputation: This is the most common technique used. A skin flap is sutured over the end of the residual limb, closing the site.

Open amputation: This technique is used when an active infection is present. A skin flap is not sutured over the end of the residual limb, allowing for drainage of infection. The skin flap is closed at a later date.

INTERPROFESSIONAL CARE

Intensive efforts by the interprofessional team are necessary to facilitate successful rehabilitation.
- A certified prosthetic orthotist fits client with prosthesis after the wound is healed and the stump has shrunk.
- A physical therapist trains the client in application and care of the prosthesis and mobility aids.
- A psychologist might need to help with adjustment to loss of the extremity.
- A social worker assists clients who have financial issues and can refer clients to resources and support groups or organizations for people who have had amputations.

COMPLICATIONS

Flexion contractures

Flexion contractures are more likely with the hip or knee joint following amputation due to improper positioning.

NURSING ACTIONS
- Prevention includes range-of-motion (ROM) exercises and proper positioning immediately after surgery.
- To prevent hip or knee flexion contracture, some providers do not advocate elevating the stump on a pillow. Other providers allow elevation for the first 24 to 48 hr to reduce swelling and discomfort.
- Have the client lie prone for 20 to 30 min several times a day to help prevent hip flexion contractures.
- Discourage prolonged sitting.
- Have a physical therapist teach the client some exercises that will prevent contractures.

CLIENT EDUCATION: Stand using good posture with the residual limb in extension. This also will aid in balance.

Application Exercises

1. A nurse is presenting information to a group of clients at a health fair about measures to reduce the risk of amputation. Which of the following information should the nurse provide? (Select all that apply.)

   A. Clients who smoke should consider smoking cessation programs.

   B. Clients who have diabetes mellitus should maintain blood glucose within the expected reference range.

   C. Unplug electrical equipment when performing repairs.

   D. Clients who have vascular disease should maintain good foot care.

   E. Wait 2 hr after taking pain medication before driving.

2. A nurse is collecting data from an older adult client who has arteriosclerosis and is scheduled for a right lower extremity amputation. Which of the following are expected findings in the affected extremity? (Select all that apply.)

   A. Skin cool to touch from mid-calf to the toes

   B. Lower leg appearing dusky when client is sitting

   C. Palpable pounding pedal pulse

   D. Lack of hair on lower leg

   E. Blackened areas on several toes

3. A nurse is caring for a client following a below-the-elbow amputation. Which of the following actions should the nurse take? (Select all that apply.)

   A. Encourage dependent positioning of the residual limb.

   B. Inspect for presence and amount of drainage on the dressing.

   C. Implement shrinkage intervention of the residual limb.

   D. Wrap the residual limb in a circular manner using gauze.

   E. Observe for body image changes.

4. A nurse is caring for a client who had an above-the-knee amputation. The client reports a sharp, stabbing type of phantom pain. Which of the following actions should the nurse take?

   A. Remove the initial pressure dressing.

   B. Encourage use of cold therapy.

   C. Question whether the pain is real.

   D. Administer an antiepileptic medication.

5. A nurse is assisting with preparing a plan of care to prevent a client from developing flexion contractures following a below-the-knee amputation 24 hr ago. Which of the following actions should the nurse include in the plan of care?

   A. Limit any type of exercise to the residual limb for the first 48 hr after surgery.

   B. Position the client prone several times each day.

   C. Wrap the stump in a figure-eight pattern.

   D. Encourage sitting in a chair during the day.

PRACTICE Active Learning Scenario

A nurse is assisting with completing discharge planning for a client who had an amputation. What members of an interprofessional team should the nurse include in the discharge planning process? Use the ATI Active Learning Template: Basic Concept to complete this item.

RELATED CONTENT: List three members of the interprofessional team and describe the principal purpose of each member.

Application Exercises Key

1. A. **CORRECT:** Smoking cessation can decrease the development of arteriosclerosis and possible amputation of a lower extremity.

   B. **CORRECT:** Regulating blood glucose levels within a normal reference range prevents the development of arteriosclerosis and possible amputation of a lower extremity.

   C. **CORRECT:** Unplugging electrical equipment when performing repairs prevents electrocution and injury to an extremity, which can lead to amputation.

   D. **CORRECT:** Maintaining good foot care prevents infection, which can result in amputation.

   E. Driving under the influence of pain medication can lead to an accident or injury to an extremity, requiring amputation.

   Ⓝ *NCLEX® Connection: Health Promotion and Maintenance, Health Promotion/Disease Prevention*

2. A. **CORRECT:** The client can have coolness of the affected extremity where decreased vascularization starts.

   B. **CORRECT:** The affected extremity can become dusky when sitting due to decreased vascularization of the extremity.

   C. The client will have a lack of or diminished pedal pulse of the affected extremity due to decreased vascularization.

   D. **CORRECT:** The client can have decreased hair growth on areas of the affected extremity due to decreased vascularization.

   E. **CORRECT:** The client can have blackened areas on several toes suggestive of gangrene due to decreased vascularization to the affected extremity.

   Ⓝ *NCLEX® Connection: Basic Care and Comfort, Mobility/Immobility*

3. A. **CORRECT:** The nurse should place the residual limb in a dependent position to improve circulation to the end of the stump and promote healing.

   B. **CORRECT:** The nurse should inspect the residual limb for the presence and amount of drainage to observe for bleeding and early manifestations of infection.

   C. **CORRECT:** The nurse should prepare the residual limb to include shrinkage interventions before fitting of the prosthesis.

   D. The nurse should wrap the residual limb with an elastic bandage in a figure-eight manner to prevent restriction of blood flow before fitting for the prosthesis.

   E. **CORRECT:** The nurse should monitor the client for feelings of depression, anger, withdrawal, and grief due to body image changes.

   Ⓝ *NCLEX® Connection: Reduction of Risk Potential, Potential for Complications from Surgical Procedures and Health Alterations*

4. A. The nurse should not remove the initial pressure dressing. The surgeon should remove the dressing in 48 to 72 hr. However, this action will not reduce phantom pain.

   B. Heat therapy, not cold therapy, to the residual limb is an alternative therapy that the nurse can implement to relieve phantom pain.

   C. Phantom pain is related to the severed nerve pathways following the amputation. The nurse should not question whether the pain is real.

   D. **CORRECT:** An antiepileptic medication can relieve a sharp, stabbing type of phantom pain.

   Ⓝ *NCLEX® Connection: Pharmacological Therapies, Pharmacological Pain Management*

5. A. The nurse should encourage the client to perform range-of-motion exercise to the residual limb to prevent flexion contractures.

   B. **CORRECT:** The nurse should position the client prone several times each day for 20 to 30 min to prevent flexion contractures of the hip.

   C. The nurse should wrap the residual limb in a figure eight to reduce edema and prepare for the prosthesis, but this action does not prevent flexion contractures.

   D. The client can develop flexion contractures by allowing the residual stump to hang in a bent position when sitting for an extended period following the amputation.

   Ⓝ *NCLEX® Connection: Reduction of Risk Potential, Potential for Complications of Diagnostic Tests/Treatments/Procedures*

PRACTICE Answer

Using the ATI Active Learning Template: Basic Concept

RELATED CONTENT
- Certified prosthetic orthotist fits the client with the prosthesis following healing and shrinking of the stump.
- Physical therapist provides training for applying the prosthesis, assists in mobility training, and reviews mobility aids.
- Psychologist assists the client and family in adjusting to the loss of an extremity.
- Social worker provides referral information for financial assistance, resources and support groups, or organizations to help adjust to life-changing physical conditions.

Ⓝ *NCLEX® Connection: Coordinated Care, Collaboration with Interdisciplinary Team*

CHAPTER 62 *Osteoporosis*

Osteoporosis is a common chronic metabolic bone disorder resulting in low bone density (decrease in bone mass). Osteoporosis occurs when the rate of bone resorption exceeds the rate of bone formation, resulting in fragile bone tissue and possible fractures. Common sites of osteoporotic fractures include the wrists, hips, and spine, but any bone can sustain a fracture.

Osteopenia, the precursor to osteoporosis, refers to low bone mineral density relative to the client's age and sex. Bone mineral density peaks between the ages of 18 to 30. After peak years, bone density decreases 1% per year. After menopause, loss of bone mass accelerates to 2% each year, with a significant increase in the rate of loss in postmenopausal clients due to estrogen loss. There is a heredity tendency for osteoporosis.

HEALTH PROMOTION AND DISEASE PREVENTION

- Ensure the diet includes adequate amounts of calcium, phosphorus and vitamin D, especially before age 35.
  - Foods rich in vitamin D are most fish, egg yolks, fortified milk, and cereal.
  - Foods rich in calcium are milk products, green vegetables, fortified orange juice and cereals, red and white beans, and figs.
- Take a calcium supplement with vitamin D if dietary intake is inadequate (lactose intolerance).
- Limit the amount of carbonated beverages, which contain phosphates and can cause calcium loss.
- Expose areas of skin to sun 5 to 30 min twice a week. Exposure to the sun for any length of time should include wearing sunscreen to avoid getting a sunburn.
- Discuss the pros and cons of postmenopausal hormone replacement therapy with the provider.
- Engage in weight-bearing exercises (walking, lifting weights, climbing stairs).

DATA COLLECTION

RISK FACTORS

- Female sex, family history, and thin, lean body build are precursors to low bone density.
- Increased bone loss can occur with the following.
  - Age older than 60
  - Postmenopausal estrogen deficiency or low levels of calcitonin
  - Testosterone hormonal changes after age 70
- History of low calcium intake with suboptimal levels of vitamin D decreases bone formation.
- Inadequate intake of calcium and vitamin D stimulates the parathyroid hormone to be released and triggers calcium to be pulled from the bone.
- A diet deficient or excessive in protein can contribute to development of osteoporosis. Clients who limit protein have a reduced ability to use calcium because up to 50% of calcium is bound to protein. Clients who follow a high-protein, low-carbohydrate diet can eliminate important nutrients, such as calcium-rich foods.
- History of smoking and high alcohol intake (three or more drinks per day) causes decreased bone formation and increased bone absorption.
- Excess caffeine consumption causes excretion of calcium in the urine.
- History of gastric bypass surgery (bypassing of the duodenum where the majority of calcium is absorbed) limits the amount of calcium available.
- Lack of physical activity or prolonged immobility places the client at risk for osteoporosis because bones need the stress of weight-bearing activity for bone rebuilding and maintenance.
- Chronic disease (liver, lung, kidney)
- Secondary osteoporosis results from medical conditions.
  - Comorbidities including hyperparathyroidism, hyperthyroidism, diabetes mellitus, Cushing's syndrome, rheumatoid arthritis, malabsorption syndrome, kidney impairment, anorexia nervosa, and chronic airway disorders (COPD, asthma) that affect calcium absorption and bone development.
  - Medication use over a prolonged period (loop diuretics, corticosteroids, thyroid medications, anticonvulsants) affects calcium absorption and bone metabolism.
  - Long-term lack of weight-bearing (spinal cord injury, sedentary lifestyle)
- Older adult clients have an increased risk of falls related to impaired balance, generalized weakness, gait changes, and impaired vision and hearing. Medication adverse effects can cause orthostatic hypotension, urinary frequency, or confusion, which can also raise the risk for falls. The body also does not absorb and use calcium as efficiently, but it does excrete calcium more readily than in younger adults. Ⓖ
- Daily weight-bearing exercise should include walking down stairs or walking for 30 min at least three times a week to decrease the chance of developing osteoporosis.

EXPECTED FINDINGS

Osteoporosis is a silent disease with no early findings until the following manifestations occur.

- Reduced height (postmenopausal)
- Acute back pain after lifting or bending (worse with activity, relieved by rest)
- Pain from a compression fracture of the spine.
- Restriction in movement and spinal deformity
- History of fractures (wrist, femur, thoracic spine)
- Thoracic (kyphosis) of the dorsal spine (62.1)
- Pain upon palpation over affected area

LABORATORY TESTS

- Serum calcium, vitamin D, phosphorus, and alkaline phosphatase levels are checked to rule out other metabolic bone diseases (Paget's disease or osteomalacia).
- 24-hr urine can evaluate the rate of calcium excretion.

DIAGNOSTIC PROCEDURES

Radiographs

Radiographs of the spine and long bones reveal low bone density and fractures.

Dual-energy x-ray absorptiometry (DXA)

- A DXA scan is used to screen for early changes in bone density and is usually done on the hip or spine.
- The client will lie on an x-ray table while a scan of a selected area is done.
- A peripheral DXA scan is used to determine the bone density of the heel, forearm, or finger.
- DXA uses two beams of radiation. Findings are analyzed by a computer and interpreted by a radiologist. Clients receive a score that indicates how much their bone density deviates from the expected bone density of a young, healthy adult.
  - Normal bone density: less than 1 standard deviation (SD) below the expected bone density
  - Osteopenia: 1 to 2.5 SD below the expected bone density
  - Osteoporosis: greater than 2.5 SD below the expected bone density

Computed tomography

Used to measure bone density, especially in the vertebral column.

PATIENT-CENTERED CARE

NURSING CARE

- Determine risk factors (family history, steroid medication use, diet and exercise pattern, history of smoking and alcohol intake).
- Encourage screening.
- Reinforce education about the benefits of a healthy lifestyle.
- Reinforce education on the harmful effects of smoking.

- Administer medications.
- Reinforce the instructions for the client and family regarding dietary calcium food sources.
- Provide information regarding calcium and vitamin D supplementation. (Take with food.)
- Reinforce instructions regarding the need for adequate amounts of protein, magnesium, vitamin K, and other trace minerals for bone formation.
- Reinforce the need for exposure to vitamin D (moderate sun exposure using sunscreen, fortified milk).
- Encourage weight-bearing exercises (at least 30 min, at least three times a week) to improve strength and reduce bone loss.

CLIENT EDUCATION

- Limit caffeine, alcohol, and carbonated beverages, which increase bone loss.
- Check the home environment for safety (remove throw rugs, provide adequate lighting, clear walkways) to prevent falls, which can result in fractures. Qs
  - Use safety equipment and assistive devices.
  - Avoid inclement weather (ice, slippery surfaces).
  - Mark clearly thresholds, doorways, and steps.

MEDICATIONS

Medications (calcium, vitamin D) can slow or prevent osteoporosis. The client can use a combination of several of the following medications to decrease the loss of bone density, increase bone formation, and decrease fractures.

Thyroid hormone

Calcitonin human, calcitonin salmon

THERAPEUTIC USES: Decreases bone resorption by inhibiting osteoclast activity for treatment of osteoporosis, hypercalcemia, and Paget's disease of the bone.

NURSING ACTIONS

- Calcitonin human can only be administered subcutaneously.
- Calcitonin salmon can be administered subcutaneously, intramuscularly, and intranasally.
- Advise the client to increase dietary intake of calcium and vitamin D to increase the effectiveness of treatment.

Teriparatide

THERAPEUTIC USES

- A parathyroid hormone that stimulates osteoblasts to increase new bone formation to increase bone mass
- Stimulates calcium absorption
- Indicated for clients who are at high risk for fractures and those who have prolonged corticosteroid use

NURSING ACTIONS

- Administered only subcutaneously
- Contraindicated for a client who has hypercalcemia, history of bone cancer, radiation, or Paget's disease
- Report leg cramps or bone pain to the provider.
- Orthostatic hypotension can occur up to 4 hr after receiving the medication.

Estrogen hormone supplements

Estrogen, medroxyprogesterone

THERAPEUTIC USES: Replaces estrogen lost due to menopause or surgical removal of ovaries

NURSING ACTIONS
- Reinforce with the client about potential complications (breast and endometrial cancers, deep-vein thrombosis [DVT]).
- Reinforce monthly breast self-examinations. Estrogen should be given along with progesterone in clients who still have their uterus.

Selective estrogen receptor modulators

Raloxifene

THERAPEUTIC USES
- Decreases osteoclast activity, subsequently decreasing bone resorption and increasing bone mineral density
- Prevents and treats postmenopausal osteoporosis and breast cancer

NURSING ACTIONS
- Avoid the medication for a client who has a history of DVT.
- Reinforce with the client to increase calcium and vitamin D supplements.
- Monitor and reinforce with the client to report to the provider unusual calf pain or tenderness, acute migraine.
- Discontinue use 72 hr before prolonged bed rest.

Calcium supplement

Calcium carbonate, calcium citrate

THERAPEUTIC USES: Supplements calcium consumed in food products to promote healthy bones (not to slow osteoporosis)

NURSING ACTIONS
- Give with food in divided doses with 6 to 8 oz of water.
- Calcium supplements can cause GI upset.
- Monitor for constipation and development of hypercalcemia.

Vitamin D

THERAPEUTIC USES
- Increases absorption of calcium from the intestinal tract and availability of calcium in the serum needed for remineralization of bone
- Needed by individuals who are not exposed to adequate amounts of sunlight or who do not meet its daily requirements
- Vitamin D is a fat-soluble vitamin, so toxicity can occur. Indications of toxicity include weakness, fatigue, nausea, constipation, and kidney stones.

62.1 Kyphosis

normal spine   kyphosis spine

Bisphosphonates

Alendronate, ibandronate, risedronate, etidronate, zoledronic acid, zoledronate, pamidronate

THERAPEUTIC USES
- Decreases number and actions of osteoclasts, subsequently inhibiting bone resorption for prevention and treatment of osteoporosis, hypercalcemia, and Paget's disease of the bone.
- Ibandronate, zoledronic acid, and pamidronate are available as IV preparations.
- Alendronate, ibandronate, and risedronate are available as oral medications.

NURSING ACTIONS
- Monitor calcium levels in clients receiving IV preparations (hypercalcemia; paresthesias, twitching, colic or laryngospasm).
- The client who is receiving IV preparations should have dental examinations and preventative treatment prior to starting therapy to minimize the risk of osteonecrosis of the jaw.
- Check bone density routinely.

CLIENT EDUCATION

- There is risk for esophagitis and esophageal ulcers with oral preparations. Report early manifestations of indigestion, chest pain, difficulty swallowing, or bloody emesis to the provider immediately.
- Take with 8 oz water upon waking, 30 to 60 min before eating.
- Remain upright for 30 min after taking oral medication.
- Take once per week or once per month as a scheduled medication.
- Do not take a missed daily dose later in the day.
- Take a missed weekly dose the next morning.
- Do not to take more than one dose per week.
- Inform the provider if pregnant or planning to become pregnant.

Denosumab

THERAPEUTIC USES

- Decreases formation and function of osteoclasts, reducing bone resorption and increases bone density
- Indicated for clients who are at a high risk for fractures

NURSING ACTIONS

- Contraindicated with hypocalcemia.
- Monitor calcium levels.
- The client should have dental examinations and preventative treatment prior to starting therapy to minimize the risk of osteonecrosis of the jaw.
- Administer subcutaneously into the upper arm, upper thigh, or abdomen.

CLIENT EDUCATION

- Take at least 1,000 mg calcium and 400 IU vitamin D daily to prevent hypocalcemia.
- Notify the provider if manifestations of infection develop.

THERAPEUTIC PROCEDURES

Orthotic devices

Orthotic devices are available for immobilization of the spine immediately after a compression fracture of the spine.
- The device provides support and decreases pain.
- A physical therapist fits and teaches how to apply the device with the client. Qтc

CLIENT EDUCATION

- How to check for skin breakdown under the orthotic device
- The importance of good posture and body mechanics
- How to log roll when getting out of bed
- Use heat and back rubs to promote muscle relaxation.

Joint repair or joint arthroplasty

Total hip arthroplasty is often necessary to repair or replace a joint weakened by osteoporosis.

NURSING ACTIONS (HIP REPAIR)

- Monitor operative site for bleeding.
- Do not cross midline with operative hip.
- Do not flex hip greater than 90%.
- Obtain a toilet riser if needed to prevent hip flexion greater than 90%.

Vertebroplasty or kyphoplasty

Minimally invasive procedures performed by a surgeon or radiologist
- Bone cement is injected into the fractured space of the vertebral column with or without balloon inflation.
- Balloon inflation of the fracture is to contain the cement and add height to the fractured vertebra.
- Mild sedation is used.
- Client lies in a supine position for 1 to 2 hr following procedure.

NURSING ACTIONS

- Monitor vital signs for shortness of breath and the puncture site for bleeding.
- Monitor the client's neurological status.
- Apply cold therapy to the injection site.

CLIENT EDUCATION

- Remain supine for 1 to 2 hr postprocedure.
- Avoid driving for 24 hr following the procedure.
- Keep the dressing dry. Remove it the day following the procedure.
- Monitor the site for manifestations of infection.
- Resume activities such as walking the day following the procedure and gradually increase activity level as tolerated.

INTERPROFESSIONAL CARE

- Physical therapy can establish an exercise regimen: 20 to 30 min of aerobic exercise (walking) three to four times per week in addition to weightlifting.
- The client can need rehabilitation if fractures cause immobilization or disability.
- Most hip fractures are due to osteoporosis. Joint repair or joint arthroplasty requires physical therapy for a full recovery.

COMPLICATIONS

Fractures

- Fractures are the leading complication of osteoporosis and are often atraumatic (occur without trauma). Early recognition and treatment is essential.
- Older adult clients (60 years and older) who have nontraumatic osteoporotic fractures can have an increase in the risk of death 5 to 10 years after the hip fracture. Additional research of the risks is needed.

NURSING ACTIONS

- Review risk factors for osteoporosis and falls.
- Check dietary intake of calcium and vitamin D.
- Reinforce daily exercise including weight-bearing activities.
- Ensure proper screening with a DXA.

Application Exercises

1. A nurse is assisting in the admission of an older adult client who has suspected osteoporosis. Which of following findings should the nurse expect? (Select all that apply.)

   A. History of consuming one glass of wine daily

   B. Loss in height of 5.1 cm (2 in)

   C. Body mass index (BMI) 21

   D. Kyphotic curve at upper thoracic spine

   E. History of lactose intolerance

2. A nurse is assisting in the care of a client immediately following vertebroplasty of the thoracic spine. Which of the following actions should the nurse take?

   A. Apply heat to the puncture site.

   B. Place the client in a supine position.

   C. Turn the client every 1 hr.

   D. Ambulate the client within the first hour postprocedure.

3. A nurse is reinforcing dietary teaching about calcium-rich foods to a client who has osteoporosis. Which of the following foods should the nurse include in the instructions?

   A. White bread

   B. White beans

   C. White meat of chicken

   D. White rice

4. A nurse is assisting with health screenings at a health fair. The nurse should identify that which of the following clients are at risk for osteoporosis? (Select all that apply.)

   A. 40-year-old client who takes prednisone for asthma

   B. 30-year-old client who jogs 3 miles daily

   C. 45-year-old client who takes phenytoin for seizures

   D. 65-year-old client who has a sedentary lifestyle

   E. 70-year-old client who has smoked for 50 years

5. A nurse is reinforcing discharge teaching on home safety for an older adult client who has osteoporosis. Which of the following information should the nurse include? (Select all that apply.)

   A. Remove throw rugs in walkways.

   B. Use prescribed assistive devices.

   C. Remove clutter from the environment.

   D. Walk with caution on icy surfaces.

   E. Maintain lighting of doorway areas.

PRACTICE Active Learning Scenario

A nurse is administering raloxifene to a client who has osteoporosis. What should the nurse consider before administering the medication? Use the ATI Active Learning Template: Medication to complete this item.

THERAPEUTIC USES: List two.

NURSING INTERVENTIONS: Describe two.

EVALUATION OF MEDICATION EFFECTIVENESS: Describe one.

Application Exercises Key

1. A. A client who consumes more than three glasses of alcohol each day is at risk for developing osteoporosis because alcohol can increase bone loss.

   B. **CORRECT:** The loss of 2 inches of height is suggestive of osteoporosis due to fractures of the vertebral column.

   C. **CORRECT:** The client who has a BMI of 21 is at risk of developing osteoporosis due to low body weight and thin body build, suggesting decreased bone mass.

   D. **CORRECT:** Kyphosis curve is highly suggestive of osteoporosis due to fractures of the vertebrae causing the curve.

   E. **CORRECT:** Lactose intolerance is highly suggestive of osteoporosis due to possible lack of calcium intake.

   Ⓝ *NCLEX® Connection: Health Promotion and Maintenance, Health Promotion/Disease Prevention*

2. A. The client should have cold therapy applied to the puncture site to decrease bleeding and swelling following the procedure.

   B. **CORRECT:** The client should remain in a supine position with bed flat for the first 1 to 2 hr following the procedure to allow for hardening of the cement.

   C. The client should remain in a supine position with bed flat for 1 to 2 hr following the procedure.

   D. The client should remain in a supine position with bed flat for 1 to 2 hr following the procedure.

   Ⓝ *NCLEX® Connection: Reduction of Risk Potential, Potential for Complications from Surgical Procedures and Health Alterations*

3. A. White bread is not a calcium-rich food, but it is a good source of carbohydrates.

   B. **CORRECT:** White beans are a good source of calcium.

   C. White meat of chicken is not a calcium-rich food, but it is a good source of protein.

   D. White rice is not a calcium-rich food, but it is a good source of carbohydrates.

   Ⓝ *NCLEX® Connection: Basic Care and Comfort, Nutrition and Oral Hydration*

4. A. **CORRECT:** Prednisone affects the absorption and metabolism of calcium and places the client at risk for osteoporosis.

   B. Weight-bearing activities decrease the risk for osteoporosis due to placing stress on bones, which promotes bone rebuilding and maintenance.

   C. **CORRECT:** Phenytoin affects the absorption and metabolism of calcium and places the client at risk for osteoporosis.

   D. **CORRECT:** A sedentary lifestyle places the client at risk for osteoporosis because bones need the stress of weight bearing activity for bone rebuilding and maintenance.

   E. **CORRECT:** Smoking increases the risk for osteoporosis because it decreases osteogenesis.

   Ⓝ *NCLEX® Connection: Health Promotion and Maintenance, Health Promotion/Disease Prevention*

5. A. **CORRECT:** Removing throw rugs in walkways can help to prevent a fall and bone fracture.

   B. **CORRECT:** Assistive devices can help to prevent a fall and bone fracture.

   C. **CORRECT:** Removing clutter from the environment can help prevent tripping, falling, and a bone fracture.

   D. The client should avoid walking on icy surfaces during inclement weather to help prevent a fall and bone fracture.

   E. **CORRECT:** Good lighting in doorway areas can prevent a fall and bone fracture.

   Ⓝ *NCLEX® Connection: Safety and Infection Control, Home Safety*

PRACTICE Answer

Using the ATI Active Learning Template: Medication

THERAPEUTIC USES
Selective estrogen receptor modulator
- Decreases bone resorption and increases bone density
- Treatment of postmenopausal osteoporosis
- Treatment of breast cancer by reducing the risk of cancer metastasis

NURSING INTERVENTIONS
- Avoid administering the medication for a client who has a history of deep vein thrombosis (DVT).
- Reinforce with the client to report unusual calf pain or tenderness, an indication of DVT.
- Review need for calcium and vitamin D supplements when taking the medication.

EVALUATION OF MEDICATION EFFECTIVENESS
- Improved bone mineral density
- No further loss in height
- No metastasis of the cancer

Ⓝ *NCLEX® Connection: Pharmacological Therapies, Medication Administration*

CHAPTER 63 *Musculoskeletal Trauma*

A fracture is a break in a bone secondary to trauma or a pathological condition. Fractures caused by trauma are the most common type of bone fracture. Pathological fractures are often caused by metastatic cancer, osteoporosis, or Paget's disease. How the injury occurred can help determine the type of fracture.

Bone is continually going through a process of remodeling as osteoclasts release calcium from the bone and osteoblasts build up the bone. Remodeling of bone occurs at equal rates until an individual reaches age 30. From this age on, the activity of the osteoclasts outpace the osteoblasts, increasing an individual's risk of osteoporosis. This process significantly increases following menopause. Subsequently, females experience fractures secondary to osteoporosis about a decade earlier than males.

FIVE STAGES OF BONE HEALING

- Hematoma forms between the two ends of broken bone (1 to 3 days).
- Granulation tissue forms a bridge between the two ends of broken bone (3 days to 2 weeks).
- New bone is formed (2 to 6 weeks).
- Mature bone cells replace immature bone cells (3 weeks to 6 months).
- Reconstruction of the medullary canal (6 weeks to 1 year).

Fractures

Closed (simple) fractures do not break through the skin surface. **Open (compound) fractures** occur when broken bone disrupts the skin integrity, causing an open wound and tissue injury and an increased risk of infection.

Complete fractures go through the entire bone, dividing it into two distinct parts. **Incomplete fractures** go through part of the bone.

Simple fractures have one fracture line. **Comminuted fractures** have multiple fracture lines splitting the bone into multiple pieces.

63.1 X-ray of leg fracture

Displaced fractures have bone fragments that are not in alignment. **Nondisplaced fractures** have bone fragments that remain in alignment.

Fatigue (stress) fractures result when excess strain occurs from recreational and athletic activities.

Pathological (spontaneous) fractures occur to bone that is weak from a disease process (bone cancer, osteoporosis).

Compression fractures occur from a loading force pressing on callus bone. This condition is common in older adult clients who have osteoporosis.

COMMON TYPES OF FRACTURES

Comminuted: Bone is fragmented.

Oblique: Fracture occurs at oblique angle and across bone.

Spiral: Fracture occurs from twisting motion (common with physical abuse).

Impacted: Fractured bone is wedged inside opposite fractured fragment.

Greenstick: Fracture occurs on one side (cortex) but does not extend completely through the bone (most often in children).

Longitudinal fracture: Linear fracture parallel to the long axis of the bone

Hip fractures are a common injury in older adults and are usually associated with falls. Ⓖ

HEALTH PROMOTION AND DISEASE PREVENTION

- Ensure recommended intake of calcium for developmental stage in life.
- Ensure adequate intake of vitamin D and exposure to sunlight.
- Monitor for development of osteoporosis, especially in clients who are postmenopausal or have a thyroid disorder.
- Engage in weight-bearing exercise on a regular basis.
- Take a bisphosphonate if prescribed to slow bone resorption and treat osteoporosis.
- Use caution to prevent falls or accidents.
- Prevent injury with the use of seat belts and helmets.

DATA COLLECTION

RISK FACTORS

- Osteoporosis
  - Excessive weight loss from dieting and malnutrition can lead to osteoporosis.
  - Clients who do not use estrogen replacement therapy after menopause lose estrogen and are unable to form strong new bone.
  - Clients on long-term corticosteroid therapy lose calcium from their bones due to direct inhibition of osteoblast function, inhibition of gastrointestinal calcium absorption, and enhancement of bone resorption.
- Falls (older adults are at increased risk due to failing vision, decreased agility, changes in balance, and decrease muscle tone) ⓒ
- Motor vehicle crashes
- Substance use disorder
- Diseases (bone cancer, Paget's disease)
- Contact sports and hazardous recreational activities (football, skiing)
- Physical abuse
- Lactose intolerance
- Age (bone becomes less dense with advancing age)
- Proton pump inhibitor use for more than 1 year

EXPECTED FINDINGS

- History of trauma, metabolic bone disorders, chronic conditions, and possible use of corticosteroid therapy
- Pain, tenderness, and reduced movement manifest at the area of fracture or the area distal to the fracture

PHYSICAL FINDINGS

- Crepitus (a grating sound created by the rubbing of bone fragments)
- Deformity (internal rotation of extremity, shortened extremity, visible bone with open fracture)
- Muscle spasms due to the pulling forces of the bone when not aligned
- Edema (swelling from trauma)
- Ecchymosis (bleeding into underlying soft tissues from trauma)

DIAGNOSTIC PROCEDURES

- Standard radiographs, computed tomography (CT) imaging scan used to detect fractures of the hip and pelvis, and magnetic resonance imagery (MRI) (63.1)
  - Identify the type of fracture and location.
  - Indicate pathological fracture resulting from tumor or mass.
  - Determine soft tissue damage around fracture (MRI).
- Bone scan using radioactive material determines hairline fractures and complications/delayed healing.

PATIENT-CENTERED CARE

NURSING CARE

- Provide emergency care at time of injury. Prevent shock or hemorrhage.
- Maintain ABCs.
- Monitor vital signs and neurological status because injury to vital organs can occur due to bone fragments (fractures of pelvis, ribs).
- Stabilize the injured area, including the joints above and below the fracture, by using a splint and avoiding unnecessary movement. Do not try to straighten or set the broken bone.
- Maintain alignment of the affected extremity.
- Elevate the limb above the heart, and apply ice.
- Check for bleeding and apply pressure, if needed.
- Cover open wounds with a sterile dressing.
- Remove clothing and jewelry near the injury or on the affected extremity.
- Keep the client warm.
- Monitor for pain frequently and follow pain management protocols, both pharmacological and nonpharmacological.
- Initiate and continue neurovascular checks at least every hour. Immediately report any change in status to the provider.
- Prepare the client for any immobilization procedure indicated for the fracture.
- If open fracture, provide tetanus immunization if indicated.

Immobilizing interventions (casts, splints, traction)

Immobilization secures the injured extremity in order to
- Prevent further injury.
- Promote healing/circulation.
- Reduce pain.
- Correct a deformity.

TYPES OF IMMOBILIZATION DEVICES

- Casts
- Splints/immobilizers
- Traction
- External fixation
- Internal fixation

Closed reduction: A pulling force (traction) is applied manually to realign the displaced fractured bone fragments. Once the fracture is reduced, immobilization is used to allow the bone to heal.

Open reduction internal fixation: A surgical incision is made, and the bone is manually aligned and kept in place with pins, nails, rods, plates, and screws. Older adults who have brittle bones benefit from internal fixation. ©

Open reduction external fixation: An external frame is attached with pins into bone fragments. This is indicated for fractures of an extremity or of the pelvis, massive open fractures, infected fractures, and multiple trauma injuries. External fixation allows the client freedom of movement and good stability.

PATIENT-CENTERED CARE

NURSING CARE

Neurovascular status

Neurovascular checks are essential throughout immobilization. Following initial trauma, neurovascular checks are performed every hour for the first 24 hr and every 1 to 4 hr thereafter to monitor neurovascular compromise related to edema or the immobilization device. Neurovascular checks include the following.

Pain: Monitor pain level, location, and frequency. Assess pain using a 0 to 10 pain rating scale, and have the client describe the pain. Immobilization, ice, and elevation of the extremity with the use of analgesics should relieve most of the pain.

Sensation: Monitor for numbness or tingling of the extremity. Loss of sensation can indicate nerve damage.

Skin temperature: Check the temperature of the affected extremity. The extremity should be warm (not cool) to touch. Cool skin can indicate decreased arterial perfusion.

Skin color: Pale (restricted blood), blue (impaired oxygenation), bruised (bleeding into tissues) or red (infection)

Capillary refill: Press nail beds of affected extremity until blanching occurs. Blood return should be within 3 seconds. Prolonged refill indicates decreased arterial perfusion. Nail beds that are cyanotic can indicate venous congestion.

Pulses: Should be palpable and strong. Pulses should be equal to the unaffected extremity. Edema can make it difficult to palpate pulses, use Doppler ultrasonography if needed.

Movement: Client should have movement of affected extremity and the area distal to the injury in active motion.

Casts

Casts are more effective than splints or immobilizers because the client is unable to remove them.

- Casts, as circumferential immobilizers, are applied once the swelling has subsided (to avoid compartment syndrome). If the swelling continues after cast application and causes unrelieved pain, the cast can be split on one side (univalve) or on both sides (bivalve).
- A window can be placed in an area of the cast to allow for skin inspection and monitoring of pulses (example: if the client has a wound under the area of the cast).
- Moleskin is used over any rough area of the cast that can rub against the skin.
- A fitted stockinette is placed under the plaster cast.

TYPES OF CASTS
- Short and long arm and leg casts
- Walking cast (a rubber walking pad on the sole of the cast assists the client in ambulating when weight-bearing is allowed)
- Spica casts (a portion of the trunk and one or two extremities; typically used on children who have congenital hip dysplasia)
- Body casts (encircle the trunk of the body)

CASTING MATERIALS
- Plaster of Paris casts are heavy, not water-resistant, and can take 24 to 72 hr to dry.
- Synthetic fiberglass casts are light, stronger, water-resistant, and dry very quickly (in 30 min).

NURSING ACTIONS
- Monitor neurovascular status every hour for first 24 hr and monitor pain. Qs
- Apply ice for 24 to 48 hr.
- Handle a plaster cast with the palms, not fingertips, until the cast is dry to prevent denting the cast.
- Avoid placing the cast on hard surfaces or sharp edges.
- Prior to casting, clean and dry the area. Place tubular cotton web roll over the affected area to maintain skin integrity. The casting material is then applied.
- After cast application, position the client so that warm, dry air circulates around and under the cast (support the casted area without pressure under or directly on the cast) for faster drying and to prevent pressure from changing the shape of the cast. Use gloves to touch the cast until it is completely dry.
- Elevate the cast above the level of the heart during the first 24 to 48 hr to prevent edema of the affected extremity. Use a cloth-covered pillow instead of plastic while cast is drying.
- Ensure that cast is not too tight; there should be room for one finger between the skin and cast. A tight cast can cause numbness, tingling, increased pain with movement of distal digits, and sharp localized pain.
- Document presence of drainage and report sudden increase in drainage. Circling drainage on cast is an unreliable indicator of drainage amount and can increase client anxiety.
- Older adult clients have an increased risk for impaired skin integrity due to the loss of elasticity of the skin and decreased sensation (comorbidities). ©
- Monitor for skin breakdown, urinary tract infections, constipation, atelectasis, and deep vein thrombosis.

CLIENT EDUCATION

- To avoid trauma to the skin, do not to place any foreign objects inside the cast. Relieve itching under the cast by blowing cool air from a hair dryer into the cast.
- Cover the cast with plastic if needed to avoid soiling from urine or feces.
- Use plastic bags to cover the cast during baths and showers to keep the cast dry.
- Report any areas under the cast that are painful, have a "hot spot," have increased drainage, are warm to the touch, or have an odor, which can indicate infection.
- Report change in mobility and complications (shortness of breath, skin breakdown, constipation).
- Increase protein intake to promote healing. Include vitamins D, B and C, and calcium in meals. Increase fiber intake and fluid intake to 2,000 to 3,000 mL/day to reduce the risk for bladder infections and constipation.
- Clients who have a spica cast should consume small, frequent meals to prevent abdominal distension.

Traction

- Traction uses a pulling force to promote and maintain alignment of the injured area.
- Traction prescriptions should include the type of traction, amount of weight, and whether the nurse can remove traction for nursing care.

GOALS OF TRACTION

- Prevent soft tissue injury.
- Realign bone fragments.
- Decrease muscle spasms and pain.
- Correct or prevent further deformities.

TYPES OF TRACTION

Manual: A pulling force is applied by the hands of the provider for temporary immobilization, usually with sedation or anesthesia, in conjunction with the application of an immobilizing device.

Straight or running: The counter traction is provided by the client's body by applying a pulling force in a straight line. Movement of the client's body can alter the traction provided.

- **Skin:** Primary purpose is to decrease muscle spasms and immobilize the extremity prior to surgery. The pulling force is applied by weights that are attached by rope to the client's skin with tape, straps, boots, or cuffs. Examples include Bryant's traction (used for congenital hip dislocation in children) and Buck's traction (used preoperatively for hip fractures for immobilization in adult clients). **(63.2)**

Balanced suspension: The counter traction is produced by devices such as slings or splints to support the fractured extremity off the bed while pulling with ropes and weights. The client's body can move without altering the traction. **(63.3)**

- **Skeletal:** Screws are inserted into the bone (Halo traction). Can use heavier weights (15 to 30 lb) and longer traction time to realign the bone. Provide frequent pin site care to prevent infection. **(63.4)** Qs

NURSING ACTIONS

- Check neurovascular status of the affected body part every hour for 24 hr and every 4 hr after that.
- Maintain body alignment and realign if the client seems uncomfortable or reports pain.
- Avoid lifting or removing weights.
- Ensure that weights hang freely and are not resting on the floor.
- If the weights are accidentally displaced, replace them. If the problem is not corrected, notify the provider.
- Ensure that pulley ropes are free of knots, fraying, loosening, and improper positioning at least every 8 to 12 hr.
- Notify the provider if the client experiences severe pain from muscle spasms unrelieved with medications or repositioning. Move the client in halo traction as a unit, without applying pressure to the rods. This will prevent loosening of the pins and pain.
- Routinely monitor skin integrity and document.
- Use heat/massage as prescribed to treat muscle spasms.
- Use therapeutic touch and relaxation techniques.
- Do not use the bars of the external fixation device to turn the client or lift the extremity.

PIN SITE CARE

- Pin care is done frequently throughout immobilization (skeletal traction and external fixation methods) to prevent and to monitor for manifestations of infection.
  - Drainage and redness (color, amount, odor)
  - Loosening of pins
  - Tenting of skin at pin site (skin rising up pin)
- Pin care protocols are based on provider preference and facility policy. A primary concept of pin care is that one cotton swab is designated for each pin to avoid cross-contamination.
- Chlorhexidine is recommended for routine cleaning of pin sites. If the client has an allergy to chlorhexidine then sterile saline is advised.
- Pin care is provided usually once a shift, one to two times per day, or per facility protocol.

MEDICATIONS

Analgesics
- Administer opioid and nonopioid analgesics as needed to control pain.
- Nonsteroidal anti-inflammatory drugs (NSAIDs) decrease associated tissue inflammation.

Muscle relaxants: To relieve muscle spasms

Stool softener: To prevent constipation

Antibiotic: Prophylactic antibiotics decrease the risk of infection for open fractures.

THERAPEUTIC PROCEDURES

Splints and mobilizers

Splints and immobilizers provide support, control movement, and prevent additional injury.

- Splints are removable and allow for monitoring of skin swelling or integrity.
- Splints can support fractured/injured areas until casting occurs and swelling is decreased. Casting is then used for post-paralysis injuries to avoid joint contracture.
- Immobilizers are prefabricated and typically fasten with hook-and-loop fastener straps.

NURSING ACTIONS: Ensure the client is aware of application protocol regarding full-time or part-time use.

CLIENT EDUCATION: Observe for skin breakdown at pressure points.

External fixation

Involves fracture immobilization using percutaneous pins and wires that are attached to a rigid external frame

USED TO TREAT

- Comminuted fracture or nonunion fractures with extensive soft tissue damage
- Leg length discrepancies from congenital defects
- Bone loss related to tumors or osteomyelitis

ADVANTAGES

- Immediate fracture stabilization
- Minimal blood loss compared to internal fixation
- Allows for early mobilization and ambulation
- Maintains alignment of closed fractures that could not be maintained in cast or splint
- Permits wound care with open fractures

DISADVANTAGES

- Risk of pin site infection leading to osteomyelitis
- Potential overwhelming appearance to client
- Noncompliance issues

NURSING ACTIONS

- Elevate extremity.
- Monitor neurovascular status and skin integrity.
- Perform pin care every 8 to 12 hr. Monitor site for drainage, color, odor, and redness.
- Observe for manifestations of fat and pulmonary embolism.
- Provide antiembolism stockings and sequential compression device to prevent deep vein thrombosis (DVT).
- Monitor for indications of body image disturbance.
- Discuss clothing and other materials that can be used to cover the device.

CLIENT EDUCATION

- Maintain proper pin care.
- If activity is restricted, perform deep breathing, leg exercises, and other techniques to prevent complications to immobilization (pneumonia, thrombus formation).

63.2 Buck's traction

63.3 Balanced suspension skeletal traction

63.4 Halo fixation device

Open reduction and internal fixation

- Open reduction is visualization of a fracture through an incision in the skin; internal fixation with plates, screws, pins, and rods; and prosthetics as needed.
- After the bone heals, the hardware is removed, depending on the location and type of hardware.
- Circular external fixation is a technique to promote new bone growth for malunion and nonunion fracture. The device is turned four times per day to pull apart the cortex of the bone and stimulate growth.

NURSING ACTIONS
- Prevent dislocation, especially of hip.
- Monitor skin integrity.
- Ensure heels are off bed at all times and inspect bony prominence every shift.
- Perform neurovascular checks.
- Observe the cast or dressing for postoperative drainage. The cast can have a window cut in it through which the incision can be viewed. An elastic wrap is used to keep the window block cover in place to decrease localized edema.
- Monitor for manifestations of fat and pulmonary embolism.
- Provide antiembolism stockings and a sequential compression device to prevent DVT and administer anticoagulants.
- Monitor the client's pain level.
  - Administer analgesics, antispasmodics, or NSAIDs, and monitor for relief.
  - Position for comfort and with ice on the surgical site.
- Monitor for manifestations of infection.
  - Monitor vital signs, observing for fever, tachycardia, incisional drainage, redness, and odor.
  - Monitor laboratory values (WBC, ESR).
  - Provide surgical aseptic wound care.
- Increase physical mobility as indicated.
  - Consult physical and occupational therapy for ambulation and activities of daily living.
  - Monitor orthostatic blood pressure when the client gets out of bed for the first time.
  - Turn and reposition the client every 2 hr.
  - Have the client get out of bed from the unaffected side.
  - Position the client for comfort (within restrictions).
- Support nutrition.
  - Encourage increased calorie intake.
  - Ensure use of calcium supplements.
  - Encourage small, frequent meals with snacks.
  - Monitor for constipation.

COMPLICATIONS

Compartment syndrome

- Compartment syndrome usually affects extremities and occurs when pressure within one or more of the muscle compartments (an area covered with an elastic tissue called fascia) of the extremity compromises circulation, resulting in an ischemia–edema cycle.
- Capillaries dilate in an attempt to pull oxygen into the tissue. Increased capillary permeability from the release of histamine leads to edema from plasma proteins leaking into the interstitial fluid space.
- Increased edema causes pressure on the nerve endings, resulting in pain. Blood flow is further reduced and ischemia persists, resulting in compromised neurovascular status.
- Pressure can result from external sources (tight cast, constrictive bulky dressing).
- Internal sources, such as accumulation of blood or fluid within the muscle compartment, can cause pressure.

MANIFESTATIONS
- Compartment syndrome is identified by using the five P's (pain, paralysis, paresthesia, pallor, and pulselessness).
  - Increased **pain** unrelieved with elevation or by pain medication. Intense pain when passively moved.
  - **Paresthesia** or numbness, burning, and tingling are early manifestations.
  - **Paralysis**, motor weakness, or inability to move the extremity indicate major nerve damage and are late manifestations.
  - Color of tissue is pale (**pallor**), and nail beds are cyanotic.
  - **Pulselessness** is a late manifestation of compartment syndrome.
  - Palpated muscles are hard and swollen from edema.
- If untreated, tissue necrosis can result. Neuromuscular damage occurs within 4 to 6 hr.
- Surgical treatment is a fasciotomy.
  - A surgical incision is made through the subcutaneous tissue and fascia of the affected compartment to relieve the pressure and restore circulation.
- After fasciotomy, open wounds require sterile packings and dressings until secondary closure occurs. Skin grafts are performed if needed. Negative-pressure wound therapy can be used to reduce edema.

NURSING ACTIONS: Prevention includes the following.
- Check neurovascular status frequently.
- Notify the provider when compartment syndrome is suspected.
- The provider will cut the cast on one side (univalve) or both sides (bivalve).
- Loosen the constrictive dressing or cut the bandage or tape.

CLIENT EDUCATION
- Report pain not relieved by analgesics or pain that continues to increase in intensity.
- Report numbness, tingling, or a change in color of the extremity.

Fat embolism

- Adults older than 70 are at a high risk of developing a fat embolism. Hip and pelvis fractures are common causes. Ⓖ
- Fat embolism can occur after the injury, usually within 12 to 48 hr following long bone fractures or with total joint arthroplasty.
- Fat globules from the bone marrow are released into the vasculature and travel to the small blood vessels (including those in the lungs), resulting in acute respiratory insufficiency and impaired organ perfusion. Careful diagnosis should differentiate between fat embolism and pulmonary embolism.

MANIFESTATIONS

Early manifestations

- Dyspnea, increased respiratory rate, decreased oxygen saturation
- Headache
- Decreased mental acuity related to low arterial oxygen level
- Respiratory distress, crackles, and wheezes on auscultation
- Tachycardia
- Confusion
- Chest pain

Late manifestation: Cutaneous petechiae are pinpoint-sized subdermal hemorrhages that occur on the neck, chest, upper arms, and abdomen (from the blockage of the capillaries by the fat globules). This is a discriminating finding from pulmonary embolism.

NURSING ACTIONS

- Remain with the client and notify the provider.
- Maintain the client on bed rest in high-Fowler's position.
- Administer high-flow oxygen.
- Prevention includes immobilization of fractures of the long bones and minimal manipulation during turning if immobilization procedure has not yet been performed.
- Treatment includes oxygen for respiratory compromise, corticosteroids for cerebral edema, vasopressors, fluid replacement for shock, and pain and antianxiety medications as needed.

Venous thromboembolism

Deep-vein thrombosis and pulmonary embolism:
Deep-vein thrombosis is a common complication following trauma, surgery, or disability related to immobility (especially hip fracture)

NURSING ACTIONS

- Encourage early ambulation.
- Apply antiembolism stockings and sequential compression device.
- Administer anticoagulants.
- Encourage intake of fluids to prevent hemoconcentration.
- Monitor for manifestations (swollen, reddened calf).

CLIENT EDUCATION: Rotate feet at the ankles and perform other lower extremity exercises as permitted by the immobilization device.

Osteomyelitis

An infection of the bone that begins as an inflammation within the bone secondary to penetration by infectious organisms (virus, bacteria, or fungi) following trauma or surgical repair of a fracture

MANIFESTATIONS

- Bone pain that is constant, pulsating, localized, and worse with movement
- Sudden onset
- Erythema and edema at the site of the infection
- Fever (older adults might not have an elevated temperature) Ⓖ
- Leukocytosis and possible elevated sedimentation rate
- Headache
- Malaise

DIAGNOSTIC PROCEDURES

- Bone scan using radioactive material to diagnose osteomyelitis and MRI can facilitate a diagnosis.
- Cultures are performed for detection of possible aerobic and anaerobic organisms.
- If septicemia develops, blood cultures will be positive for offending microbes.
- Necrosis is identified in a bone biopsy.

TREATMENT

- Long course (3 months) of IV and oral antibiotic therapy.
- Surgical debridement can be indicated. If a significant amount of the bone requires removal, the client might need a bone graft
- Hyperbaric oxygen treatments can promote healing in chronic cases of osteomyelitis.
- Surgically implanted antibiotic beads in bone cement are packed into the wound as a form of antibiotic therapy.
- Unsuccessful treatment can result in amputation.

NURSING ACTIONS

- Administer antibiotics to maintain a constant blood level.
- Administer analgesics.
- Conduct neurovascular checks if debridement is done.

Avascular necrosis

- Avascular necrosis results from the circulatory compromise that occurs after a fracture. Blood flow is disrupted to the fracture site and the resulting ischemia leads to tissue (bone) necrosis.
- Commonly found in hip fractures or in fractures with displacement of a bone.
- Clients receiving long-term corticosteroid therapy are at greater risk for developing avascular necrosis.
- Replacement of damaged bone with a bone graft or prosthetic replacement is often necessary.

Failure of fracture to heal

A fracture that has not healed within 6 months of injury is considered a delayed union.
- **Malunion:** Fracture heals incorrectly.
- **Nonunion:** Fracture never heals.
  - Electrical bone stimulation and bone grafting can treat nonunion.
  - Low intensity pulse ultrasound can promote healing to treat nonunion.
  - Can occur more frequently in older adult clients due to impaired healing process. ⑥
- Malunion or nonunion can cause immobilizing deformity of the bone involved.

Carpal tunnel syndrome

Compression of the median nerve in the wrist from swollen or thickened synovium, causing pain and numbness in the hands and wrists

DATA COLLECTION

RISK FACTORS

- Some metabolic and connective tissue diseases
  - Rheumatoid arthritis (synovitis)
  - Diabetes mellitus (reduced circulation)
- Occupational injury from repetitive stress of hand activities such as pinching or grasping during wrist flexion (computer users)
- Repetitive sports injury (tennis)
- Children and adolescents due to use of computers and handheld devices
- Growth of a space occupying lesion (ganglia, lipoma)

EXPECTED FINDINGS

- The provider makes a diagnosis based on history and report of pain and numbness in affected hand, compression test, electromyography.
- Pain is often worse at night and can radiate to the arm, shoulder, neck, or chest.
- Paresthesia (painful tingling): Sensory changes occur weeks or months before motor.
- Phalen's maneuver (positive in most clients who have carpal tunnel syndrome): Ask the client to place the back of his hands together and flex both wrists at the same time.
- Tinel's sign: Tap lightly over the median nerve area of the wrist. A positive result is paresthesia in the median nerve distribution (palmar side of thumb, index, middle and half of ring finger).

PATIENT-CENTERED CARE

NURSING CARE

- Medication therapy
  - NSAIDs for relief of pain and inflammation
  - Corticosteroid injections directly into the carpal tunnel
- Splint or hand brace to immobilize the wrist can be used during the day and/or night
- Laser or ultrasound therapy
- Yoga and exercise
- Surgery to relieve pressure by decompressing the pressure on the nerve
  - Endoscopic carpal tunnel release: less invasive but a longer recovery period of postoperative pain and numbness
  - Open carpal tunnel release

POSTOPERATIVE CARE
- Monitor vital signs.
- Check dressing for drainage and tightness.
- Elevate hand above the heart to reduce swelling.
- Check neurovascular status of fingers every hour and encourage the client to move them frequently.
- Offer pain medications.

CLIENT EDUCATION
- Hand movements (gripping, pinching) and heavy lifting are often restricted for 4 to 6 weeks.
- Expect weakness and discomfort for weeks or months.
- Report any changes in neurovascular status, including increase in pain, to surgeon immediately.

Sprains and strains

Strain

- Excessive stretching or pulling of a muscle or tendon that is weak or unstable
- Often occurs in back muscles, hamstrings, quadriceps, and calf muscles
- Often caused by falls, lifting heavy items, and exercise

CLASSIFICATIONS
- **First-degree (mild) strain** causes mild inflammation and little bleeding. There can be swelling, ecchymosis, and tenderness.
- **Second-degree (moderate) strain** involves partial tearing of the muscle or tendon fibers. Involves impaired muscle function.
- **Third-degree (severe) strain** involves a ruptured muscle or tendon with separation of muscle from muscle, tendon from muscle, or tendon from bone. Causes severe pain and immobility.

MANIFESTATIONS
- Soft-tissue swelling and pain
- Report of excessive use of a joint
- Ecchymosis if there is a muscle tear

Sprain

Excessive stretching of a ligament.
- Twisting motions from a fall or sports activity are often the cause of the injury.
- The ankle, knee, and wrist are the most commonly sprained joints.

PATIENT-CENTERED CARE

Management of strain

- Cold and heat application
- Exercise and activity limitations
- Elevation and rest
- Neurovascular checks
- Anti-inflammatory medications to decrease inflammation and pain
- Muscle relaxants
- Surgical repair if needed for third-degree strains to repair ruptured muscle or tendon
- Education of proper body mechanics

Management of sprain

- Treatment involves protecting the ligament until it heals.
- RICE (rest, ice, compression, elevation) for mild sprains.
- Elevate.
- Apply ice for the first 24 to 72 hr after injury.
- Second-degree sprains require immobilization and partial weight-bearing while the tear heals.
- Immobilization for 4 to 6 weeks is necessary for third-degree sprains.
- Administer NSAIDs.

PRACTICE Active Learning Scenario

A nurse is performing a neurovascular check on a client who has a cast applied following a right arm fracture. What interventions should the nurse take? Use the ATI Active Learning Template: Basic Concept to complete this item:

RELATED CONTENT: Identify the purpose of neurovascular check.

UNDERLYING PRINCIPLES: Identify the components of a neurovascular check.

NURSING INTERVENTIONS: Describe a nursing intervention related to each of the components.

Application Exercises

1. A nurse is reinforcing teaching with a client about how to manage an external fixation device upon discharge. Which of the following client statements indicate understanding? (Select all that apply.)
   - A. "I will clean the pins twice a day."
   - B. "I will use a separate cotton swab for each pin."
   - C. "I will report loosening of the pins to my doctor."
   - D. "I will clean the pins with tap water and antibacterial soap."
   - E. "I will report increased redness at the pin sites."

2. A nurse is collecting data from a client who has a casted compound fracture of the femur. The nurse should identify which of the following findings as a manifestation of fat emboli?
   - A. Altered mental status
   - B. Reduced bowel sounds
   - C. Swelling of the toes distal to the injury
   - D. Pain with passive movement of the foot distal to the injury

3. A nurse is collecting data from a client who had an external fixation device applied 2 hr ago for a fracture of the left tibia and fibula. The nurse should identify which of the following findings as manifestations of compartment syndrome? (Select all that apply.)
   - A. Intense pain when the left foot is passively moved
   - B. Capillary refill of 3 sec on the left toes
   - C. Hard, swollen muscle in the left leg
   - D. Burning and tingling of the left foot
   - E. Client report of minimal pain relief following a second dose of opioid medication

4. A nurse is reinforcing discharge teaching with a client who had a wound debridement for osteomyelitis. Which of the following information should the nurse include?
   - A. Antibiotic therapy should continue for 3 months.
   - B. Relief of pain indicates the infection is eradicated.
   - C. Airborne precautions are used during wound care.
   - D. Expect paresthesia distal to the wound.

5. A nurse is caring for a client who has a right hip fracture. Which of the following immobilization devices should the nurse anticipate?
   - A. Skeletal traction
   - B. Buck's traction
   - C. Halo traction
   - D. Bryant's traction

Application Exercises Key

1. A. **CORRECT:** Clean the external fixation pins one or two times each day to remove exudate that can harbor bacteria.

   B. **CORRECT:** Using a separate cotton swab on each pin will decrease the risk of cross-contamination, which could cause pin site infection.

   C. **CORRECT:** Notify the provider if a pin is loose so the provider can tighten the pin to prevent damage to the tissue and bone.

   D. Chlorhexidine or sterile saline is recommended for cleansing pin sites. Tap water is not sterile and increases the risk of infection at pin sites.

   E. **CORRECT:** The client should report redness, heat, and drainage at the pin sites, which can indicate an infection that can lead to osteomyelitis.

   Ⓝ *NCLEX® Connection: Basic Care and Comfort, Mobility/Immobility*

2. A. **CORRECT:** Altered mental status is an early manifestation of fat emboli. Other manifestations include dyspnea, chest pain, and hypoxemia.

   B. **CORRECT:** Reduced bowel sounds is an adverse effect of opioid narcotics and can result in constipation.

   C. Swelling of the toes distal to the injury is a manifestation of reduced circulation and is often the result of a tight cast. The nurse should elevate the extremity and apply ice.

   D. Pain with passive movement of the foot distal to the injury is an expected finding. Severe pain or pain unrelieved by narcotics is a manifestation of compartment syndrome.

   Ⓝ *NCLEX® Connection: Reduction of Risk Potential, Potential for Complications from Surgical Procedures and Health Alterations*

3. A. **CORRECT:** Intense pain of the left foot when passively moved can indicate pressure from edema on nerve endings and is a manifestation of compartment syndrome.

   B. Capillary refill of 3 seconds is within the expected reference range. Prolonged refill greater than 3 seconds is an indication of decreased arterial perfusion.

   C. **CORRECT:** A hard, swollen muscle on the affected extremity indicates edema build-up in the area of injury and is a manifestation of compartment syndrome.

   D. **CORRECT:** Burning and tingling of the left foot indicates pressure from edema on nerve endings and is an early manifestation of compartment syndrome.

   E. **CORRECT:** Minimal pain relief after receiving opioid medication can indicate pressure from edema on nerve endings and is an early manifestation of compartment syndrome.

   Ⓝ *NCLEX® Connection: Physiological Adaptation, Unexpected Response to Therapies*

4. A. **CORRECT:** Treatment of osteomyelitis includes continuing antibiotic therapy for 3 months.

   B. Relief of pain does not indicate that osteomyelitis is resolved. The client should continue antibiotic therapy as prescribed.

   C. When performing wound care, contact precautions are implemented to prevent spread of the organism.

   D. The client should monitor and report manifestations of neurovascular compromise, such as paresthesia.

   Ⓝ *NCLEX® Connection: Physiological Adaptation, Alterations in Body Systems*

5. A. Skeletal traction is an immobilization device applied surgically to a long bone (femur, tibia) and cervical spine. It is not used for a hip fracture.

   B. **CORRECT:** Buck's traction is a temporary immobilization device applied to a client who has a femur or hip fracture to diminish muscle spasms and immobilize the affected extremity until surgery is performed.

   C. Halo traction immobilizes the cervical spine when a cervical fracture occurs.

   D. Bryant's traction is used for congenital hip dislocation in children.

   Ⓝ *NCLEX® Connection: Basic Care and Comfort, Mobility/Immobility*

PRACTICE Answer

Using the ATI Active Learning Template: Basic Concept

RELATED CONTENT: Neurovascular check is performed to monitor for any compromise in the affected extremity caused by edema and or immobilization device.

UNDERLYING PRINCIPLES
- Pain: Monitor pain level, location, and frequency. Monitor pain using a 0 to 10 pain rating scale, and have the client describe the pain. Immobilization, ice, and elevation of the extremity with the use of analgesics should relieve most of the pain.
- Sensation: Monitor for numbness or tingling of the extremity. Loss of sensation can indicate nerve damage.
- Skin temperature: Check the temperature of the affected extremity. The extremity should be warm to the touch. Cool skin can indicate decreased arterial perfusion.
- Skin color: Pale (restricted blood), blue (impaired oxygenation), bruised (bleeding into tissues) or red (infection)
- Capillary refill: Press nail beds of affected extremity until blanching occurs. Blood return should be within 3 seconds. Prolonged refill indicates decreased arterial perfusion. Nail beds that are cyanotic can indicate venous congestion.
- Pulses: Should be palpable and strong. Pulses should be equal to the unaffected extremity. Edema can make it difficult to palpate pulses, use Doppler ultrasonography if needed.
- Movement: Client should have movement of affected extremity and the area distal to the injury in active motion.

NURSING INTERVENTIONS: Immobilize, apply ice, and elevate the extremity to reduce swelling, relieve pain, increase sensation, improve circulation, and increase movement.

Ⓝ *NCLEX® Connection: Reduction of Risk Potential, Potential for Alterations in Body Systems*

CHAPTER 64 *Osteoarthritis and Low-Back Pain*

Osteoarthritis (OA), or degenerative joint disease (DJD), is a disorder characterized by progressive deterioration of the articular cartilage. It is a noninflammatory (unless localized), nonsystemic disease. OA usually affects only one or two joints on one side of the body. OA tends to occur in clients who don't produce sufficient collagen to provide adequate joint protection and strength. Over time, joints thicken and damage occurs as the joints are unable to withstand weight. Changes within the joints can lead to pain, immobility, muscle spasms, and inflammation. Early in the disease process of OA, it can be difficult to distinguish from rheumatoid arthritis (RA). **(64.1)**

Low-back pain (LBP) occurs along the lumbosacral area of the vertebral column. LBP can be acute (self-limiting) or chronic (longer than 3 months or repeated episodes of pain). In addition to back pain, the client can experience foot, ankle, and leg weakness or burning/stabbing pain radiating to the leg or foot. LBP can be related to an injury, fall, or heavy lifting. LBP is the leading cause of work disability. It is most prevalent between ages 30 and 60. Smoking and obesity contribute to LBP.

HEALTH PROMOTION AND DISEASE PREVENTION

Osteoarthritis

- Increase balance exercise and gentle exercises (walking, knitting, swimming), which are important in maintaining joint mobility and decreasing pain.
- Avoid placing stress on affected joints.
- Use joint-saving measures (good body mechanics, labor-saving devices).
- Maintain a healthy weight to decrease joint degeneration of the hips and knees.
- Stop smoking to reduce cartilage loss, especially if there is a family history of OA.
- Avoid or limit repetitive strain on joints (jogging, contact sports, risk-taking activities).
- Wear well-fitted shoes with supports to prevent falls.

Low-back pain

- Exercise to keep back healthy and strong.
- Use body mechanics and proper lifting techniques (ergonomics).
- Maintain correct posture.
- Wear low-heeled shoes.
- Maintain a healthy weight.
- Smoking cessation, as smoking is linked to disk degeneration. Q EBP
- Avoid prolonged sitting/standing.
- Healthy diet including adequate calcium and vitamin D.

64.1 Characteristics of osteoarthritis and rheumatoid arthritis

	Osteoarthritis	Rheumatoid arthritis
DISEASE PROCESS	Cartilage destruction with bone spur growth at joint ends; degenerative	Synovial membrane inflammation resulting in cartilage destruction and bone erosion; inflammatory
FINDINGS	Pain with activity that improves at rest	Swelling, redness, warmth, pain at rest or after immobility (morning stiffness)
EFFUSIONS	Localized inflammatory response	All joints
BODY SIZE	Usually overweight	Usually underweight
NODES	Heberden's and Bouchard's nodes	Swan neck and boutonnière deformities of hands
SYSTEMIC INVOLVEMENT	No: articular	Yes: lungs, heart, skin, and extra-articular
SYMMETRICAL	No	Yes
DIAGNOSTIC TESTS	X-rays	X-rays and positive rheumatoid factor

DATA COLLECTION

RISK FACTORS

Osteoarthritis

- Aging: Majority of adults older than 60 have joint changes on x-ray.
- Genetic factors
- Joint injury due to acute or repetitive stress on joints predisposes to later OA.
- Obesity: OA affects weight-bearing joints (knees, hips) in clients who are overweight.
- Metabolic disorders (such as diabetes) and blood disorders (such as sickle cell disease) predispose clients to joint degeneration.

Low-back pain

- Can occur at any time but most prevalent from ages 30 to 60
- Family history of back pain or history of a back injury
- Being pregnant (changes in posture and weight distribution)
- History of spine problems, back surgery, or compression fracture
- Job or occupation that requires heavy lifting, twisting, or repetitive motion
- Smoking (linked to disk degeneration)
- Overweight
- Having poor posture

CAUSES OF LOW-BACK PAIN
- Muscle strain/spasm
- Ligament sprain
- Osteoarthritis
- Osteoporosis
- Scoliosis
- Compression fracture

64.2 Heberden's and Bouchard's nodes

Bouchard's

Heberden's

- Defect of a vertebrae (spondylolysis)
- A vertebra that slips forward on the one below it (spondylolisthesis)
- Narrowing of the spinal canal (spinal stenosis)
- Herniated disk (herniated nucleus pulposus), which can cause sciatic nerve involvement with burning or stabbing pain into one leg or foot

EXPECTED FINDINGS

Osteoarthritis

- Joint pain and stiffness
- Pain with joint palpation or range of motion (muscle atrophy, loss of function, limp when walking, restricted activity due to pain)
- Crepitus in one or more of the affected joints
- Enlarged joint related to bone hypertrophy
- Heberden's nodes enlarged at the distal interphalangeal joints (64.2)
- Bouchard's nodes located at the proximal interphalangeal joints
  - OA is not a symmetrical disease, but these nodes can occur bilaterally.
  - These nodes can be inflamed and painful.
- Inflammation resulting from secondary synovitis, indicating advanced disease
- Joint effusion (excess joint fluid) that is easily moved from one area of the joint to another area
- Vertebral radiating pain affected by cervical or lumbar compression of nerve roots
- Limping gait due to hip or knee pain
- Back pain due to OA of the spine

Low-back pain

- Dull or sharp low back pain
- Pain aggravated by coughing, sneezing, or straining
- Muscle spasms, cramping, and stiffness
- Pain in the buttock
- Sciatic nerve compression (causes severe pain when leg is straightened and held up)
- Numbness/tingling of the leg (paresthesia); burning or stabbing pain in the leg or foot

NURSING ACTIONS: Report chills/fever, bowel or bladder incontinence, progression of decreased ability to move, and paresthesias to the provider promptly (can indicate a more serious condition). Qs

LABORATORY TESTS

OA: Laboratory test results are usually within expected reference ranges. Erythrocyte sedimentation rate (ESR) and high-sensitivity C-reactive protein can be increased slightly related to secondary synovitis.

LBP: CBC, ESR, and urinalysis may be checked with LBP to rule out cancer or infection. Serum electrophoresis can help to rule out multiple myeloma.

DIAGNOSTIC PROCEDURES

X-rays to rule out fracture, spondylosis (spinal degeneration), or neoplasm

Magnetic resonance imaging with or without contrast shows soft tissue structures of the back (intervertebral disks, spinal cord, spinal nerves)

Computed tomography (CT) scan
- Shows injuries or pathology that involves bone
- Can be done with or without contrast

Nuclear bone scan
- Provides ability to scan entire skeleton
- Detects tumors, arthritis, osteomyelitis, osteoporosis, vertebral compression fractures, and unexplained bone pain

CT myelogram
- Uses x-ray and contrast, which is put into the subarachnoid space with a thin needle (lumbar puncture).
- The contrast moves through the space so the nerve roots and spinal cord can be visualized.

Electromyogram (EMG) and nerve conduction
- Measures electrical impulses produced by nerves and muscle response
- Looks for bone, nerve or muscle problems that might be causing pain

Arthrogram
- X-ray study of a joint after contrast medium has been injected to enhance visualization.
- Bone chips, torn ligaments, or other loose bodies within a joint can be visualized.

PATIENT-CENTERED CARE

NURSING CARE

PAIN ASSESSMENT/MONITORING
- Location, characteristics, quality, severity, precipitating or relieving factors
- Sciatic nerve pain becomes worse when the leg is held straight and lifted upward

MUSCULOSKELETAL DATA COLLECTION
Muscle tone and strength
- Inspect back for vertebral alignment and tenderness
- Degree of functional limitation; ability to perform ADLs
- Gait ability and characteristics
- Proper functional/joint alignment (OA), vertebral alignment (LBP)
- Levels of fatigue and pain after activity
- Range of motion

NEUROLOGICAL DATA COLLECTION
Sensory perception
- Genitourinary: bowel or bladder problems
- Home barriers

PSYCHOSOCIAL DATA COLLECTION Qᴘᴄᴄ
- Pain interference with sexuality
- Depression related to pain
- Anxiety related to pain
- Alteration in self-esteem and body image due to joint deformities and nodules in OA

CLIENT EDUCATION
- Acute LBP often resolves spontaneously.
- Positioning (Williams position: semi-Fowler's with a pillow under flexed knees) can alleviate pain associated with LBP from a herniated disk. Qᴇʙᴘ
- Use analgesics and NSAIDs prior to activity and around the clock as needed.
- Balance rest with activity.
- Use correct body mechanics to decrease stress on back muscles.
- Use thermal applications: heat (dry or moist) to alleviate pain and ice for acute inflammation.
- Consider complementary and alternative therapies (tai chi, acupuncture, hypnosis, magnets, music therapy).
- Use splinting for joint protection, and use larger joints.
- Use assistive devices to promote safety and independence (elevated toilet seat, shower bench, long-handled reacher, shoe horn).
- Use a daily schedule of activities that promote independence (high-energy activities in the morning).
- Maintain a well-balanced diet and ideal body weight. Consult a dietitian to provide meal planning for balanced nutrition.

MEDICATIONS

Analgesic therapy

Acetaminophen does not provide anti-inflammatory benefits, which might not be needed if synovitis is not present

NURSING ACTIONS
- Limit administration of acetaminophen to a maximum of 4,000 mg/24 hr. Some experts recommend a maximum daily dose of 2,500 to 3,000 mg/day when used long-term to prevent liver toxicity. Qꜱ
- Make sure clients are aware of opioids that contain acetaminophen, such as hydrocodone bitartrate 5 mg/acetaminophen 500 mg.
- Monitor liver function tests.

Nonsteroidal anti-inflammatory drugs (NSAIDs)

- Analgesics and anti-inflammatories (celecoxib, naproxen, ibuprofen) are used to relieve pain and synovitis if present.
- Baseline liver and kidney function tests and CBC are needed if NSAIDs are to be given.
- Acetaminophen can be replaced with an NSAID if adequate relief is not obtained.
- Topical NSAID (diclofenac epolamine patch) may be used and is nonsystemic.
- Older adult clients can have increased adverse effects and more medication interactions when taking NSAIDs, especially when taking ACE inhibitors

NURSING ACTIONS: Monitor kidney function (BUN, creatinine).

CLIENT EDUCATION
- NSAIDs are nephrotoxic and should be taken as prescribed. Qs
- Report evidence of black tarry stool, indigestion, and shortness of breath.

Muscle relaxants

- Cyclobenzaprine hydrochloride may be given for muscle spasms due to LBP.
- Can cause acute confusion in older adults. Ⓖ
- Do not drive or operate dangerous equipment.

Opioids

Opioid analgesics (hydrocodone, oxycodone) are indicated for treating moderate to severe pain.
- Tramadol is a weak opioid that can be used for OA.
- Monitor and intervene for adverse effects of opioid use, especially for older adults.
- Opioids should be taken only on a short-term basis by most clients. Some clients who have chronic back pain may receive prescriptions for opioids for long-term use. QEBP

Topical analgesics

Trolamine salicylate: Can provide varying amounts of temporary pain relief, depending on client response.
- Apply topically over the area of involvement.
- Contains salicylate.

Lidocaine 5% patch: Can be helpful for nerve pain and OA of knees for short-term use.
- Apply to clean, dry, intact skin for 12 hr each day.
- Can cause skin irritation.
- Contraindicated with class I antidysrhythmic medications.

Capsaicin: Can provide varying amounts of temporary pain relief depending on client response.
- Apply topically over an area of involvement.
- Use gloves for application; wash hands thoroughly to prevent burning of eyes.
- Made from alkaloid that is derived from hot peppers.
- Thought to prevent transmission of pain sensations from peripheral neural transmitters.
- CLIENT EDUCATION
  ○ Wear gloves during application. QPcc
  ○ Wear nitrile gloves when applying capsaicin patch.
  ○ Avoid applying tight dressings to area where capsaicin cream was applied, to prevent skin irritation.
  ○ Wash hands immediately after applying capsaicin, and avoid touching eyes or applying over broken skin areas, which can cause painful burning.
  ○ A burning sensation of the skin after application is normal and should subside.
  ○ Apply frequently (up to four times per day) for maximum benefit.

Intra-articular injections

- Glucocorticoids are used to treat localized inflammation. One joint may be injected no more than 4 times a year.
- Hyaluronic acid is used to replace the body's natural hyaluronic acid, which is destroyed by joint inflammation. It is currently only approved for treatment of hip and knee joints.

CLIENT EDUCATION: For hyaluronic acid, notify the provider of allergy to birds, feathers, or eggs because this medication is made from combs of chickens.

COMPLEMENTARY AND ALTERNATIVE THERAPIES

- Chiropractic or spinal manipulation
- Imagery, acupuncture, acupressure, music therapy, massage, biofeedback, and herbal medicines
- Yoga
- Massage

Glucosamine supplements

- Glucosamine is a naturally occurring chemical involved in the makeup of cartilage. Glucosamine sulfate is believed to aid in the synthesis of synovial fluid and rebuild cartilage.
- Glucosamine can decrease the cells that cause joint inflammation and degradation of cartilage.
- Glucosamine is often taken in combination with chondroitin and might not have a pain reduction effect.

NURSING ACTIONS: Question clients about concurrent use of chondroitin, NSAIDs, heparin, and warfarin.

CLIENT EDUCATION
- Consult the provider regarding use and dosage. Qs
- Chondroitin is contraindicated with hypertension, pregnancy, and breastfeeding.
- Chondroitin can cause bleeding, especially if taking anticoagulants.
- Chondroitin can cause mild GI upset (nausea, heartburn).
- Use with caution with shellfish allergy.

INTERPROFESSIONAL CARE

Physical therapy: A physical therapist can instruct the client on muscle strengthening exercises, application of heat, diathermy (treatment with electrical currents), ultrasonography (treatment with sound waves), or stretching and strengthening exercises. QTc
- Phonophoresis: A physical therapist may apply a topical medication, such as lidocaine, followed by ultrasound or iontophoresis (using heat and dexamethasone) to force medication into subcutaneous tissue and increase relief of pain.
- A provider may prescribe a transcutaneous electrical nerve stimulation (TENS) unit to be applied by a physical therapist with client instruction on how to use it.

A **nutritionist** may assist the client in diet for weight loss in relation to reduced activity level, providing teaching regarding a balanced diet and foods high in calcium and vitamin D.

Occupational therapy: to increase independent function such as personal care or home skills.

THERAPEUTIC PROCEDURES

Conservative therapy includes the following.
- Balancing rest with activity
- Exercising with water therapy
- Practicing proper joint positioning
- Using bracing, splints, canes, and proper posture
- Wearing supportive shoes
- Applying thermal therapies (heat or cold)

Osteoarthritis

Total joint arthroplasty or total joint replacement: When all other conservative measures fail, the client may choose to undergo total joint arthroplasty to relieve the pain and improve mobility and quality of life.
- Joint replacement is contraindicated with any type of infection.
- A dental exam and dental procedures should be done before surgery to decrease risk of infection.
- Uncontrolled diabetes or hypertension increase the risk of postoperative complications.

Low-back pain

MINIMALLY INVASIVE SURGERY
- **Microscopic endoscopic diskectomy or percutaneous endoscopic diskectomy:** Fluoroscopy is used to guide a tubular device through which the herniated disk is removed by cutting it out, or suctioning out the center of the disk.
- **Laser-assisted laparoscopic lumbar diskectomy:** Laparoscope and laser are used to treat the herniated disks.
- **Kyphoplasty:** A needle is inserted into the back to inflate a balloon to help the vertebra regain its shape. Then a cement substance is injected into the space. Vertebroplasty is very similar, but a balloon is not used.

OPEN SURGICAL PROCEDURES
- **Open diskectomy:** removal of the herniated disk
- **Laminectomy:** removal of part of the laminae and facet joints
- **Surgery for tumors or infection**
- **Arthrodesis/spinal fusion:** surgery to join or fuse two or more vertebrae
  - A bone graft from the pelvic bone or bone bank is used to make a bridge between vertebrae that are next to each other.
  - Metal implants can also be used.

Application Exercises

1. A nurse is collecting data from a client who has osteoarthritis of the knees and fingers. Which of the following manifestations should the nurse expect to find? (Select all that apply.)

   A. Heberden's nodes
   B. Swelling of all joints
   C. Small body frame
   D. Enlarged joint size
   E. Limp when walking

2. A nurse is reviewing information with a client who has osteoarthritis of the hip and knee. Which of the following instructions should the nurse reinforce? (Select all that apply.)

   A. Apply heat to joints to alleviate pain.
   B. Ice inflamed joints following activity.
   C. Install an elevated toilet seat.
   D. Take tub baths.
   E. Complete high-energy activities in the morning.

3. A nurse is reviewing information about capsaicin cream with a client who reports continuous knee pain from osteoarthritis. Which of the following information should the nurse reinforce?

   A. Continuous pain relief is provided.
   B. Inspect for skin irritation and cuts prior to application.
   C. Cover the area with tight bandages after application.
   D. Apply the medication every 2 hr during the day.

4. A nurse is caring for a client who injured her lower back during a fall and describes sharp pain in her back and down her left leg. In which of the following positions should the nurse plan to place the client to attempt to decrease her pain?

   A. Prone without use of pillows
   B. Semi-Fowler's with a pillow under the knees
   C. High-Fowler's with the knees flat on the bed
   D. Supine with the head flat

5. A nurse is reinforcing teaching with a client who has a history of low-back injury. Which of the following instructions should the nurse reinforce with the client to prevent low-back pain? (Select all that apply)

   A. Engage in regular exercise, including walking.
   B. Sit for up to 10 hr each day to rest the back.
   C. Maintain weight within 25% of ideal body weight.
   D. Create a smoking cessation plan.
   E. Wear low-heeled shoes.

Application Exercises Key

1. A. **CORRECT:** Heberden's nodes are enlarged nodules on the distal interphalangeal joints of the hands and feet of a client who has osteoarthritis.

   B. Swelling and pain of all joints is a manifestation of rheumatoid arthritis. A local inflammation of a joint is related to osteoarthritis.

   C. A small body frame is a risk factor for rheumatoid arthritis. Obesity is a risk factor for osteoarthritis.

   D. **CORRECT:** A client can manifest enlarged joints due to bone hypertrophy.

   E. **CORRECT:** A client can manifest a limp when walking due to pain from inflammation in the localized joint.

   Ⓝ *NCLEX® Connection: Physiological Adaptation, Basic Pathophysiology*

2. A. **CORRECT:** Applying heat to joints can provide temporary relief of pain.

   B. **CORRECT:** Applying ice to inflamed joints following activity can decrease edema.

   C. **CORRECT:** An elevated toilet seat can decrease strain and pain of the affected joints.

   D. Taking a tub bath places the client at risk for increased strain and pain on the affected joints when getting in and out of the tub and increases the risk for falls.

   E. **CORRECT:** Encouraging high-energy activity in the morning is recommended as part of a daily routine to promote independence.

   Ⓝ *NCLEX® Connection: Physiological Adaptation, Alterations in Body Systems*

3. A. Capsaicin cream provides temporary relief of pain rather than continuous relief when applied several times daily.

   B. **CORRECT:** Inspect the skin for irritation and cuts before applying capsaicin cream, because hot peppers in the cream can cause a painful burning sensation in areas of skin breakdown.

   C. After capsaicin cream is applied, avoid covering the area with a tight bandage, which can cause increased skin irritation.

   D. For maximum pain relief benefit, apply capsaicin cream up to four times a day.

   Ⓝ *NCLEX® Connection: Pharmacological Therapies, Medication Administration*

4. A. Prone position without use of pillows has not been found to decrease acute low-back pain.

   B. **CORRECT:** Williams position (semi-Fowler's position with the knees flexed by pillows) has been found to relieve low-back pain caused by a bulging disk and nerve root involvement.

   C. High-Fowler's position with the knees flat has not been found to decrease acute low back pain.

   D. Supine position with the head flat has not been found to decrease acute low back pain.

   Ⓝ *NCLEX® Connection: Basic Care and Comfort, Nonpharmacological Comfort Interventions*

5. A. **CORRECT:** Regular exercise, including walking or swimming, is a strategy that can prevent low-back pain.

   B. Long periods of sitting or standing can cause low-back pain. Advise the client to use footstools or ergonomic chairs when sitting is necessary.

   C. The client should maintain weight within 10% of ideal body weight, as obesity can cause low-back pain.

   D. **CORRECT:** Stopping or cutting down on smoking can decrease low-back pain, as smoking can cause disk degeneration.

   E. **CORRECT:** Wearing low-heeled, well-fitting shoes can prevent low back pain. The nurse should instruct the client to avoid high-heeled shoes.

   Ⓝ *NCLEX Connection: Basic Care and Comfort, Nonpharmacological Comfort Interventions*

PRACTICE Active Learning Scenario

A nurse is reviewing information on collaborative and nonpharmacologic therapies with a client who is having continual joint pain from osteoarthritis. What information should the nurse review? Use the ATI Active Learning Template: Basic Concept to complete this item.

RELATED CONTENT: Describe two activities each for collaborative care involving physical therapy and nutrition therapy.

NURSING INTERVENTIONS: Describe three actions the nurse could recommend for this client.

PRACTICE Answer

Using the ATI Active Learning Template: Basic Concept

RELATED CONTENT
- Physical therapy
  - Apply heat, diathermy, and ultrasound.
  - Perform stretching and strengthening exercises.
  - Use transcutaneous electrical nerve stimulation (TENS).
- Nutritional therapy
  - Provide nutritional information on weight loss.
  - Provide nutritional information on a balanced diet.
  - Provide information on use of vitamin D and calcium.

NURSING INTERVENTIONS
- Balance rest with activity.
- Use braces, splints, and cane.
- Apply thermal therapies (heat or cold).
- Use assistive devices such as a long-handled reacher and an elevated toilet seat.
- Plan high-energy activities in the morning when feeling most rested.

Ⓝ *NCLEX® Connection: Basic Care and Comfort, Nonpharmacological Comfort Interventions*

NCLEX® Connections

When reviewing the following chapters, keep in mind the relevant topics and tasks of the NCLEX outline, in particular:

Basic Care and Comfort

MOBILITY/IMMOBILITY: Use measures to maintain or improve the client's skin integrity.

NUTRITION AND ORAL HYDRATION
Monitor and provide for the client's nutritional needs.

Monitor the impact of disease/illness on the client's nutritional status.

Reduction of Risk Potential

POTENTIAL FOR ALTERATIONS IN BODY SYSTEMS:
Reinforce client teaching on methods to prevent complications associated with activity level/diagnosed illness/disease (such as foot care for client with diabetes mellitus).

POTENTIAL FOR COMPLICATIONS OF DIAGNOSTIC TESTS/ TREATMENTS/PROCEDURES: Implement measures to prevent complication of the client's condition or procedure (circulatory complication, seizure, aspiration, potential neurological disorder).

Physiological Adaptation

ALTERATIONS IN BODY SYSTEMS
Identify signs and symptoms of an infection (temperature changes, swelling, redness, mental confusion, foul smelling urine).

Perform wound care and/or dressing change.

BASIC PATHOPHYSIOLOGY: Consider general principles of the client's disease process when providing care (injury and repair, immunity, cellular structure).

FLUID AND ELECTROLYTE IMBALANCES: Identify signs and symptoms of the client's fluid and/or electrolyte imbalances.

CHAPTER 65 *Integumentary Diagnostic Procedures*

Integumentary diagnostic procedures involve identification of pathogenic micro-organisms. The most accurate and definitive way to identify micro-organisms and cell characteristics is by examining blood, body fluids, and tissue samples under a microscope.

Skin lesions or changes in the skin can need confirmation by microscope to determine if the cause is viral, fungal, or bacterial.

Skin diagnostic studies

Wood's light examination

- Ultraviolet light is used to produce specific colors to reveal a skin infection.
- Useful in the diagnosis of fungal infections of the scalp and chronic bacterial infections of the major skin folds.

Diascopy

A glass slide or lens is pressed down over the area to be examined to test for blanchability. It is used to determine whether the lesion is vascular (inflammatory) or nonvascular (nevus) or hemorrhagic (petechiae or purpura). Hemorrhagic and nonvascular lesions do not blanch, but inflammatory lesions do.

Skin culture and sensitivity

- **Culture** refers to isolation of the pathogen on culture media. Qᴇʙᴘ
- **Sensitivity** refers to the effect that antimicrobial agents have on the micro-organism.
  - If the micro-organism is killed by the antimicrobial, the microbe is sensitive to that medication.
  - If tolerable levels of the medication are unable to kill the microbe, the microbe is resistant to that medication.

- Culture and sensitivity can be done on a sample of purulent drainage from a skin lesion.
- Cultures should be done prior to initiating antimicrobial therapy.
- Preliminary results of a culture and sensitivity test are usually available within 24 to 48 hr, and final results in 72 hr.

INDICATIONS

CLIENT PRESENTATION

- Skin lesions can be infectious, raised, reddened, edematous, and warm.
- There can be purulent drainage and fever.

CONSIDERATIONS

PREPROCEDURE

NURSING ACTIONS
- Use standard precautions when collecting and handling specimens. Qs
- Most specimens are collected by the nurse or provider.

INTRAPROCEDURE

Bacterial or viral specimens

NURSING ACTIONS
- Express material from the lesion by lifting or puncturing the crusted or scabbed area over the lesion using a small-gauge sterile needle or 0.9% sodium chloride and a sterile cotton swab.
- Culturette tubes are specific for specimen collection and contain a sterile cotton-tipped applicator and a fixative that is released after the infectious exudate is applied to the applicator and inserted in the tube.
- A specimen obtained for a viral culture is immediately placed on ice and sent to the laboratory.

Fungal specimen

NURSING ACTIONS
- Requires a sufficient quantity of scales collected using a wooden tongue depressor and placing the specimen in a clean container to be sent to the laboratory.
- If a fungal culture is needed because of inconclusive results due to a deeper fungal infection, a punch biopsy is performed.
- Specimens must be properly labeled and delivered to the laboratory promptly for appropriate storage and analysis.

POSTPROCEDURE

CLIENT EDUCATION: Measures to prevent the spread of an infectious skin disorder include the following.

- **Bacterial infection:** Bathe daily using an antibacterial soap.
  - Do not squeeze bacterial lesions but remove the crusted exudate so the antibacterial topical medication can penetrate into the lesion.
  - Apply warm compresses twice daily for comfort to furuncles or areas where cellulitis is present. Qpcc
- **Viral lesion:** Apply compress of Burow's solution (aluminum acetate in water) for 20 min, three times a day to promote the formation of a crust and healing.
  - Avoid tight, restrictive clothing that can irritate a lesion.
  - Allow a lesion to dry between treatments, and avoid lying on the lesion to promote circulation and comfort.
  - Use good hand hygiene to prevent cross-contamination of the infection.
  - Avoid sharing personal items (combs, brushes, clothing, footwear).

Medication therapy for bacterial infections

- Superficial skin infections are treated with topical antibacterial cream or ointment.
- Extensive bacterial skin infections involving the lymphatic system, or if cellulitis is present, are treated with systemic antibiotic therapy (cephalosporins or penicillins).
- If the client is allergic to cephalosporins and penicillins, the provider can prescribe tetracycline, erythromycin, azithromycin, or tobramycin.
- If the skin lesion is cultured as having methicillin-resistant *Staphylococcus aureus*, IV vancomycin or oral linezolid or clindamycin is used.

Medication for viral infections

Topical treatment with acyclovir, valacyclovir, or famciclovir decreases the number of active viruses on the surface of the skin and reduces the discomfort associated with a herpetic infection or lesion.

Medication for fungal infections

- Yeast and dermatophyte infections are treated with topical cream or powder. For example, clotrimazole cream is applied to the infected skin twice a day and for 1 to 2 weeks after the lesions are no longer present, or as prescribed.
- Skin must be clean and dry before applying topical ointments or creams.

INTERPRETATION OF FINDINGS

BACTERIAL INFECTION
- The microbe responsible for the infection is identified in the culture, and the antimicrobials that are sensitive to that microbe are listed.
- Heavy growth of greater than 100,000 colonies definitively diagnoses an infection.
- Indeterminate results are 10,000 to 100,000 colonies.
- Negative results are less than 10,000 colonies.
- Appropriate medications have three to four degrees of sensitivity.

VIRAL INFECTION (HERPES VIRUS): A cotton-tipped applicator is used to obtain vesicle fluid from intact lesions for culture.

Tzanck smear

A microscopic cytology examination is completed after extracting cells from the base of a lesion. Microscopic examination reveals multinucleated giant cells to confirm the lesion is viral.

Potassium hydroxide (KOH) test

- The test confirms a fungal skin lesion.
- A microscopic examination of specimens from hair, nails or the scales scraped off a lesion is mixed with KOH. Specimen is positive for fungus if there is the presence of fungal hyphae (threadlike filaments).

Biopsy

- Biopsy is the removal of a sample of tissue by excision or needle aspiration for cytological (histological) examination.
- Biopsy confirms or rules out malignancy.
- Skin biopsies are performed under local anesthesia.
- Biopsy for skin lesions can be a punch biopsy, shave biopsy, or excisional biopsy.

Punch biopsy: A plug of tissue approximately 2 to 6 mm is removed with a specific cutting instrument, with or without sutures to close the site.

Shave biopsy: Only the part of the lesion that is raised above the surrounding tissue is removed using a scalpel or razor blade with no suturing.

Excisional biopsy: A larger and deeper specimen is obtained, and suturing is required.

INDICATIONS

POTENTIAL DIAGNOSES: A biopsy is commonly performed to establish an exact diagnosis or to rule out diseases such as cancer.

CLIENT PRESENTATION: Evidence of skin lesion can include an area of discoloration that is thickened, thinned, raised, flat, rough, painful, open, dry, or itchy.

CONSIDERATIONS

PREPROCEDURE

NURSING ACTIONS
- Ensure that the client has signed the informed consent form.
- Inform the client about what to expect in regard to the formation of a scar.
- Instruct the client about what to expect about the test or procedure.

INTRAPROCEDURE

NURSING ACTIONS
- Review with the client what to expect according to the type of biopsy.
- Assist the provider with the test or procedure as needed, and assist with local anesthesia.
- Establish a sterile field. Qs
- Place the tissue sample in a container containing appropriate solution, label, and send to the laboratory.
- Apply pressure to the biopsy site to control bleeding as appropriate.
- Place a sterile dressing over the biopsy site if needed.

POSTPROCEDURE

Postbiopsy discomfort usually is relieved by mild analgesics.

NURSING ACTIONS: Monitor the biopsy site as appropriate.

CLIENT EDUCATION
- Report excessive bleeding or evidence of infection (redness, warmth, drainage, fever) to the provider. Qs
- Check the incision daily. The incision should be clean, dry, and intact.
- Dressings may be removed after 8 hr. Use tap water or 0.9% sterile sodium chloride to clean the biopsy site of dried blood or crusts.
- If prescribed, apply an antibacterial topical medication to prevent infection.
- If sutures are used, return to the provider for removal in 7 to 10 days

INTERPRETATION OF FINDINGS

After a biopsy is completed, the tissue sample is sent to pathology for interpretation.

Application Exercises

1. A nurse is caring for a client who has a suspected viral skin lesion. Which of the following laboratory findings should the nurse anticipate the provider reviewing to confirm this diagnosis?

   A. Potassium hydroxide (KOH)

   B. Diascopy

   C. Tzanck smear report

   D. Biopsy

2. A nurse in a clinic is preparing to obtain a skin specimen from a client who has a suspected herpes infection. Which of the following actions should the nurse take? (Select all that apply.)

   A. Scrape the site with a wooden tongue depressor.

   B. Puncture the crusted area with a sterile needle.

   C. Swab the crusted area with a sterile cotton-tipped applicator.

   D. Place cotton-tipped applicator in culturette tube.

   E. Place culturette tube in ice.

3. A nurse is reinforcing teaching with a client on home care after a culture for a bacterial infection and cellulitis. Which of the following information should the nurse include?

   A. Bathe daily with moisturizing soap.

   B. Apply antibacterial topical medication to the crusted exudate.

   C. Apply warm compresses to the affected area.

   D. Cover affected area with snug-fitting clothing.

4. A nurse is reinforcing discharge instructions with a client who had a skin biopsy with sutures. Which of the following client statements indicates that the teaching has been effective?

   A. "I can expect redness around the site for 5 to 7 days."

   B. "I will most likely have a fever for the first few days."

   C. "I should apply an antibiotic ointment to the area."

   D. "I will make a return appointment in 3 days for removal of my sutures."

5. A nurse is reinforcing teaching with a client about a new prescription for clotrimazole topical cream. Which of the following statements should the nurse include in the teaching?

   A. "It reduces the discomfort of a herpetic infection but does not cure the infection."

   B. "This is a cream to treat a bacterial infection."

   C. "I will apply the topical medication for up to 2 weeks after the lesions are gone."

   D. "I will apply the cream to lesions while they are moist."

Application Exercises Key

1. A. Findings of a potassium hydroxide (KOH) test reveal if skin lesions are fungal in origin.

   B. Diascopy provides increased visibility of a skin lesion by blanching the skin over the lesion, eliminating erythema, which can obscure findings.

   C. **CORRECT:** A Tzanck smear report confirms whether a skin lesion is viral in origin.

   D. Findings of a biopsy report confirm or rule out if a lesion is malignant.

   Ⓝ *NCLEX® Connection: Reduction of Risk Potential, Laboratory Values*

2. A. A wooden tongue depressor is used to scrape cells of a skin lesion to test for a fungus.

   B. **CORRECT:** Exudate under the crusted area should be collected. The crust or scab should be punctured or lifted to obtain a reliable specimen.

   C. Swab the moist lesion bed under the crust with a sterile cotton-tipped applicator to obtain a reliable specimen.

   D. **CORRECT:** The cotton-tipped applicator is placed in liquid fixative within the culturette tube.

   E. **CORRECT:** The culturette tube is immediately placed in ice when obtaining a viral specimen.

   Ⓝ *NCLEX® Connection: Reduction of Risk Potential, Diagnostic Tests*

3. A. The client should use antibacterial soap to reduce the bacteria count on the skin.

   B. The client should apply topical medication directly to the moist lesion bed. The medication will not penetrate the crusted exudate.

   C. **CORRECT:** The client should apply warm compresses to the affected area to promote comfort.

   D. The client should wear loose-fitting clothes to avoid irritating the lesion.

   Ⓝ *NCLEX® Connection: Physiological Adaptation, Alterations in Body Systems*

4. A. The client should report redness, pain, drainage, or warmth at the biopsy site to the provider.

   B. A fever is an indication of an infection, and the provider should be notified.

   C. **CORRECT:** Antibiotic ointment is applied as prescribed to prevent infection.

   D. Sutures are removed 7 to 10 days following a biopsy.

   Ⓝ *NCLEX® Connection: Physiological Adaptation, Alterations in Body Systems*

5. A. Clotrimazole is not an antiviral medication.

   B. Clotrimazole is not an antibacterial medication.

   C. **CORRECT:** Clotrimazole is a medication used to treat a fungal infection and is applied for 1 to 2 weeks after the infection is resolved.

   D. Clotrimazole should be applied to clean, dry skin. Wash the skin gently and pat dry before applying.

   Ⓝ *NCLEX® Connection: Pharmacological Therapies, Medication Administration*

PRACTICE Active Learning Scenario

A nurse is caring for a client who will have a biopsy of a skin lesion. What should the nurse consider in planning for the procedure? Use the ATI Active Learning Template: Basic Concept to complete this item.

UNDERLYING PRINCIPLES: Describe the three types of integumentary biopsies.

NURSING INTERVENTIONS: Describe two intraprocedure nursing actions.

PRACTICE Answer

Using the ATI Active Learning Template: Basic Concept

UNDERLYING PRINCIPLES
- Punch biopsy: A 2 to 6 mm plug of tissue is removed from the skin lesion, with or without suturing.
- Shave biopsy: A scalpel or razor blade removes only the raised area of the lesion, with no suturing.
- Excisional biopsy: A large, deep specimen of tissue is obtained, followed with suturing.

NURSING INTERVENTIONS
- Assist with setting up materials for placement of a local anesthetic.
- Apply pressure to the biopsy site to control bleeding.
- Place a sterile dressing over the biopsy site if needed.

Ⓝ *NCLEX® Connection: Reduction of Risk Potential, Therapeutic Procedures*

UNIT 11　NURSING CARE OF CLIENTS WHO HAVE
INTEGUMENTARY DISORDERS
SECTION: INTEGUMENTARY DISORDERS

CHAPTER 66　*Skin Disorders*

Psoriasis is a skin disorder characterized by scaly, dermal patches and caused by overproduction of keratin. This overproduction can occur at a rate up to seven times the rate of normal cells. It is thought to be an autoimmune disorder and has periods of exacerbations and remissions. Although lesions can appear anywhere, they are commonly present on the elbows, knees, trunk, scalp, sacrum, and the lateral aspects of extremities. Psoriasis can be classified as psoriasis vulgaris, exfoliative, or palmoplantar pustulosis. In some clients, psoriasis affects the joints, causing arthritis-type changes and pain.

Dermatitis is an inflammation of the skin resulting from exposure to allergens (internal or external) that causes changes in the skin structure or tissue destruction. Manifestations of dermatitis can be nonspecific (itching, lesions without distinct borders, different distribution patterns). Rashes can evolve from acute to chronic, and place the client at increased risk for bacterial infection resulting from breaks in the skin caused by scratching. Dermatitis can be classified as eczematous, contact, or atopic.

Psoriasis

DATA COLLECTION

RISK FACTORS

- Infections (severe streptococcal throat infection, Candida infection, upper respiratory infection)
- Skin trauma (recent surgery, sunburn)
- Genetics
- Stress (related to overstimulation of the immune system)
- Seasons (warm weather improves manifestations)
- Hormones (puberty or menopause)
- Medications (lithium, beta blockers, indomethacin)
- Obesity
- Female sex

EXPECTED FINDINGS

- **Psoriasis vulgaris** presents as reddened, thickened skin with silvery white scales with bilateral distribution.
- **Exfoliative psoriasis** displays as erythema and scaling from a severe inflammatory reaction with no obvious lesions. The reaction can cause dehydration and hypothermia or hyperthermia.
- **Palmoplantar pustulosis** manifests as reddened hyperkeratotic areas (accelerated maturation of epidermal cells) due to an inflammatory disorder. Plaques form and pustules turn brown, peel, and form a crust on the palms of the hands and soles of the feet. The course of the disease is cyclic.
- Exacerbation and remission of pruritic lesions

66.1　Psoriasis

psoriasis skin lesions

common psoriasis locations

PHYSICAL FINDINGS
- Scaly patches (66.1)
- Bleeding stimulated by removal of scales
- Skin lesions primarily on the scalp, elbows and knees, sacrum, and lateral areas of the extremities (psoriasis vulgaris)
- Pitting, crumbling nails

PATIENT-CENTERED CARE

MEDICATIONS

Topical therapies

Corticosteroids (triamcinolone, betamethasone) reduce secondary inflammatory response of lesions and suppresses cellular division/proliferation.
- NURSING ACTIONS
  - Observe skin for thinning, striae, or hypopigmentation with high-potency corticosteroids.
  - Instruct clients about proper application.
- CLIENT EDUCATION
  - Apply high-potency corticosteroids as prescribed to prevent adverse effects and take periodic medication vacations.
  - Use warm, moist, occlusive dressings of plastic wrap (gloves, plastic garments, booties) after applying the topical medication. These can be left in place up to 8 hr each day. Q**EBP**
  - Avoid application of medication on face or into skin folds. Medication may be applied to the scalp.

Tar preparations: coal tar and tars made from trees (juniper, birch, and pine) that suppress cellular division/proliferation and reduces inflammation
- NURSING ACTIONS
  - Monitor skin for irritation.
  - Instruct the client on proper application
- CLIENT EDUCATION
  - Tar applications can cause stinging and burning.
  - Tar applications can cause staining of the skin and hair.
  - Due to odor and staining, apply this product at night and cover areas of body with old pajamas, gloves, and socks.

Vitamin D analogs (calcipotriene, calcitriol) prevents cellular proliferation
- NURSING ACTIONS
  - Monitor for itching, irritation, and erythema.
  - Monitor for hypercalcemia (elevated serum calcium, muscle weakness, fatigue, anorexia).
  - Instruct clients on proper application.
  - Instruct clients on recognition of cancerous lesions.
  - Inform the medication is available in a topical solution for scalp lesions.
- CLIENT EDUCATION
  - Limit sun exposure due to increased risk of developing skin cancer.
  - Take a pregnancy test prior to application of the medication.
  - Expect some burning or stinging following application.
  - Do not apply the medication to the face or skin folds.

Vitamin A (tazarotene) slows cellular division and reduces inflammation
- NURSING ACTIONS
  - Contraindicated during pregnancy. Q**s**
  - Monitor for localized reactions, inflammation, and desquamation of the skin.
  - Instruct clients on proper application.
- CLIENT EDUCATION
  - Avoid exposure to sun or artificial UV light.
  - Use reliable forms of birth control.
  - Discontinue use and notify provider if pregnancy occurs.

Systemic medications

Cytotoxic medications (methotrexate, acitretin) reduce turnover of epidermal cells
- Used for severe, intractable cases
- Contraindicated during pregnancy (can cause fetal death or congenital anomalies).
- NURSING ACTIONS
  - Monitor liver function tests for liver toxicity if methotrexate or acitretin therapy is being used.
  - Methotrexate can cause bone marrow suppression (leukopenia, thrombocytopenia, anemia).
- CLIENT EDUCATION
  - Avoid alcohol while taking these medications.
  - Monitor for fever, sore throat, increased bleeding or bruising, and fatigue.
  - These medications can decrease the effectiveness of contraceptives.

Biologic agents: first-line treatment for moderate to severe plaque psoriasis that suppress immune function (adalimumab, etanercept, ustekinumab, alefacept, infliximab)
- NURSING ACTIONS
  - Evaluate for latent tuberculosis and hepatitis B virus.
  - Inspect prefilled syringe for particles or discoloration.
  - Rotate injection sites, and do not rub after administration.
  - Protect medication from light.
  - Instruct the client how to administer subcutaneous medication.
  - Inform the client about the need for lifelong treatment and the increased risk of cancer.
- CLIENT EDUCATION
  - Do not take if pregnant or breastfeeding.
  - Report manifestations of infection.
  - Do not receive any live vaccines while taking the medication.

Cyclosporine and azathioprine
- Immunosuppressant medications are administered when lesions do not respond to other therapies.
- Nephrotoxicity occurs and increases the risk of infections.

THERAPEUTIC PROCEDURES

Photochemotherapy and ultraviolet light (PUVA therapy)
- A psoralen photosensitizing medication (methoxsalen) is administered followed by long-wave ultraviolet A (UVA) to decrease proliferation of epidermal cells.
- Methoxsalen is given orally 2 hr before UV treatments.
- Treatments are given two to three times per week, avoiding consecutive days.

- NURSING ACTIONS
  - ○ Monitor the skin's response to light (redness, tenderness, tanning).
  - ○ Ensure that the client wears eye protection during treatment and for 24 hr following a treatment (indoors and outside). Qs
- CLIENT EDUCATION
  - ○ Notify the provider of extreme redness, swelling, and discomfort.
  - ○ Long-term effects include premature skin aging, cataracts, and skin cancer.

Narrow-band ultraviolet B light therapy can be implemented without medication application, and requires fewer treatments.

Dermatitis

HEALTH PROMOTION AND DISEASE PREVENTION

- If the cause is identified, avoidance therapy is used.
- Do not scratch affected areas because it can cause secondary skin infections.
- Use products (soap, laundry detergent, cosmetics) that do not contain fragrance.
- Avoid the use of fabric softener dryer sheets.
- Wash skin thoroughly after exposure to irritants.

DATA COLLECTION

RISK FACTORS

- External skin exposure to allergens
- Internal exposure to allergens and irritants
- Stress (eczematous dermatitis)
- Genetic predisposition (eczematous dermatitis)
- Specific cause not always known

EXPECTED FINDINGS

Eczematous dermatitis

- Development of thickened areas of skin
- Can appear dry or moist and crusted
- Pruritus
- Symmetrical involvement usually of face, neck, arms, legs, and feet

Contact dermatitis

- Caused by exposure to allergen, chemical, or mechanical irritation.
- Rash is well-demarcated.
- Distribution varies depending upon the cause and the exposure to the allergen.

Atopic dermatitis

- Chronic rash
- Can be caused by allergens or chronic skin disease.
- Development of thickened areas of skin along with scaling and desquamation.
- Pruritus can be intense.
- Distribution includes face, neck, and upper torso along with skin folds (antecubital, popliteal).

PATIENT-CENTERED CARE

- Avoidance therapy if cause identified
- Apply cool, damp compresses to rash to decrease inflammation.
- Use colloidal oatmeal baths to relieve itching.

MEDICATIONS

Steroid therapy: topical, intralesional, systemic (hydrocortisone, betamethasone, triamcinolone, prednisone)
- Reduce secondary inflammatory response of lesions.
- NURSING ACTIONS
  - ○ Monitor for adrenal suppression.
  - ○ Instruct clients about proper application.
- CLIENT EDUCATION Qpcc
  - ○ Avoid using topical steroids on lesions that are infected.
  - ○ If using steroids for long periods, taper doses when discontinuing medication.
  - ○ Warm, moist dressings may be used over topical application to increase absorption of medication.
  - ○ Avoid the use of occlusive dressings over rash after applying topical steroid medications.

Antihistamines: topical, systemic (diphenhydramine, cetirizine, fexofenadine)
- Relief of redness, pruritus, and edema
- NURSING ACTIONS: Monitor for urinary retention with the use of systemic medications.
- CLIENT EDUCATION
  - ○ Product can cause photosensitivity.
  - ○ Avoid operating machinery and driving while taking systemic antihistamine.
  - ○ Take systemic form at bedtime, as product can cause drowsiness.

Topical immunosuppressants: tacrolimus, pimecrolimus
- For use in treatment of eczematous dermatitis that has been resistant to glucocorticoid treatment
- Relieves inflammation
- NURSING ACTIONS
  - ○ Instruct clients on application of medication.
  - ○ Monitor for erythema, burning sensation.
  - ○ Avoid the use of occlusive dressings.
- CLIENT EDUCATION
  - ○ Avoid use if infection is present.
  - ○ Discontinue use when rash clears.
  - ○ Avoid direct sunlight and the use of tanning beds.

Application Exercises

1. A nurse is reviewing information about a new prescription for corticosteroid cream with a client who has mild psoriasis. Which of the following instructions should the nurse include? (Select all that apply.)

    A. Apply an occlusive dressing after application.

    B. Apply three to four times per day.

    C. Wear gloves after application to lesions on the hands.

    D. Avoid applying in skin folds.

    E. Use medication continuously over a period of several months.

2. A nurse is reinforcing teaching with a client who has a history of psoriasis about photochemotherapy and ultraviolet light (PUVA) treatments. Which of the following instructions should the nurse include in the teaching?

    A. Apply vitamin A cream before each treatment.

    B. Administer a psoralen medication before the treatment.

    C. Use the treatment every evening.

    D. Remove the scales gently following each treatment.

3. A nurse is reinforcing teaching with a female client on the use of calcipotriene topical medication for the treatment of psoriasis. Which of the following information should the nurse include? (Select all that apply.)

    A. Recommended for facial lesions.

    B. Expect a stinging sensation upon application.

    C. Apply to the scalp.

    D. Obtain a pregnancy test.

    E. Limit application to skin folds.

4. A nurse is reinforcing teaching with the parent of a child who has contact dermatitis. Which of the following information should the nurse include?

    A. Use fabric softener dryer sheets when drying the child's clothing.

    B. Apply a warm, dry compress to the rash area.

    C. Place the child in a bath with colloidal oatmeal.

    D. Leave the child's hands uncovered during the night.

5. A nurse caring for a client who has contact dermatitis and a new prescription for diphenhydramine. For which of the following adverse effects should the nurse monitor?

    A. Elevated blood glucose levels

    B. Urinary retention

    C. Hyperpigmentation of the skin

    D. Insomnia

PRACTICE Active Learning Scenario

A nurse is reviewing information with a client who has a prescription for pimecrolimus to treat severe eczematous dermatitis. What information should the nurse include? Use the ATI Active Learning Template: Medication to complete this item.

THERAPEUTIC USES

NURSING INTERVENTIONS: Describe two.

CLIENT EDUCATION: Describe two teaching points.

Application Exercises Key

1. A. **CORRECT:** An occlusive dressing can enhance the efficacy of the topical corticosteroid on the exposed lesions.

   B. Corticosteroid cream is applied twice daily to prevent development of local and systemic adverse effects.

   C. **CORRECT:** Wearing gloves after applying the medication can enhance the efficacy of the topical corticosteroid on the exposed lesions of the hands.

   D. **CORRECT:** Applying corticosteroid cream to lesions in skin folds increases the risk of yeast infections.

   E. The client should take periodic medication vacations to minimize the risk for development of local and systemic adverse effects.

   Ⓝ *NCLEX® Connection: Pharmacological Therapies, Expected Actions/Outcomes*

2. A. PUVA treatment does not involve the use of vitamin A cream.

   B. **CORRECT:** PUVA treatment involves the administration of a medication, such as a psoralen, to enhance photosensitivity.

   C. PUVA treatments are completed two to three times each week and not on consecutive days.

   D. Removal of scales can cause bleeding and is not recommended when treating psoriasis.

   Ⓝ *NCLEX® Connection: Reduction of Risk Potential, Therapeutic Procedures*

3. A. Applying calcipotriene to the face is not recommended because it can cause facial dermatitis.

   B. **CORRECT:** Calcipotriene causes stinging and burning sensations when applied to the lesions.

   C. **CORRECT:** Calcipotriene solution is applied to scalp lesions.

   D. **CORRECT:** Calcipotriene can cause birth defects. Clients should obtain a pregnancy test before using the medication.

   E. **CORRECT:** Applying calcipotriene to skin folds can cause a possible local reaction of itching, irritation, and erythema.

   Ⓝ *NCLEX® Connection: Pharmacological Therapies, Expected Actions/Outcomes*

4. A. The parent should avoid fabric softener dryer sheets when cleaning the child's clothing. Liquid fabric softener may be used.

   B. The parent should apply a cool, moist compress to the rash area to decrease inflammation.

   C. **CORRECT:** A colloidal oatmeal bath will relieve the child's itching.

   D. The parent should apply mittens on the child's hands at night to decrease unconscious scratching of the rash, which can lead to a secondary infection.

   Ⓝ *NCLEX® Connection: Pharmacological Therapies, Expected Actions/Outcomes*

5. A. Glucocorticoids such as prednisone can increase blood glucose levels. However, this is not an adverse effect of diphenhydramine.

   B. **CORRECT:** The nurse should monitor the client's urinary output, as retention is a possible adverse effect of diphenhydramine.

   C. Hyperpigmentation of the skin can be seen in clients who have adrenal insufficiency, but is not associated with the use of diphenhydramine.

   D. Diphenhydramine is a first-generation antihistamine and can cause excessive drowsiness rather than insomnia.

   Ⓝ *NCLEX® Connection: Pharmacological Therapies, Adverse Effects/Contraindications/Side Effects/Interactions*

PRACTICE Answer

Using the ATI Active Learning Template: Medication

THERAPEUTIC USES: Relieve itching and inflammation

NURSING INTERVENTIONS
- Instruct clients on application of medication.
- Monitor for erythema and burning sensation.
- Avoid the use of occlusive dressings.

CLIENT EDUCATION
- Avoid use if infection is present.
- Discontinue use when rash clears.
- Avoid direct sunlight and the use of tanning beds.

Ⓝ *NCLEX® Connection: Pharmacological Therapies, Expected Actions/Outcomes*

CHAPTER 67 *Burns*

Dry heat, moist heat, direct contact with hot surfaces, chemicals, electricity, and ionizing radiation can cause burns, which result in cellular destruction of the skin layers and underlying tissue. The type and severity of the burn affect the treatment plan.

In addition to destruction of body tissue, a burn injury results in the loss of temperature regulation, sweat and sebaceous gland function, and sensory function. Metabolism increases to maintain body heat as a result of burn injury and tissue damage.

TYPES OF BURNS

Dry heat injuries result from open flames and explosions.

Moist heat injuries result from contact with hot liquid or steam. Scald injuries are more common in older adults and younger children.

Contact burns occur when hot metal, tar, or grease contacts the skin

Chemical burns result from exposure to a caustic agent. Cleaning agents in the home (drain cleaner, oven cleaner, bleach) and agents in the industrial setting (caustic soda, sulfuric acid) can cause chemical burns.

Electrical burns result when an electrical current passes through the body and can cause severe damage, including loss of organ function, tissue destruction with subsequent need for amputation of a limb, and cardiac or respiratory arrest.
- **Thermal burns** result when clothes ignite from heat or flames that electrical sparks produce.
- **Flash (arc) burns** result from contact with electrical current that travels through the air from one conductor to another.
- **Conductive electrical injury** results when a person touches electrical wiring or equipment.

Radiation burns most often result from therapeutic treatment for cancer or from sunburn.

SEVERITY OF THE BURNS

Percentage of total body surface area (TBSA): Use standardized charts for age groups to identify the extent of the injury and calculate medication doses, fluid replacement volumes, and caloric needs. Q̲EBP

Depth of the burn: Classify burns according to the layers of skin and tissue involved: superficial, partial, full, and deep full thickness. **(67.1)**

Body location of the burn: In areas where the skin is thinner, there is more damage to underlying tissue (any part of the face, hand, perineum, feet).

67.1 Depth of injury

	Superficial thickness	Superficial partial thickness	Deep partial thickness	Full thickness	Deep full thickness
AREA INVOLVED	Damage to epidermis	Damage to the entire epidermis and some parts of the dermis	Damage to entire epidermis and deep into the dermis	Damage to the entire epidermis and dermis. Can extend into the subcutaneous tissue. Nerve damage	Damage to all layers of skin. Extends to muscle, tendons, and bones
APPEARANCE	Pink to red. No blisters. Mild edema. No eschar	Pink to red. Blisters. Mild to moderate edema. No eschar	Red to white. No blisters. Moderate edema. Eschar soft and dry	Red, black, brown, yellow, or white. No blisters. Severe edema. Eschar hard and inelastic	Black. No blisters. No edema. Eschar hard and inelastic
SENSATION/ HEALING	Painful/tender. Sensitive to heat. Heals within 3 to 6 days. No scarring	Painful. Heals within 3 weeks. No scarring, but minor pigment changes	Painful and sensitive to touch. Heals in 2 to 6 weeks. Scarring likely. Possible grafting	Sensation minimal or absent. Heals within weeks to months. Scarring. Grafting	Heals within weeks to months. Scarring. Grafting
EXAMPLE	Sunburn. Flash burn (sudden intense heat)	Flash flame and scalds. Brief contact with hot object	Flame and scalds. Grease, tar, or chemical burns. Prolonged exposure to hot objects	Scalds. Grease, tar, chemical, or electrical burns. Prolonged exposure to hot objects	Electrical burns. Flames

Age: Young clients and older adult clients have less reserve capacity to deal with a burn injury. Skin thins with aging, so more damage to underlying tissue can occur. ©

Causative agent: Thermal, chemical, electrical, or radioactive

Presence of other injuries: Fractures and other injuries increase the risk of complications.

Involvement of the respiratory system: Inhalation of deadly fumes, smoke, steam, and heated air can cause respiratory failure or airway edema. Carbon monoxide poisoning also can occur, especially if the injury took place in an enclosed area.

Overall health of the client: A client who has a chronic illness has a greater risk of complications and a worse prognosis.

METHODS TO ASSESS BURNS

Rule of Nines: Quick method to approximate the extent of burns by dividing the body into multiples of nine. The sum equals the TBSA.

Lund and Browder Method: A more exact method estimating the extent of burn by the percentage of surface area of specific anatomic parts, particularly the head and legs.

THREE PHASES OF BURN CARE

Emergent (resuscitative phase)

- Begins with the injury and continues for 24 to 48 hr.
- Priorities include securing the airway, supporting circulation and organ perfusion by fluid replacement, managing pain, preventing infection through wound care, maintaining body temperature, and providing emotional support.

Acute

- Begins 36 to 48 hr after injury when the fluid shift resolves.
- Ends with closure of the wound.
- Priorities include data collection and maintenance of the cardiovascular, respiratory, and gastrointestinal systems (including nutrition); wound care; pain control; and psychosocial interventions.

Rehabilitative

- Begins when most of the burn area has healed.
- Ends when the client achieves the highest level of functioning possible.
- Priorities include psychosocial support; prevention of scars and contractures; and resumption of activities, including work, family, and social roles.
- This phase can last for years.

HEALTH PROMOTION AND DISEASE PREVENTION

- Ensure that the number and placement of fire extinguishers and smoke alarms in the home is adequate and operable. Family members should know how to use the extinguishers.
- Keep emergency numbers near the phone. Qs
- Have a family exit and meeting plan for fires. No one should ever re-enter a burning building.
- In the event that clothing or skin is on fire, "stop, drop, and roll" to extinguish the fire.
- Store matches and lighters out of reach and out of sight of children and adults who lack the ability to protect themselves.
- Reduce the setting on water heaters to 48.9° C (120° F).
- Have an annual professional inspection and cleaning of the chimney and fireplace.
- Turn handles of pots and pans to the side, or use back burners.
- Don't leave hot cups on the edge of the counter.
- Cover electrical outlets.
- Keep flammable objects away from space heaters.
- Wear gloves when handling chemicals.
- Wear protective clothing during sun exposure and to use sunscreen.
- Avoid using tanning beds.
- Avoid smoking in bed and when under the influence of alcohol or sedating medications.
- Do not smoke or have open flames in a room where oxygen is in use.
- Never add flammable substances (gasoline, lighter fluid, kerosene) to an open flame.

DATA COLLECTION

RISK FACTORS

Inhalation injury

OLDER ADULTS ©
- Higher risk for damage to subcutaneous tissue, muscle, connective tissue, and bone because of thinner skin
- Higher risk for complications from burns due to chronic illnesses (diabetes mellitus, cardiovascular disease)

EXPECTED FINDINGS

- Report of burn agent (dry heat, moist heat, chemical, electrical, ionizing radiation)
- Duration of contact
- Body area of the burn
- Demographic data: age, weight, height
- Health history, including pre-existing illnesses

PHYSICAL FINDINGS (67.2)

67.2 Burn staging

epidermis

dermis

subcutaneous tissue

muscle

bone

superficial

superficial partial thickness

deep partial thickness

full thickness

deep full thickness

Levels of care

Inhalation damage findings include singed nasal hair, eyebrows, and eyelashes; sooty sputum; hoarseness; wheezing; edema of the nasal septum; and smoky-smelling breath. Indications of the impending loss of the airway include hoarseness, brassy cough, drooling or difficulty swallowing, and audible wheezing, crowing, and stridor. Qs

Carbon monoxide inhalation (from burns in an enclosed area) findings include headache, weakness, dizziness, confusion, erythema (pink or cherry red skin) and upper airway edema, followed by sloughing of the respiratory tract mucosa.

Hypovolemia and shock can result from fluid shifts from the intercellular and intravascular space to the interstitial space. Additional findings include hypotension, tachycardia, and decreased cardiac output.

LABORATORY TESTS

Resuscitation phase

Initial fluid shift (occurs in the first 12 hr and continues for 24 to 36 hr)
- **CBC** with differential
  - **Hct and Hgb** elevated (hemoconcentration) due to the loss of fluid volume and the fluid shift into the interstitial space (third spacing)
- **Glucose** elevated due to stress
- **BUN** elevated due to fluid loss
- **Carboxyhemoglobin** more than 10% strongly indicates smoke inhalation

ELECTROLYTES
- **Sodium** decreased due to third spacing (hyponatremia)
- **Potassium** increased due to cell destruction (hyperkalemia)

OTHER: total protein, albumin, ABGs, liver enzymes, urinalysis, and clotting studies

Fluid remobilization

Starts at about 24 hr; diuretic stage begins at 48 to 72 hr after injury
- **Hgb and Hct** decreased (hemodilution) due to the fluid shift from the interstitial space back into vascular fluid
- **WBC count**: initial increase then decrease with left shift
- **Blood glucose** elevated due to the stress response
- **ABGs:** slight hypoxemia and metabolic acidosis
- **Total protein and albumin** low due to fluid loss

ELECTROLYTES
- **Sodium** remains decreased due to kidney and wound loss
- **Potassium** decreased due to kidney loss and movement back into cells (hypokalemia)

DIAGNOSTIC PROCEDURES

Diagnostic studies can include kidney scans, computed tomography, ultrasonography, bronchoscopy, and magnetic resonance imaging to determine extent of the burn injury.

PATIENT-CENTERED CARE

NURSING CARE

Minor burns

- Stop the burning process. Q︎EBP
  - Remove clothing or jewelry that might conduct heat.
  - Apply cool water soaks or run cool water over injury; do not use ice.
  - Flush chemical burns with a large volume of water.
  - Cover the burn with a clean cloth to prevent contamination and hypothermia.
  - Provide warmth.
- Provide analgesics.
- Cleanse with mild soap and tepid water. (Avoid excess friction.)
- Use antimicrobial ointment.
- Apply a dressing (nonadherent, hydrocolloid) if clothing is irritating the burn.
- Instruct the family to avoid using greasy lotions or butter on the burn.
- Instruct the family to observe for evidence of infection.
- Determine the need for a tetanus immunization.

Moderate and major burns

During the initial (resuscitation) phase (from the time of injury to 12 to 48 hr later) following a major burn, sympathetic nervous system manifestations such as tachycardia, increased respiratory rate, decreased gastrointestinal motility, and increased blood glucose are expected findings.

Cardiovascular system: Presence of edema, central and peripheral pulses, capillary refill, pulse oximetry, invasive or noninvasive blood pressure, and electrocardiographic changes

Respiratory system
- Monitor respiratory rate and depth.
- Upper airway edema becomes pronounced 8 to 12 hr after the beginning of fluid resuscitation. Crowing, stridor, or dyspnea requires nasal or oral intubation.
- Provide humidified supplemental oxygen.
- Support the airway and ventilation. Mechanical ventilation and paralytic medications (atracurium or vecuronium) can become necessary.
- Provide care for tracheotomy when long-term intubation is expected.
- Monitor and maintain chest tubes.
- Instruct the client to cough, breathe deeply, and use incentive spirometry every hour.
- Suction (endotracheal or nasotracheal) every hour or as needed. Consider the need for additional analgesics.

Gastrointestinal system
- Clients at risk for aspiration might need nasogastric tube insertion. Some clients experience gastroparesis and vomiting.
- Monitor stool, vomitus, and gastric secretions for blood.
- Keep the head of the bed elevated at all times.

Urinary system
- Insert an indwelling urinary catheter.
- Monitor I&O.
- Monitor urine characteristics, specific gravity, BUN, creatinine, and sodium.

Fluid replacement to maintain cardiac output
- Hypovolemic shock is a common cause of death in the resuscitation phase.
- Ensure IV access is initiated using a large-bore needle. If burns cover a large area of the body, the client requires insertion of a central venous catheter or intraosseous catheter.
- Fluid replacement is important during the first 24 hr.
- Third spacing (capillary leak syndrome) is a continuous leak of plasma from the vascular space into the interstitial space, which results in electrolyte imbalance and hypotension.
- Rapid fluid replacement during the emergent phase maintains tissue perfusion and prevents hypovolemic (burn) shock.
- Fluid resuscitation meets individual client needs (TBSA of burn, burn depth, inhalation injury, associated injuries, age, urine output, cardiac output, blood pressure, status of electrolytes).
- Ensure administration of half of the total 24-hr IV fluid volume within the first 8 hr and the remaining volume over the next 16 hr. Q︎EBP
- Monitor infusion of isotonic crystalloid solutions (0.9% sodium chloride, lactated Ringer's).
- Monitor infusion of colloid solutions (albumin, synthetic plasma expanders) after the first 24 hr of burn recovery.
- Monitor vital signs.
- Monitor for fluid overload (edema, engorged neck veins, rapid and thready pulse, lung crackles, wheezes).
- Weigh the client daily.
- Maintain urine output of 0.5 mL/kg/hr, which is around 30 mL/hr for the average client.
- Prepare to assist with the administration and monitoring of blood products.
- Monitor for manifestations of shock.
  - Alterations in sensorium (confusion)
  - Increased capillary refill time
  - Urine output less than 30 mL/hr
  - Rapid elevations of temperature
  - Decreased bowel sounds
  - Decreased blood pressure
- Maintain thermoregulation.

Hypothermia
- The skin helps control the body's temperature. With skin injury, the body loses heat.
- Use warm, inspired air; a warm room; and warming blankets. Ensure the use of warmers for infusing fluids.

Hyperthermia
- Hypermetabolic conditions increase core body temperature.
- Low-grade temperature develops as a compensatory mechanism.

Pain management

- Monitor pain and the effectiveness of pain treatment.
- Ensure that routes other than IV are avoided during the resuscitation phase due to decreased absorption from other routes.
- Request opioid analgesics (morphine, hydromorphone, fentanyl) or anesthetics (ketamine, nitrous oxide). QEBP
- Monitor for respiratory depression in clients who receive opioid analgesics. Qs
- The use of patient-controlled analgesia (PCA) is appropriate for some clients. PCA helps manage pain, and the client benefits from having a sense of control.
- Administer pain medication prior to dressing changes and procedures.
- Use nonpharmacologic methods for pain control (guided imagery, music therapy, therapeutic touch) to enhance the effects of analgesic medications and manage pain more effectively.

Infection prevention

- Maintain a protective environment.
- Restrict plants and flowers due to the risk of contact with *Pseudomonas aeruginosa*.
- Restrict consumption of fresh fruits and vegetables.
- Limit visitors.
- Monitor for manifestations of infection and report them to the provider.
- Use client-dictated equipment (blood pressure cuffs, thermometers).
- Administer tetanus toxoid.
- Administer antibiotics to treat infection. Monitor peak and trough levels.
- Use strict asepsis with wound care.

Nutritional support

- Large burn areas create a hypermetabolic and hypercatabolic state. The client can require 50% to 150% increased calorie intake, which may be more than 5,000 calories/day.
- Increase caloric intake to meet increased metabolic demands and prevent hypoglycemia.
- Increase protein intake to prevent tissue breakdown and promote healing.
- Decreased gastrointestinal motility and increased caloric needs require enteral therapy or total parenteral nutrition.

Restoration of mobility

- Maintain correct body alignment, splint extremities, and facilitate position changes to prevent contractures.
- Maintain active and passive range of motion.
- Assist with ambulation as soon as the client is stable.
- Apply pressure dressings to prevent contractures and scarring.
- Monitor areas at high risk for pressure sores (heels, sacrum, back of the head).

Psychological support of client and family

- Provide emotional support. QPCC
- Assist with coping.

MEDICATIONS

Apply topical agents (antimicrobial creams, ointments, solutions).

Silver nitrate 0.5%

Apply with a gauze dressing.

ADVANTAGES
- Reduces fluid evaporation
- Bacteriostatic
- Inexpensive

DISADVANTAGES
- Does not penetrate eschar
- Stains clothing and linen
- Depletes sodium and potassium

Silver sulfadiazine 1%

- Collect data regarding allergies to sulfonamides.
- Apply a thin layer with a clean glove.

ADVANTAGES
- Usually pain-free
- Effective against gram-negative bacteria, gram-positive bacteria, and yeast

DISADVANTAGES
- Can cause transient neutropenia
- Contraindicated with sulfa allergy
- Penetrates eschar minimally
- Can cause a gray or blue-green discoloration
- Decreases granulocyte formation

Mafenide acetate

- Collect data regarding client allergies to sulfonamides.
- Apply twice daily.

ADVANTAGES
- Penetrates eschar and goes into underlying tissues
- Bacteriostatic against gram-negative and gram-positive bacteria

DISADVANTAGES
- Painful to apply and remove
- Can cause metabolic acidosis

Polymyxin B/bacitracin

Apply every 2 to 8 hr to keep the burn moist.

ADVANTAGES
- Bacteriostatic against gram-positive organisms
- Painless and easy to apply

DISADVANTAGES: Hypersensitivity can develop.

Gentamicin topical

Aminoglycoside anti-infective agent

ADVANTAGES: Bactericidal aminoglycoside

DISADVANTAGES
- Nephrotoxic: Monitor kidney function.
- Ototoxic: Monitor for hearing loss weekly.

THERAPEUTIC PROCEDURES

Escharotomy

Incision through the eschar relieves pressure from the constricting force of fluid buildup under circumferential burns on the extremity or chest and improves circulation.

Fasciotomy

Incision through eschar and fascia relieves tissue pressure when escharotomy alone does not.

Wound care

Nonsurgical management, such as hyperbaric oxygen therapy

NURSING ACTIONS QPCC
- Premedicate the client with an analgesic.
- Remove all previous dressings.
- Monitor for odors, drainage, and discharge. Monitor for sloughing, eschar, bleeding, and new skin-cell regeneration.
- Cleanse the wound thoroughly, removing all previous ointments.
- Assist with debridement.
  - **Mechanical:** Use scissors and forceps to cut away the dead tissue during the hydrotherapy treatment.
  - **Hydrotherapy:** Assist the client into a warm tub of water or use warm running water, as if to shower, to cleanse the wound.
    - Use mild soap or detergent to wash burns gently, and then rinse with room-temperature water.
    - Encourage the client to exercise his joints during the hydrotherapy treatment.
  - **Enzymatic:** Apply a topical enzyme to break down and remove dead tissue.
  - Apply topical enzyme agents, such as collagenase, to the wound during a daily dressing change.
- Ensure that the client does not become hypothermic during the treatment.
- Use surgical asepsis while applying a thin layer of topical antibiotic ointment and cover it with a dressing.

Skin coverings

Biologic skin coverings temporarily promote healing of large burns. Additionally, biologic skin coverings promote the retention of water and protein and provide coverage of nerve endings, thus reducing pain. The provider stipulates whether to leave skin coverings open or protect them with a dressing.
- Allograft (homograft): Skin donations from human cadavers for partial- and full-thickness burn wounds
- Xenograft (heterograft): Skin from animals, such as pigs, for partial-thickness burn wounds
- Amnion: From human placenta; requires frequent changes
- Cultured skin: Grows from a small specimen of epidermal cells from an unburned area
- Artificial skin: Two layers of skin made beef collagen and shark cartilage
- Synthetic skin coverings: For partial-thickness burn wounds

Permanent skin coverings can be the treatment of choice for burns covering large areas of the body.
- Autografts: Skin from another area of the client's body
  - Sheet graft: Sheet of skin for covering the wound
  - Mesh graft: Sheet of skin in which a mesher has created small slits, so the graft can stretch over large areas of the burn
- Artificial skin: Synthetic product for faster healing of partial- and full-thickness burns
- Cultured epithelium: Epithelial cells to use for clients who have few grafting sites

NURSING ACTIONS
- Maintain immobilization of graft sites.
- Elevate extremities.
- Provide wound care to the donor site.
- Administer analgesics.
- Monitor for infection before and after applying skin coverings or grafts. QEBP
  - Discoloration of unburned skin surrounding burn wound
  - Green subcutaneous fat
  - Degeneration of granulation tissue
  - Development of subeschar hemorrhage
  - Hyperventilation indicating systemic involvement of infection
  - Unstable body temperature
- Determine the client's level of pain. Provide additional measures to control donor site pain.

CLIENT EDUCATION
- Keep the extremity elevated.
- Report manifestations of infection.
- Continue to perform range-of-motion exercises, and work with a physical therapist to prevent contractures.
- Observe the wound for infection and perform wound care.

INTERPROFESSIONAL CARE

- Recommend referrals to a dietitian, social worker (for community support services), psychological counselor, and physical therapist.
- Respiratory therapy can help improve pulmonary function.
- Consult a case manager to coordinate the client's postdischarge care.
- Recommend a referral for home health nursing care. QTC
- Recommend a referral to occupational therapy for evaluation of the home environment and assistance to relearn how to perform ADLs.

COMPLICATIONS

Airway injury

- Thermal injuries to the airway can result from steam or chemical inhalation, aspiration of scalding liquid, and external explosion while breathing. If the injury took place in an enclosed space, suspect carbon monoxide poisoning.
- Effects might not manifest for 24 to 48 hr. They include progressive hoarseness, brassy cough, difficulty swallowing, drooling, copious secretions, adventitious breath sounds, and expiratory sounds that include audible wheezes, crowing, and stridor.

NURSING ACTIONS
- Support the airway and ventilation, and administer supplemental oxygen.
- Instruct the client and family about airway management, such as deep breathing, coughing, and elevating the head of the bed.

Fluid and electrolyte imbalances

NURSING ACTIONS
- Monitor fluid volume status. Weigh the client daily, and document I&O.
- Monitor laboratory results and compare them to previous data.
- Ensure the administration of IV fluids and electrolytes.

CLIENT EDUCATION: Alert the provider immediately of manifestations of electrolyte imbalances.

Wound infections

Burns can leave skin vulnerable to bacterial infection and increase risk of infection and sepsis.

NURSING ACTIONS
- Monitor for discoloration, edema, odor, and drainage.
- Monitor for fluctuations in temperature and heart rate.
- Obtain specimens for wound culture.
- Administer antibiotics.
- Monitor laboratory results, observing for anemia and infection.
- Use surgical aseptic technique with dressing changes.
- Instruct the client and family about the importance of infection control.

Muscle and joint mobility

Scarring and contractures: Deep burns can limit movement of bones and joints. Scar tissue can form and cause shortening and tightening of skin, muscles, and tendons (contractures).

NURSING ACTIONS
- Assist with active or passive range-of-motion exercises at least three times daily.
- Encourage neutral positions with limited flexion. Encourage the use of splints.
- Encourage ambulation as soon as possible.
- Use compression dressings for up to 24 months to increase mobility and reduce scarring.

Application Exercises

1. A nurse in a provider's office is collecting data from a client who has a severe sunburn. Which of the following classifications should the nurse use to document this burn?
   - A. Superficial thickness
   - B. Superficial partial thickness
   - C. Deep partial thickness
   - D. Full thickness

2. A nurse is caring for a client who has sustained burns over 35% of his total body surface area. Most of the burns are full-thickness burns on the arms, face, neck, and shoulders. The client's voice has become hoarse. He has a brassy cough and is drooling. These findings are indications of which of the following?
   - A. Pulmonary edema
   - B. Bacterial pneumonia
   - C. Inhalation injury
   - D. Carbon monoxide poisoning

3. A nurse is collecting data from a client who sustained deep partial-thickness and full-thickness burns over 40% of his body 24 hr ago. Which of the following findings should the nurse expect? (Select all that apply.)
   - A. Dyspnea
   - B. Bradycardia
   - C. Hyperkalemia
   - D. Hyponatremia
   - E. Decreased hematocrit

4. A nurse is assisting with the care of a client who sustained deep partial-thickness and full-thickness burns over 60% of his body 24 hr ago and is requesting pain medication. The nurse should ensure the medication is administered using which of the following routes to administer the medication?
   - A. Subcutaneous
   - B. Oral
   - C. Intravenous
   - D. Transdermal

5. A nurse is assisting with the plan of care for an adult client who sustained severe burn injuries. Which of the following interventions should the nurse include in the plan of care? (Select all that apply.)
   - A. Limit visitors in the client's room.
   - B. Encourage fresh vegetables in the diet.
   - C. Increase protein intake.
   - D. Instruct the client to consume 2,000 calories/day.
   - E. Restrict fresh flowers in the room.

Application Exercises Key

1. A. **CORRECT:** A sunburn is a superficial thickness burn. Superficial burns damage the top layer of the skin.

   B. A superficial partial-thickness burn results from flames or scalds. This damages the entire epidermis layer of the skin.

   C. A deep partial-thickness burn can result from contact with hot grease. This affects the deep layers of the skin.

   D. A full-thickness burn can result from contact with hot tar. This affects the dermis and sometimes the subcutaneous fat layer.

   Ⓝ *NCLEX® Connection: Physiological Adaptation, Basic Pathophysiology*

2. A. Difficulty breathing and production of pink frothy sputum indicate pulmonary edema.

   B. Productive cough and fever are indicative of a bacterial infection.

   C. **CORRECT:** Wheezing and hoarseness indicate inhalation injury with impending loss of the airway. These require immediate reporting to the provider.

   D. Confusion and headaches indicate carbon monoxide poisoning.

   Ⓝ *NCLEX® Connection: Physiological Adaptation, Basic Pathophysiology*

3. A. **CORRECT:** Dyspnea can occur during the initial phase following a burn due to airway injury and fluid shifts.

   B. Tachycardia occurs during the initial phase following a burn due to sympathetic nervous system compensation.

   C. **CORRECT:** Hyperkalemia occurs during the initial phase following a burn as a result of leakage of fluid from the intracellular space.

   D. **CORRECT:** Hyponatremia occurs during the initial phase of a burn as a result in sodium retention in the interstitial space.

   E. Hematocrit increases during the initial phase of a burn due to hemoconcentration.

   Ⓝ *NCLEX® Connection: Physiological Adaptation, Basic Pathophysiology*

4. A. The nurse should ensure the medication is not given by a subcutaneous injection due to the difficulty of absorption from tissue during the resuscitation phase.

   B. The nurse should ensure the medication is not given orally (including buccal, sublingual) due to decreased motility in the gastrointestinal tract during the resuscitation phase.

   C. **CORRECT:** The nurse should ensure the use of the IV route for the administration of pain medication for rapid absorption and fast pain relief during the resuscitation phase.

   D. The nurse should ensure the medication is not given using the transdermal route of administration due to delays in absorption during the resuscitation phase.

   Ⓝ *NCLEX® Connection: Physiological Adaptation, Basic Pathophysiology*

5. A. **CORRECT:** The nurse should limit the number of visitors and the amount of time they can visit to decrease the risk of infection.

   B. The client should restrict consumption of fresh vegetables due to the presence of bacteria on the surface and the increased risk for infection.

   C. **CORRECT:** The client should increase protein consumption, which promotes wound healing and prevents tissue breakdown.

   D. The client should consume up to 5,000 calories/day because caloric needs double or triple beginning 4 to 12 days following the burn.

   E. **CORRECT:** Flowers should not be in the client's room due to the bacteria they carry, which increase the risk for infection.

   Ⓝ *NCLEX® Connection: Basic Care and Comfort, Nutrition and Oral Hydration*

PRACTICE Active Learning Scenario

A nurse is reviewing the plan of care of a client who has an autograft skin covering over a burn injury with a nurse who will assume care of the client at the end of the day. What should the nurse include in the review? Use the ATI Active Learning Template: Therapeutic Procedure to complete this item.

DESCRIPTION OF PROCEDURE

NURSING INTERVENTIONS: Describe at least four.

PRACTICE Answer

Using the ATI Active Learning Template: Therapeutic Procedure

DESCRIPTION OF PROCEDURE: An autograft is donor skin from another area of the client's body. This is a permanent skin covering and used for burns on larger areas of the body.

NURSING INTERVENTIONS
- Maintain immobilization of the graft site.
- Elevate the extremity.
- Provide wound care to the donor site.
- Administer analgesics.
- Monitor for evidence of infection before and after skin coverings or grafts are applied.
  - Discoloration of unburned skin surrounding burn wound
  - Green color to subcutaneous fat
  - Degeneration of granulation tissue
  - Development of subeschar hemorrhage
  - Hyperventilation indicating systemic involvement of infection
  - Unstable body temperature

Ⓝ *NCLEX® Connection: Physiological Adaptation, Basic Pathophysiology*

When reviewing the following chapters, keep in mind the relevant topics and tasks of the NCLEX outline, in particular:

Pharmacological Therapies

ADVERSE EFFECTS/CONTRAINDICATIONS/SIDE EFFECTS/ INTERACTIONS: Monitor the client for actual and potential adverse effects of medications (prescribed, over-the-counter, herbal supplements).

DOSAGE CALCULATIONS: Use clinical decision making when calculating dosages.

MEDICATION ADMINISTRATION
Collect required data prior to medication administration.

Reinforce client teaching on self-administration of medications (insulin, subcutaneous insulin pump).

Reduction of Risk Potential

DIAGNOSTIC TESTS: Perform diagnostic testing (blood glucose, oxygen saturation, testing for occult blood).

LABORATORY VALUES
Perform blood glucose monitoring.

Reinforce client teaching on the purposes of laboratory tests.

Monitor diagnostic or laboratory test results.

Notify the primary health care provider about the client's laboratory test results.

Physiological Adaptation

ALTERATIONS IN BODY SYSTEMS
Identify and/or intervene to control signs of hypoglycemia or hyperglycemia.

Provide care to correct the client's alteration in body systems.

Reinforce education to the client regarding care and condition.

BASIC PATHOPHYSIOLOGY: Apply knowledge of pathophysiology to monitoring the client for alterations in body systems.

FLUID AND ELECTROLYTE IMBALANCES: Provide interventions to restore the client's fluid and/or electrolyte balance.

CHAPTER 68   *Endocrine Diagnostic Procedures*

Disorders of the endocrine system relate to an excess or deficiency of a hormone, or to a defect in a receptor site for a hormone. Laboratory tests for evaluating endocrine function vary according to the organ or system under analysis.

Many of these are blood, urine, or saliva tests that determine an excess or lack of a particular hormone in the body. Some of these tests stimulate a reaction in the body that can facilitate diagnosis of a particular disorder.

Stimulation testing involves giving hormones to stimulate the target gland to determine if the gland is capable of adequate hormone production. Suppression testing involves giving medications or substances to evaluate the body's ability to suppress excessive hormone production.

Posterior pituitary gland

The posterior pituitary gland secretes the hormone vasopressin (antidiuretic hormone [ADH]). ADH increases permeability of the renal distal tubules, causing the kidneys to reabsorb water.

- A deficiency of ADH causes diabetes insipidus, which is the excretion of a large quantity of dilute urine.
- Excessive secretion of ADH causes the syndrome of inappropriate antidiuretic hormone (SIADH). With SIADH, the kidneys retain water, urine becomes concentrated, urinary output decreases, and extracellular fluid volume increases.
- Diagnostic tests for the posterior pituitary gland include the water deprivation test, ADH level, serum and urine electrolytes and osmolality, and urine specific gravity.

INDICATIONS

Water deprivation test

The water or fluid deprivation test measures the kidneys' ability to concentrate urine in light of an increased plasma osmolality and a low plasma vasopressin level. It requires a controlled setting with careful observation of the client for complications of dehydration.

- This test helps identify causes and types of diabetes insipidus (DI).
- Osmolality increases with dehydration and decreases with overhydration, so it provides information about fluid and electrolyte balance.
- Contraindications include impaired kidney function, uncontrolled diabetes mellitus, hypovolemia, and adrenal or thyroid hormone deficiency.

Tests that diagnose SIADH

- ADH level
- Serum and urine electrolytes and osmolality
- Urine specific gravity

CONSIDERATIONS

Water deprivation test

PREPROCEDURE
- Begin the test by withholding fluids for a specific number of hours, or until the client loses a specific amount of body weight.
- Ensure the client has an IV access.

INTRAPROCEDURE
- The test involves ADH administration.
- The client requires hourly urine tests for specific gravity and osmolality, hourly weights, and ongoing vital sign monitoring.
- Monitor closely to identify and intervene for severe dehydration.
  - Poor skin turgor
  - Dizziness and weakness
  - Orthostatic hypotension
  - Flat neck veins
  - Tachycardia
  - Dry skin and mucous membranes

POSTPROCEDURE
- Promote client rehydration.
- Monitor for indications of orthostatic hypotension and protect the client from falls. Qs

ADH level

- The client should fast and avoid stress for 12 hr prior to the test.
- Some medications (acetaminophen, antidepressants, diuretics, opioids, phenytoin) can interfere with the test. Review medications with the provider.
- Collect a blood sample and transport it to the laboratory within 10 min.

Electrolytes

- No preprocedure or postprocedure care is necessary.
- The laboratory analyzes samples of blood for electrolyte components.

Urine electrolytes and osmolality

- No preprocedure or postprocedure care is necessary.
- The laboratory analyzes samples of urine for electrolyte components.

Urine specific gravity

The laboratory usually performs this test. Nurses can use a calibrated hydrometer or a temperature-compensated refractometer to perform it on a clinical unit.

INTERPRETATION OF FINDINGS

Water deprivation test

Based on the change in urine osmolality during the test the provider can determine the type of DI the client has.

ADH

Increased ADH indicates SIADH.

EXPECTED REFERENCE RANGE: 1 to 5 pg/mL (1 to 5 ng/L)

Electrolytes

Low serum sodium is an expected finding with SIADH.

EXPECTED REFERENCE RANGE: Sodium: 136 to 145 mEq/L

Urine electrolytes and osmolality

- High urine sodium content is an expected finding of SIADH.
- Increased urine osmolality is an expected finding of SIADH.
- Decreased urine osmolality is an expected finding of diabetes insipidus.

EXPECTED REFERENCE RANGE
- **Urine sodium**: 40 to 220 mEq/24 hr in a 24-hr collection or greater than 20 mEq/L in a random urine collection
- **Urine potassium:** 25 to 100 mEq/L/24 hr, depending on potassium intake
- **Urine chloride:** 110 to 250 mEq/24 hr
- **Urine osmolality:** 50 to 1,200 mOsm/kg H_2O, depending on fluid intake

Urine-specific gravity

A decrease in urine output and an increase in urine specific gravity occur as a result of excess production of ADH.

EXPECTED REFERENCE RANGE: 1.010 to 1.025

COMPLICATIONS

Water deprivation test

Dehydration can occur due to a decrease in vascular volume.

NURSING ACTIONS
- Monitor closely for early indications of dehydration, including postural hypotension, tachycardia, and dizziness.
- Discontinue the test if the client loses more than 2 kg (or a prescribed amount) of body weight.

Adrenal cortex

- A hyperfunctioning adrenal cortex and an excess production of cortisol characterize Cushing's disease and Cushing's syndrome (hypercortisolism).
- Hypofunctioning of the adrenal cortex and a consequent lack of adequate amounts of serum cortisol characterize Addison's disease.
- Diagnostic tests for the adrenal cortex include the dexamethasone suppression test, plasma and salivary cortisol, 24-hr urine for cortisol, adrenocorticotropic hormone (ACTH), and ACTH stimulation tests.
- A CT scan and an MRI identify atrophy of the adrenal glands causing hypofunction.

INDICATIONS

Dexamethasone suppression test

Determines whether dexamethasone (a synthetic steroid similar to cortisol) has an effect on cortisol levels

CONSIDERATIONS

Dexamethasone suppression test

- Typically, the client takes a dose of dexamethasone by mouth. A blood sample the next morning determines whether cortisol is present.
- A low dose of dexamethasone screens for Cushing's disease; high doses help determine the cause of the disease.
- The client should stop taking some medications (diuretics, antibiotics, oral contraceptives) and try to reduce stress prior to and during testing, as these can affect the test results.

Plasma cortisol

The provider determines the best time for testing, usually with blood sampling at 0800 and again at 1600.

Salivary cortisol

A salivary cushion pad inside the cheek, directly over the salivary gland, collects the sample.

Urinary cortisol

The laboratory measures cortisol in a 24-hr urine collection.

ACTH

- ACTH is most accurate with morning blood samples.
- Place the venous blood sample in an ice water bath immediately after obtaining the sample. Q EBP

ACTH stimulation test

Blood sampling for plasma cortisol levels occurs 30 min and 1 hr after cosyntropin IV administration.

INTERPRETATION OF FINDINGS

Dexamethasone suppression test

- When the pituitary gland produces decreased amounts of ACTH, the adrenal glands release decreased amounts of cortisol.
- When clients who have Cushing's disease receive dexamethasone, there is no decrease in the production of ACTH and cortisol.

Plasma cortisol

High levels can indicate hypercortisolism (Cushing's disease). Low levels can indicate hypocortisolism (Addison's disease).

EXPECTED REFERENCE RANGE
- Expected range varies according to the following times.
  - 0800: 5 to 23 mcg/dL
  - 1600: 3 to 13 mcg/dL
- Range is slightly decreased for children.
- Cortisol levels vary according to the time of day. Because it has a diurnal (daily) pattern, higher levels are present in the early morning.
- Expected values are transposed for clients who consistently work at night and sleep during the day.

Salivary cortisol

High levels indicate hypercortisolism.

EXPECTED REFERENCE RANGE
- Expected range varies according to the following times.
  - 0700 to 0900: 100 to 750 ng/dL
  - 1500 to 1700: less than 401 ng/dL
  - 2300 to 2400: less than 100 ng/d
- Salivary cortisol is at its lowest point around midnight and at its highest point in the early morning.

Urinary cortisol

High levels can indicate hypercortisolism (Cushing's disease). Low levels can indicate hypocortisolism (Addison's disease).

EXPECTED REFERENCE RANGE: Less than 100 mcg/day in a 24-hr urine collection

ACTH

ACTH increases with Addison's disease and either increases or decreases with Cushing's disease (depending on the cause of the syndrome).

ACTH stimulation test

- An increase in cortisol after administration of ACTH is expected.
- If cortisol does not increase after administration of cosyntropin (an ACTH-like medication), the test is positive for Addison's disease or hypocortisolism.
- The ACTH stimulation test determines the functioning of the pituitary gland in relation to stimulating the secretion of adrenal hormones of cortisol.
- A 24-hr or 3-day test is an option with IV infusions of cosyntropin over several hours.

Adrenal medulla

- Disorders of the adrenal medulla, such as a tumor, can cause hypersecretion of catecholamines, resulting in stimulation of a sympathetic response, such as tachycardia, hypertension, and diaphoresis. These tests determine whether the cause of a client's unrelieved hypertension is a pheochromocytoma.
- Diagnostic tests for the adrenal medulla include plasma-free metanephrine testing.

INDICATIONS

Plasma-free metanephrine test

- Identification of a pheochromocytoma
- The laboratory tests blood samples for both metanephrine and normetanephrine.

CONSIDERATIONS

Plasma-free metanephrine test

PREPROCEDURE
- Caffeine, alcohol, and several medications interfere with the test results. Review the client's medications, including acetaminophen, with the provider. The client should stop taking a acetaminophen for 48 hr prior to test.
- Physical exercise and increased stress can interfere with test results.
- Determine the client's stress level. Having the client lie down and rest for 30 min prior to the test can reduce stress.
- Notify the provider about any interfering factors before obtaining a blood sample for the test.

CLIENT EDUCATION
- Maintain a moderate level of activity.
- Restrict caffeine and alcohol.

INTERPRETATION OF FINDINGS

Plasma-free metanephrine test

- Elevation of both metanephrine and normetanephrine above the expected reference range indicates a pheochromocytoma.
- If only one of these catecholamines is elevated, pheochromocytoma is probable.

Carbohydrate metabolism

- Insulin deficiency (as in type 1 diabetes mellitus) and insulin resistance (as in type 2 diabetes mellitus) can alter carbohydrate metabolism, resulting in hyperglycemia.
- Diagnostic tests to evaluate carbohydrate metabolism include fasting (no caloric intake for 8 hr) blood glucose, oral glucose tolerance testing, and glycosylated hemoglobin (HbA1c).

CONSIDERATIONS

Fasting blood glucose

- Ensure that the client has fasted (no food or beverages other than water) for the 8 hr prior to blood sampling.
- The client should postpone taking antidiabetic medications until after the blood sampling.

Random (casual) blood glucose

- Refers to any time of day without regard to mealtime.
- No preprocedure or postprocedure care is necessary. The test requires obtaining a random blood sample.

Oral glucose tolerance test

- Instruct the client to consume a balanced diet for 3 days prior to the test and fast for 10 to 12 hr prior to the test.
- The technician will obtain a blood specimen for a fasting blood glucose level at start of the test.
- The client then consumes a specific amount of glucose.
- The technician obtains blood samples at 30 min, 1 hr, 2 hr, 3 hr, and sometimes 4 hr after the client consumes glucose. Monitor for hypoglycemia throughout the procedure.

Glycosylated hemoglobin (HbA1c)

- No preprocedure or postprocedure care is necessary. The test requires obtaining a random blood sample.
- Fasting is not necessary.

INTERPRETATION OF FINDINGS

Fasting blood glucose

- Determines blood glucose when the client has consumed no foods or fluids (other than water) for the past 8 hr.
- Fasting blood glucose greater than 126 mg/dL on two occasions can indicate diabetes mellitus.

- Fasting blood glucose levels 100 to 125 mg/dL can indicate prediabetes.

EXPECTED REFERENCE RANGE
- 70 to 110 mg/dL for adults and children older than 2 years
- Slightly increased for adults older than 50 years

Random (casual) blood glucose

EXPECTED REFERENCE RANGE: Less than 200 mg/dL

Oral glucose tolerance test

- Blood glucose greater than 200 mg/dL at 2 hr following glucose ingestion can indicate diabetes. The provider might repeat the test on another day to check results.
- Determines the ability to metabolize a standard amount of glucose.

EXPECTED REFERENCE RANGE
- Less than 200 mg/dL 1 hr following glucose ingestion
- Less than 140 mg/dL 2 hr following glucose ingestion
- 70 to 115 mg/dL 3 or 4 hr following glucose ingestion

Glycosylated hemoglobin (HbA1c)

- HbA1c is the best indicator of an average blood glucose level for the past 120 days.
- Assists in evaluating treatment effectiveness and adherence to the diet plan, medication regimen, and exercise schedule.
- 6.5% to 8% indicates diabetes.
- Greater than 8% indicates poor control of diabetes.

EXPECTED REFERENCE RANGE: 5.7% or less indicates that the client does not have diabetes mellitus.

Thyroid and anterior pituitary gland

Hyperthyroidism and hypothyroidism are disorders in which there are inappropriate amounts of the thyroid hormones triiodothyronine (T_3) and thyroxine (T_4) circulating. These inappropriate amounts of T_3 and T_4 cause an increase or decrease in metabolic rate that affects all body systems.
- The anterior pituitary gland secretes thyroid stimulating hormone (TSH). Hyposecretion of TSH can lead to secondary hypothyroidism, and hypersecretion of TSH can cause secondary hyperthyroidism.
- Diagnostic tests to evaluate the function of the thyroid and anterior pituitary glands include T_3, T_4, TSH, thyrotropin-releasing hormone (TRH) stimulation test, and radioactive iodine uptake.
- Ultrasounds and CT scans determine the size, shape, and presence of nodules and masses on these glands.

INDICATIONS

TSH

Results help monitor thyroid replacement therapy and differentiate types of thyroid disorders.

Thyroid scan

- A noninvasive gamma probe over the thyroid measures the amount of ^{123}I the gland absorbed.
- Evaluates size, shape, position and ability of the thyroid gland to function following an oral dose of ^{123}I

CONSIDERATIONS

T_3 and T_4

- No preprocedure or postprocedure care is necessary.
- The laboratory requires a random blood sample.

TSH

- No preprocedure or postprocedure care is necessary.
- The laboratory requires a random blood sample.
- TSH stimulates the release of thyroid hormone by the anterior pituitary gland.

TRH

Requires giving a bolus of thyrotropin-releasing hormone, and then assessing serum concentrations of TSH at intervals.

Thyroid scan

- The client receives an oral radioactive dose of ^{123}I, and a scintillation counter measures the amount the thyroid absorbed.

- Pregnancy and recent exposure to iodine-containing dye are contraindications. **Qs**

CLIENT EDUCATION: ^{123}I has a very short half life. Thus radiation precautions are not necessary for this test.

INTERPRETATION OF FINDINGS

T_3 and T_4

- Low levels indicate hypothyroidism.
- High levels indicate and hyperthyroidism.
- A high level of T_3 is a better indicator of hyperthyroidism than is T_4.

EXPECTED REFERENCE RANGE
- **T³:** 70 to 205 ng/dL
- **T⁴ (total):** 4.0 to 12.0 mcg/dL

TSH

- An increased value indicates primary hypothyroidism due to thyroid dysfunction or thyroiditis.
- A decreased value indicates hyperthyroidism (Graves' disease) or secondary hypothyroidism (due to pituitary or hypothalamus dysfunction).

TRH

- The expected reference range is relative to baseline.
- The TSH should double the baseline value shortly after administration of thyrotropin-releasing hormone.
- TSH that increases twofold or more above baseline indicates hypothyroidism.

Thyroid scan

Clients who have hyperthyroidism absorb high amounts (greater than 35%) of ^{123}I.

PRACTICE Active Learning Scenario

A nurse is contributing to the plan of care for a client who is scheduled for an oral glucose tolerance test. What interventions should the nurse recommend?

Use the ATI Active Learning Template: Diagnostic Procedure to complete this item to include the following.

INDICATIONS

INTERPRETATION OF FINDINGS

NURSING ACTIONS: Describe one preprocedure.

PRACTICE Answer

Using the ATI Active Learning Template: Diagnostic Procedure

INDICATIONS: The test determines the ability to metabolize a standard amount of glucose.

INTERPRETATION OF FINDINGS: Blood glucose greater than 200 mg/dL at 2 hr following glucose ingestion can indicate diabetes. The provider might repeat the test on another day to check results.

NURSING ACTIONS: Instruct the client to consume a balanced diet for 3 days prior to the test and fast for 10 to 12 hr prior to the test.

Ⓝ *NCLEX® Connection: Reduction of Risk Potential, Laboratory Values*

Application Exercises

1. A nurse is caring for a client who asks why the provider bases the medication regimen on the HbA1c instead of the log of morning fasting blood glucose results. Which of the following responses should the nurse make?

   A. "HbA1c measures how well insulin is regulating your blood glucose between meals."

   B. "HbA1c indicates how well you have regulated your blood glucose over the past 120 days."

   C. "HbA1c is the first test your provider prescribed to determine that you have diabetes."

   D. "HbA1c determines if you need an additional dose of insulin at this time."

2. A nurse is reviewing the laboratory findings for a client who might have hyperthyroidism. The nurse should identify that an elevation in which of the following substances indicates hyperthyroidism?

   A. Triiodothyronine

   B. Plasma-free metanephrine

   C. Urine cortisol

   D. Urine osmolality

3. A nurse is reviewing the medical record of a client who has syndrome of inappropriate antidiuretic hormone (SIADH). Which of the following laboratory findings should the nurse expect? (Select all that apply.)

   A. Low sodium

   B. High potassium

   C. Increased urine osmolality

   D. High urine sodium

   E. Increased urine specific gravity

4. A nurse is caring for a client who has primary adrenal insufficiency and is preparing to undergo an ACTH stimulation test. Which of the following findings should the nurse expect after an IV injection of cosyntropin?

   A. No change in plasma cortisol

   B. Elevated fasting blood glucose

   C. Decrease in sodium

   D. Increase in urinary output

5. A nurse is collecting data from a client during a water deprivation test. Which of the following manifestations should the nurse identify as a indicating dehydration?

   A. Bradycardia

   B. Orthostatic hypotension

   C. Neck vein distention

   D. Crackles in lungs

Application Exercises Key

1. A. Capillary glucose monitoring evaluates how well insulin is regulating blood glucose between meals.

   B. **CORRECT:** HbA1c measures blood glucose control over the past 120 days

   C. A fasting blood glucose is the first test providers prescribe to diagnose diabetes mellitus. HbA1c is not a screening test.

   D. Capillary glucose monitoring identifies the client's current blood glucose level and if an additional dose of insulin is needed at the present time.

   Ⓝ NCLEX® Connection: Reduction of Risk Potential, Laboratory Values

2. A. **CORRECT:** Increased triiodothyronine (T₃) indicates hyperthyroidism.

   B. An increase in plasma-free metanephrine indicates the presence of a pheochromocytoma (tumor of the cells of the adrenal medulla).

   C. A high cortisol level indicates hyperfunction of the adrenal cortex and can indicate that the client has Cushing's disease.

   D. Increased urine osmolality indicates SIADH.

   Ⓝ NCLEX® Connection: Reduction of Risk Potential, Laboratory Values

3. A. **CORRECT:** SIADH results in water retention, causing a low sodium level.

   B. SIADH does not affect potassium levels.

   C. **CORRECT:** SIADH results in an increase in urine osmolality due to the decreased urine volume.

   D. **CORRECT:** SIADH results in water retention, causing a high urine sodium level.

   E. **CORRECT:** SIADH results in water retention, causing an increase in urine specific gravity.

   Ⓝ NCLEX® Connection: Reduction of Risk Potential, Laboratory Values

4. A. **CORRECT:** No change in plasma cortisol indicates primary adrenal insufficiency (Addison's disease or hypocortisolism) after an IV injection of cosyntropin during an ACTH stimulation test due to an inadequate production of cortisol.

   B. An elevated fasting blood glucose helps identify diabetes mellitus.

   C. An increase in sodium indicates primary adrenal insufficiency.

   D. A decrease in urinary output indicates primary adrenal insufficiency.

   Ⓝ NCLEX® Connection: Pharmacological Therapies, Pharmacological Pain Management

5. A. The nurse should monitor for tachycardia during a water deprivation test due to dehydration.

   B. **CORRECT:** The nurse should identify orthostatic hypotension as a manifestation of dehydration, which can occur during a water deprivation test.

   C. Flat neck veins are likely during a water deprivation test due to dehydration.

   D. The nurse should monitor the client for dizziness rather than lung crackles during a water deprivation test.

   Ⓝ NCLEX® Connection: Physiological Adaptation, Fluid and Electrolyte Imbalances

CHAPTER 69 *Pituitary Disorders*

The pituitary gland (hypophysis) is known as the "master gland" due to its regulation of many bodily functions. The hypothalamus, at the base of the skull, sits above the pituitary gland and regulates its function. Two lobes make up the gland: the anterior (adenohypophysis) and posterior (neurohypophysis), which secrete regulatory hormones. The anterior pituitary gland secretes six hormones while the posterior pituitary secretes two hormones.

The hypothalamus produces the hormones associated with the posterior pituitary. The posterior pituitary stores and releases them into circulation as needed.

HORMONES

Anterior pituitary

Thyroid-stimulating hormone (TSH): Stimulation of the thyroid gland

Adrenocorticotropic hormone (ACTH): Stimulation of the adrenal glands to secrete glucocorticoids

Luteinizing hormone
- FEMALES: stimulates maturation of ova and ovulation
- MALES: stimulates production of testosterone

Follicle-stimulating hormone (FSH)
- FEMALES: stimulates growth of ovarian follicles and estrogen secretion
- MALES: stimulates sperm production

Prolactin: Stimulates breast milk production during lactation

Growth hormone (GH): Stimulates protein synthesis and growth of muscle and bone

Posterior pituitary

Antidiuretic hormone (ADH) (vasopressin): Increases resorption of water in the kidneys

Oxytocin (OT)
- Stimulates contraction of uterus following delivery
- Stimulates ejection of breast milk during lactation

DISORDERS

Disease of the pituitary gland or the hypothalamus, trauma, tumor, or vascular lesion can cause altered pituitary gland function. Hyperfunction or hypofunction of the anterior and posterior pituitary gland can occur independently of one another.

- Oversecretion of ACTH from the anterior pituitary gland results in Cushing's disease.
- Oversecretion of GH results in gigantism in children and acromegaly in adults. In adult clients, acromegaly manifests as enlargement of body parts without affecting height.
- Undersecretion of GH in children results in dwarfism.
- Insufficient secretion of hormones in the anterior pituitary typically affects all the hormones, known as panhypopituitarism. It affects the target organs of the hormones produced in the anterior pituitary (thyroid, adrenal cortex, gonads).
- A deficiency of ADH causes diabetes insipidus (DI). Excretion of a large quantity of diluted urine is characteristic of DI.
- Excessive secretion of ADH causes the syndrome of inappropriate antidiuretic hormone (SIADH). In SIADH, the kidneys retain water, urine output decreases, and extracellular fluid volume is increased.
- Posterior pituitary disorders result in fluid and electrolyte imbalances.

Acromegaly

- Characterized by excess growth hormone in adults, which causes an increase in size of body parts but not height.
- Manifestations are widespread.
  - Overgrowth of skin; bones of the forehead, jaw, feet, and hands
  - Enlargement of organs (liver, heart)
- If left untreated, can cause hypertension, diabetes mellitus, and heart problems.
- Onset is gradual and can progress for years before becoming noticeable.

DATA COLLECTION

RISK FACTORS

- Age (adulthood)
- Benign tumors (pituitary adenoma)

EXPECTED FINDINGS

- Severe headaches
- Visual disturbances (diplopia, decreased visual acuity)
- Thick lips with coarse facial structures
- Joint pain
- Decreased libido
- Enlarged hands and feet
- Hyperglycemia
- Barrel-shaped chest

- Lower-jaw protrusion
- Increasing head size
- Change in voice characteristics
- Change in menstrual pattern
- Sleep apnea
- Increases in intracranial pressure (decreased level of consciousness, pupillary changes, severe hypertension, widened pulse pressure, bradycardia, seizures) Qs

LABORATORY TESTS

Growth hormone suppression test

Client will have baseline GH, then GH and blood glucose levels at 10, 60, and 120 min after glucose administration.
- Elevated glucose levels should suppress GH.
- Clients who have acromegaly show only a slight decrease or no decrease in GH levels.

CLIENT EDUCATION: Consume nothing but water for 6 to 8 hr preceding the test.

DIAGNOSTIC PROCEDURES

X-rays of the skull: Identify abnormalities of the sella turcica (location of the pituitary gland within the skull).

CT or MRI of the head: Identify soft tissue lesions.

Cerebral angiography: Evaluates for the presence of vascular malformation or aneurysms.

PATIENT-CENTERED CARE

NURSING CARE

Use therapeutic communication to discuss body image concerns with the client.

MEDICATIONS

Dopamine agonists (bromocriptine mesylate, cabergoline) inhibit the release of GH.
CLIENT EDUCATION: Notify the provider immediately if chest pain, dizziness, or watery nasal discharge occurs while taking bromocriptine. This can indicate cardiac dysrhythmia, coronary artery spasms, or leakage of CSF. Qs

Somatostatin analogs (octreotide, lanreotide) inhibit GH release.

Growth hormone receptor blocker (pegvisomant) prevents GH receptor activity and blocks production of insulin-like growth factor.

THERAPEUTIC PROCEDURES

Hypophysectomy: Removal of the pituitary gland through an endoscopic transnasal (most common) or oronasal (transsphenoidal) approach. If these approaches do not provide access to the tumor, a craniotomy is indicated.

Radiation therapy: Shrinks pituitary tumor over a period of time.

CLIENT EDUCATION

- Hormone replacement therapy is lifelong.
- Rinse mouth frequently to minimize effects of mouth breathing.
- Use oral rinses and flossing to clean teeth. Avoid brushing teeth due to risk of trauma to the operative site.
- Consume a diet high in fiber to minimize straining to defecate.

Diabetes insipidus

- Diabetes insipidus results from a deficiency of ADH. The posterior lobe of the pituitary gland secretes ADH (the neurohypophysis).
- Decreased ADH reduces the ability of the distal renal tubules in the kidneys to collect and concentrate urine, resulting in excessive diluted urination, excessive thirst, electrolyte imbalance, and excessive fluid intake.

TYPES OF DIABETES INSIPIDUS

Neurogenic (central): Caused by damage or defect of the hypothalamus or pituitary.

Nephrogenic: Inherited; renal tubules do not react to ADH.

DATA COLLECTION

RISK FACTORS

- Head injury
- Tumor or lesion
- Surgery or irradiation near the pituitary gland
- Infection (meningitis, encephalitis)
- Taking lithium carbonate or demeclocycline
- Older adult clients are at higher risk for dehydration Ⓖ
  - Lower water content of the body
  - Decreased thirst response
  - Decreased ability of the kidneys to concentrate urine
  - Increased use of diuretics
  - Swallowing difficulties
  - Inadequate food intake

EXPECTED FINDINGS

- Polyuria (abrupt onset of excessive urination, urinary output of 4 to 30 L/day of dilute urine): failure of the renal tubules to collect and reabsorb water
- Polydipsia (excessive thirst: 2 to 20 L/day)
- Nocturia
- Fatigue
- Dehydration evidenced by extreme thirst, weight loss, muscle weakness, headache, constipation, and dizziness

PHYSICAL FINDINGS
- Sunken eyes
- Tachycardia
- Hypotension
- Loss or absence of skin turgor

- Dry mucous membranes
- Weak, poor peripheral pulses
- Decreased cognition

LABORATORY TESTS

Electrolyte imbalances: such as increased sodium

Urine chemistry: Think DILUTE.
- Decreased urine specific gravity (less than 1.005)
- Decreased urine osmolality (less than 200 mOsm/L)
- Decreased urine pH
- Decreased urine sodium
- Decreased urine potassium
- As urine volume increases, urine osmolality decreases.

Serum chemistry: Think CONCENTRATED.
- Increased serum osmolality (greater than 300 mOsm/L)
- Increased serum sodium
- Increased serum potassium
- As serum volume decreases, the serum osmolality increases.

DIAGNOSTIC PROCEDURES

Water deprivation test (ADH stimulation test)

- This is an easy and reliable diagnostic test. Withholding fluids leads to dehydration.
- The test is positive for nephrogenic DI if the kidneys are unable to concentrate urine despite increased plasma osmolarity.
- A subcutaneous injection of vasopressin produces urine output with an increased specific gravity if the client has neurogenic diabetes insipidus.

NURSING ACTIONS
- Obtain baseline weight, vital signs, serum electrolytes and osmolarity, and urine specific gravity and osmolarity.
- Monitor hourly vital signs, urine specific gravity, osmolarity, and body weight. Discontinue the test and rehydrate the client for a loss of more than 2 kg in body weight. Q**EBP**
- Monitor for severe dehydration. Early indications of dehydration can include orthostatic hypotension, tachycardia, and dizziness. Be prepared to discontinue the test if these indicators develop.
- Explain the test procedure to the client.

CLIENT EDUCATION: Report dizziness, headache, or nausea.

PATIENT-CENTERED CARE

NURSING CARE

- Monitor vital signs, urinary output, I&O, specific gravity, and laboratory results (potassium, sodium, BUN, creatinine, specific gravity, osmolarity).
- Weigh the client daily.
- Promote the prescribed diet (regular diet with restriction of foods that exert a diuretic effect, such as caffeine).

- Assist with IV therapy
  - Hydration and electrolyte replacement
  - Provide intake to match output to prevent dehydration.
- Promote safety.
  - Keep bedside rails up while client is in bed.
  - Provide assistance with ambulation due to dizziness or muscle weakness.
  - Ensure easy access to a bathroom or bedpan. Q**s**
- Add bulk foods and fruit juices to the diet if constipation develops. The client might require a laxative.
- Observe skin turgor and mucous membranes.
- Provide skin and mouth care, and apply a lubricant to cracked or sore lips. Use a soft toothbrush and mild mouthwash to avoid trauma to the oral mucosa. Use alcohol-free skin care products, and apply emollient lotion after baths.

CLIENT EDUCATION: Drink fluids in response to thirst.

MEDICATIONS

ADH replacement agents

- Desmopressin (a synthetic ADH) or aqueous vasopressin is administered intranasally, orally, or parenterally.
- Results in increased water absorption from kidneys and decreased urine output

NURSING ACTIONS
- Monitor vital signs, urinary output, I&O, specific gravity, and laboratory values (potassium, sodium, BUN, creatinine, specific gravity, osmolarity).
- Dose is titrated depending on urine output.
- Give vasopressin cautiously to clients who have coronary artery disease because the medication can cause vasoconstriction.
- Monitor for headache, confusion, or other indications of water intoxication.

CLIENT EDUCATION
- Self-administration of vasopressin therapy is lifelong. Q**PCC**
- For an intranasal dose, clear nasal passage and sit upright prior to inhalation.
- Monitor weight daily and notify the provider of a gain greater than 0.9 kg (2 lb) in 24 hr.
- Restrict fluids if directed.
- Notify the provider of headache or confusion.

INTERPROFESSIONAL CARE

Home health care services can help with fluid, medication, and dietary management. Q**TC**

CLIENT EDUCATION

- Take medications at home as prescribed.
- Weigh daily, eat a high-fiber diet, wear a medical alert wristband, and monitor fluid I&O.
- Monitor for indications of dehydration (weight loss; dry, cracked lips; confusion; weakness).
- Drink adequate fluids as prescribed to maintain fluid and electrolyte balance.

COMPLICATIONS

Untreated DI can cause hypovolemia, hyperosmolarity, hypernatremia, circulatory collapse, unconsciousness, central nervous system damage, and seizures. Excessive urine output causing severe dehydration can lead to these complications.

NURSING ACTIONS: Monitor fluid balance. Prevent dehydration by providing proper fluid intake.

CLIENT EDUCATION: Seek early medical attention for any indications of DI. Follow care instructions.

Syndrome of inappropriate antidiuretic hormone

SIADH, or Schwartz-Bartter syndrome, is an excessive release of ADH (vasopressin) secreted by the posterior lobe of the pituitary gland (neurohypophysis).

Excess ADH leads to kidney reabsorption of water and suppression of renin-angiotensin mechanism, causing excretion of sodium leading to water intoxication, cellular edema, and dilutional hyponatremia. Fluid shifts within compartments causes decreased serum osmolarity.

DATA COLLECTION

RISK FACTORS

Conditions that stimulate the hypothalamus to hypersecrete ADH include malignant tumors, increased intrathoracic pressure (such as with positive pressure ventilation), head injury, meningitis, stroke, tuberculosis, and medications (chemotherapy agents, TCAs, SSRIs, opioids, fluoroquinolone antibiotics).

EXPECTED FINDINGS

- Early manifestations include headache, weakness, anorexia, muscle cramps, and weight gain (without edema because water, not sodium, is retained).
- As the serum sodium level decreases, the client experiences personality changes, hostility, sluggish deep tendon reflexes, nausea, vomiting, diarrhea, and oliguria with dark yellow concentrated appearance.

PHYSICAL FINDINGS
- Confusion, lethargy, and Cheyne-Stokes respirations are indications of an impending crisis. When the serum sodium level drops further, seizures, coma, and death can occur.
- Manifestations of fluid volume excess include tachycardia, bounding pulses, possible hypertension, crackles in lungs, distended neck veins, taut skin, and weight gain without edema. Intake is greater than output.

LABORATORY TESTS

Urine chemistry: Think CONCENTRATED.
- Increased urine sodium
- Increased urine osmolarity
- As urine volume decreases, urine osmolarity increases.

Blood chemistry: Think DILUTE.
- Decreased serum sodium (dilutional hyponatremia)
- Decreased serum osmolarity (less than 270 mEq/L)
- As serum volume increases, serum osmolarity decreases.

PATIENT-CENTERED CARE

NURSING CARE

- Restrict oral fluids to 500 to 1,000 mL/day to prevent further hemodilution (first priority). During fluid restriction, provide comfort measures for thirst (mouth care, ice chips, lozenges, staggered water intake).
- Flush all enteral and gastric tubes with 0.9% sodium chloride (instead of water) to replace sodium and prevent further hemodilution. Q EBP
- Monitor I&O. Report decreased urine output.
- Monitor vital signs for increased blood pressure, tachycardia, and hypothermia.
- Auscultate lung sounds to monitor for pulmonary edema (can develop rapidly and is a medical emergency).
- Monitor for decreased serum sodium/osmolarity and elevated urine sodium/osmolarity.
- Weigh the client daily. A weight gain of 1 kg (2.2 lb) indicates a gain of 1 L of fluid. Report this to the provider.
- Report altered mental status (headache, confusion, lethargy, seizures, coma).
- Reduce environmental stimuli and position the client as needed.
- Provide a safe environment for clients who have altered levels of consciousness. Maintain seizure precautions. Qs
- Monitor for indications of heart failure, which can occur from fluid overload. The client might require a loop diuretic.

MEDICATIONS

Tetracycline derivative (demeclocycline)

- Unlabeled use to correct fluid and electrolyte imbalances by stimulating urine flow.
- Contraindicated in clients who have impaired kidney function.

NURSING ACTIONS: Monitor for effective treatment (increased serum sodium/osmolarity, decreased urine sodium osmolarity).

CLIENT EDUCATION

- Avoid taking demeclocycline at the same time as calcium, iron, magnesium supplements, antacids containing aluminum, or milk products.
- Monitor for indications of a yeast infection, such as a white, cheese-like film inside the mouth.
- Avoid prolonged exposure to sunlight. Wear protective clothing and sunscreen.
- Notify the provider if diarrhea develops.

Vasopressin antagonists (tolvaptan, conivaptan)

- Use to promote water excretion without causing sodium losses.
- Administration is initiated in the acute care setting.

NURSING ACTIONS Qpcc

- Monitor blood glucose levels.
- Monitor serum sodium levels.
- Monitor intake and output.
- Monitor bowel patterns.

CLIENT EDUCATION

- Perform frequent oral care.
- Monitor for indications of dehydration, such as weakness.

Loop diuretic (furosemide)

Used to increase water excretion from the kidneys

NURSING ACTIONS: Use with caution because loop diuretics cause sodium excretion and can worsen hyponatremia.

CLIENT EDUCATION

- Change positions slowly in case of orthostatic hypotension.
- Notify the provider of findings of hyponatremia (nausea, decreased appetite, vomiting).

THERAPEUTIC PROCEDURES

Hypertonic sodium chloride IV fluid

The goal is to elevate the sodium level enough to alleviate neurologic compromise.

NURSING ACTIONS

- In severe hyponatremia/water intoxication, 200 to 300 mL hypertonic IV fluid (3% to 5% sodium chloride) is administered.
- Monitor for fluid overload and heart failure (distended neck veins, crackles in lungs).

CLIENT EDUCATION

- Follow discharge instructions for medications.
- Report difficulty breathing or shortness of breath, which can indicate heart failure.
- Obtain daily weights and restrict fluid intake.
- Wear a medical alert wristband.
- Monitor for indications of hypervolemia (weight gain, difficulty breathing) and neurological changes (tremors, disorientation), which can lead to seizures.
- Notify the provider of indications of hyponatremia (nausea, decreased appetite, vomiting).
- Avoid consumption of alcohol.

INTERPROFESSIONAL CARE

Home health care services can help with fluid, medication, and dietary management.

COMPLICATIONS

Water intoxication, cerebral/pulmonary edema, severe hyponatremia

Without prompt treatment, SIADH can lead to these complications, which can result in coma and death.

NURSING ACTIONS

- Monitor for early manifestations of water intoxication (lung crackles, distended neck veins, changes in neurological state [confusion, headaches, twitching, disorientation], edema, decreased urinary output).
- Monitor neurologic status frequently.
- Maintain seizure precautions.
- Administer medications.
- Monitor serum sodium level.
- Instruct the client and family about fluid restrictions and offer information about the condition and treatment.
- Provide support to ease the client's fears.

Application Exercises

1. A nurse is caring for a client who has syndrome of inappropriate antidiuretic hormone (SIADH). Which of the following findings should the nurse expect? (Select all that apply.)

   A. Decreased serum sodium

   B. Decreased urine specific gravity

   C. Decreased serum osmolarity

   D. Polyuria

   E. Increased thirst

2. A nurse is caring for a client who has diabetes insipidus. Which of the following urinalysis laboratory findings should the nurse anticipate?

   A. Presence of glucose

   B. Decreased specific gravity

   C. Presence of ketones

   D. Presence of red blood cells

3. A nurse is reinforcing teaching with a client who has a new diagnosis of diabetes insipidus. Which of the following client statements indicates an understanding of the teaching?

   A. "I can drink up to 2 quarts of fluid a day."

   B. "I will need to use insulin to control my blood glucose levels."

   C. "I should expect to gain weight during this illness."

   D. "Muscle weakness is a symptom of diabetes insipidus."

4. A nurse is caring for client who has acromegaly. Which of the following findings should the nurse expect?

   A. Muscle rigidity

   B. Sunken eyes

   C. Sluggish deep tendon reflexes

   D. Visual disturbances

PRACTICE Active Learning Scenario

A nurse is reinforcing teaching with a client who has SIADH and a new prescription for demeclocycline. What should the nurse include?

Use the ATI Active Learning Template: Medication to complete this item.

THERAPEUTIC USES

NURSING INTERVENTIONS: Describe one.

CLIENT EDUCATION: Describe two.

Application Exercises Key

1. A. **CORRECT:** A decrease in serum sodium is caused by an increase in the secretion of ADH.

   B. A urine specific gravity greater than 1.030 follows increased secretion of ADH in SIADH.

   C. **CORRECT:** A decrease in serum osmolarity is caused by an increase in the secretion of ADH.

   D. Reduced urine output follows the increased secretion of ADH in SIADH.

   E. Increased thirst is an expected finding in a client who has diabetes insipidus.

   Ⓝ *NCLEX® Connection: Physiological Adaptation, Basic Pathophysiology*

2. A. Glucose in the urine is an expected finding of diabetes mellitus.

   B. **CORRECT:** The urine of a client who has diabetes insipidus will be dilute with a urine specific gravity of less than 1.005.

   C. Ketones in the urine is an expected finding of diabetes mellitus.

   D. Red blood cells in the urine is an expected finding of a urinary tract infection.

   Ⓝ *NCLEX® Connection: Reduction of Risk Potential, Laboratory Values*

3. A. Excessive thirst is a manifestation of diabetes insipidus. The client might consume 4 to 30 L and should take in sufficient fluid to match output.

   B. Elevated blood glucose levels are a manifestation of diabetes mellitus.

   C. Weight loss is a manifestation of diabetes insipidus.

   D. **CORRECT:** Muscle weakness, weight loss, extreme thirst, headache, constipation, and dizziness are manifestations of dehydration that occur with diabetes insipidus.

   Ⓝ *NCLEX® Connection: Physiological Adaptation, Alterations in Body Systems*

4. A. The nurse should expect a client who has acromegaly to report joint pain.

   B. Sunken eyes are a manifestation of diabetes insipidus following dehydration. The nurse should expect a client who has acromegaly to have an increased head size and coarse facial structures.

   C. Sluggish deep tendon reflexes are a manifestation of hyponatremia, common in clients who have SIADH. The nurses should expect a client who has acromegaly to have enlarged hands and feet.

   D. **CORRECT:** The nurse should expect a client who has acromegaly to report visual changes such as double vision and to have decreased visual acuity.

   Ⓝ *NCLEX Connection: Physiological Adaptation, Basic Pathophysiology*

PRACTICE Answer

Using the ATI Active Learning Template: Medication

THERAPEUTIC USES: Demeclocycline is a derivative of tetracycline and is used to treat SIADH.

NURSING INTERVENTIONS: Monitor effectiveness of treatment (increased serum sodium/osmolarity, decreased urine sodium osmolarity).

CLIENT EDUCATION
- Avoid taking demeclocycline at the same time as calcium, iron, magnesium supplements, antacids containing aluminum, or milk products.
- Monitor for indications of a yeast infection, such as a white, cheese-like film inside the mouth.
- Avoid prolonged exposure to sunlight. Wear protective clothing and sunscreen.
- Notify the provider if diarrhea develops.

Ⓝ *NCLEX® Connection: Physiological Adaptation, Basic Pathophysiology*

UNIT 12   NURSING CARE OF CLIENTS WHO
HAVE ENDOCRINE DISORDERS
SECTION: THYROID DISORDERS

CHAPTER 70 *Hyperthyroidism*

The thyroid gland produces three hormones: thyroxine (T_4), triiodothyronine (T_3), and thyrocalcitonin (calcitonin). The anterior pituitary gland regulates the secretion of T_3 and T_4 through a negative feedback mechanism.

The anterior pituitary releases thyroid-stimulating hormone (TSH) when serum levels of T_3 and T_4 decrease. This stimulates the thyroid gland to secrete more hormones until normalization of T_3 and T_4 levels occur. T_3 and T_4 affect all body systems by regulating overall body metabolism and energy production, and controlling tissue use of fats, proteins, and carbohydrates.

Calcitonin inhibits mobilization of calcium from bone and reduces blood calcium levels. Dietary intake of protein and iodine is necessary for the production of thyroid hormones.

Hyperthyroidism is a syndrome caused by excessive circulating thyroid hormones. Because thyroid activity affects all body systems, excessive thyroid hormone exaggerates normal body functions and produces a hypermetabolic state.

HEALTH PROMOTION AND DISEASE PREVENTION

- Take all medications as directed.
- Check with the provider prior to taking over-the-counter medications.
- Keep all follow-up appointments.
- Adjust diet to increased metabolism when needed.
- Seek measures to reduce stress, and get rest as needed.
- Notify the provider of fever, increased restlessness, palpitations, or chest pain.

DATA COLLECTION

RISK FACTORS

CAUSES OF HYPERTHYROIDISM

- **Primary hyperthyroidism** results from dysfunction of the thyroid gland. The most common cause is Graves' disease, an autoimmune disorder.
- **Secondary hyperthyroidism** results from dysfunction of another gland. Excessive secretion of thyroid hormone can result from an overproduction of TSH from the pituitary gland.
- Other risk factors of hyperthyroidism include medications that contain iodine, infections, and cigarette smoking.
- Hyperthyroidism occurs most often in women.

EXPECTED FINDINGS

- Nervousness, irritability, hyperactivity, emotional lability, decreased attention span
- Crying or laughing without cause
- Change in mental or emotional status
- Weakness, easy fatigability, exercise intolerance
- Muscle weakness
- Heat intolerance
- Weight change (usually loss) and increased appetite
- Insomnia and interrupted sleep
- Frequent stools and diarrhea
- Menstrual irregularities (amenorrhea, decreased menstrual flow) and decreased fertility
- Libido initially increased in both men and women, followed by a decrease as the condition progresses
- Warm, sweaty, flushed skin with velvety smooth texture
- Hair thinning and developing a fine, soft, silky texture
- Tremor, hyperkinesia, hyperreflexia
- Pretibial myxedema: dry waxy swelling of the front surfaces of the lower legs that resembles benign tumors (Graves' disease only)

- Vision changes
  - Eyelid retraction (lag): movement of the eyelid is delayed when the eye moves downward
  - Globe (eyeball) lag: upper eyelid pulls back faster than the eyeball when the client gazes upward
  - Exophthalmos (Graves' disease only) due to edema in the extraocular muscles and increased fatty tissue behind the eye (70.1)
  - Blurred or double vision and tiring of eyes due to pressure on the optic nerve
  - Photophobia (sensitivity to light)
  - Excessive tearing and bloodshot appearance of eyes
- Hair thinning or loss
- Goiter
- Bruit over the thyroid gland
- Elevated systolic blood pressure and widened pulse pressure
- Tachycardia, palpitations, dysrhythmias
- Dyspnea
- Findings in older adult clients are often more subtle than those in younger clients. Ⓖ
  - Occasionally, older adult clients who have hyperthyroidism demonstrate apathy or withdrawal instead of the more typical hypermetabolic state.
  - Older adult clients who have hyperthyroidism often present with heart failure, angina, and atrial fibrillation.

LABORATORY TESTS

Serum TSH test: Decreased in the presence of Graves' disease (can be elevated in secondary or tertiary hyperthyroidism)

Free T_4 index, T_4 (total) T_3: Elevated in the presence of disease

Thyroid-stimulating immunoglobulins: Elevated in Graves' disease; normal in other types of hyperthyroidism

Thyrotropin receptor antibodies: Elevation is most indicative of Graves' disease.

DIAGNOSTIC PROCEDURES

Ultrasound: Used to produce images of the thyroid gland and surrounding tissue

Electrocardiogram: Used to evaluate the effects of excessive thyroid hormone on the heart (tachycardia, dysrhythmias). ECG changes include atrial fibrillation, and changes in the P and T waveforms.

Radioactive iodine uptake: Nuclear medicine test
- Clarifies size and function of the gland.
- Contraindicated in pregnant clients.
- Data collection prior to testing should include determination of an allergy to iodine or shellfish.
- The uptake of radioactive iodine, administered orally 24 hr prior to the test, is measured.
- An elevated uptake of iodine is indicative of hyperthyroidism.

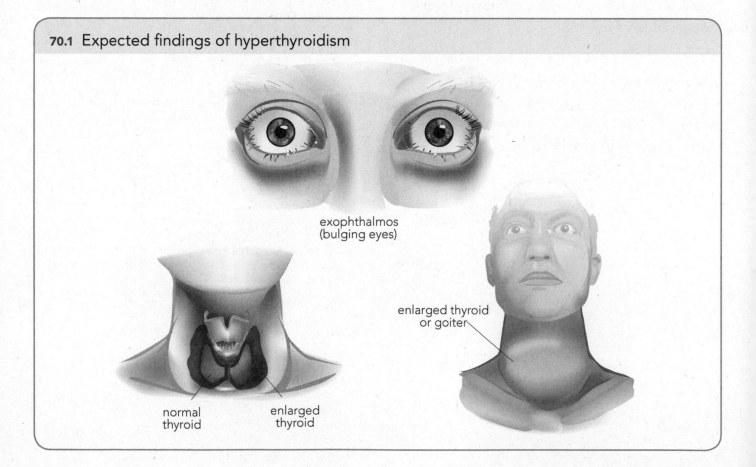

70.1 Expected findings of hyperthyroidism

exophthalmos (bulging eyes)

normal thyroid   enlarged thyroid

enlarged thyroid or goiter

NURSING ACTIONS

- Confirm that the client is not pregnant prior to the scan.
- Take a medication history to determine the use of iodides.
- Recent use of contrast media and oral contraceptives can cause falsely elevated serum thyroid hormone levels.
- Severe illness; malnutrition; and the use of aspirin, corticosteroids, or phenytoin sodium can cause a false decrease in serum thyroid hormone levels.
- Inform the provider if the client received iodine contrast recently.

CLIENT EDUCATION

- Avoid foods high in iodine for 1 week prior to the test.
- Use noniodized salt, and avoid fish, shellfish, and medications that contain iodine.

PATIENT-CENTERED CARE

NURSING CARE

- Minimize the client's energy expenditure by assisting with activities as necessary and by encouraging the client to alternate periods of activity with rest.
- Promote a calm environment.
- Monitor mental status and decision-making ability. Intervene as needed to ensure safety.
- Monitor nutritional status. Provide increased calories, protein, and other nutritional support as necessary.
- Monitor I&O and weight.
- Provide eye protection (patches, eye lubricant, tape to close eyelids) for a client who has exophthalmos.
- Monitor vital signs
- Reduce room temperature.
- Provide cool shower or sponge bath to promote comfort.
- Provide linen changes as necessary.
- Report a temperature increase of 1° F or greater to the provider immediately, because this can be indicative of an impending thyroid crisis.
- Monitor ECG for dysrhythmias.
- Assure the family that any abrupt changes in the client's behavior are likely disease-related and should subside with antithyroid therapy.
- Avoid excessive palpation of the thyroid gland.
- Administer antithyroid medications.
- Prepare the client for a total/subtotal thyroidectomy if the client is unresponsive to antithyroid medications or has an airway-obstructing goiter.

MEDICATIONS

Thionamides

- Methimazole and propylthiouracil inhibit the production of thyroid hormone.
- The use of thionamides includes the treatment of Graves' disease (as an adjunct to radioactive iodine therapy) to decrease hormone levels in preparation for surgery and to treat thyrotoxicosis.

NURSING ACTIONS

- Monitor for manifestations of hypothyroidism (intolerance to cold, edema, bradycardia, increase in weight, depression).
- Monitor CBC for leukopenia or thrombocytopenia.
- Monitor for indications of hepatotoxicity.

CLIENT EDUCATION

- Take the medication with meals.
- Take the medication in divided doses at regular intervals to maintain an even therapeutic medication level.
- Report fever, sore throat, or bruising to the provider.
- Report any evidence of jaundice (yellowing of skin or eyes, darkening of urine).
- Follow the provider's instructions about dietary intake of iodine.
- Inform the provider of pregnancy.

Beta adrenergic blockers

Propranolol, atenolol, and metoprolol treat sympathetic nervous system effects (tachycardia, palpitations). These medications counteract the effects of increased thyroid hormones but do not alter the levels of the hormones.

NURSING ACTIONS

- Monitor blood pressure, heart rate, and ECG.
- Monitor for hypoglycemia in clients who have diabetes mellitus.

CLIENT EDUCATION

- The medication can cause dizziness. Sit on the side of the bed for a few minutes before standing.
- Check pulse prior to each dose. Notify the provider if heart rate falls below 60/min.
- Discontinue the medication only on the advice of the provider.

Iodine solutions

Lugol's solution is a nonradioactive 5% elemental iodine in 10% potassium iodine that inhibits the release of thyroid hormone.

CLIENT EDUCATION

- These medications are only for short-term use (taken for 10 days followed by surgery).
- Administer 1 hr after an antithyroid medication.
- Pregnancy is a contraindication to the use of these medications.
- Medication is available as a solution. Mix with juice or other liquid to mask the taste. Use a straw to avoid staining teeth. Take with food.
- These medications pass into breast milk and can have undesirable effects on a nursing infant.
- Use during pregnancy is contraindicated.
- Notify the provider of fever, sore throat, and mouth ulcers.

THERAPEUTIC PROCEDURES

Radioactive iodine therapy

Following uptake by the thyroid, radioactive iodine destroys some of the hormone-producing cells (^{131}I).

- One dose can be sufficient, but it can be necessary to administer a second or third dose.
- The degree of thyroid destruction varies and can require lifelong thyroid replacement.

NURSING ACTIONS

- Radioactive iodine therapy is contraindicated in clients who are pregnant
- Monitor for manifestations of hypothyroidism (edema, intolerance to cold, bradycardia, increase in weight, depression).

CLIENT EDUCATION Qᵒⁱ

- Effects of therapy might not be evident for 6 to 8 weeks.
- Continue to take the medication as directed.
- Stay away from pregnant people, infants, and small children for the first week following treatment. Avoid contact closer than 3 feet (1 meter) and limit contact to 1 hr daily.
- Although a low dose of radiation is used, take precautions to prevent radiation exposure to others. Follow directions from provider, which can include the following.
  - Do not use same toilet as others for 2 weeks.
  - Sit down to urinate.
  - Flush the toilet three times after use.
  - Take a laxative 2 to 3 days after treatment to help rid the body of stool contaminated with radiation.
  - Wear clothing that is washable, wash clothing separate from clothing of others, and run the washing machine for a full cycle after washing contaminated clothing.
  - Avoid contamination from saliva, do not share a toothbrush, and use disposable food service items (paper plates).

Thyroidectomy

Surgical removal of part or all of the thyroid gland

- The provider performs a subtotal thyroidectomy if medication therapy fails or radiation therapy is contraindicated. Subtotal thyroidectomy is also used to correct diffuse goiter and thyroid cancer. After a subtotal thyroidectomy, the remaining thyroid tissue usually supplies enough thyroid hormone for normal function.
- The client will need thyroid hormone replacement therapy following a total thyroidectomy.

PREPROCEDURE NURSING ACTIONS

- Explain the purpose of the thyroidectomy. Tell the client that there will be an incision in the neck, a dressing, and possibly a drain in place. Some hoarseness and a sore throat from intubation and anesthesia is expected. Qᴾᶜᶜ
- The client usually receives propylthiouracil or methimazole for 4 to 6 weeks before surgery.
- The client should receive iodine for 10 to 14 days before surgery. This reduces the gland's size and prevents excess bleeding.
- Beta blockers can be given to control hypertension, dysrhythmias, or tachycardia.
- The client should follow a high-protein, high-carbohydrate diet prior to surgery
- Instruct the client to support the neck when performing deep breathing and coughing exercises postoperatively.
- Notify the provider immediately if the client does not follow the medication regimen.

POSTPROCEDURE NURSING ACTIONS

- Keep the client in a semi-Fowler's position. Support head and neck with pillows. Avoid neck extension. Qᵒⁱ
- Following protocols, monitor vital signs (typically every 15 min until stable then every 30 min).
- Assist with deep breathing exercises every 30 to 60 min.
- Provide oral and tracheal suction as needed.
- Check the surgical dressing and back of the neck for excessive bleeding. Respiratory distress can occur from compression of trachea due to hemorrhage, which is most likely to occur in the first 24 hr.
- Respiratory distress also can occur due to edema. Ensure that tracheostomy supplies are immediately available. Humidify air, assist to cough and deep breathe, and provide oral and tracheal suction if needed.
- Check for laryngeal nerve damage by asking the client to speak as soon as awake from anesthesia and every 2 hr thereafter.
- Administer medication to manage pain. Reassure the client that discomfort will resolve within a few days.
- The damage or removal of the parathyroid glands can cause hypocalcemia and tetany. Check for positive Chvostek's and Trousseau's signs. Ensure that IV calcium gluconate or calcium chloride is immediately available.
  - Keep emergency equipment near the bedside. Qˢ
  - Monitor for evidence of hypocalcemia (tingling, muscle twitching, numbness of mouth or distal extremities).
  - Advise the client to notify the nurse of any muscle twitching or tingling sensation of the mouth or distal extremities.

CLIENT EDUCATION

- Cough and breathe deeply while stabilizing the neck. Qᴘᴄᴄ
- Change positions while supporting the back of the neck.
- Be careful of the incisional drain.
- The voice will become hoarse. Expect pain.
- Notify the nurse of any tingling sensation of the mouth, tingling of the distal extremities, or muscle twitching.
- Talk at intervals to check for nerve damage.
- Notify the surgeon of incisional drainage, swelling, or redness that can indicate infection.
- Monitor for manifestations of hypothyroidism (hypothermia, lethargy, weight gain).
- Take all medications as directed.
- Following a total thyroidectomy, lifelong thyroid replacement medications will be required.
- Check with the provider prior to taking over-the-counter medications.
- Keep all follow-up appointments.
- Notify the surgeon of fever, increased restlessness, palpitations, or chest pain.

INTERPROFESSIONAL CARE

An endocrinologist, radiologist, pharmacist, and dietitian can collaborate in providing care for the client.

COMPLICATIONS

Hemorrhage at the incision site

Due to a loosened surgical tie, excessive coughing, or movement

NURSING ACTIONS

- Inspect the surgical incision and dressing for drainage and bleeding, especially at the back of the neck. Change the dressing as directed.
- Expect only scant drainage after 24 hr.
- Support the client's head and neck with pillows or sandbags. Maintain the client's head and neck in good body alignment if it is necessary to transfer the client from a stretcher to the bed.

CLIENT EDUCATION

- To avoid pressure on the suture line, avoid neck flexion or extension. Qᴘᴄᴄ
- Cough and deep breathe while supporting the neck.
- Change positions while supporting the back of the neck.

Thyroid storm/crisis

Results from a sudden surge of large amounts of thyroid hormones into the bloodstream, causing an even greater increase in body metabolism

- This is a medical emergency with a high mortality rate.
- Precipitating factors include uncontrolled hyperthyroidism occurring most often with Graves' disease, infection, trauma, emotional stress, diabetic ketoacidosis, and digitalis toxicity, all of which increase demands on body metabolism. It also can occur following a surgical procedure or a thyroidectomy because of manipulation of the gland during surgery.
- Findings are hyperthermia, hypertension, delirium, vomiting, abdominal pain, tachydysrhythmias, chest pain, dyspnea, and palpitations.

NURSING ACTIONS

- Maintain a patent airway.
- Provide continuous cardiac monitoring for dysrhythmias.
- Administer acetaminophen to decrease temperature.
- It is a contraindication to administer salicylate antipyretics (aspirin) for fever because they release thyroxine from protein-binding sites and increase free thyroxine levels.
- Provide cool sponge baths, or apply ice packs to decrease fever. If fever continues, obtain a prescription for a cooling blanket for hyperthermia.
- Administer thionamides (methimazole or propylthiouracil) to prevent further synthesis and release of thyroid hormones.
- Administer sodium iodide 1 hr after administering thionamide medication.
- Administer beta adrenergic blocking agents (such as propranolol) to block sympathetic nervous system effects.
- Administer glucocorticoids if adrenal insufficiency is suspected or to treat shock.
- Monitor for therapeutic effect of administration of IV fluids to provide adequate hydration and prevent vascular collapse. Fluid volume deficit can occur due to increased fluid excretion by the kidneys or excessive diaphoresis. Monitor I&O hourly to prevent fluid overload or inadequate replacement.
- Administer supplemental oxygen to meet increased oxygen demands.
- Provide support and information to the client and family about the condition and all procedures. Qᴘᴄᴄ

CLIENT EDUCATION: Notify the provider of fever, increased restlessness, palpitations, or chest pain.

Airway obstruction

Hemorrhage, tracheal collapse, tracheal mucus accumulation, laryngeal edema, and vocal cord paralysis can cause respiratory obstruction, with sudden stridor and restlessness.

NURSING ACTIONS
- Keep a tracheostomy tray near the client at all times during the immediate recovery period. Qs
- Maintain the bed in a high-Fowler's position to decrease edema and swelling of the neck.
- If the client reports that the dressing feels tight, alert the provider immediately.
- Listen for respiratory stridor.
- Provide humidified air.
- Have suction equipment at the bedside.
- Medicate to reduce swelling.

CLIENT EDUCATION: Notify the nurse of tightness or difficulty breathing.

Hypocalcemia and tetany

Damage to parathyroid gland causes hypocalcemia and tetany.

NURSING ACTIONS
- Monitor for indications of hypocalcemia (tingling of the fingers and toes, carpopedal spasms, convulsions).
- Monitor for Chvostek's and Trousseau's signs, which are indicators of neuromuscular irritability from hypocalcemia.
- Have IV calcium gluconate available for emergency administration. Qs
- Maintain seizure precautions.

CLIENT EDUCATION: Notify the nurse of any tingling sensation of the mouth, tingling of distal extremities, or muscle twitching.

Nerve damage

- Nerve damage can lead to vocal cord paralysis and vocal disturbances.
- Incisional damage or swelling can cause nerve damage.
- Clients will be hoarse, able to speak only rarely, and need to rest their voice for several days.

NURSING ACTIONS
- After the procedure, monitor the client's ability to speak every 2 hr and document any changes.
- Monitor voice tone and quality, and compare it with the preoperative voice.

CLIENT EDUCATION: After resting the voice for a few days, talk at intervals to check for nerve damage. A hoarse voice is not typically permanent.

Application Exercises

1. A nurse in a provider's office is reviewing the health record of a client who is undergoing evaluation for Graves' disease. Which of the following laboratory results is an expected finding?

   A. Decreased thyrotropin receptor antibodies (TRAb)

   B. Decreased thyroid-stimulating hormone (TSH)

   C. Decreased free thyroxine index (T_4)

   D. Decreased triiodothyronine (T_3)

2. A nurse is reviewing manifestations of hyperthyroidism with a client. Which of the following findings should the nurse include? (Select all that apply.)

   A. Anorexia

   B. Heat intolerance

   C. Constipation

   D. Palpitations

   E. Weight loss

   F. Bradycardia

3. A nurse is reinforcing instructions with a client who has Graves' disease and a new prescription for propranolol. Which of the following information should the nurse include?

   A. "An adverse effect of this medication is jaundice."

   B. "Take your pulse before each dose."

   C. "The purpose of this medication is to decrease production of thyroid hormone."

   D. "You should stop taking this medication if you have a sore throat."

4. A nurse is preparing to receive a client from the PACU who is postoperative following a thyroidectomy. The nurse should ensure that which of the following equipment is available? (Select all that apply.)

   A. Suction equipment

   B. Humidified oxygen

   C. Flashlight

   D. Tracheostomy tray

   E. Chest tube tray

5. A nurse in a provider's office is assisting with the plan of care for a client who has a new diagnosis of Graves' disease and a new prescription for methimazole. Which of the following interventions should the nurse include? (Select all that apply.)

   A. Monitor CBC.

   B. Monitor triiodothyronine (T_3).

   C. Instruct the client to increase consumption of shellfish.

   D. Advise the client to take the medication at the same time every day.

   E. Inform the client that an adverse effect of this medication is iodine toxicity.

6. A nurse is caring for a client who is 12 hr postoperative following a thyroidectomy. Which of the following findings indicate that the client is experiencing thyroid crisis? (Select all that apply.)

   A. Bradycardia

   B. Hypothermia

   C. Dyspnea

   D. Abdominal pain

   E. Mental confusion

PRACTICE Active Learning Scenario

A nurse is reinforcing teaching with a client who will have radioactive iodine therapy. What information should the nurse include? Use the ATI Active Learning Template: Therapeutic Procedure to complete this item.

DESCRIPTION OF PROCEDURE: Provide a brief description of the procedure.

CLIENT EDUCATION: Identify five client instructions the nurse should include.

Application Exercises Key

1. A. In the presence of Graves' disease, elevated TRAb is an expected finding.

   B. **CORRECT:** In the presence of Graves' disease, low TSH is an expected finding. The pituitary gland decreases the production of TSH when thyroid hormone levels are elevated.

   C. In the presence of Graves' disease, elevated free T₄ index is an expected finding.

   D. In the presence of Graves' disease, elevated T₃ is an expected finding.

   Ⓝ *NCLEX® Connection: Reduction of Risk Potential, Laboratory Values*

2. A. The client who has hyperthyroidism has an increased metabolic rate, resulting in increased hunger.

   B. **CORRECT:** Hyperthyroidism increases metabolism, causing heat intolerance.

   C. Diarrhea is an expected finding for the client who has hyperthyroidism.

   D. **CORRECT:** Hyperthyroidism increases metabolism, causing palpitations.

   E. **CORRECT:** Hyperthyroidism increases metabolism, causing weight loss.

   F. Hyperthyroidism increases metabolism, causing tachycardia.

   Ⓝ *NCLEX® Connection: Physiological Adaptation, Alterations in Body Systems*

3. A. Yellowing of the skin is an adverse effect of methimazole.

   B. **CORRECT:** Propranolol can cause bradycardia. Clients should take their pulse before each dose. If there is a significant change, withhold the dose and consult the provider.

   C. The purpose of propranolol is to suppress tachycardia, diaphoresis, and other effects of Graves' disease.

   D. Sore throat is not an adverse effect of this medication. The client should not discontinue taking this medication because this action can result in tachycardia and dysrhythmias.

   Ⓝ *NCLEX® Connection: Pharmacological Therapies, Expected Actions/Outcomes*

4. A. **CORRECT:** The client can require oral or tracheal suctioning. The nurse should ensure that suctioning equipment is available.

   B. **CORRECT:** The client can require supplemental oxygen due to respiratory complications. Humidified oxygen thins secretions and promotes respiratory exchange. This equipment should be available.

   C. A flashlight assists in measuring the reaction of the pupils to light for a client who has an intracranial disorder. It is not necessary to check pupil reaction with a flashlight for this client.

   D. **CORRECT:** The client can experience respiratory obstruction. A tracheostomy tray should be available at the bedside.

   E. A chest tube tray is necessary for a client who develops a hemothorax or pneumothorax. This is not an expected complication of a thyroidectomy.

   Ⓝ *NCLEX® Connection: Reduction of Risk Potential, Potential for Complications of Diagnostic Tests/Treatments/Procedures*

5. A. **CORRECT:** Methimazole can cause hematologic effects, including leukopenia and thrombocytopenia. The nurse should monitor CBC.

   B. **CORRECT:** Methimazole reduces thyroid hormone production. The nurse should monitor T₃.

   C. Methimazole reduces thyroid hormone production by blocking iodine. The client should limit iodine-containing foods such as shellfish.

   D. **CORRECT:** Methimazole should be taken at the same time every day to maintain blood levels.

   E. Iodine toxicity is an adverse effect of potassium iodide solution.

   Ⓝ *NCLEX® Connection: Pharmacological Therapies, Expected Actions/Outcomes*

6. A. When thyroid crisis occurs, the client experiences an extreme rise in metabolic rate, which results in tachycardia.

   B. When thyroid crisis occurs, the client experiences an extreme rise in metabolic rate, which results in a high fever.

   C. **CORRECT:** Excessive levels of thyroid hormone can cause the client to experience dyspnea.

   D. **CORRECT:** When thyroid crisis occurs, the client can experience gastrointestinal conditions, such as vomiting, diarrhea, and abdominal pain.

   E. **CORRECT:** Excessive thyroid hormone levels can cause the client to experience confusion.

   Ⓝ *NCLEX® Connection: Physiological Adaptation, Basic Pathophysiology*

PRACTICE Answer

Using the ATI Active Learning Template: Therapeutic Procedure

DESCRIPTION OF PROCEDURE: Radioactive iodine (¹³¹I) is administered orally 24 hr prior to a thyroid scan. The thyroid absorbs the radiation, which results in destruction of cells that produce thyroid hormone.

CLIENT EDUCATION

- The effects of the therapy might not be evident for 6 to 8 weeks.
- Take medication as directed.
- Practice precautions to prevent radiation exposure to others.
- Take a laxative 2 to 3 days after treatment to help rid the body of stool contaminated with radiation.
- Stay away from pregnant people, infants, or small children for the first week following treatment. Avoid contact closer than 1 meter (3 feet) and limit contact to 1 hr daily.

- Follow directions from the provider, which can include the following.
  ○ Do not use same toilet as others for 2 weeks.
  ○ Sit down to urinate.
  ○ Flush the toilet three times after use.
  ○ Wear clothing that is washable, wash clothing separate from clothing of others, and run the washing machine for a full cycle after washing contaminated clothing.
  ○ Avoid infants or small children for 2 to 4 days after the procedure.
  ○ Avoid contamination from saliva, do not share a toothbrush, and use disposable food service items (paper plates).

Ⓝ *NCLEX® Connection: Reduction of Risk Potential, Therapeutic Procedures*

CHAPTER 71 *Hypothyroidism*

Hypothyroidism is a condition in which there is an inadequate amount of circulating thyroid hormones triiodothyronine (T_3) and thyroxine (T_4), causing a decrease in metabolic rate that affects all body systems.

Because hypothyroidism can have manifestations that mimic the aging process, it is often undiagnosed in older adult clients. This can lead to potentially serious adverse effects from medications (sedatives, opiates, anesthetics). Ⓒ

CLASSIFICATIONS BY ETIOLOGY

Primary hypothyroidism stems from dysfunction of the thyroid gland. This is the most common type of hypothyroidism. Causes include the following.
- Disease (autoimmune thyroiditis)
- Use of medications that decrease the synthesis of thyroid hormone
- Loss of the thyroid gland (iodine deficiency, radioactive iodine treatment, surgical removal of the gland)

Secondary hypothyroidism results from a failure of the anterior pituitary gland to stimulate the thyroid gland or failure of the target tissues to respond to the thyroid hormones (pituitary tumors).

Tertiary hypothyroidism results from a failure of the hypothalamus to produce thyroid-releasing hormone.

DATA COLLECTION

RISK FACTORS

- Females 30 to 60 years old are affected seven to 10 times more often than males.
- Many individuals who have mild hypothyroidism are frequently undiagnosed, but the hormone disturbance can contribute to an acceleration of atherosclerosis or complications of medical treatment (intraoperative hypotension, cardiac complications following surgery).
- Use of some medications (lithium, amiodarone)
- Inadequate intake of iodine
- Radiation therapy to the head and neck

EXPECTED FINDINGS

Hypothyroidism findings are often vague and develop slowly over time. Manifestations can vary and relate to the severity of the condition.
- Fatigue, lethargy
- Irritability
- Intolerance to cold
- Constipation
- Weight gain without an increase in caloric intake
- Pale skin
- Thick, brittle fingernails
- Depression and apathy
- Periorbital edema
- Joint or muscle pain
- Bradycardia, hypotension, dysrhythmias
- Slow thought processes and speech
- Hypoventilation, pleural effusion
- Thickening of the skin
- Thinning of hair on the eyebrows
- Dry, flaky skin
- Swelling in face, hands, and feet (myxedema [nonpitting, mucinous edema])
- Decreased acuity of taste and smell
- Hoarse, raspy speech
- Abnormal menstrual periods (menorrhagia/amenorrhea)
- Decreased libido

LABORATORY TESTS

T_3 expected reference range
- 70 to 205 ng/dL in clients age 20 to 50
- 40 to 180 ng/dL in clients older than 50

T_4 expected reference range
- 4 to 12 mcg/dL in male clients
- 5 to 12 mcg/dL in female clients

EXPECTED RESULTS WITH HYPOTHYROIDISM
- **T_4:** Decreased
- **Serum thyroid-stimulating hormone (TSH)**
  - Increased with primary hypothyroidism
  - Decreased or within the expected reference range in secondary hypothyroidism
- **Free thyroxine index and T_4 levels:** Decreased
- **T_3 resin uptake:** Decreased
- **Thyrotropin receptor antibodies:** No response
- **Serum cholesterol:** Increased

DIAGNOSTIC PROCEDURES

Radioisotope (^{123}I) scan and uptake: Clients who have hypothyroidism have a low uptake of the iodine preparation.

ECG: Sinus bradycardia, dysrhythmias

PATIENT-CENTERED CARE

NURSING CARE

- Monitor for cardiovascular changes (low blood pressure, bradycardia, dysrhythmias).
- Monitor the client's weight. Inspect for peripheral edema.
- If mental status compromise occurs, orient the client periodically and provide safety measures. Qs
- Increase the client's activity level gradually, and provide frequent rest periods to avoid fatigue and decrease myocardial oxygen demands.
- Apply antiembolism stockings, and elevate the client's legs to assist venous return.
- Monitor respiratory status including rate, depth, pattern, oximetry, and arterial blood gases. Encourage the client to cough and breathe deeply to prevent pulmonary complications.
- Consult with a dietitian. Provide a low-calorie, high-bulk diet, and encourage fluids and activity to prevent constipation and promote weight loss. Administer cathartics and stool softeners as needed. Avoid fiber laxatives, which interfere with absorption of levothyroxine. Qtc
- Provide meticulous skin care. Turn and reposition the client every 2 hr if the client is on extended bed rest. Use alcohol-free skin care products and an emollient lotion after bathing.
- Provide extra clothing and blankets for clients who have decreased cold tolerance. Dress the client in layers, adjust room temperature, and encourage intake of warm liquids if possible.
- Caution the client against using electric blankets or other electric heating devices because the combination of vasodilation, decreased sensation, and decreased alertness can result in unrecognized burns. Qs
- Encourage the client to verbalize feelings and fears about changes in body image. Return to the euthyroid (normal thyroid gland function) state takes time. The client might need frequent reassurance that most physical manifestations are reversible.
- Use caution with medications due to alteration in metabolism. Qs
  - Use central nervous system (CNS) depressants (barbiturates, sedatives) cautiously due to the risk of respiratory depression.
  - Dosages of CNS depressants should be significantly less than for a client who does not have hypothyroidism.
  - Hypothyroidism alters metabolism and excretion of medications. The provider uses caution in prescribing medications to clients who have this condition.

MEDICATIONS

Thyroid hormone replacement therapy

Levothyroxine

- Thyroid hormone replacement therapy is the treatment of choice.
- Levothyroxine increases the effects of warfarin and can increase the need for insulin and digoxin.
- Medications that decrease the absorption of levothyroxine include cimetidine, lansoprazole, sucralfate, and colestipol. Instruct the client to separate administration of these medications from levothyroxine by at least 4 hr.
- Medications that can accelerate the metabolism of levothyroxine include phenytoin, carbamazepine, rifampin, sertraline, and phenobarbital, thus requiring an increase in dosage of levothyroxine to achieve therapeutic levels.
- Use caution when starting thyroid hormone replacement with older adult clients and those who have coronary artery disease to avoid coronary ischemia because of increased oxygen demands of the heart. It is preferable to start with much lower doses and increase gradually, taking 1 to 2 months to reach full replacement doses. Ⓖ

NURSING ACTIONS

- Administer thyroid hormone replacement therapy.
- Monitor for cardiovascular compromise (chest pain, palpitations, rapid heart rate, shortness of breath).

CLIENT EDUCATION

- Treatment begins slowly. The provider will increase the dosage every 2 to 3 weeks to obtain the desired response. Monitoring of serum TSH should occur at scheduled times to ensure correct dosage.
- Take the dose prescribed. Do not stop taking the medication or change the dose.
- Take the medication on an empty stomach, typically 30 to 60 min before breakfast.
- Fiber supplements, calcium, iron, and antacids interfere with absorption. Consult with the provider before taking any over-the-counter medications.
- Monitor for and report manifestations of hyperthyroidism (irritability, tremors, tachycardia, palpitations, heat intolerance, rapid weight loss).
- The treatment is lifelong, requiring ongoing medical assessment of thyroid function.

INTERPROFESSIONAL CARE

A home health nurse might need to visit the client and monitor for adverse effects during the first few weeks of therapy.

COMPLICATIONS

Myxedema

Myxedema coma is a life-threatening condition that occurs when hypothyroidism is untreated or when a stressor (acute illness, surgery, chemotherapy, discontinuing thyroid replacement therapy, sedative/opioid use) affects a client who has hypothyroidism.

MANIFESTATIONS
- Respiratory failure
- Hypotension
- Hypothermia
- Bradycardia, dysrhythmia
- Hyponatremia
- Hypoglycemia
- Coma

NURSING ACTIONS
- Monitor airway and respirations. Monitor mental status.
- Cover the client with warm blankets.
- Monitor body temperature hourly until stable.
- Observe for therapeutic effect of fluid administration and thyroid hormone replacement.
- Monitor vital signs because rapid correction of hypothyroidism can cause adverse cardiac effects.
- Monitor I&O and daily weights. With treatment, urine output should increase, and body weight should decrease. Report a lack of increase in urine output to the provider.
- Treat hypoglycemia with glucose.
- Observe for therapeutic effect of corticosteroid administration.
- Initiate aspiration precautions.
- Check for possible sources of infection (blood, sputum, urine) that might have precipitated the coma. Treat any underlying illness.

PRACTICE Active Learning Scenario

A nurse is reinforcing teaching with a client who has hypothyroidism. What information should the nurse include in the teaching? Use the ATI Active Learning Template: System Disorder to complete this item.

ALTERATION IN HEALTH (DIAGNOSIS): Provide a brief description of the disorder.

RISK FACTORS: Identify two risk factors.

DIAGNOSTIC PROCEDURES: Identify two laboratory tests that are used to diagnose hypothyroidism and the expected findings.

Application Exercises

1. A nurse in a provider's office is reviewing laboratory results for a client who has secondary hypothyroidism. Which of the following findings should the nurse expect?
   - A. Elevated serum T₄
   - B. Decreased serum T₃
   - C. Elevated serum thyroid-stimulating hormone
   - D. Decreased serum cholesterol

2. A nurse is collecting an admission history from a female client who has hypothyroidism. Which of the following findings should the nurse expect? (Select all that apply.)
   - A. Diarrhea
   - B. Menorrhagia
   - C. Dry skin
   - D. Increased libido
   - E. Hoarseness

3. A nurse is reinforcing teaching with a client who has a new prescription for levothyroxine to treat hypothyroidism. Which of the following information should the nurse include? (Select all that apply.)
   - A. Weight gain will occur while taking this medication.
   - B. Do not discontinue medication without the advice of the provider.
   - C. Have follow-up serum TSH levels performed.
   - D. Take the medication on an empty stomach.
   - E. Use fiber laxatives for constipation.

4. A nurse is assisting in planning care for a client who has myxedema coma. Which of the following actions should the nurse include? (Select all that apply.)
   - A. Monitor daily weights.
   - B. Observe for evidence of urinary tract infection.
   - C. Record input and output.
   - D. Initiate aspiration precautions.
   - E. Provide warmth using a heating pad.

5. A nurse in a provider's office is collecting data from a client who has hypothyroidism and recently began treatment with thyroid hormone replacement therapy. Which of the following findings indicate that the client might need a decrease in the dosage of the medication?
   - A. Hand tremors
   - B. Bradycardia
   - C. Pallor
   - D. Slow speech

Application Exercises Key

1. A. Decreased serum T_4 is an expected finding for a client who has hypothyroidism.

   B. **CORRECT:** Decreased serum T_3 is an expected finding for a client who has hypothyroidism.

   C. Decreased TSH level is an expected finding for a client who has secondary hypothyroidism.

   D. Elevated serum cholesterol is an expected finding for a client who has hypothyroidism.

   Ⓝ *NCLEX® Connection: Reduction of Risk Potential, Laboratory Values*

2. A. Constipation is a manifestation of hypothyroidism.

   B. **CORRECT:** Abnormal menstrual periods, including menorrhagia and amenorrhea, are manifestations of hypothyroidism.

   C. **CORRECT:** Dry skin is a manifestation of hypothyroidism.

   D. Decreased libido is a manifestation of hypothyroidism.

   E. **CORRECT:** Hoarseness is a manifestation of hypothyroidism.

   Ⓝ *NCLEX® Connection: Physiological Adaptation, Basic Pathophysiology*

3. A. Levothyroxine speeds up metabolism. Weight loss is an expected effect.

   B. **CORRECT:** The provider carefully titrates the dosage of this medication, increasing it slowly until the client reaches a euthyroid state. The client should not discontinue the medication unless directed by the provider.

   C. **CORRECT:** Serum TSH levels monitor the effectiveness of the medication.

   D. **CORRECT:** Taking the medication on an empty stomach promotes absorption.

   E. The client should avoid fiber laxatives, which reduce absorption of the medication.

   Ⓝ *NCLEX® Connection: Pharmacological Therapies, Expected Actions/Outcomes*

4. A. **CORRECT:** The nurse should monitor the client's daily weight because decreasing weight is an indication of effective therapy.

   B. **CORRECT:** An infection, such as in the urinary tract, can precipitate myxedema coma. The nurse should observe the client for manifestations of infection and treat any underlying illness.

   C. **CORRECT:** The nurse should record daily I&O because increased urine output is an indication of effective therapy.

   D. **CORRECT:** The nurse should initiate aspiration precautions, because myxedema coma is a severe complication of hypothyroidism that can lead to a compromised airway.

   E. The nurse should provide warmth with extra clothing and blankets. The nurse should avoid using electric heating devices because the combination of vasodilation, decreased sensation, and decreased alertness places the client at risk for burns.

   Ⓝ *NCLEX® Connection: Reduction of Risk Potential, Potential for Complications from Surgical Procedures and Health Alterations*

5. A. **CORRECT:** Hand tremors are a manifestation of hyperthyroidism that can result from thyroid hormone replacement therapy. The nurse should report this finding to the provider for a possible decrease in the medication dosage.

   B. Bradycardia is an expected finding for hypothyroidism. This finding indicates the need for continued thyroid hormone replacement therapy with a possible increase in dosage.

   C. Pallor is an expected finding for hypothyroidism. This finding indicates the need for continued thyroid hormone replacement therapy with a possible increase in dosage.

   D. Slow thought processes and speech are expected findings for hypothyroidism. This finding indicates the need for continued thyroid hormone replacement therapy with a possible increase in dosage.

   Ⓝ *NCLEX® Connection: Pharmacological Therapies, Expected Actions/Outcomes*

PRACTICE Answer

Using the ATI Active Learning Template: System Disorder

ALTERATION IN HEALTH (DIAGNOSIS):
Hypothyroidism is a condition in which there is an inadequate amount of circulating thyroid hormones triiodothyronine (T_3) and thyroxine (T_4), causing a decrease in metabolic rate that affects all body systems.

RISK FACTORS
- Female clients age 30 to 60 years
- Use of lithium or amiodarone

DIAGNOSTIC PROCEDURES
- Serum T_3: Decreased
- Serum thyroid-stimulating hormone (TSH)
  - Increased with primary hypothyroidism
  - Decreased or within the expected reference range in secondary hypothyroidism
- Free T_4 index: Decreased
- T_3 resin uptake: Decreased
- Serum cholesterol: Increased

Ⓝ *NCLEX® Connection: Physiological Adaptation, Alterations in Body Systems*

CHAPTER 72 *Adrenal Disorders*

Cushing's disease (hypercortisolism) and Cushing's syndrome are caused by an oversecretion of the hormones the adrenal cortex produces.

A tumor in the pituitary gland resulting in release of the hormone ACTH can cause Cushing's disease. The ACTH then stimulates the adrenal cortex to increase the secretion of the glucocorticoid hormone cortisol. Hyperplasia of the adrenal cortex is another cause of Cushing's disease.

Cushing's syndrome results from long-term use of glucocorticoids to treat other conditions, such as asthma or rheumatoid arthritis.

Addison's disease is an adrenocortical insufficiency caused by damage or dysfunction of the adrenal cortex. The production of mineralocorticoids and glucocorticoids is diminished, resulting in decreased aldosterone and cortisol.

Acute adrenal insufficiency, also known as Addisonian crisis, has a rapid onset and is a medical emergency. If it is not quickly diagnosed and properly treated, the prognosis is poor.

Older adult clients are less able to tolerate complications of Addison's disease and acute adrenal insufficiency and need more frequent monitoring. ©

Cushing's Disease/ Syndrome

ADRENAL CORTEX HORMONES

Mineralocorticoids: Aldosterone increases sodium reabsorption and potassium excretion in the kidney.

Glucocorticoids: Cortisol affects glucose, protein, and fat metabolism; the body's response to stress; and the body's immune function.

Sex hormones: Androgens and estrogens

HEALTH PROMOTION AND DISEASE PREVENTION

Take medications that can lead to Cushing's disease as a complication as directed and watch for adverse reactions. The need for medication therapy is often lifelong.

DATA COLLECTION

RISK FACTORS

Females age 30 to 50 years are at increased risk for Cushing's syndrome.

Cushing's disease

ENDOGENOUS CAUSES OF INCREASED CORTISOL
- Adrenal hyperplasia
- Adrenocortical carcinoma
- Pituitary carcinoma that secretes adrenocorticotropic hormone (ACTH)
- Carcinomas of the lung, gastrointestinal (GI) tract, or pancreas (these tumors can secrete ACTH)

Cushing's syndrome

EXOGENOUS CAUSES OF INCREASED CORTISOL:
Therapeutic use of glucocorticoids for the following.
- Organ transplant
- Chemotherapy
- Autoimmune diseases
- Asthma
- Allergies
- Chronic inflammatory diseases

EXPECTED FINDINGS

- Weakness, fatigue, sleep disturbances
- Back and joint pain
- Altered emotional state (irritability, depression)
- Decreased libido

PHYSICAL FINDINGS

- Evidence of decreased immune function and decreased inflammatory response (infections without fever, swelling, drainage, redness)
- Thin, fragile skin
- Bruising and petechiae (fragile blood vessels)
- Hypertension (sodium and water retention)
- Tachycardia
- Gastric ulcers due to oversecretion of hydrochloric acid
- Weight gain and increased appetite
- Irregular menses
- Dependent edema: Changes in fat distribution (characteristic fat distribution of moon face, truncal obesity, fat collection on back of neck [buffalo hump])
- Bone pain and fractures due to osteoporosis, with an increased risk for falls Qs
- Muscle wasting (particularly in the extremities)
- Impaired glucose tolerance
- Frequent infections, poor wound healing
- Hirsutism
- Acne
- Red cheeks
- Striae (reddened lines on abdomen, upper arms, thighs)
- Clitoral hypertrophy
- Thinning, balding hair
- Hyperglycemia
- Emotional lability

LABORATORY TESTS

Elevated plasma cortisol in the absence of acute illness or stress indicate Cushing's disease/syndrome. Urine (24-hr collection) contains elevated levels of free cortisol.

Plasma adrenocorticotropic hormone (ACTH) levels
- Hypersecretion of ACTH by the anterior pituitary results in elevated ACTH levels.
- Disorders of the adrenal cortex or medication therapy result in decreased ACTH levels.

Salivary cortisol elevations confirm the diagnosis of Cushing's disease.

Potassium and calcium: Decreased

Glucose: Increased

Sodium: Increased

Lymphocytes: Decreased

Dexamethasone suppression tests vary in length and amount of dexamethasone to administer.
- 24-hr urine collections show suppression of cortisol excretion in clients who do not have Cushing's disease.
- Nonsuppression of cortisol excretion indicates Cushing's disease.
- Clients should stop taking medications and try to reduce stress prior to and during testing.
- False positive results can result for clients who have acute illnesses and alcohol use disorder.

DIAGNOSTIC PROCEDURES

- X-ray, magnetic resonance imaging, and CT scans identify lesions of the pituitary gland, adrenal gland, lung, GI tract, and pancreas.
- Radiological imaging determines the source of adrenal insufficiency (tumor, adrenal atrophy).

NURSING ACTIONS
- Ensure the client has IV access.
- Determine allergies.
- Reinforce teaching about the procedure.
- Provide padding, pillows, and blankets for comfort. Qs

CLIENT EDUCATION: Tests are noninvasive and not painful.

PATIENT-CENTERED CARE

NURSING CARE

- Monitor I&O and daily weight.
- Monitor for indications of hypervolemia (edema, distended neck veins, shortness of breath, adventitious breath sounds, hypertension, tachycardia).
- Maintain a safe environment to minimize the risk of pathological fractures and skin trauma.
- Prevent infection by performing frequent hand hygiene.
- Encourage physical activity within the client's limitations.
- Provide meticulous skin care.
- Change the client's position at least every 2 hr.
- Monitor for and protect against skin breakdown and infection.
- Use surgical asepsis when performing dressing changes and any invasive procedures.
- Monitor WBC count with differential daily.

MEDICATIONS

- Treatment depends on the cause.
- For Cushing's syndrome, taper glucocorticoids and manage manifestations if possible.

Ketoconazole

- Ketoconazole is an antifungal agent that also inhibits adrenal corticosteroid synthesis in high dosages.
- Ketoconazole supplements radiation or surgery.

NURSING ACTIONS
- Monitor liver enzymes and for indications of liver toxicity (yellow sclera, dark-colored urine).
- Monitor fluids and electrolytes for clients who have gastric effects.

CLIENT EDUCATION
- The medication can cause nausea, vomiting, and dizziness.
- Relief is temporary. Manifestations will return if the medication is stopped.
- Take the medication with food to relieve gastric effects. Qs

Mitotane

Produces selective destruction of adrenocortical cells

NURSING ACTIONS
- Mitotane treats inoperable adrenal carcinoma.
- Monitor for indications of shock, renal damage, and hepatotoxicity.
- Monitor for orthostatic hypotension.

CLIENT EDUCATION
- The purpose of the medication is to reduce the size of the tumor.
- Notify the provider of weakness, dizziness, nausea, vomiting, or weight loss.
- Use caution when driving or operating heavy machinery.
- Lifelong replacement with glucocorticoids is needed.

Hydrocortisone

For replacement therapy for clients who have adrenocortical insufficiency

NURSING ACTIONS
- Monitor potassium and glucose levels.
- Measure daily weight. Notify the provider of weight gain greater than 2.3 kg (5 lb)/week.
- Monitor blood pressure and pulse.
- Monitor for manifestations of infection (increased temperature, increased WBC).

CLIENT EDUCATION
- Carry emergency identification about corticosteroid use.
- Report abdominal pain or black, tarry stools.
- Notify the provider for any manifestations of infection.
- Take the medication without skipping any doses.
- Consume a diet high in calcium and vitamin D.
- Consult the provider before taking any OTC medications or supplements.

THERAPEUTIC PROCEDURES

Chemotherapy

With cytotoxic agents for Cushing's disease resulting from a tumor

NURSING ACTIONS
- Monitor for adverse effects (thrombocytopenia, nausea, vomiting) and other effects specific to the chemotherapeutic agent.
- Monitor WBC, absolute neutrophil count, platelet count, Hgb, and Hct.
- Monitor for bruising and bleeding gums.
- Administer an antiemetic.

CLIENT EDUCATION
- Avoid crowds and contact with individuals who have infections.
- Watch for bleeding, such as tarry stools or coffee-ground emesis.
- Some hair loss can occur.

Radiation therapy

NURSING ACTIONS: Provide skin care and monitor for skin damage. Q_{EBP}

CLIENT EDUCATION
- Remove radiation markings.
- Avoid applying lotions, other than those the radiologist prescribes, to affected areas.
- Avoid exposing irradiated areas to sunlight.
- Expect fatigue and altered taste due to radiation.

Hypophysectomy

Surgical removal of the pituitary gland (depending on the cause of Cushing's disease)
- The surgeon will perform a transsphenoidal hypophysectomy through the sphenoid sinus via the nasal cavity or under the upper lip and place packing in the nares. The client will have a drip pad under the nose for bloody drainage and will need to breathe through the mouth.
- Immediate postoperative care requires intensive care unit monitoring for increased intracranial pressure, cerebrospinal fluid (CSF) leak, and cardiopulmonary status.

NURSING ACTIONS
- Monitor and correct electrolytes, especially sodium, potassium, and chloride.
- Monitor and adjust glucose levels.
- Protect the client from developing an infection by using good hand hygiene and making sure the client avoids contact with individuals who have infections.
- Use caution to prevent a fracture by providing assistance getting out of bed and raising side rails.
- Monitor for bleeding.
- Monitor nasal drainage for a possible CSF leak.
- Monitor drainage for the presence of glucose or a halo sign (yellow on the edge and clear in the middle), which can indicate CSF.
- Monitor neurologic status every hour for the first 24 hr and then every 4 hr.
- Administer glucocorticoids to prevent an abrupt drop in cortisol level.
- Administer stool softeners to prevent straining.

CLIENT EDUCATION
- Avoid coughing, blowing the nose, and sneezing.
- Use caution preoperatively to prevent infection or fractures.
- There might be numbness at the surgical site and a diminished sense of smell for 3 to 4 months after surgery.
- Avoid bending over at the waist and straining to prevent increased intracranial pressure. If bending to pick up an object or to tie shoes is needed, bend at the knees.
- Avoid brushing teeth for 2 weeks. Floss and rinse mouth. Q[EBP]
- Notify the provider of sweet-tasting drainage, drainage that makes a halo, or clear drainage from the nose, which can indicate a CSF leak. Another indication is a headache.
- Notify the provider of excessive bleeding, confusion, or headache.
- Eat high-fiber food and take docusate to avoid constipation, which contributes to increased intracranial pressure.

Adrenalectomy

Surgical removal of the adrenal gland
- Unilateral (one gland)
- Bilateral (both glands)

Immediate postoperative care requires intensive care unit monitoring for acute adrenal insufficiency and cardiopulmonary status.

NURSING ACTIONS
- Provide glucocorticoid and hormone replacement.
- Monitor for adrenal crisis due to an abrupt drop in cortisol level. Findings include hypotension, tachycardia, tachypnea, nausea, and headache.
- Monitor vital signs frequently.
- Monitor fluids and electrolytes.
- Monitor the incision site for bleeding.
- Monitor bowel sounds.
- Provide pain medication. Administer stool softeners.
- Slowly reintroduce foods.
- Monitor the abdomen for distention and tenderness
- Monitor the incision site for redness, discharge, and swelling.
- Reinforce to the client about postoperative pain management, deep breathing, and antiembolism care.

CLIENT EDUCATION: Take glucocorticoids, mineralocorticoids, and hormone replacements.

INTERPROFESSIONAL CARE

Request a dietary consult. Dietary alterations include decreased sodium intake and increased intake of potassium, protein, calcium, and vitamin D.

COMPLICATIONS

Perforated viscera/ulceration

Decreases production of protective mucus in the lining of the stomach due to an increase in cortisol

NURSING ACTIONS
- Monitor for evidence of GI bleeding (tarry, black stool; coffee-ground emesis).
- Administer antiulcer medications.

CLIENT EDUCATION
- Monitor for GI bleeding.
- Avoid alcohol, caffeine, and smoking.

Bone fractures due to hypocalcemia

NURSING ACTIONS
- Use caution when moving the client. Q[s]
- Provide assistance when the client is ambulating.
- Clear floors to prevent falls.

CLIENT EDUCATION
- Consume a diet high in calcium and vitamin D.
- Avoid dangerous activities.

Infection due to immunosuppression

Immunosuppression and reduced inflammatory response occur due to elevated glucocorticoid levels.

NURSING ACTIONS: Monitor for subtle indications of infection (fatigue, fever, localized swelling or redness).

CLIENT EDUCATION
- Minimize exposure to infectious organisms. (Avoid people who are ill. Avoid crowds. Use hand hygiene.) Q[s]
- Report indications of infection to the provider.

Adrenal crisis (acute adrenal insufficiency)

Sudden drop in corticosteroids is due to the following.
- Sudden tumor removal
- Stress of illness, trauma, surgery, or dehydration
- Abrupt withdrawal of steroid medication

NURSING ACTIONS
- Transfer client to intensive care unit for monitoring of cardiopulmonary status.
- Manifestations include hypotension, hypoglycemia, hyperkalemia, abdominal pain, weakness, and weight loss.
- Administration of glucocorticoids treats acute adrenal insufficiency.
- The provider might prescribe insulin with dextrose, a potassium-binding and -excreting resin (sodium polystyrene sulfonate), or loop or thiazide diuretics to treat hyperkalemia.
- The provider might prescribe glucagon or glucose to treat hypoglycemia.
- Monitor vital signs and glucose levels.
- Monitor electrolytes.

CLIENT EDUCATION
- Taper the medication.
- During times of stress, additional glucocorticoids might be needed to prevent adrenal crisis.

Addison's Disease and Acute Adrenal Insufficiency (Addisonian Crisis)

DATA COLLECTION

RISK FACTORS

CAUSES OF PRIMARY ADDISON'S DISEASE
- Idiopathic autoimmune dysfunction (majority of cases)
- Tuberculosis
- Histoplasmosis
- Adrenalectomy
- Cancer
- Radiation therapy of the abdomen

CAUSES OF SECONDARY ADDISON'S DISEASE
- Steroid withdrawal
- Hypophysectomy
- Pituitary neoplasm
- High-dose radiation of pituitary gland or entire brain

ACUTE ADRENAL INSUFFICIENCY is a life-threatening event that if left untreated can lead to death. Factors that precipitate acute adrenal insufficiency are the following.
- Sepsis
- Trauma
- Stress (myocardial infarction, surgery, anesthesia, hypothermia, volume loss, hypoglycemia)
- Adrenal hemorrhage
- Steroid withdrawal

EXPECTED FINDINGS

Manifestations of chronic Addison's disease develop slowly. Manifestations of acute adrenal insufficiency develop rapidly.
- Weight loss
- Craving for salt
- Hyperpigmentation
- Weakness and fatigue
- Nausea and vomiting
- Abdominal pain
- Constipation or diarrhea
- Dizziness with orthostatic hypotension
- Severe hypotension (acute adrenal insufficiency)
- Dehydration

LABORATORY TESTS

Serum electrolytes: Increased K+, decreased Na+, and increased calcium

BUN and creatinine: Increased

Serum glucose: Within expected reference range or decreased

Serum cortisol: Decreased

WBCs: Increased

Adrenocorticotropic hormone (ACTH) stimulation test: ACTH is infused, and the cortisol response is measured 30 min and 1 hr after the injection.
- With primary adrenal insufficiency, plasma cortisol levels do not rise.
- With secondary adrenal insufficiency, plasma cortisol levels are decreased.

DIAGNOSTIC PROCEDURES

Electrocardiogram (ECG)

Used to monitor for ECG changes or dysrhythmias associated with electrolyte imbalance.

NURSING ACTION: Explain procedures to the client.

X-ray, CT scan, MRI scan

Radiological imaging to determine source of adrenal insufficiency, such as a tumor or adrenal atrophy

CLIENT EDUCATION: Tests are noninvasive and not painful.

PATIENT-CENTERED CARE

NURSING CARE

- Monitor for fluid deficits and electrolyte imbalances. The provider might prescribe saline infusions to restore fluid volume.
- Observe for dehydration.
- Obtain orthostatic vital signs.
- The provider might prescribe hydrocortisone
- Monitor for and treat hyperkalemia.
  - Obtain serum potassium and ECG.
  - The provider might prescribe sodium polystyrene sulfonate, insulin, calcium, glucose, and sodium bicarbonate.
  - Monitor vital signs frequently, and assist with monitoring for dysrhythmias.
- Monitor for and treat hypoglycemia:
  - Perform frequent checks of neurologic status, monitor for hypoglycemia, and check serum glucose.
  - Administer food and/or supplemental glucose.
- Maintain a safe environment. Qs
  - Provide assistance ambulating.
  - Prevent falls by keeping floors clear.

MEDICATIONS

Hydrocortisone, prednisone, cortisone

Glucocorticoids are used as adrenocorticoid replacement for adrenal insufficiency and as an anti-inflammatory.

NURSING ACTIONS
- Monitor weight, blood pressure, and electrolytes.
- Increase dosage during periods of stress or illness if necessary.
- Taper dose if discontinuing to avoid acute adrenal insufficiency.
- Administer with food to reduce gastric effects.

CLIENT EDUCATION Qpcc
- Take medication as directed.
- Avoid discontinuing the medication abruptly.
- Report manifestations of Cushing's syndrome (round face, edema, weight gain).
- Take the medication with food.
- Report manifestations of adrenal insufficiency (fever, fatigue, muscle weakness, anorexia).

Fludrocortisone

A mineralocorticoid used as a replacement in adrenal insufficiency

NURSING ACTIONS
- Monitor weight, blood pressure, and electrolytes.
- Hypertension is a potential adverse effect.
- Increase dosage as needed during periods of stress or illness.

CLIENT EDUCATION
- Take the medication as directed.
- Mild peripheral edema is expected.

INTERPROFESSIONAL CARE

Home assistance for fluid, medication, and dietary management as required.

CLIENT EDUCATION

- Take medications as prescribed and monitor for adverse reactions. Qpcc
- Avoid consuming alcohol and caffeine.
- Monitor for indications of gastric bleeding (coffee-ground emesis; tarry, black stool).
- Monitor for hypoglycemia (diaphoresis, shaking, tachycardia, headache).
- Report manifestations of adrenal insufficiency (fever, fatigue, muscle weakness, dizziness, anorexia).
- To prevent acute adrenal insufficiency, increase corticosteroid doses as prescribed during times of stress.
- Medication therapy is often lifelong.

COMPLICATIONS

Adrenal crisis (acute adrenal insufficiency)

- Sudden drop in corticosteroids is due to
  - Sudden tumor removal
  - Stress of illness, trauma, surgery, or dehydration
  - Abrupt withdrawal of steroid medication
- Manifestations include hypotension, hypoglycemia, hyperkalemia, abdominal pain, weakness, and weight loss.

NURSING ACTIONS
- Transfer client to intensive care unit for close monitoring of cardiopulmonary status.
- Administer glucocorticoids to treat acute adrenal insufficiency.
- The provider might prescribe insulin with dextrose, a potassium-binding and -excreting resin (sodium polystyrene sulfonate), or loop or thiazide diuretics to treat hyperkalemia.
- The provider might prescribe glucagon or glucose to treat hypoglycemia.
- Monitor vital signs and glucose levels.
- Monitor electrolytes.

CLIENT EDUCATION
- Taper the medication.
- During times of stress, additional glucocorticoids might be needed to prevent adrenal crisis.

Hypoglycemia

Insufficient glucocorticoid causes increased insulin sensitivity and decreased glycogen, which leads to hypoglycemia.

NURSING ACTIONS: Monitor glucose levels.

CLIENT EDUCATION
- Monitor for hypoglycemia. Manifestations can include diaphoresis, shaking, tachycardia, and headache.
- Have a 15 g carbohydrate snack readily available. Qebp

Hyperkalemia/Hyponatremia

Decrease in aldosterone levels can cause an increased excretion of sodium and a decreased excretion of potassium.

NURSING ACTIONS: Monitor electrolytes and ECG.

CLIENT EDUCATION
- Take the medications as directed.
- Report indications of hyperkalemia (muscle weakness, tingling sensation, irregular heartbeat). Qs

Application Exercises

1. A nurse is caring for a client who has Cushing's disease. Clients who have Cushing's disease are at increased risk for which of the following? (Select all that apply.)

   A. Infection

   B. Gastric ulcer

   C. Renal calculi

   D. Bone fractures

   E. Dysphagia

2. At the beginning of a shift, a nurse is collecting data on a client who has Cushing's disease. Which of the following findings is the nurse's priority?

   A. Weight gain

   B. Fatigue

   C. Fragile skin

   D. Joint pain

3. A nurse is reinforcing discharge teaching with a client who had a transsphenoidal hypophysectomy. Which of the following instructions should the nurse include? (Select all that apply.)

   A. Brush teeth after every meal or snack.

   B. Avoid bending at the knees.

   C. Eat a high-fiber diet.

   D. Notify the provider of any sweet-tasting drainage.

   E. Notify the provider of a diminished sense of smell.

4. A nurse is reinforcing teaching with a client who has Addison's disease and is taking hydrocortisone. Which of the following instructions should the nurse include? (Select all that apply.)

   A. Take the medication on an empty stomach.

   B. Notify the provider of any illness or stress.

   C. Report any manifestations of weakness or dizziness.

   D. Do not discontinue the medication suddenly.

   E. Eat a low-sodium diet.

5. A nurse is planning to reinforce teaching with a client who is being evaluated for Addison's disease about the adrenocorticotropic hormone (ACTH) stimulation test. The nurse should base her instructions to the client on which of the following information?

   A. The ACTH stimulation test measures the response by the kidneys to ACTH.

   B. In the presence of primary adrenal insufficiency, plasma cortisol levels rise in response to administration of ACTH.

   C. ACTH is a hormone produced by the pituitary gland.

   D. The client will take a dose of ACTH by mouth the evening before the test.

PRACTICE Active Learning Scenario

A nurse is reinforcing teaching with a client who had a bilateral adrenalectomy for adrenal hyperplasia and has a new prescription for hydrocortisone. Use the ATI Active Learning Template: Medication to complete this item.

THERAPEUTIC USES: Explain why the client needs to take this medication.

CLIENT EDUCATION: Identify three instructions to include about this medication.

Application Exercises Key

1. A. **CORRECT:** Suppression of the immune system places the client at risk for infection.

   B. **CORRECT:** Overproduction of cortisol inhibits the production of a protective mucus lining in the stomach and causes an increase in the amount of gastric acid. These factors place clients who have Cushing's disease at increased risk for gastric ulcers.

   C. Clients who have Cushing's disease are not at risk for renal calculi, but they are at risk for neurological and cardiovascular problems.

   D. **CORRECT:** Clients who have Cushing's disease are at risk for bone fractures because decreased calcium reabsorption can lead to osteoporosis.

   E. Clients who have Cushing's disease are not at risk for dysphagia, but they are at risk for other gastrointestinal problems, including anorexia, nausea, vomiting, and abdominal pain.

   Ⓝ *NCLEX® Connection: Physiological Adaptation, Basic Pathophysiology*

2. A. **CORRECT:** The greatest risk to a client who has Cushing's disease is fluid retention, which can lead to pulmonary edema, hypertension, and heart failure.

   B. The client is at risk for inability to perform self-care due to fatigue. However, another finding is the priority.

   C. The client is at risk for skin tears and breakdown due to fragile skin. However, another finding is the priority.

   D. The client is at risk for impaired mobility due to joint pain. However, another finding is the priority.

   Ⓝ *NCLEX® Connection: Physiological Adaptation, Basic Pathophysiology*

3. A. The client should avoid brushing his teeth for 2 weeks to allow time for the incision to heal.

   B. The client should avoid bending at the waist. If bending is necessary, he should bend at the knees.

   C. **CORRECT:** The client should eat a high-fiber diet and take docusate to avoid constipation, which contributes to increased intracranial pressure when straining to have a bowel movement.

   D. **CORRECT:** Sweet-tasting fluid is an indication of a cerebrospinal fluid leak. The client should notify the provider.

   E. Diminished sense of smell is an expected finding after surgery.

   Ⓝ *NCLEX® Connection: Physiological Adaptation, Alterations in Body Systems*

4. A. The client should take hydrocortisone with food to decrease GI distress.

   B. **CORRECT:** Physical and emotional stress increase the need for hydrocortisone. The provider might increase the dosage when stress occurs.

   C. **CORRECT:** Weakness and dizziness are indications of adrenal insufficiency. The client should report these indications to the provider.

   D. **CORRECT:** Rapid discontinuation can result in adverse effects, including acute adrenal insufficiency. If hydrocortisone is discontinued, the dose is tapered.

   E. Clients who have Addison's disease have hyponatremia. A low-sodium diet is not advised.

   Ⓝ *NCLEX® Connection: Pharmacological Therapies, Expected Actions/Outcomes*

5. A. The ACTH stimulation test measures the response by the adrenal glands to ACTH.

   B. In the presence of primary adrenal insufficiency, plasma cortisol levels do not rise in response to administration of ACTH.

   C. **CORRECT:** Secretion of corticotropin-releasing hormone from the hypothalamus prompts the pituitary gland to secrete ACTH.

   D. ACTH is administered IV during the testing process. Plasma cortisol levels are measured 30 min and 1 hr after the injection.

   Ⓝ *NCLEX® Connection: Pharmacological Therapies, Expected Actions/Outcomes*

PRACTICE Answer

Using the ATI Active Learning Template: Medication

THERAPEUTIC USES: Hydrocortisone is a glucocorticoid that treats adrenal insufficiency resulting from adrenalectomy surgery.

CLIENT EDUCATION
- Carry emergency identification about corticosteroid use.
- Report abdominal pain or black, tarry stools.
- Notify the provider for any manifestations of infection.
- Take the medication without skipping any doses.
- Consume a diet high in calcium and vitamin D.
- Consult the provider before taking any OTC medications or supplements.

Ⓝ *NCLEX® Connection: Pharmacological Therapies, Expected Actions/Outcomes*

CHAPTER 73 *Diabetes Mellitus Management and Complications*

Diabetes mellitus is a metabolic disorder resulting from either an inadequate production of insulin (type 1) or an inability of the body's cells to respond to insulin that is present (type 2).

Type 1 diabetes mellitus is an autoimmune dysfunction involving the destruction of beta cells, which produce insulin in the islets of Langerhans of the pancreas. Immune system cells and antibodies are present in circulation and can also be triggered by certain genetic tissue types or viral infections.

Type 2 diabetes mellitus is a progressive condition due to increasing inability of cells to respond to insulin (insulin resistance) and decreased production of insulin by the beta cells. It is linked to obesity, sedentary lifestyle, and heredity. Metabolic syndrome often precedes type 2 diabetes mellitus.

Diabetes mellitus has wide ranging systemic effects and is a contributing factor to development of cardiovascular disease, hypertension, kidney disease, neuropathy, retinopathy, peripheral vascular disease, and stroke.

Diabetes mellitus is significantly more prevalent in African American, Native American, and Hispanic populations and is more common in males than females.

Acute complications of diabetes mellitus include diabetic ketoacidosis (DKA) and hyperglycemic hyperosmolar state (HHS).

Chronic complications of diabetes mellitus include cardiovascular and cerebrovascular disease, diabetic retinopathy, diabetic neuropathy, and diabetic nephropathy.

HEALTH PROMOTION AND DISEASE PREVENTION

The American Diabetes Association recommends screening a client who has a BMI greater than 25 and age greater than 45 years, or if a child is overweight and has additional risk factors.

CLIENT EDUCATION
- Exercise regularly, and follow recommendations for preventing or controlling diabetes.
  - Carbohydrates: 45% of total daily intake
  - Protein: 15% to 20% of total daily intake, depending upon kidney function
  - Unsaturated and polyunsaturated fats: 20% to 35% of total daily intake
- Consistency in the amount of food consumed and regularity in meal times promotes blood glucose control.
- Consume a diet low in saturated fats to decrease low-density lipoprotein (LDL), assist with weight loss for secondary prevention of diabetes, and reduce risk of heart disease.
- Include omega-3 fatty acids and fiber in the diet to lower cholesterol, improve blood glucose control, prevent diabetes mellitus, and reduce the risk of heart disease.
- Engage in physical activity at least three times per week.

DATA COLLECTION

RISK FACTORS

- Metabolic syndrome: A collection of manifestations that predispose an individual to the development of diabetes mellitus including abdominal obesity, insulin resistance, sedentary lifestyle, hypertension, and elevated lipid and triglyceride levels. It also has an associated risk of cardiovascular disease.
- Prediabetes: Impaired fasting glucose levels 100 to 125 mg/dL, impaired glucose tolerance 140 to 199 mg/dL, or A1C level 5.7% to 6.40%.
- Pancreatitis and Cushing's syndrome: Secondary causes of diabetes
- Obesity
- Age 45 years or older
- Hypertension (140/90 mm Hg or greater)
- History of gestational diabetes, polycystic ovary disease, or delivering an infant larger than 4,000 g (9 lb)
- Smoking

EXPECTED FINDINGS

Hyperglycemia: Blood glucose level usually greater than 250 mg/dL (**73.1**)

Polyuria: Excess urine production and frequency from osmotic diuresis

Polydipsia: Excessive thirst due to dehydration
- Loss of skin turgor, skin warm and dry
- Dry mucous membranes
- Weakness and malaise
- Rapid weak pulse and hypotension

Polyphagia: Excessive hunger and eating caused from inability of cells to receive glucose (because of a lack of insulin or cellular resistance to available insulin) and the body's use of protein and fat for energy (which causes ketosis)
- Possible weight loss

LABORATORY TESTS

Diagnostic criteria for diabetes include two findings (on separate days) of at least one of the following.
- Manifestations of diabetes plus casual blood glucose concentration greater than 200 mg/dL (without regard to time since last meal)
- Fasting blood glucose greater than 126 mg/dL
- 2-hr glucose greater than 200 mg/dL with oral glucose tolerance test
- Glycosylated hemoglobin (A1C) greater than 6.5%

Fasting blood glucose

NURSING ACTIONS: Postpone administration of antidiabetic medication until after the level is drawn.

CLIENT EDUCATION: Fast (no food or drink other than water) for the 8 hr prior to the blood test.

Oral glucose tolerance test

- Often used to diagnose gestational diabetes mellitus
- Not generally used for routine diagnosis
- A fasting blood glucose level is drawn at the start of the test. The client is then instructed to consume a specified amount of glucose. Blood glucose levels are obtained every 30 min for 2 hr. The client must be checked for hypoglycemia throughout the procedure.

CLIENT EDUCATION
- Consume a balanced diet for 3 days prior to the test. Then fast for 10 to 12 hr prior to the test.
- Only water may be consumed during the testing period. Food and other liquids affect test results.

Glycosylated hemoglobin (HbA1c)

- HbA1c is the best indicator of the average blood glucose level for the past 120 days. It assists in evaluating treatment effectiveness and compliance
- The expected reference range is 4% to 5.7%, but an acceptable reference range for clients who have diabetes can be 6.5% to 8%, with a target goal of less than 7%.

CLIENT EDUCATION
- The test evaluates treatment effectiveness and compliance.
- The test is recommended quarterly or twice yearly depending on the glycemic levels.

Urine ketones

High ketones in the urine associated with hyperglycemia (exceed 300 mg/dL) is a medical emergency.

73.1 Hypoglycemia and hyperglycemia manifestations and management

Hypoglycemia

NURSING ACTIONS
- If the client is unconscious or unable to swallow, administer glucagon subcutaneous or IM (repeat in 10 min if still unconscious) and notify the provider. Place the client into a lateral position to prevent aspiration.
- In acute care, monitor the infusion of 50% dextrose. Consciousness should occur within 20 min.
- Once consciousness occurs and the client is able to swallow, have the client ingest oral carbohydrates.

CLIENT EDUCATION
- Follow recommendations for treatment of hypoglycemia (mild shakiness, confusion, sweating, palpitations, headache, lack of coordination, blurred vision, seizures, coma).
- Hypoglycemia preventive measures include avoiding excess insulin, exercise, and alcohol consumption on an empty stomach.
- A decrease in food intake or delay in food absorption can also cause hypoglycemia.
- Check blood glucose level.
- Follow guidelines outlined by the provider or diabetes educator.
- For hypoglycemia (glucose 70 mg/dL or less), take 15 to 20 g of a readily absorbable carbohydrate (4 to 6 oz fruit juice or regular soft drink, glucose tablets or glucose gel per package instructions, 6 to 10 hard candies, or 1 tbsp honey) and recheck blood glucose in 15 min.
- Repeat the administration of carbohydrates if not within normal limits, and recheck blood glucose in 15 min.
- If blood glucose is within normal limits, have a snack containing a carbohydrate and protein (if the next meal is more than 1 hr away). Blood glucose increases approximately 40 mg/dL over 30 min following ingestion of 10 g of absorbable carbohydrate.

Hyperglycemia

CLIENT EDUCATION
- Manifestations of hyperglycemia include hot, dry skin and fruity breath. Follow recommendations for treatment of hyperglycemia.
- Encourage oral fluid intake of sugar-free fluids to prevent dehydration.
- Administer insulin.
- When blood glucose levels are greater than 240 mg/dL, test urine for ketones.
- If ketones are present, do not exercise and report if outside of the expected reference range.
- Consult the provider if manifestations progress.

DIAGNOSTIC PROCEDURES

Self-monitored blood glucose (SMBG)

NURSING ACTION: Ensure that the client follows the proper procedure for blood sample collection and use of a glucose meter. Supplemental short-acting insulin may be prescribed for elevated pre-meal glucose levels.

CLIENT EDUCATION
- Check the accuracy of the strips with the control solution provided.
- Use the correct code number in the meter to match the strip bottle number.
- Store strips in the closed container in a dry location.
- Obtain an adequate amount of blood sample when preforming the test.
- Use appropriate hand hygiene.
- Use fresh lancets, and avoid sharing glucose monitoring equipment to prevent infection.
- Keep a record of SMBG levels that includes time, date, serum glucose level, insulin dose, food intake, and other events that can alter glucose metabolism (activity level, illness).

MEDICATIONS

- Insulin regimens are established for clients who have type 1 diabetes mellitus
  - Types of insulin: rapid-, short-, intermediate-, and long-acting
  - Given one or more times a day based on blood glucose results
- Insulin can be required by some clients who have type 2 diabetes or gestational diabetes if glycemic control is not obtained with diet, exercise, and oral hypoglycemic agents.
  - Continuous infusion of insulin can be accomplished using a small pump that is worn externally. The pump is programmed to deliver insulin through a needle in subcutaneous tissue. The needle should be changed at least every 2 to 3 days to prevent infection.
  - Complications of the insulin pump are accidental cessation of insulin administration, obstruction of the tubing/needle, pump failure, and infection.
- Insulin pens are prefilled cartridges of 150 to 300 units of insulin in a programmable device with disposable needles.
  - Convenient for travel
  - Used for clients who have vision impairment or problems with dexterity
- Oral hypoglycemics are used by clients who have type 2 diabetes, along with diet and exercise, to regulate blood glucose.

INSULIN

Also see the **PN PHARMACOLOGY REVIEW MODULE: CHAPTER 34 DIABETES MELLITUS.**

Rapid-acting insulin

Insulin lispro, insulin aspart, insulin glulisine
- Administer before meals to control postprandial rise in blood glucose.
- Onset is rapid (10 to 30 min), depending on which insulin the nurse administers.
- Administer in conjunction with intermediate- or long-acting insulin to provide glycemic control between meals and at night.

Short-acting insulin

Regular insulin
- Administer 30 to 60 min before meals to control postprandial hyperglycemia.
- Regular insulin is available in two concentrations.
  - U-500 is reserved for the client who has insulin resistance. It is never administered IV.
  - U-100 is prescribed for most clients and may be administered IV.

Intermediate-acting insulin

NPH insulin
- Administered for glycemic control between meals and at night.
- Contains protamine (a protein), which causes a delay in the insulin absorption or onset and extends the duration of action of the insulin.
- Administer NPH insulin subcutaneous only and as the only insulin to mix with short-acting insulin.

Long-acting insulin

Insulin glargine, insulin detemir
- Administered once daily, anytime during the day but always at the same time each day.
- Glargine insulin forms microprecipitates that dissolves slowly over 24 hr and maintains a steady blood sugar level with no peaks or troughs.
- Insulin detemir has an added fatty-acid chain that delays absorption. Although it does not have a peak, duration is dose-dependent (12 to 24 hr).
- Administer glargine insulin and insulin detemir subcutaneous only.
- Dosage can be adjusted when the client is scheduled for procedures that require fasting.

NURSING ACTIONS
- Observe the client perform self-administration of insulin, and reinforce instruction as needed.
- Monitor for hypoglycemic reactions (sweating, weakness, dizziness, confusion, headache, tachycardia, slurred speech) at insulin peak times.

CLIENT EDUCATION
- **Self-administration of insulin**
  - Rotate injection sites (to prevent lipohypertrophy) within one anatomic site (to prevent day-to-day changes in absorption rates).
  - Inject subcutaneously at a 90° angle (45° angle if the client is thin). Aspiration for blood is not necessary.
  - When mixing a rapid- or short-acting insulin with a longer-acting insulin, draw up the shorter-acting insulin into the syringe first and then the longer-acting insulin. This reduces the risk of introducing the longer-acting insulin into the shorter-acting insulin vial.
- Eat at regular intervals, avoid alcohol intake, and adjust insulin to exercise and diet to avoid hypoglycemia.
- Wear a medical identification wristband.

ORAL HYPOGLYCEMICS

Also see the **PN PHARMACOLOGY REVIEW MODULE: CHAPTER 34 DIABETES MELLITUS**.

Biguanides

Metformin
- Reduces the production of glucose by the liver (gluconeogenesis)
- Increases tissue sensitivity to insulin
- Slows carbohydrate absorption in the intestines

NURSING ACTIONS
- Monitor significance of gastrointestinal (GI) effects (flatulence, anorexia, nausea, vomiting).
- Monitor for lactic acidosis, especially in clients who have kidney disorders or liver dysfunction.
- Stop medication for 48 hr before any type of elective radiographic test with iodinated contrast dye and restart 48 hr after (can cause lactic acidosis due to acute kidney injury).

CLIENT EDUCATION
- Take with food to decrease adverse GI effects.
- Take vitamin B_{12} and folic acid supplements.
- Contact the provider if manifestations of lactic acidosis develop (myalgia, sluggishness, somnolence, hyperventilation).
- Biguanides may be taken for gestational diabetes.
- Never crush or chew the medication.

Second-generation sulfonylureas

Glipizide, glimepiride, glyburide
- Stimulates insulin release from the pancreas, causing a decrease in blood sugar levels
- Increases tissue sensitivity to insulin

NURSING ACTIONS
- Monitor for hypoglycemia.
- Beta blockers can mask tachycardia typically seen during hypoglycemia.

CLIENT EDUCATION
- Administer 30 min before meals.
- Monitor for hypoglycemia and report frequent episodes to the provider.
- Avoid alcohol due to disulfiram effect.

Meglitinides

Repaglinide, nateglinide
- Stimulates insulin release from pancreas.
- Administered for post-meal hyperglycemia.

NURSING ACTIONS
- Monitor for hypoglycemia.
- Monitor HbA1c every 3 months to determine effectiveness.

CLIENT EDUCATION
- Administer 15 to 30 min before a meal.
- Eat with 30 min of administration.
- Omit the dose if a meal is skipped, to prevent hypoglycemic crisis.

Thiazolidinediones

Pioglitazone
- Reduces the production of glucose by the liver (gluconeogenesis)
- Increases tissue sensitivity to insulin

NURSING ACTIONS
- Monitor for fluid retention, especially in clients who have a history of heart failure.
- Monitor for elevation of ALT, LDH, and triglycerides levels.

CLIENT EDUCATION
- Report rapid weight gain, shortness of breath, or decreased exercise tolerance.
- Use additional contraception methods because the medication reduces the blood levels of oral contraceptives, which could allow ovulation to occur.
- Have liver function tests at baseline and every 3 to 6 months thereafter.

Alpha-glucosidase inhibitors

Acarbose, miglitol
- Slow carbohydrate absorption from the intestinal tract
- Reduces post-meal hyperglycemia

NURSING ACTIONS
- Monitor liver function every 3 months.
- Treat hypoglycemia with dextrose, not table sugar (prevents table sugar from breaking down).

CLIENT EDUCATION
- GI discomfort (abdominal distention, cramps, excessive gas, diarrhea) is common with these medications.
- Have liver function tests performed every 3 months or as prescribed.
- Take the medication with the first bite of each meal in order for the medication to be effective.
- Have available dextrose paste to treat hypoglycemia.

Dipeptidyl peptidase-4 (DPP-4) inhibitors

Sitagliptin, saxagliptin, linagliptin, alogliptin
- Augments naturally occurring intestinal incretin hormones, which promote release of insulin and decrease secretion of glucagon
- Lowers fasting and postprandial glucose levels
- Few adverse effects, but upper respiratory manifestations (nasal and throat inflammation) and pancreatitis can occur

CLIENT EDUCATION
- GI discomforts are possible (nausea, vomiting, diarrhea).
- Report persistent upper respiratory manifestations.
- Report severe abdominal pain, with or without emesis.
- Medication only works when blood sugar is rising.

Incretin mimetic

Exenatide, liraglutide
- Mimics the function of intestinal incretin hormone by decreasing glucagon secretion and gastric emptying.
- Decrease insulin demand by reducing fasting and postprandial hyperglycemia.

NURSING ACTIONS
- Administer subcutaneously 60 min before morning and evening meal.
- Monitor for gastrointestinal distress.

CLIENT EDUCATION
- Do not administer after a meal.
- Do not take oral antibiotics, oral contraceptives, or acetaminophen within 1 hr of oral exenatide or 2 hr after an injection of exenatide.
- Incretin mimetics can cause decreased appetite and weight loss.
- Wait for the next scheduled dose if the scheduled medication is missed.
- Report severe abdominal pain, with or without emesis.

Amylin mimetic

Pramlintide
A synthetic amylin hormone found in the beta cells of the pancreas, it suppresses glucagon secretion and controls postprandial blood glucose levels. Clients can take pramlintide in addition to insulin or hypoglycemic agent therapy.

NURSING ACTIONS
- Administer subcutaneously immediately before each major meal.
- Do not administer if client has hypoglycemia unawareness, or noncompliance/poor adherence to treatment regimens and self-monitoring blood glucose.
- Pre-meal doses of rapid- or short-acting insulins should be reduced by 50% to reduce risk of hypoglycemia.

CLIENT EDUCATION
- Monitor and report frequent periods of hypoglycemia.
- Monitor for injection site reactions.

Sodium-glucose cotransporter 2 inhibitors

Canagliflozin, dapagliflozin
Blocks reabsorption of glucose from the kidneys

NURSING ACTIONS
- Monitor for development of urinary tract infections and genital yeast infections in females.
- Monitor for postural hypotension in older adult clients.

CLIENT EDUCATION
- Take the medication before the first meal of the day.
- Change positions slowly.
- Monitor and report genital burning, itching, increased drainage.

PATIENT-CENTERED CARE

NURSING CARE

- Monitor the following.
  - Blood glucose levels and factors affecting levels (other medications)
  - I&O and weight
  - Skin integrity and healing status of any wounds for presence of recurrent infections (feet and folds of the skin should be monitored)
  - Sensory alterations (tingling, numbness)
  - Visual alterations
  - Dietary practices
  - Exercise patterns
  - SMBG skill proficiency
  - Self-medication administration proficiency
- Instruct the client about the management of hypoglycemia and hyperglycemia
- Vision and hearing deficits can impair communication between the nurse and client regarding diabetes mellitus and treatment. Use additional communication methods as needed to facilitate client understanding (written materials, interpreter).
- Provide information regarding self-administration of insulin. **(73.2)**

73.2 Insulin subcutaneous injection site

- Tissue deterioration secondary to aging can affect the client's ability to prepare food, care for self, perform ADLs, perform foot/wound care, and perform glucose monitoring.
- A fixed income can mean that there are limited funds for buying diabetic supplies, wound care supplies, insulin, and medications. This can result in complications.
- Older adult clients might not be able to drive to the provider's office, grocery store, or pharmacy. Inquire about support systems available for older adult clients. ©
- Older adults are at risk for altered metabolism of medication due to decreased kidney and liver function because of the aging process.
- Older adults can have vision alterations (yellowing of lens, decreased depth perception, cataracts), which can affect ability to read information and administer medication.

CLIENT EDUCATION
- Use appropriate techniques for SMBG, including obtaining blood samples, recording and responding to results, and correctly handling supplies and equipment.
- Rotate injection sites to prevent lipohypertrophy (increased swelling of fat) or lipoatrophy (loss of fat tissue) within one anatomic site (prevents day-to-day changes in absorption rates).

Foot care

- Inspect feet daily. Wash feet daily with mild soap and warm water. Test water temperature with hands before washing feet.
- Pat feet dry gently, especially between the toes, and avoid lotions between toes to decrease excess moisture and prevent infection.
- Use mild foot powder with cornstarch on sweaty feet.
- Do not use commercial remedies for the removal of calluses or corns, which can increase the risk for tissue injury and infection.
- Consult a podiatrist.
- The best time to perform nail care is after a bath/shower, when toenails are soft and easier to trim.
- Separate overlapping toes with cotton or lamb's wool.
- Avoid open-toe, open-heel shoes. Leather shoes are preferred to plastic. Wear shoes that fit correctly. Wear slippers with soles. Do not go barefoot.

CLIENT EDUCATION
- Wear clean, absorbent socks or stockings that are made of cotton or wool and have not been mended.
- Do not use hot water bottles or heating pads to warm feet. Wear socks for warmth.
- Avoid prolonged sitting, standing, and crossing of legs.
- Follow recommendations from a podiatrist for nail care. Some protocols allow for trimming toenails straight across with clippers and filing edges with an emery board or nail file to prevent soft tissue injury. If clippers or scissors are contraindicated, file the nails straight across.
- Cleanse cuts with warm water and mild soap, gently dry, and apply a dry dressing. Monitor healing and seek intervention promptly.

Nutritional guidelines

Participate in referring clients and their family to a dietitian for collaborative education on meal planning to include food intake, weight management, and lipid and glucose management. Qtc

CLIENT EDUCATION
- Plan meals to achieve appropriate timing of food intake, activity, onset, and peak of insulin. Calories and food composition should be similar each day. Eat at regular intervals, and do not skip meals.
- Count grams of carbohydrates consumed for glycemic control.
- Recognize that 15 g carbohydrates is equal to 1 carbohydrate exchange.
- Restrict calories and increase physical activity as appropriate to facilitate weight loss (for clients who are obese) or to prevent obesity.
- Include fiber in the diet to increase carbohydrate metabolism and to help control cholesterol levels.
- To sweeten food and beverages, use artificial sweeteners following FDA recommendations for acceptable quantities.
- Read and interpret fat content information on food labels to keep saturated fats within 7% of the recommendations of the daily total caloric intake.

Illness

CLIENT EDUCATION: Guidelines to follow when sick
- Monitor blood glucose every 3 to 4 hr.
- Continue to take insulin or oral hypoglycemic agents.
- Consume 4 oz of sugar-free, noncaffeinated liquid every 30 min to prevent dehydration.
- Meet carbohydrate needs through soft food (custard, cream soup, gelatin, graham crackers) six to eight times per day, if possible. If not, consume liquids equal to usual carbohydrate content.
- Test urine for ketones and report to provider if they are outside the expected reference range. (The level should be negative to small.)
- Rest.
- Call the provider for the following.
  - Blood glucose greater than 240 mg/dL (Test urine for ketones, if prescribed.)
  - Fever greater that is than 38.6° C (101.5° F), does not respond to acetaminophen, or lasts more than 24 hr
  - Feeling disoriented or confused
  - Experiencing rapid breathing
  - Vomiting that occurs more than once
  - Diarrhea that occurs more than five times or for longer than 24 hr
  - Inability to tolerate liquids
  - Illness that lasts longer than 2 days

INTERPROFESSIONAL CARE

Recommend a referral for the client to a diabetes educator for comprehensive education in diabetes management.

CHRONIC COMPLICATIONS

Consistent maintenance of blood glucose within the expected reference range is the best protection against the complications of diabetes mellitus. Expected reference ranges can vary.

Cardiovascular and cerebrovascular disease

Hypertension, myocardial infarction, stroke

NURSING ACTIONS
- Monitor blood pressure.
- Encourage a dietary consult.

CLIENT EDUCATION
- Get checks of cholesterol (HDL, LDL, triglycerides) yearly, and monitoring of blood pressure (less than 130/80 mm Hg) and HbA1c every 3 months.
- Participate in regular activity for weight loss and control.
- Consume a diet of low-fat meals that are high in fruits, vegetables, and whole grains.
- Report shortness of breath, headaches (persistent and transient), numbness in distal extremities, swelling of feet, infrequent urination, and changes in vision.

Diabetic retinopathy

Impaired vision and blindness (73.3)

CLIENT EDUCATION
- Get yearly eye exams to ensure the health of the eyes and to protect vision.
- Manage blood glucose levels.

Diabetic neuropathy

- Caused from damage to sensory nerve fibers resulting in numbness and pain
- Is progressive, can affect every aspect of the body, and can lead to ischemia and infection (73.4)

NURSING ACTIONS
- Monitor blood glucose to keep within the range prescribed by the provider to slow progression.
- Provide foot care.

CLIENT EDUCATION
- Get annual exams by a podiatrist.
- Follow-up regularly with provider to treat neuropathy.

Diabetic nephropathy

Damage to the kidneys from prolonged elevated blood glucose levels and dehydration

NURSING ACTIONS
- Monitor hydration and kidney function (I&O, serum creatinine).
- Report an hourly output less than 30 mL/hr.
- Monitor blood pressure.

CLIENT EDUCATION
- Have yearly urine analysis, BUN, microalbumin, and serum creatinine.
- Avoid soft drinks, alcohol, and toxic levels of acetaminophen or NSAIDs.
- Consume 2 to 3 L/day of fluid from food and low calorie beverages, and to drink an adequate amount of water.
- Report decrease in output to the provider.

73.3 Diabetic retinopathy

normal retina

diabetic retinopathy

hemorrhages

"cotton-wool" spots

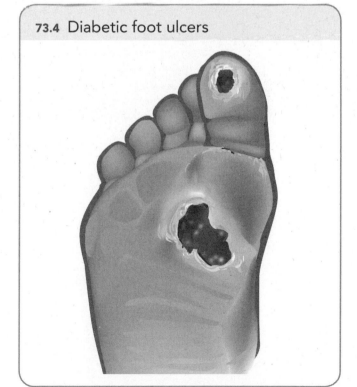

73.4 Diabetic foot ulcers

Acute complications

- Diabetic ketoacidosis (DKA) is an acute, life-threatening condition characterized by uncontrolled hyperglycemia. This leads to the breakdown of body fat for energy, dehydration, metabolic acidosis, and an accumulation of ketones in the blood and urine. The onset is rapid, and the mortality rate is up to 10%.
- Hyperglycemic-hyperosmolar state (HHS) is an acute, life-threatening condition characterized by profound hyperglycemia, hyperosmolarity that leads to dehydration, and an absence of ketosis. Onset generally occurs gradually over several days, and if left untreated can lead to coma and death.

DATA COLLECTION

RISK FACTORS

Diabetic ketoacidosis

- Lack of sufficient insulin related to undiagnosed or untreated type 1 diabetes mellitus or inadequate disease management.
- Any condition that increases carbohydrate metabolism and increases the body's need for insulin, such as physical or emotional stress, illness, surgery, or trauma. Infection is the leading cause of DKA.
- Increased production of some hormones (cortisol, glucagon, epinephrine) stimulates the liver to produce glucose and decreases the effect of insulin.

Hyperglycemic–hyperosmolar state

- Lack of sufficient insulin related to undiagnosed diabetes mellitus. There is sufficient endogenous insulin present to prevent the development of ketosis, but not enough to prevent hyperglycemia.
- Inadequate fluid intake or poor kidney function contribute to the development of HHS.
- Most common in older adult clients (50 to 70 years). Mortality rates in these clients are 40% to 70% because older clients seek medical attention later and are sicker than younger clients.
- Medical conditions (myocardial infarction, cerebral vascular injury, sepsis)
- Some medications (glucocorticoids, thiazide diuretics, phenytoin, beta blockers, calcium channel blockers)
- Infection or stress

EXPECTED FINDINGS

	DKA	HHS
Polyuria: Osmotic diuresis resulting in excess urine production	✓	✓
Polydipsia (excess thirst): Osmotic diuresis causing excess loss of fluids resulting in dehydration and increased thirst	✓	✓
Polyphagia: Cell starvation due to inability to receive glucose resulting in increased appetite	✓	✓
Weight loss: Cells are unable to use glucose because of insulin deficiency. The body is placed in a catabolic state.	✓	✓
GI effects (nausea, vomiting, abdominal pain): Increased ketones and acidosis lead to nausea, vomiting, and abdominal pain	✓	✓
Blurred vision, headache, weakness: Fluid volume depletion caused from osmotic diuresis resulting in dehydration	✓	✓
Orthostatic hypotension: Fluid volume depletion caused by osmotic diuresis resulting in dehydration	✓	✓
Fruity odor of breath: Elevated ketone bodies (small fatty acids) used for energy that collect in the blood, which leads to metabolic acidosis	✓	
Kussmaul respirations: Deep rapid respirations occur in an attempt to excrete carbon dioxide and acid when in metabolic acidosis	✓	
Metabolic acidosis: Breakdown of stored glucose, protein, and fat to produce ketone bodies	✓	
Mental status changes: Lack of glucose circulating to the brain can cause neuron dysfunction and even cell death in the brain.	✓	✓
Seizures, myoclonic jerking: Related to serum osmolarity greater than 350 mOsm/L		✓
Reversible paralysis: Related to how elevated the serum osmolarity becomes (coma occurs once serum osmolarity is greater than 350 mOsm/L)		✓

LABORATORY TESTS

Therapeutic management is guided by serial laboratory analysis.

Serum glucose

DKA: Greater than 300 mg/dL

HHS: Greater than 600 mg/dL

Serum electrolytes: Sodium (Na⁺) and potassium (K⁺)

DKA
- **Na⁺:** low, normal, or high
- **K⁺:** initial levels depend on how long DKA existed prior to treatment, then decrease with treatment

HHS
- **Na⁺:** normal or low
- **K⁺:** normal to high as a result of dehydration; must monitor for decrease when treatment started

Serum kidney studies: BUN and creatinine

DKA AND HHS
- Increased secondary to dehydration
- BUN greater than 30 mg/dL
- Creatinine greater than 1.5 mg/dL

Ketones: Serum and urine

DKA: Present in serum and urine

HHS: Absent in serum and urine

Serum osmolarity

DKA: High

HHS: Greater than 320 mOsm/L

Serum pH (ABG)

DKA
- Metabolic acidosis with respiratory compensation (Kussmaul respirations)
- pH less than 7.3

HHS
- Absence of acidosis
- pH greater than 7.4

PATIENT-CENTERED CARE

NURSING CARE

- Always treat the underlying cause (infectious process).
  - Monitor clients receiving rapid isotonic fluid (0.9% sodium chloride) replacement to maintain perfusion to vital organs. Monitor for evidence of fluid volume excess (increased urine output, dyspnea and lung crackles, jugular venous distention, and increased body weight) due to the need for large quantities of fluid.
  - Physiological changes in cardiac and pulmonary function can place older adult clients at greater risk for fluid overload (precipitate heart failure exacerbation) from fluid replacement therapy. Ⓖ
- Ensure the next solution is a hypotonic fluid (0.45% sodium chloride) to continue replacing losses to total body fluid.
- When serum glucose levels approach 250 mg/dL, add glucose to IV fluids to minimize the risk of cerebral edema associated with drastic changes in serum osmolarity and prevent hypoglycemia.
- Monitor the client receiving regular insulin 0.1 to 0.15 unit/kg as an IV bolus dose and then follow with a continuous IV infusion of regular insulin at 0.1 unit/kg/hr.

- Insulin is administered IV rather than subcutaneously to provide immediate treatment. The client who has DKA will absorb subcutaneous insulin slowly and erratically, making it difficult to adjust dosages of insulin appropriately. Monitor blood glucose hourly. Blood glucose of less than 200 mg/dL is the goal for resolution.
- Monitor serum potassium levels. Potassium levels will initially be increased, but with insulin therapy potassium will shift into cells, and the client will need to be monitored for hypokalemia.
  - Provide potassium replacement therapy in all replacement IV fluids, as indicated by laboratory values.
  - Monitor cardiac rhythm constantly.
  - Make sure urinary output is adequate before administering potassium.
- Ask the charge nurse to administer sodium bicarbonate by slow IV infusion for severe acidosis (pH less than 7.0). Infuse potassium along with bicarbonate because bicarbonate promotes hypokalemia, unless the client has hyperkalemia.
- Monitor for and report changes in neurological status in clients who have HHS. Ⓠs
- Reinforce education to prevent reoccurrence.

CONSIDERATIONS FOR OLDER ADULT CLIENTS Ⓖ
- Encourage older adult clients to monitor blood glucose every 1 to 4 hr when ill.
- Emphasize the importance of not skipping an insulin dose when ill.
- Maintain hydration because older adult clients can have a diminished thirst sensation.
- Changes in mental status can prevent older adult clients from seeking treatment.

CLIENT EDUCATION

- Wear a medical alert bracelet.
- Take measures to decrease the risk of dehydration.
  - Unless contraindicated by other health problems, consume 2 to 3 L/day of fluid from food and sugar-free beverages, and drink an adequate amount of water.
  - If blood glucose levels are low, consume liquids with sugar.
- Monitor glucose every 4 hr when ill and continue to take insulin.
- Check urine for ketones if blood glucose is greater than 240 mg/dL.
- Consume liquids with carbohydrates and electrolytes (sports drinks) when unable to eat solid food.
- Notify the provider for the following.
  - Illness that lasts longer than 24 hr
  - Blood glucose greater than 250 mg/dL
  - Inability to tolerate food or fluids
  - Ketones in urine for more than 24 hr
  - Temperature of 38.6° C (101.5° F) for 24 hr

Application Exercises

1. A nurse is preparing to administer a morning dose of insulin aspart to a client who has type 1 diabetes mellitus. Which of the following actions should the nurse take?

   A. Check blood glucose immediately after breakfast.

   B. Administer insulin when breakfast arrives.

   C. Hold breakfast for 1 hr after insulin administration.

   D. Clarify the prescription because insulin should not be administered at this time.

2. A nurse is assisting with a presentation about nutrition habits that prevent type 2 diabetes mellitus for a group of clients. Which of the following should the nurse include? (Select all that apply.)

   A. Eat less meat and processed foods.

   B. Decrease intake of saturated fats.

   C. Increase daily fiber intake.

   D. Limit unsaturated fat intake to 15% of daily caloric intake.

   E. Include omega-3 fatty acids in the diet.

3. A nurse is reinforcing teaching about foot care with a client who has diabetes mellitus. Which of the following information should the nurse include in the teaching? (Select all that apply.)

   A. Remove calluses using over-the-counter remedies.

   B. Apply lotion between toes.

   C. Perform nail care after bathing.

   D. Trim toenails straight across.

   E. Wear closed-toe shoes.

4. A nurse is reviewing the health record of a client who has hyperglycemic-hyperosmolar state (HHS). Which of the following factors can cause HHS? (Select all that apply.)

   A. Evidence of recent myocardial infarction

   B. BUN 35 mg/dL

   C. Takes a calcium channel blocker

   D. Age 77 years

   E. Fluid volume excess

5. A nurse is collecting data from a client who has diabetic ketoacidosis and ketones in the urine. The nurse should expect which of the following findings? (Select all that apply.)

   A. Weight gain

   B. Fruity odor of breath

   C. Abdominal pain

   D. Kussmaul respirations

   E. Metabolic acidosis

PRACTICE Active Learning Scenario

A nurse is reviewing guidelines with a client who has type 1 diabetes mellitus about self-care during illness. What information should the nurse include? Use the ATI Active Learning Template: System Disorder to complete this item.

LABORATORY TESTS: Discuss parameters for testing urine and notifying the provider.

CLIENT EDUCATION: Describe six teaching points.

Application Exercises Key

1. A. Blood glucose should be checked prior to insulin administration to prevent an episode of hypoglycemia.

   B. **CORRECT:** Administering insulin aspart when breakfast arrives can prevent a hypoglycemic episode. Insulin aspart is rapid-acting, and should be administered 5 to 10 min before breakfast.

   C. Insulin aspart is rapid-acting and is administered 5 to 10 min before breakfast. Breakfast should be available at the time of the injection.

   D. Insulin aspart is administered at breakfast time and may be prescribed for administration 2 to 3 times a day.

   Ⓝ NCLEX® Connection: Pharmacological Therapies, Medication Administration

2. A. **CORRECT:** Healthy nutrition should include decreasing the consumption of meats and processed foods, which can prevent diabetes and hyperlipidemia.

   B. **CORRECT:** Healthy nutrition should include lowering LDL by decreasing intake of saturated fats, which can prevent diabetes and hyperlipidemia.

   C. **CORRECT:** Healthy nutrition should include increasing dietary fiber to control weight gain and decrease the risk of diabetes and hyperlipidemia.

   D. The recommended unsaturated fat intake is 20% to 35% of total daily caloric intake.

   E. **CORRECT:** Healthy nutrition should include omega-3 fatty acids for secondary prevention of diabetes and heart disease.

   Ⓝ NCLEX® Connection: Reduction of Risk Potential, Potential for Alterations in Body Systems

3. A. A podiatrist should remove calluses or corns. Over-the-counter remedies can increase the risk for tissue injury and an infection.

   B. Applying lotion between the toes increases moisture for growth of micro-organisms, which can lead to infection.

   C. **CORRECT:** The client should perform nail care after bathing, when toenails are soft and easier to trim.

   D. **CORRECT:** The client should trim toenails straight across to prevent injury to soft tissue of the toes.

   E. **CORRECT:** The client should wear closed-toe shoes to prevent injury to soft tissue of the toes and feet.

   Ⓝ NCLEX® Connection: Reduction of Risk Potential, Potential for Alterations in Body Systems

4. A. **CORRECT:** The client who has type 2 diabetes mellitus and had a myocardial infarction is at risk for developing HHS. This is due to the increased hormone production during illness or stress, which can stimulate the liver to produce glucose and decrease the effects of insulin.

   B. **CORRECT:** The client who has type 2 diabetes mellitus can be at risk for developing HHS when the BUN is 35 mg/dL because it is an indication of decreased kidney function and inability of the kidney to filter high levels of blood glucose into the urine.

   C. **CORRECT:** A calcium channel blocker is one of several medications that increase the risk for HHS in a client who has type 2 diabetes mellitus.

   D. **CORRECT:** The older adult client is at risk for developing type 2 diabetes mellitus and can be unaware of associated manifestations, increasing the risk for HHS.

   E. The nurse should recognize that inadequate fluid intake is a risk factor for HHS.

   Ⓝ NCLEX® Connection: Physiological Adaptation, Basic Pathophysiology

5. A. Weight loss occurs when the cells are unable to use glucose because of insulin deficiency and places the body in a catabolic state.

   B. **CORRECT:** Fruity odor of breath is a manifestation of elevated ketone levels that lead to metabolic acidosis.

   C. **CORRECT:** Abdominal pain is a GI manifestation of increased ketones and acidosis.

   D. **CORRECT:** Kussmaul respirations are an attempt to excrete carbon dioxide and acid when in metabolic acidosis.

   E. **CORRECT:** Metabolic acidosis is caused by glucose, protein, and fat breakdown, which produces ketones.

   Ⓝ NCLEX® Connection: Physiological Adaptation, Basic Pathophysiology

---

PRACTICE Answer

Using the ATI Active Learning Template: System Disorder

LABORATORY TESTS: Test urine for ketones and report to the provider if ketones are present.

CLIENT EDUCATION
- Monitor blood glucose every 3 to 4 hr and call the provider for a level greater than 240 mg/dL.
- Continue to take insulin as prescribed.
- Prevent dehydration by consuming 2 to 3 L/day of fluid obtained from food and sugar-free beverages and drinking an adequate amount of water.
- Call the provider if unable to tolerate liquids.
- If unable to eat soft foods, consume liquids equal to usual carbohydrate content.
- Call the provider for illness longer than 2 days, or diarrhea more than five episodes or for longer than 24 hr.
- Call the provider for fever that is greater than 38.6° C (101.5° F), does not respond to acetaminophen, or lasts more than 24 hr.

Ⓝ NCLEX® Connection: Reduction of Risk Potential, Laboratory Values

When reviewing the following chapters, keep in mind the relevant topics and tasks of the NCLEX outline, in particular:

Safety and Infection Control

STANDARD PRECAUTIONS/TRANSMISSION-BASED PRECAUTIONS/SURGICAL ASEPSIS: Protect immunocompromised client from exposure to infectious diseases/organisms.

Health Promotion and Maintenance

HEALTH PROMOTION/DISEASE PREVENTION

Gather data on the client's health history and risk for disease (lifestyle, family and genetic history).

Check the results of the client's health screening tests (Papanicolaou [Pap] test or smear, stool occult blood test).

Assist the client in disease prevention activities.

Monitor the client's actions to maintain health and prevent disease (smoking cessation, exercise, diet, stress management).

Monitor incorporation of healthy behaviors into lifestyle by the client (screening examinations, immunizations, limiting risk-taking behaviors).

Psychosocial Integrity

COPING MECHANISMS: Monitor the client's progress toward achieving improved body image (mastectomy, colostomy).

Basic Care and Comfort

NONPHARMACOLOGICAL COMFORT INTERVENTIONS

Identify the client's need for palliative/comfort care.

Provide nonpharmacological measures for pain relief (imagery, massage, repositioning).

Provide palliative/comfort care interventions to the client.

Evaluate pain using a standardized rating scale.

Pharmacological Therapies

PHARMACOLOGICAL PAIN MANAGEMENT: Monitor and document client response to pharmacological interventions (pain rating scale, verbal reports).

Physiological Adaptation

ALTERATIONS IN BODY SYSTEMS

Identify signs and symptoms of an infection (temperature changes, swelling, redness, mental confusion, foul smelling urine).

Perform care for the client after a surgical procedure.

Reinforce education to the client regarding care and condition.

Notify the primary health care provider of a change in the client's status.

CHAPTER 74

UNIT 13 NURSING CARE OF CLIENTS WHO HAVE IMMUNE SYSTEM AND CONNECTIVE TISSUE DISORDERS
SECTION: DIAGNOSTIC AND THERAPEUTIC PROCEDURES

CHAPTER 74 *Immune and Infectious Disorders Diagnostic Procedures*

Diagnostic procedures for immune and infectious disorders involve identification of pathogenic micro-organisms. The most accurate and definitive way to identify micro-organisms and cell characteristics is by examining blood, body fluids, and tissue samples under a microscope. Effective treatment of infectious disease begins with identification of the pathogenic micro-organism.

White blood cells

- WBCs (also known as leukocytes) stimulate the inflammatory response and offer protection against various types of infection and foreign antigens.
- There are five types of WBCs. Laboratory analysis of circulating WBCs is the differential, which lists the percentages of the types of WBCs for a total of 100%. The percentages represent the proportion of each type of cell in a sample of WBCs. If the percentage of one type of cell increases, the percentages of other types decrease accordingly.

INTERPRETATION OF FINDINGS

The expected reference range for WBCs is 5,000 to 10,000/mm³.

Leukopenia is a total WBC count less than 4,000/mm³. It can indicate drug toxicity, autoimmune disease, bone marrow failure, and some overwhelming infections.

Leukocytosis is a total WBC count greater than 10,000/mm³. It can indicate inflammation, infection, some malignancies, trauma, dehydration, stress, steroid use, and thyroid storm.
- A client who has had a splenectomy can have a persistently increased WBC count.
- Older adult clients can have a severe bacterial infection without leukocytosis. Manifestations of infection, such as fever, can be absent in an older adult who has an infection. The nurse should monitor older adult clients carefully for infection risks. Ⓖ

Neutropenia is a neutrophil count less than 2,000/mm³. Neutropenia occurs in clients who have viral or overwhelming bacterial infections, or are undergoing radiation or chemotherapy. A client who has neutropenia is at an increased risk for infection.
- The absolute neutrophil count (ANC) of a client who has neutropenia can help determine the client's real risk for infection. Multiplying the total WBC count by the percentage of neutrophils plus the percentage of bands determines the ANC.
- An ANC less than 1,000 means that neutropenic precautions are essential.
- Neutropenic precautions (a protective environment) include the following.
  ○ Restricting visitors
  ○ Prohibiting visits by individuals who have an infection
  ○ Restricting exposure to live plants
  ○ Restricting ingestion of fresh fruits and vegetables
  ○ Avoiding contamination from the client's own bacterial flora by avoiding the measurement of rectal temperature and limiting IM injections Ⓠpcc

Left shift is an increase in immature neutrophils (bands or stabs) that occurs with an acute infection. Neutrophil production increases, allowing the release of immature neutrophils that are not capable of phagocytosis (ingesting and destroying bacteria).

TYPES OF WBCS

Neutrophils

The majority of neutrophils are segmented (mature) with others being banded (not fully mature).

PERCENT OF CIRCULATING NEUTROPHILS: 55% to 70%

INCREASED WITH
- Acute bacterial infection
- Myelocytic leukemia
- Trauma
- Rheumatoid arthritis

DECREASED WITH
- Sepsis
- Radiation therapy, aplastic anemia, chemotherapy
- Influenza

Lymphocytes (T cells and B cells)

- T-lymphocytes initiate cell-mediated immunity.
- B-lymphocytes initiate humoral immunity.

PERCENT OF CIRCULATING LYMPHOCYTES: 20% to 40%

INCREASED WITH
- Chronic bacterial or viral infection
- Viruses (mononucleosis, mumps, measles)
- Bacteria such as hepatitis
- Lymphocytic leukemia, multiple myeloma

DECREASED WITH
- Leukemia
- Sepsis

Monocytes

PERCENT OF CIRCULATING MONOCYTES: 2% to 8%

INCREASED WITH
- Chronic inflammation
- Protozoal infections
- Tuberculosis
- Viral infections such as mononucleosis

DECREASED WITH
- Corticosteroid therapy
- Aplastic anemia
- Hairy cell leukemia

Eosinophils

PERCENT OF CIRCULATING EOSINOPHILS: 1% to 4%

INCREASED WITH
- Allergic reactions
- Parasitic infection
- Eczema
- Leukemia
- Autoimmune diseases

DECREASED WITH
- Stress
- Corticosteroids

Basophils

PERCENT OF CIRCULATING BASOPHILS: 0.5% to 1%

INCREASED WITH: Leukemia

DECREASED WITH
- Acute allergic/hypersensitivity reactions
- Hyperthyroidism
- Stress reactions

Radioallergosorbent test

A radioallergosorbent test (RAST) is a blood test to determine sensitivity to various allergens. It can complement skin testing or be an alternative when the risk of a hypersensitivity reaction to an allergen exists.

ADVANTAGES
- Will not precipitate a dangerous allergic reaction
- Quicker than skin testing

DISADVANTAGES
- Available for fewer antigens
- Can be less sensitive than skin testing

INDICATIONS

POTENTIAL DIAGNOSES: Environmental and food allergies

CLIENT PRESENTATION
- Report of hypersensitivity reactions
- Hives, asthma, gastrointestinal (GI) dysfunction, rhinitis, dermatitis, angioedema

CONSIDERATIONS

INTRAPROCEDURE: Obtain a blood sample.

INTERPRETATION OF FINDINGS

The technician mixes specific allergens with the blood and incubates it with radiolabeled anti-IgE antibodies. Results reflect allergen-specific IgE levels and thus the degree of sensitivity on a 0 to 6 scale.

Skin testing for allergens

- Skin testing for allergens involves the use of intradermal injections or scratching the superficial layer (scratch or prick test) of the skin with small amounts of potential allergens.
- Intradermal testing runs a higher risk of hypersensitivity reactions and follows inconclusive scratch-test results.

INDICATIONS

POTENTIAL DIAGNOSES: Environmental and food allergies

CLIENT PRESENTATION: Hives, asthma, GI dysfunction, rhinitis, dermatitis, angioedema

INTERPRETATION OF FINDINGS

- A localized reaction (wheal and flare) to an allergen is a positive reaction to that allergen.
- The larger the reaction, the more severe the allergy.

CONSIDERATIONS

PREPROCEDURE

NURSING ACTIONS
- Prepare the skin on the client's back or forearm for application of various allergens using soap and water.
- Use alcohol to remove any oil.
- Have equipment available to treat anaphylaxis. Q_QI

CLIENT EDUCATION: Avoid taking corticosteroids and antihistamines from 48 hr to 2 weeks, depending on various factors, prior to testing.

INTRAPROCEDURE

NURSING ACTIONS
- Scratch or prick the skin with a needle after applying a drop of an allergen.
- Use a standard pattern of application to help identify the allergen. Q_EBP
- Apply control drops (substances that should not produce a reaction, such as 0.9% sodium chloride irrigation) and substances that should produce a reaction (such as histamine).
- Monitor for reactions after 15 to 20 min.

POSTPROCEDURE

NURSING ACTIONS
- Monitor skin for areas of reaction, and document the allergen that is responsible.
- Remove all solutions from the skin.
- Recommend an antihistamine or topical corticosteroid if skin itches after testing.
- Reinforce teaching about desensitizing options and avoidance therapies for allergens.

CLIENT EDUCATION: Consume a diet that eliminates allergens (gluten-free). Qpcc

Application Exercises

1. A nurse is caring for a client who has a WBC count of 20,000/mm³. Which of the following WBC abnormalities is consistent with this finding?

    A. Neutropenia

    B. Leukocytosis

    C. Left shift

    D. Leukopenia

2. A nurse is reviewing the laboratory findings of a client who has measles. The nurse should expect an increase in which of the following types of WBCs?

    A. Neutrophils

    B. Basophils

    C. Lymphocytes

    D. Eosinophils

3. A nurse is preparing to administer a scratch test to a client who has possible food and environmental allergies. Which of the following actions should the nurse perform prior to the procedure? (Select all that apply.)

    A. Cleanse the client's skin with povidone-iodine.

    B. Ask the client about previous reactions to allergens.

    C. Ask the client about medications taken the past several days.

    D. Inform the client to expect itching at one site.

    E. Obtain emergency resuscitation equipment.

Application Exercises Key

1. A. Neutropenia is a neutrophil count less than 2,000/mm³.

    B. **CORRECT:** Leukocytosis is a WBC count greater than 10,000/mm³, which can indicate inflammation or infection.

    C. A left shift is an increase in immature neutrophils (bands or stabs) that occurs with acute infection.

    D. Leukopenia is a total WBC count less than 4,000/mm³, which can indicate overwhelming infection or drug toxicity.

    Ⓝ *NCLEX® Connection: Reduction of Risk Potential, Laboratory Values*

2. A. Neutrophils increase with an acute bacterial infection. Measles is a viral infection.

    B. Basophils increase with leukemia.

    C. **CORRECT:** Lymphocytes increase with viral infections, such as measles, mumps, and mononucleosis.

    D. Eosinophils increase with allergic reactions, leukemia, eczema, and parasitic infections.

    Ⓝ *NCLEX® Connection: Reduction of Risk Potential, Laboratory Values*

3. A. The nurse should use soap and water to cleanse the skin. Povidone-iodine could interfere with an allergen and elicit a response.

    B. **CORRECT:** The nurse should ask the client about any previous reactions to allergens, which could indicate increased risk of an anaphylactic reaction.

    C. **CORRECT:** The nurse should ask the client about medications taken over the past several days. Antihistamines and corticosteroids can suppress reactions.

    D. **CORRECT:** The nurse will apply histamine at a control site so the client will probably have itching at this site.

    E. **CORRECT:** Emergency equipment should be available, even if the client denies previous anaphylactic reactions.

    Ⓝ *NCLEX® Connection: Pharmacological Therapies, Expected Actions/Outcomes*

PRACTICE Answer

Using the ATI Active Learning Template: Diagnostic Procedure

INDICATIONS
- Possible environmental and food allergies
- Report of hypersensitivity reactions
- Hives, asthma, gastrointestinal dysfunction, rhinitis, dermatitis, angioedema

INTERPRETATION OF FINDINGS: The technician mixes specific allergens with the blood and incubates it with anti-IgE antibodies. Results reflect allergen-specific IgE levels and thus the degree of sensitivity on a 0 to 6 scale.

NURSING INTERVENTIONS (PRE, INTRA, POST): Obtain a blood sample.

Ⓝ *NCLEX® Connection: Pharmacological Therapies, Expected Actions/Outcomes*

CHAPTER 75 *Immunizations*

Administration of a vaccine causes production of antibodies that prevent illness from a specific microbe. Vaccines originate from killed viruses or live attenuated (weakened) viruses.

IMMUNITY

ACTIVE IMMUNITY is an adaptive process that allows the body to make antibodies in response to the entry of antigens into the body.

- **Active-natural immunity** develops when the body produces antibodies in response to exposure to a live pathogen that enters the body naturally. Q**EBP**
- **Active-artificial immunity** develops when a vaccine is given and the body produces antibodies in response to exposure to a killed or attenuated virus.

PASSIVE IMMUNITY develops when antibodies from another human or animal are transferred to the client. Because the client does not independently develop antibodies, passive immunity is temporary.

- **Passive-natural immunity** occurs when antibodies pass from the mother to the fetus/newborn through the placenta and breast milk.
- **Passive-artificial immunity** occurs after administration of antibodies in the form of immune globulins to an individual who requires immediate protection against a disease where exposure has already occurred, such as following a bite from a poisonous snake or an animal who has rabies. The individual's protection from the disease will only extend for several weeks or months.

ADMINISTRATION

The 2016 Centers for Disease Control and Prevention (CDC) immunization recommendations for adults (19 years and older) follows. Immunization recommendations change periodically. Check the CDC website for current recommendations.

Tetanus, diphtheria (Td) booster: Give booster every 10 years. For adults 19 and older who did not receive a dose of tetanus, diphtheria, pertussis (Tdap) previously, substitute one dose with Tdap.

- Pregnant clients should receive the vaccine between 27 and 36 weeks gestation. Pregnant clients should get Tdap vaccine with each pregnancy to protect the fetus from pertussis. Q**s**

Measles, mumps, and rubella (MMR) vaccine: Follow recommendations for administering one or two doses to clients between the ages of 19 and 49 who lack documentation of immunization or prior infection, or laboratory proof of immunity. The CDC considers people born before 1957 immune to measles and mumps.

Varicella vaccine: Give two doses to adults who do not have evidence of a previous infection. Adults who have had only one previous dose should receive a second dose. Pregnant clients should not receive a varicella immunization.

Pneumococcal vaccine: Two types are available: 13-valent pneumococcal conjugate vaccine (PCV13) and 23-valent pneumococcal polysaccharide vaccine (PPSV23).

- Follow recommendations for administration to adults who are immunocompromised, have specific chronic diseases, smoke cigarettes, or live in long-term care facilities.
- For adults 65 years and older who have not been immunized with PCV13 or PPSV23, administer PCV13 first and then give PPSV23 in 6 to 12 months; do not administer both during the same visit.
- No additional dose is required for adults who received a dose of PPSV23 at age 65 or older. C

Hepatitis A: Two doses for high-risk individuals.

Hepatitis B: Administer three doses to high-risk individuals who lack completion of the series. There must be at least 1 month between doses one and two, and at least 2 months between doses two and three. A minimum of 4 months are required between doses one and three.

Influenza vaccine
- Recommended for all adults annually.
- Pregnant clients should receive inactivated influenza vaccine (IIV)
- Recombinant influenza vaccine (RIV) is approved for adults 18 years and older.
- The live attenuated vaccine (LAIV) is available as a nasal spray.

Meningococcal polysaccharide vaccine (MPSV4) and Meningococcal 4-valent conjugate (MenACWY) vaccine
- Administer a dose of MenACWY to students up to age 21 years entering college and living in dormitories who did not receive a dose on or after the 16th birthday. The CDC recommends for individuals who have anatomical or functional asplenia to have two doses of MenACWY at least 2 months apart. Military recruits and those traveling to or living in areas of hyperendemic or epidemic rates of meningococcal disease should receive one dose of MenACWY.
- MPSV4 is preferred for adults who are 56 years of age or older, require a single dose, and have not had MenACWY previously.
- Reimmunization with MenACWY should occur every 5 years for adults who remain at high risk for infection and for those who were previously immunized with MenACWY or MPSV4.
- Adults who are at high risk for serogoup B meningococcal infection should receive immunization with MenB. The CDC also recommendations immunization with MenB for those individuals who have anatomical or functional asplenia.

Human papilloma virus (HPV2, HPV4, or HPV9)
- Recommendations are three doses for female clients up to age 26 years who were not immunized as children. Female clients can receive HPV2, HPV4, or HPV9.
- Male clients age 19 to 21 years who did not receive immunization as children should receive HPV4 or HPV9. Male clients age 22 to 26 years with no previous immunization and who have a high risk for human papilloma virus should also receive HPV4 or HPV9. **Qs**

Zoster vaccine: Recommended as a one-time dose for all adults older than 60 years. **ⓒ**

PURPOSE

EXPECTED PHARMACOLOGICAL ACTION

Immunizations produce antibodies that provide active immunity. Immunizations can take months to have an effect, but they provide long-lasting protection against infectious diseases.

THERAPEUTIC USES

- Eradication of infectious diseases
- Prevention of childhood and adult infectious diseases and their complications (tetanus, pneumococcal pneumonia, hepatitis)

CONTRAINDICATIONS/PRECAUTIONS

- An anaphylactic reaction to a vaccine is a contraindication to further doses of that vaccine. **Qs**
- An anaphylactic reaction to a vaccine is a contraindication to use of other vaccines containing the same substance.
- Moderate or severe illnesses with or without fever are precautions to receiving immunizations. The common cold and other minor illnesses are not contraindications.
- Do not administer live virus vaccines (varicella, MMR) to a client who is severely immunocompromised. Severe febrile illness is a contraindication to all immunizations.
- Precautions to immunizations require the provider to analyze data and weigh the risks that come with and without immunizations.

Td, DTaP

ADVERSE EFFECTS
- **Mild:** Redness, swelling, and tenderness at the injection site; low fever; behavioral changes (drowsiness, irritability, anorexia)
- **Moderate:** Temperature 40.6° C (105° F) or greater; seizures (with or without fever); shock-like state
- **Severe:** Acute encephalopathy (rare)

CONTRAINDICATIONS: Encephalopathy within 7 days following prior dose of the vaccine

PRECAUTIONS
- Guillain-Barré syndrome within 6 weeks of prior dose of tetanus toxoid
- Progressive neurologic disorders; uncontrolled seizures
- Temperature 40.6° C (105° F) or greater within 48 hr of prior dose
- Shock-like state within 48 hr of prior dose
- Seizures within 3 days of prior dose

MMR

ADVERSE EFFECTS
- **Mild:** Local reactions (rash; fever; swollen glands in cheeks or neck)
- **Moderate:** Joint pain and stiffness lasting for days to weeks, febrile seizure, low platelet count
- **Severe:** Transient thrombocytopenia, deafness, long-term seizures, brain damage

CONTRAINDICATIONS: Pregnancy

PRECAUTIONS
- History of thrombocytopenia or thrombocytopenic purpura
- Anaphylactic reaction to eggs, gelatin, or neomycin
- Transfusion with blood product containing antibodies within the prior 11 months
- Simultaneous tuberculin skin testing

Varicella

ADVERSE EFFECTS
- **Mild:** Tenderness and swelling at injection site, fever, rash (mild) for up to 1 month after immunization
- **Moderate:** Seizures
- **Severe:** Pneumonia, low blood count (extremely rare), severe brain reactions (extremely rare)

CONTRAINDICATIONS
- Pregnancy
- Anaphylactic reaction to gelatin or neomycin

PRECAUTIONS
- Transfusion with blood product containing antibodies within the prior 11 months
- Treatment with antiviral medication within 24 hr prior to immunization (avoid taking antivirals for 14 days following immunization)
- Extended use (2 weeks or longer) of corticosteroids or other medications that affect the immune system
- Cancer

Pneumococcal conjugate vaccine

ADVERSE EFFECTS
- Swelling, redness and tenderness at site of injection
- Fever
- Irritability
- Drowsiness
- Anorexia

CONTRAINDICATIONS: Anaphylactic reaction to any vaccine containing diphtheria toxoid

Pneumococcal polysaccharide vaccine

ADVERSE EFFECTS
- Redness and tenderness at site of injection
- Fever
- Myalgia

PRECAUTION: Pregnancy

Hepatitis A

ADVERSE EFFECTS
- Local reaction at injection site
- Headache
- Loss of appetite
- Mild fatigue

CONTRAINDICATIONS: Severe allergy to latex

PRECAUTION: Pregnancy

Hepatitis B

ADVERSE EFFECTS
- Local reaction at injection site
- Temperature of 37.7° C (99.9° F) or greater

CONTRAINDICATIONS: Severe allergy (anaphylaxis) to yeast

Inactivated influenza vaccine

ADVERSE EFFECTS
- Swelling, redness, and tenderness at the injection site
- Hoarseness
- Fever
- Malaise
- Headache
- Cough
- Aches
- Increased risk for Guillain-Barré syndrome

PRECAUTIONS: Guillain-Barré syndrome within 6 weeks of prior influenza vaccine

Live attenuated influenza vaccine

ADVERSE EFFECTS
- Vomiting, diarrhea
- Cough
- Fever
- Headache
- Myalgia
- Nasal congestion/runny nose

CONTRAINDICATIONS
- Age 50 years or older
- Pregnancy

PRECAUTIONS
- Guillain-Barré syndrome within 6 weeks of prior influenza vaccine
- Treatment with antiviral medication within 48 hr prior to immunization (avoid taking antivirals for 14 days following immunization)
- Some chronic conditions

Meningococcal ACWY

ADVERSE EFFECTS
- Mild local reaction and rare risk of allergic response
- Possible mild fever

Zoster

ADVERSE EFFECTS
- Local reaction at injection site
- Headache

CONTRAINDICATIONS
- Clients who are immunocompromised
- Pregnancy
- Treatment with medications that alter the immune system

Human papilloma virus (HPV4, HPV9)

ADVERSE EFFECTS
- Mild local reaction and fever
- Mild to moderate fever
- Headache
- Fainting has occurred shortly after receiving vaccine

CONTRAINDICATIONS
- Pregnancy
- Severe allergy (anaphylaxis) to yeast

Human papilloma virus (HPV2)

ADVERSE EFFECTS
- Redness, swelling, and tenderness at the injection site
- Temperature 37.7° C (99.9° F) or greater
- Headache
- Fatigue
- Nausea, vomiting, abdominal pain
- Myalgia
- Fainting (shortly after receiving the vaccine)

CONTRAINDICATIONS
- Pregnancy
- Severe allergy to latex

INTERACTIONS

None significant

NURSING ADMINISTRATION

- Have emergency medications and equipment on standby in case the client experiences an allergic response such as anaphylaxis (rare) or serious reaction at injection site. Qs
- Follow storage and reconstitution directions.
- Provide written, vaccine information sheets (VISs), and review the content with clients. Document the publication date of each VIS given to the client.
- Administer antipyretic for fever, apply cool compress for localized tenderness, and mobilize the affected extremity.
- Instruct clients to observe for complications and notify the provider if adverse effects occur.
- Document administration of vaccines (date, route, site, type, manufacturer, lot number, expiration date). Also document the client's name, address, and signature. Include the name, title of the person administering the vaccine, and the address of the facility where the permanent record is located. Qʟ

ADULTS

- Give subcutaneous immunizations in outer aspect of the upper arm or anterolateral thigh.
- Give IM immunizations into the deltoid muscle.

NURSING EVALUATION OF MEDICATION EFFECTIVENESS

Depending on therapeutic intent, evidence of effectiveness includes the following.

- Improvement of local reaction to immunization with absence of pain, fever, and swelling at the site of injection
- Development of immunity

Application Exercises

1. A nurse is preparing to administer an IM injection of immune globulin to a client following exposure to hepatitis A. Which of the following statements should the nurse make?

   A. "This medication offers permanent immunity to hepatitis A."

   B. "This medication involves three injections over several months."

   C. "This medication provides an immune response more quickly than the body can produce it."

   D. "This medication contains an attenuated virus to help the body create antibodies."

2. A nurse is preparing to administer a varicella immunization to a client. Which of the following questions should the nurse ask?

   A. "Are you allergic to eggs?"

   B. "Are you allergic to baker's yeast?"

   C. "Are you pregnant?"

   D. "Do you have a history of Guillain-Barré syndrome?"

3. A nurse is reviewing strategies to promote comfort with a client who received an immunization. Which of the following information should the nurse include? (Select all that apply.)

   A. Massage the injection site.

   B. Apply a cool compress to the injection site.

   C. Take acetaminophen or ibuprofen.

   D. Use the affected extremity.

   E. Apply an antimicrobial ointment to the injection site.

4. A nurse is preparing to document administration of a meningococcal vaccine to a client. Which of the following information should the nurse include in the documentation? (Select all that apply.)

   A. Age of client receiving the vaccine

   B. Name of vaccine manufacturer

   C. Vaccine expiration date

   D. Date of administration

   E. Serial number of the vaccine

5. A nurse in a clinic is caring for a client who is to receive an immunization. The client asks about contraindications to immunizations. Which of the following responses should the nurse make?

   A. "The use of insulin is a contraindication."

   B. "An anaphylactic reaction is a contraindication for administration of any type of immunization."

   C. "The common cold is a contraindication for receiving an immunization."

   D. "The provider will weigh the risks if you have experienced any adverse effects."

PRACTICE Active Learning Scenario

A nurse at a community health clinic is administering influenza vaccines to a group of clients. What information should the nurse take into consideration when selecting the type of vaccine to administer? Use the ATI Active Learning Template: Medication to complete this item.

NURSING INTERVENTIONS: Identify the two types of influenza vaccine and which clients should receive each of the two types.

Application Exercises Key

1. A. Hepatitis A immune globulin produces passive-artificial immunity that lasts only several weeks or months.

   B. Immune globulins are not given in a series, but as a treatment following exposure to an infectious disease.

   C. **CORRECT:** Hepatitis A immune globulin produces passive-artificial immunity and contains antibodies to help protect against the disease for several weeks or months.

   D. Hepatitis A immune globulin contains antibodies, not an attenuated virus.

   (N) *NCLEX® Connection: Pharmacological Therapies, Medication Administration*

2. A. The nurse should question a client who is receiving an influenza immunization about an allergy to eggs.

   B. The nurse should question a client who is receiving an HPV immunization about an allergy to yeast.

   C. **CORRECT:** The nurse should ask whether the client is pregnant because pregnancy is a contraindication to receiving the varicella immunization.

   D. Guillain-Barré syndrome is not a contraindication for varicella immunization.

   (N) *NCLEX® Connection: Pharmacological Therapies, Medication Administration*

3. A. Massaging the injection site for any extended period of time can increase localized discomfort.

   B. **CORRECT:** Applying a cool compress to the injection site can relieve discomfort from the localized reaction.

   C. **CORRECT:** Taking an antipyretic can relieve a low-grade fever and localized discomfort at the injection site.

   D. **CORRECT:** Mobilizing the affected extremity will help relieve discomfort due to a localized reaction.

   E. It is not necessary to apply an antimicrobial ointment at the injection site.

   (N) *NCLEX® Connection: Pharmacological Therapies, Expected Actions/Outcomes*

4. A. Age of the person receiving an immunization is not included.

   B. **CORRECT:** The nurse should document the name of the vaccine manufacturer.

   C. **CORRECT:** The nurse should document the expiration date of the vaccine.

   D. **CORRECT:** The nurse should document the date of administration of the vaccine.

   E. The nurse should document the lot number (not the serial number) of the vaccine.

   (N) *NCLEX® Connection: Health Promotion and Maintenance, Data Collection Techniques*

5. A. The client who takes insulin can receive immunizations unless other contraindications are present.

   B. The client who has experienced an anaphylactic reaction to one immunization can receive other immunizations that contain different substances.

   C. The client who has a common cold may receive an immunization because the client is not immunosuppressed.

   D. **CORRECT:** The client who has experienced adverse effects should inform the provider, who can weigh the risks of an immunization.

   (N) *NCLEX® Connection: Pharmacological Therapies, Adverse Effects/Contraindications/Side Effects/Interactions*

PRACTICE Answer

Using the ATI Active Learning Template: Medication

NURSING INTERVENTIONS
- Inactivated influenza vaccine (IIV) is approved for clients who are pregnant.
- Recombinant influenza vaccine (RIV) is approved for adults 18 years of age and older.

(N) *NCLEX® Connection: Pharmacological Therapies, Adverse Effects/Contraindications/Side Effects/Interactions*

CHAPTER 76 *HIV/AIDS*

Human immunodeficiency virus (HIV) is a retrovirus that is transmitted through blood and body fluids (semen, vaginal secretions).

HIV targets CD4+ lymphocytes, also known as T-cells or T-lymphocytes. T-cells work in concert with B-lymphocytes. Both are part of specific acquired (adaptive) immunity. HIV integrates its RNA into host cell DNA through reverse transcriptase, reshaping the host's immune system.

HIV is found in feces, urine, tears, saliva, cerebrospinal fluid, cervical cells, lymph nodes, corneal tissue, and brain tissue, but epidemiologic studies indicate that these are unlikely sources of infection.

All clients who are pregnant are screened for HIV. Q_{EBP}

DISEASE PROCESS STAGES

HIV infection is one continuous disease process with three stages. **(76.1)**

Progression of HIV infection

- Manifestations occur within 2 to 4 weeks of infection.
- Manifestations are similar to those of influenza and can include a rash, night sweats, and a sore throat.
- This stage is marked by a rapid rise in the HIV viral load, decreased CD4+ cells, and increased CD8 cells.
- The resolution of manifestations coincides with the decline in viral HIV copies.
- Lymphadenopathy persists throughout the disease process.

Chronic asymptomatic infection

- This stage can be prolonged and asymptomatic.
- The client can remain asymptomatic for 10 years or more, but can develop generalized lymphadenopathy.
- Anti–HIV antibodies are produced (HIV positive).
- Over time, the virus begins active replication using the host's genetic machinery.
  - CD4+ cells are destroyed.
  - The viral load increases.
  - Dramatic loss of immunity begins.

AIDS

- This stage is characterized by life–threatening opportunistic infections.
- This is the end stage of HIV infection. Without treatment, death occurs within 5 years.

> All people with AIDS have HIV, but not all people who have HIV have AIDS.

76.1 HIV infection stages

A confirmed case classification meets the laboratory criteria for a diagnosis of HIV infection and one of the four HIV infection stages.

To read more about HIV, go to www.cdc.gov.

Stage 1

DEFINING CONDITIONS: None

CD4+ T-LYMPHOCYTE COUNT:
500 cells/mm³ or more

CD4+ T-LYMPHOCYTE PERCENTAGE
OF TOTAL LYMPHOCYTES: 29% or more

Stage 2

DEFINING CONDITIONS: None

CD4+ T-LYMPHOCYTE COUNT:
200 to 499 cells/mm³

CD4+ T-LYMPHOCYTE PERCENTAGE
OF TOTAL LYMPHOCYTES: 14% to 28%

Stage 3 (AIDS)

Documentation of an AIDS-defining condition supersedes a CD4+ T-lymphocyte count of 200 cells/mm³ or more and a CD4+ T-lymphocyte percentage of total lymphocytes of more than 14%.

DEFINING CONDITIONS: One or more of the following

- Candidiasis of the esophagus, bronchi, trachea, or lungs
- Herpes simplex: Chronic ulcers (more than 1 month duration)
- HIV-related encephalopathy
- Disseminated or extrapulmonary histoplasmosis
- Kaposi's sarcoma

- Burkitt's lymphoma
- Mycobacterium tuberculosis of any site
- *Pneumocystis jirovecii* pneumonia
- Recurrent pneumonia
- Progressive multifocal leukoencephalopathy
- Recurrent salmonella septicemia
- Wasting syndrome attributed to HIV

CD4+ T-LYMPHOCYTE COUNT: Less than 200 cells/mm³

CD4+ T-LYMPHOCYTE PERCENTAGE OF TOTAL LYMPHOCYTES: Less than 14%

Stage 4

No information available

HEALTH PROMOTION AND DISEASE PREVENTION

- The virus is transmitted through blood and body fluids. Ways to prevent infection include the use of condoms, abstinence, and avoiding sharing needles.
- Maintain up-to-date immunizations, including yearly seasonal influenza and pneumococcal polysaccharide vaccine.
- Providers should use standard precautions when caring for the client.

DATA COLLECTION

RISK FACTORS

- Unprotected sex (vaginal, anal, oral)
- Multiple sex partners
- Occupational exposure (health care workers)
- Perinatal exposure
- Blood transfusions (not a significant source of infection in the U.S.)
- IV drug use with a contaminated needle

Older adult clients ©

- HIV infection can go undiagnosed in older adult clients due to the similarity of its manifestations to other illnesses that are common in this age group.
- Older adults are more susceptible to fluid and electrolyte imbalances, malnutrition, skin alterations, and wasting syndrome than younger adults.
- Older adult women experience vaginal dryness and thinning of the vaginal wall, increasing their susceptibility to HIV infection.

EXPECTED FINDINGS

- Chills
- Rash
- Anorexia, nausea, weight loss
- Weakness and fatigue
- Headache and sore throat
- Night sweats

LABORATORY TESTS

CBC and differential: Abnormal (anemia, thrombocytopenia, leukopenia)

Platelet count: Less than 150,000/mm³

DIAGNOSTIC PROCEDURES

- Positive result from an HIV antibody screening test (enzyme-linked immunosorbent assay [ELISA]) confirmed by a positive result from a supplemental HIV antibody test (Western blot or indirect immunofluorescence assay [IFA])
- Home test kits are also available using a drop of blood. These provide anonymous registration and counseling before the test via a telephone call.
- Two noninvasive tests are available using either mucosal fluid or urine.
- Client who has a positive result from a confirmatory test, such as Western blot, should then be tested for viral load.

HIV RNA quantification (HIV viral load test)

- Determines viral load before beginning treatment
- Can be repeated at intervals to monitor disease progression, identify compliance with treatment and determine HIV medication resistance
- Treatment is needed for levels greater than 5,000 to 10,000 copies/mL depending on CD4 counts.

HIV drug resistance testing (HIV genotype or HIV tropism)

- Guides changes in medication therapy when resistance occurs
- Useful with CD4 counts fall despite therapy

Liver profile, biopsies, and testing of stool for parasites

NURSING ACTIONS
- Prepare the client for the test.
- Inform the client about the details of the test (length, what to expect).
- Allow the client time to ask questions or express emotions.

CLIENT EDUCATION Qᴾᶜᶜ
- A positive Western blot or IFA test means the AIDS virus is in the body but does not mean the client has clinical AIDS.
- Use safe sexual practices.

Brain or lung MRI or CT scan

Detailed image of the brain or lung to detect abnormalities

NURSING ACTIONS: Prepare the client for the procedure.

CLIENT EDUCATION: The test takes up to 1 hr.

CD4+ cell count

- Used to confirm progression from HIV infection to AIDS.
- The expected reference range for the CD4+ count is 800 to 1,200 mm³. A CD4+ count less than 200/mm³ or a percentage of CD4 lymphocytes less than 14% indicates AIDS.

PATIENT-CENTERED CARE

NURSING CARE

- Collect data on risk factors (sexual practices, IV drug use).
- Monitor fluid intake/urinary output.
- Obtain daily weights to monitor weight loss.
- Monitor nutritional intake.
- Monitor electrolytes.
- Monitor skin integrity (rashes, open areas, bruising).
- Monitor pain status.
- Monitor vital signs (especially temperature).
- Check lung sounds/respiratory status (diminished lung sounds).
- Check neurological status (confusion, dementia, visual changes).
- Encourage activity alternated with rest periods.
- Administer supplemental oxygen as needed.
- Provide analgesia as needed.
- Provide skin care as needed.
- Reinforce client teaching. Q PCC
  - Transmission, infection control measures, and safe sex practices
  - Importance of maintaining a well-balanced diet
  - Self-administration of prescribed medications and potential adverse effects
  - Findings that need to be reported immediately (infection)
- Assist the client with identifying primary support systems.

MEDICATIONS

Highly active antiretroviral therapy involves using three to four HIV medications in combination with other antiretroviral medications to reduce medication resistance, adverse effects, and dosages.

Fusion inhibitors: Enfuvirtide blocks the fusion of HIV with the host cell

Entry inhibitors: Maraviroc

Nucleoside reverse transcriptase inhibitors: Zidovudine interferes with the virus's ability to convert RNA into DNA.

Non-nucleoside reverse transcriptase inhibitors: Delavirdine and efavirenz inhibit viral replication in cells.

Protease inhibitors: Atazanavir, nelfinavir, saquinavir, and indinavir inhibit an enzyme needed for the virus to replicate.

Integrase inhibitors: Raltegravir

Antineoplastic medication: Interleukin is an immunostimulant that enhances the immune response and reduces the production of cancer cells (used commonly with Kaposi's sarcoma).

NURSING ACTIONS

- Monitor laboratory results (CBC, WBC, liver function tests). Antiretroviral medications can increase alanine aminotransferase, aspartate aminotransferase, bilirubin, mean corpuscular volume, high-density lipoproteins, total cholesterol, and triglycerides. Q EBP
- Monitor total CD4+ T lymphocyte count, CD4 percentage, and ratio of CD4 to CD8 cells.
  - Normal CD4-to-CD8 ratio is 2. A ratio less than 1 indicates more severe disease manifestations
  - Low CD4 T lymphocyte counts and steadily decreasing counts indicate poor prognosis or medication resistance.
- Reinforce teaching to the client about the adverse effects of the medications and ways to decrease the severity of adverse effects.

CLIENT EDUCATION: Take medications on a regular schedule and do not miss doses. Missed medication doses can cause medication resistance. Q PCC

INTERPROFESSIONAL CARE

- Infectious disease services can manage HIV.
- Respiratory services can improve respiratory status and provide portable oxygen.
- Nutritional services can be consulted for dietary supplementation. Food services are indicated for clients who are homebound and need meals prepared.
- Rehabilitation services can be consulted for strengthening and improving the client's level of energy.
- Refer the client to local AIDS support groups as indicated. Q TC
- Home health service are indicated for clients who need help with strengthening and assistance regarding ADLs. Home health services can also provide assistance with IVs, dressing changes, and total parenteral nutrition (TPN).
- Long-term care facilities can be indicated for clients who have chronic HIV.
- Hospice services are usually indicated for clients who have a late stage of HIV.

Alternative therapy

Vitamins, herbal products, and shark cartilage can help alleviate manifestations of HIV. Ask if the client is taking herbal products. These can alter the effects of prescribed medications.

CLIENT EDUCATION

- Practice good hygiene (including frequent hand hygiene) to reduce the risk of infection.
- Avoid crowded areas or traveling to countries with poor sanitation.
- Avoid raw foods (fruits, vegetables) and undercooked foods (meat, fish, eggs).
- Avoid cleaning pet litter boxes to reduce the risk of toxoplasmosis.
- Keep the home environment clean and avoid being exposed to family and friends who have colds or flu viruses.
- Wash dishes in hot water using a dishwasher if available.
- Bathe daily using antimicrobial soap.
- Adhere to the antiretroviral dosing schedules.
- Frequent follow-up monitoring of CD4+ and viral load counts is needed.
- Use constructive coping mechanisms.
- Report manifestations of infection immediately to the provider.

COMPLICATIONS

Opportunistic infections

- **Bacterial diseases,** such as tuberculosis, bacterial pneumonia, and septicemia (blood poisoning)
- **HIV-associated malignancies,** such as Kaposi's sarcoma, lymphoma, and squamous cell carcinoma
- **Viral diseases,** such as those caused by cytomegalovirus, herpes simplex, and herpes zoster virus
- **Fungal diseases,** such as *Pneumocystis jirovecii* pneumonia (PCP), candidiasis, cryptococcosis, and penicilliosis
- **Protozoal diseases,** such as PCP, toxoplasmosis, microsporidiosis, cryptosporidiosis, isosporiasis, and leishmaniasis

NURSING ACTIONS

- Implement and maintain antiretroviral medication therapy.
- Administer antineoplastics, antibiotics, analgesics, antifungals, and antidiarrheals.
- Administer appetite stimulants (to enhance nutrition).
- Monitor for skin breakdown.
- Maintain fluid intake.
- Maintain nutrition.

CLIENT EDUCATION: Report indications of infection immediately to the provider. Qpcc

Wasting syndrome

NURSING ACTIONS

- Maintain nutrition orally or by TPN.
- Monitor weight, calorie counts, and I&O.
- Provide between-meal supplements/snacks.
- Decrease fat content of foods to prevent complications of fat intolerance.
- Rinse the client's mouth several times daily with saline or sodium bicarbonate and sterile water to reduce mouth pain and increase appetite.
- Serve at least six small feedings with high protein value per day. QEBP

Fluid/electrolyte imbalance

NURSING ACTIONS

- Monitor fluid/electrolyte status.
- Report abnormal laboratory data promptly.
- Encourage the client to drink 2,000 to 3,000 mL fluid daily.
- Make dietary adjustments to reduce diarrhea.

Seizures (HIV encephalopathy)

NURSING ACTIONS

- Maintain client safety.
- Implement seizure precautions. Qs

Application Exercises

1. A nurse in an outpatient clinic is collecting data from a client who reports night sweats and fatigue. The client's temperature is 38.1° C (100.6° F) orally. The client is afraid he has HIV. Which of the following actions should the nurse take? (Select all that apply.)

   A. Measure vital signs.

   B. Determine when manifestations began.

   C. Weigh the client.

   D. Reinforce teaching about opportunistic infections.

   E. Obtain a sexual history.

2. A nurse is caring for a client who is suspected of having HIV. Which of the following diagnostic tests and laboratory values are used to confirm HIV infection? (Select all that apply.)

   A. Western blot

   B. Indirect immunofluorescence assay

   C. CD4+ T-lymphocyte count

   D. HIV RNA quantification test

   E. Cerebrospinal fluid (CSF) analysis

3. A nurse is reinforcing teaching with a client who has stage 3 HIV. Which of the following statements by the client should indicate understanding?

   A. "I will wear gloves while changing the litter box."

   B. "I will rinse raw fruits with water before eating them."

   C. "I will wear a mask when around family members who are ill."

   D. "I will cook vegetables before eating them."

4. A nurse is collecting data from a client to identify risk factors for HIV. Which of the following are risk factors associated with this virus? (Select all that apply.)

   A. Perinatal exposure

   B. Pregnancy

   C. Monogamous sex partner

   D. Older adult woman

   E. Occupational exposure

5. A nurse is reinforcing teaching with a client who has stage 2 HIV and is having difficulty maintaining a normal weight. Which of the following client statements indicates understanding?

   A. "I will choose a diet high in fat to help gain weight."

   B. "I will be sure to eat three large meals daily."

   C. "I will drink up to 1 liter of liquid each day."

   D. "I will add high-protein foods to my diet."

PRACTICE Active Learning Scenario

A nurse is assisting in planning care for a client who has AIDS. Use the ATI Active Learning Template: System Disorder to complete this item.

NURSING CARE: Describe at least three nursing actions.

Application Exercises Key

1. A. **CORRECT:** The nurse should measure vital signs to gather data about the client's condition.

   B. **CORRECT:** The nurse should gather more data to determine whether the manifestations are acute or chronic.

   C. **CORRECT:** The nurse should weigh the client to gather data and monitor the client's condition.

   D. The nurse should not reinforce teaching with the client about opportunistic infections until a diagnosis is determined.

   E. **CORRECT:** The nurse should obtain a sexual history to determine how the virus was transmitted.

   Ⓝ *NCLEX® Connection: Health Promotion and Maintenance, Health Promotion/Disease Prevention*

2. A. **CORRECT:** Positive results of a Western blot test confirm the presence of HIV infection.

   B. **CORRECT:** Positive results of an indirect immunofluorescence assay confirm the presence of HIV infection.

   C. CD4+ T-lymphocyte count assists with classifying the stage of HIV infection.

   D. HIV RNA quantification tests are used to determine viral level and to monitor treatment.

   E. CSF analysis is used to confirm meningitis.

   Ⓝ *NCLEX® Connection: Physiological Adaptation, Basic Pathophysiology*

3. A. A client who has AIDS should avoid changing the litter box to prevent acquiring toxoplasmosis.

   B. A client who has AIDS should avoid consuming raw fruits due to the presence of bacteria that can cause opportunistic infections.

   C. Due to compromised immune response, a client who has AIDS should avoid contact with family members who are ill.

   D. **CORRECT:** A client who has AIDS should cook vegetables before eating to kill bacteria that cause opportunistic infections.

   Ⓝ *NCLEX® Connection: Physiological Adaptation, Alterations in Body Systems*

4. A. **CORRECT:** Perinatal exposure is a risk factor associated with HIV. Clients who are pregnant should take precautionary measures to prevent HIV exposure.

   B. Clients who are pregnant are tested for HIV, but pregnancy is not a risk factor associated with this virus.

   C. Having a monogamous sex partner is not a risk factor associated with the HIV virus.

   D. **CORRECT:** Being an older adult female is a risk factor associated with the HIV virus due vaginal dryness and the thinning of the vaginal wall.

   E. **CORRECT:** Occupational exposure, such as being a health care worker, is a risk factor associated with the HIV virus.

   Ⓝ *NCLEX® Connection: Health Promotion and Maintenance, Health Promotion/Disease Prevention*

5. A. The client should avoid high-fat foods to gain weight because fat intolerance causing flatus, bloating, and diarrhea is common in clients who have HIV/AIDS.

   B. The client should eat small, frequent meals (such as six meals per day) to promote weight gain.

   C. The client should drink 2 to 3 L of liquids daily to maintain hydration, not gain weight.

   D. **CORRECT:** The client should add high-protein, high-calorie foods to the diet daily to gain weight and maintain health.

   Ⓝ *NCLEX® Connection: Basic Care and Comfort, Nutrition and Oral Hydration*

PRACTICE Answer

Using ATI Active Learning Template: System Disorder

NURSING CARE
- Collect data about risk factors (sexual practices, IV drug use).
- Monitor fluid intake/urinary output.
- Obtain daily weights to monitor weight loss.
- Monitor nutritional intake.
- Monitor electrolytes.
- Check skin integrity (rashes, open areas, bruising).
- Check pain status.
- Monitor vital signs (especially temperature).
- Monitor lung sounds/respiratory status (diminished lung sounds).
- Monitor neurological status (confusion, dementia, vision changes).

Ⓝ *NCLEX® Connection: Reduction of Risk Potential, Potential for Complications from Surgical Procedures and Health Alterations*

CHAPTER 77 *Lupus Erythematosus, Gout, and Fibromyalgia*

Lupus erythematosus (lupus) is an autoimmune disorder in which an atypical immune response results in chronic inflammation and destruction of healthy tissue. Other autoimmune disorders include rheumatoid arthritis (RA), vasculitis, multiple sclerosis, scleroderma (including Raynaud's phenomenon), and psoriasis.

In autoimmune disorders, small antigens can bond with healthy tissue. The body then produces antibodies that attack the healthy tissue. This can be triggered by toxins, medications, bacteria, and viruses. Control of manifestations and a decrease in the number and frequency of exacerbations is the goal of treatment, because there is no cure for autoimmune disorders.

Gout, also known as gouty arthritis, is a systemic disorder caused by hyperuricemia (increase in serum uric acid). Urate levels can be affected by medications, diet, and overproduction in the body. This can cause uric crystal deposits to form in the joints, and a gout attack can occur.

Fibromyalgia is a chronic pain syndrome that involves stiffness, sleep disturbance, generalized muscle weakness and chronic fatigue. It is estimated that 25% to 65% of people who have fibromyalgia have another form of a rheumatologic disorder, such as RA or systemic lupus erythematosus.

Occurrence of autoimmune disorders increases with age. ©

M◊ *Online Image: Raynaud's Syndrome*

Lupus erythematosus

- Lupus varies in severity and progression. It is generally characterized by periods of exacerbations (flares) and remissions.
- Lupus is classified as discoid or systemic. A temporary form of lupus can be medication-induced.
  - **Discoid lupus erythematosus (DLE)** only affects the skin.
  - **Systemic lupus erythematosus (SLE)** affects connective tissues of multiple organ systems and can lead to major organ failure.
  - **Medication-induced lupus erythematosus** can be caused by medications (procainamide, hydralazine, isoniazid). Findings resolve when the medication is discontinued.
- Lupus can be difficult to diagnose because of the vague nature of early manifestations.

DATA COLLECTION

RISK FACTORS

- Females age 20 to 40 years
- African American, Asian, or Native American descent
- The incidence of lupus declines in females following menopause but remains steady in males.
- Diagnosis of lupus can be delayed in older adult clients because many of the manifestations mimic other disorders or can be associated with reports common to the normal aging process. ©
  - Joint pain and swelling can significantly limit ADLs in older adult clients who have comorbidities.
  - Older adult clients are at an increased risk for fractures if corticosteroid therapy is used.

EXPECTED FINDINGS

- Fatigue/malaise
- Alopecia
- Blurred vision
- Pleuritic pain
- Anorexia/weight loss
- Depression
- Joint pain, swelling, tenderness

PHYSICAL FINDINGS ○EBP
- Fever (also a major indication of exacerbation)
- Anemia
- Lymphadenopathy
- Pericarditis (presence of a cardiac friction rub or pleural friction rub)
- Raynaud's phenomenon (arteriolar vasospasm in response to cold/stress)
- Findings consistent with organ involvement (kidney, heart, lungs, vasculature)
- Erythematous "butterfly" rash over the nose and cheeks (raised, dry, scaly) (77.1)
- Alopecia

LABORATORY TESTS

Skin biopsy: Used to diagnose DLE by confirming the presence of lupus cells and cellular inflammation

Immunologic tests: Used to diagnose SLE
- Antinuclear antibodies (ANAs): antibodies produced against one's own DNA; positive titers in 95% of clients who have lupus
  - SLE prep
  - dsDNA (very specific for SLE; assists with differentiation between SLE and medication-induced lupus)
  - ssDNA
  - Anti-DNP
  - SS-A
- Serum complement (C3, C4): decreased
  - The complement system is made of proteins (there are nine major complement proteins). These proteins work with the immune system and play a role in the development of inflammation. C3 and C4 are diagnostic for SLE because they decrease due to depletion secondary to an exaggerated inflammatory response.
- Erythrocyte sedimentation rate (ESR): elevated due to systemic inflammation

BUN and serum creatinine: Increased (with kidney involvement)

Urinalysis: Positive for protein and RBCs (kidney involvement)

CBC: Pancytopenia

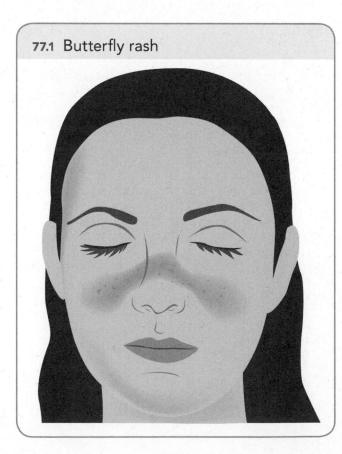

77.1 Butterfly rash

PATIENT-CENTERED CARE

NURSING CARE

- Monitor the following.
  - Pain, mobility, and fatigue
  - Vital signs (especially blood pressure)
  - Systemic manifestations
    - Hypertension and edema (renal compromise)
    - Urine output (renal compromise)
    - Diminished breath sounds (pleural effusion)
    - Tachycardia and sharp inspiratory chest pain (pericarditis)
    - Rubor, pallor, and cyanosis of hands/feet (vasculitis/vasospasm, Raynaud's phenomenon)
    - Arthralgias, myalgias, and polyarthritis (joint and connective tissue involvement)
    - Changes in mental status that indicate neurologic involvement (psychoses, paresis, seizures)
    - BUN, serum creatinine, and urinary output for renal involvement
    - Nutritional status
- Provide small, frequent meals if anorexia is a concern. Offer between-meal supplements. **Qᴇʙᴘ**
- Encourage the client to limit salt intake for fluid retention secondary to steroid therapy.
- Provide emotional support to the client and family.
- Inform clients of childbearing age regarding risks of pregnancy with lupus and treatment medications. **Qs**

MEDICATIONS

NSAIDs

- Used to reduce inflammation and arthritic pain.
- Contraindicated for clients who have impaired kidney function

NURSING ACTIONS: Monitor for NSAID-induced hepatitis.

Corticosteroids

Prednisone used for immunosuppression and to reduce inflammation.

NURSING ACTIONS: Monitor for fluid retention, hypertension, and impaired kidney function.

CLIENT EDUCATION: Do not stop taking steroids abruptly. Gradually taper the dosage as prescribed.

Immunosuppressant agents

Methotrexate and azathioprine used to suppress the immune response. **Qᴘᴄᴄ**

NURSING ACTIONS: Monitor for toxic effects (bone marrow suppression, increased liver enzymes).

Antimalarial

Hydroxychloroquine used for suppression of synovitis, fever, and fatigue.

NURSING ACTIONS: Encourage frequent eye examinations.

INTERPROFESSIONAL CARE

- Physical and occupational therapy services can be used for strengthening exercises and adaptive devices as needed.
- Refer clients to support groups as appropriate.

CLIENT EDUCATION

- Avoid UV and prolonged sun exposure. Use sunscreen when outside and exposed to sunlight.
- Use mild protein shampoo and avoid harsh hair treatments.
- Use steroid creams for skin rash.
- Report peripheral and periorbital edema promptly.
- Report evidence of infection related to immunosuppression.
- Avoid crowds and individuals who are sick, because illness can precipitate an exacerbation.

COMPLICATIONS

Lupus nephritis

Clients whose SLE cannot be managed with immunosuppressants and corticosteroids can experience chronic kidney disease resulting in the possible need for a kidney transplant. Lupus nephritis is the leading cause of death related to SLE.

NURSING ACTIONS: Monitor for periorbital and lower extremity swelling and hypertension. Monitor renal status (creatinine, BUN).

CLIENT EDUCATION
- Take immunosuppressants and corticosteroids as prescribed.
- Avoid stress and illness.

Pericarditis and myocarditis

Inflammation of the heart, its vessels, and the surrounding sac can occur secondary to SLE.

NURSING ACTIONS: Monitor for chest pain, fatigue, arrhythmias, and fever.

CLIENT EDUCATION
- Report chest pain.
- Take immunosuppressants and corticosteroids as prescribed.
- Avoid stress and illness.
- Report chest pain to the provider.

Gout

Gout or gouty arthritis is the most common inflammatory arthritis. Gout is a systemic disease caused by a disruption in purine metabolism in which uric acid crystals are deposited in joints and body tissues. Gout is classified as either primary or secondary.

Primary gout

- Most common
- Can have genetic component
- Uric acid production is greater than excretion of it by the kidneys.
- Middle- and older-adult males (peak onset between ages 40 and 50), as well as postmenopausal women are commonly affected.

Secondary gout

- Caused by another disease or condition (chronic kidney failure, excessive diuretic use) that causes excessive uric acid in the blood
- Treatment based on treating the underlying condition
- Can affect people of any age

DATA COLLECTION

RISK FACTORS

- Obesity
- Cardiovascular disease
- Trauma
- Alcohol ingestion
- Starvation dieting
- Diuretic use
- Some chemotherapy agents
- Chronic kidney failure

EXPECTED FINDINGS

- Severe joint pain, especially in the metatarsophalangeal joint of the great toe
- Redness, swelling, and warmth of affected joint

PHYSICAL FINDINGS
- Painful, swollen joint that is very painful if touched or moved
- Appearance of tophi (chronic gout)

LABORATORY TESTS

Erythrocyte sedimentation rate (ESR): Elevated

Serum uric acid: Repeated measurements obtained due to effect of dietary intake on results. Consistent elevation above 6.5 mg/dL is associated with gout.

Urinary uric acid: Elevated

Blood urea nitrogen (BUN), serum creatinine: Elevated

PATIENT-CENTERED CARE

NURSING CARE

Monitor the following.
- Pain
- Redness/swelling of affected joint
- Serum uric acid levels

MEDICATIONS

Acute gout

Antigout agent
- Colchicine (PO or parenteral) is used to decrease pain and inflammation.
- NURSING ACTIONS: Use cautiously in clients who have impaired kidney function.

NSAIDs
- Indomethacin or ibuprofen is used to decrease pain and inflammation.
- Contraindicated for clients who have impaired kidney function.
- CLIENT EDUCATION: Do not take on an empty stomach.

Corticosteroids
- Prednisone used to treat inflammation.
- NURSING ACTIONS: Monitor for fluid retention, hypertension, and impaired kidney dysfunction.
- CLIENT EDUCATION: Do not stop taking the medication abruptly. Gradually taper dosage as prescribed.

Chronic gout

Xanthine oxidase inhibitor
- Allopurinol is used as a maintenance medication to promote uric acid excretion and decrease its production.
- NURSING ACTIONS: Increase fluid intake.
- CLIENT EDUCATION: Take after meals and with a full glass of water.

Uricosuric
- Probenecid is used as a maintenance medication to promote uric acid excretion.
- NURSING ACTIONS: Monitor uric acid levels.
- CLIENT EDUCATION: Do not use aspirin because it will decrease the effectiveness of the medication.

CLIENT EDUCATION

- Stay on a low-purine diet (no organ meats or shellfish). Q_{EBP}
- Limit alcohol intake.
- Avoid starvation diets, aspirin, and diuretics.
- Limit physical or emotional stress.
- Increase fluid intake.
- Adhere to medication.

Fibromyalgia

- Fibromyalgia, also known as fibromyalgia syndrome, is a chronic pain syndrome which manifests as pain, stiffness, and tenderness at certain "trigger points" in the body.
- The pain is typically described as a burning a gnawing pain that can be elicited by palpating trigger points.
- The client can also experience chronic fatigue, sleep disturbances, and functional impairment.
- Pain and tenderness vary depending on stress, activity, and weather conditions.

DATA COLLECTION

RISK FACTORS

- Females age 30 to 50 years
- History of rheumatologic conditions, chronic fatigue syndrome, or Lyme disease
- Deep sleep deprivation

EXPECTED FINDINGS

- Mild to severe fatigue
- Sleep disturbances
- Numbness/tingling of extremities
- Sensitivity to noxious smells, loud noises, and bright lights
- Headaches
- Jaw pain
- Depression
- Concentration and memory difficulties
- GI manifestations: abdominal pain, heartburn, constipation, diarrhea
- Genitourinary manifestations (frequency, urgency, dysuria, pelvic pain)
- Vision changes

PATIENT-CENTERED CARE

NURSING CARE

- Monitor pain, mobility, and fatigue.
- Provide emotional support to the client and family

MEDICATIONS

Serotonin-norepinephrine reuptake inhibitors (SNRIs) and anticonvulsants

- Pregabalin (anticonvulsant) and duloxetine (SNRI) are used to increase the release of serotonin and norepinephrine, resulting in decreased nerve pain.
- Can cause drowsiness/sleepiness.

CLIENT EDUCATION: Do not drink alcohol while on this medication.

NSAIDs

- Used to decrease pain and inflammation
- Contraindicated for clients who have impaired kidney function

CLIENT EDUCATION: Do not take on an empty stomach.

Tricyclic antidepressants

- Amitriptyline, nortriptyline, and trazodone are used to help induce sleep and decrease pain.
- Amitriptyline and nortriptyline can cause confusion and orthostatic hypotension in older adult clients. Trazodone is often the medication of choice for the older adult clients due to decreased adverse effects. ©

INTERPROFESSIONAL CARE

- Physical therapy can be helpful to decrease pain.
- Recommend a referral for the client to national foundations and local support groups.
- Complementary and alternative therapies can be helpful (acupuncture, stress management).

CLIENT EDUCATION

- Limit intake of caffeine, alcohol, and other substances that interfere with sleep.
- Develop a routine for sleep.

Application Exercises

1. A nurse is reviewing the plan of care for a client who has systemic lupus erythematosus (SLE). The client reports fatigue, joint tenderness, swelling, and difficulty urinating. Which of the following laboratory findings should the nurse expect? (Select all that apply.)
   - A. Positive ANA titer
   - B. Increased hemoglobin
   - C. 2+ urine protein
   - D. Increased serum C3 and C4
   - E. Elevated BUN

2. A nurse is reinforcing teaching about self-care with a client who has SLE. Which of the following statements by the client indicates understanding?
   - A. "I should limit my time to 10 minutes in the tanning bed."
   - B. "I will apply powder to any skin rash."
   - C. "I should use a mild hair shampoo."
   - D. "I will inspect my skin once a month for rashes."

3. A nurse is discussing gout with a client who is concerned about developing the disorder. Which of the following findings should the nurse identify as risk factors? (Select all that apply.)
   - A. Diuretic use
   - B. Obesity
   - C. Deep sleep deprivation
   - D. Depression
   - E. Cardiovascular disease

4. A nurse is collecting data from a client who has SLE. Which of the following findings should the nurse expect?
   - A. Weight gain
   - B. Petechiae on thighs
   - C. Systolic murmur
   - D. Alopecia

5. A nurse is caring for a client who has SLE and is experiencing an episode of Raynaud's phenomenon. Which of the following findings should the nurse anticipate?
   - A. Swelling of joints of the fingers
   - B. Pallor of toes with cold exposure
   - C. Feet that become reddened with ambulation
   - D. Client report of intense feeling of heat in the fingers

---

PRACTICE Active Learning Scenario

A nurse is reinforcing teaching with a client who has a new diagnosis of fibromyalgia. What should the nurse include in the teaching? Use the ATI Active Learning Template: System Disorder to complete this item.

ALTERATION IN HEALTH (DIAGNOSIS)

RISK FACTORS: Describe two.

EXPECTED FINDINGS: Include three findings.

MEDICATIONS: Identify two types of medications used to treat fibromyalgia along with their purpose and specific nursing considerations.

Application Exercises Key

1. A. **CORRECT:** A positive antinuclear antibody (ANA) titer is an expected finding in a client who has SLE. The ANA test identifies the presence of antibodies produced against the client's own DNA.

   B. Pancytopenia, rather than an elevated hemoglobin, is an expected finding in a client who has SLE.

   C. **CORRECT:** Increased urine protein is an expected finding due to kidney injury as a result of SLE.

   D. The client who has SLE is expected to have a decreased level of serum C3 and C4.

   E. **CORRECT:** Elevated BUN is an expected finding due to kidney injury in a client who has SLE.

   (N) *NCLEX® Connection: Reduction of Risk Potential, Laboratory Values*

2. A. A client who has SLE should avoid the use of tanning beds and prolonged sun exposure.

   B. A client who has SLE should apply steroid-based creams (not powder) to skin rashes.

   C. **CORRECT:** A client who has SLE should use a mild hair shampoo that does not irritate the scalp.

   D. A client who has SLE should inspect her skin daily for any open areas or rashes.

   (N) *NCLEX® Connection: PReduction of Risk Potential, Potential for Alterations in Body Systems*

3. A. **CORRECT:** The use of diuretics is a risk factor for gout.

   B. **CORRECT:** Obesity is a risk factor for gout.

   C. Deep sleep deprivation is a manifestation of fibromyalgia and is not a risk factor for gout.

   D. Depression is a manifestation of SLE and is not a risk factor for gout.

   E. **CORRECT:** Cardiovascular disease is a risk factor for gout.

   (N) *NCLEX® Connection: Health Promotion and Maintenance, High Risk Behaviors*

4. A. Weight loss, rather than weight gain, is an expected finding in a client who has SLE.

   B. A butterfly rash on the face is a finding in a client who has lupus.

   C. A cardiac friction rub is an expected finding of SLE.

   D. **CORRECT:** Alopecia (hair loss) is an expected finding of SLE.

   (N) *NCLEX® Connection: Health Promotion and Maintenance, Data Collection Techniques*

5. A. Swelling, pain, and joint tenderness are findings of SLE and are not specific to an episode of Raynaud's phenomenon.

   B. **CORRECT:** Pallor of the extremities occurs in Raynaud's phenomenon in a client who has SLE and has been exposed to cold or stress.

   C. The extremities becoming red, white, and blue when exposed to cold or stress is characteristic of an episode of Raynaud's phenomenon in a client who has SLE.

   D. A client report of intense pain in the hands and feet is characteristic of an episode of Raynaud's phenomenon in a client who has SLE.

   (N) *NCLEX® Connection: Physiological Adaptation, Basic Pathophysiology*

PRACTICE Answer

Using the ATI Active Learning Template: System Disorder

ALTERATION IN HEALTH (DIAGNOSIS)
- Fibromyalgia, also known as fibromyalgia syndrome, is a chronic pain syndrome that manifests as pain, stiffness, and tenderness at certain trigger points in the body.
- The pain is typically described as a burning or gnawing pain that can be elicited by palpating trigger points.
- The client can also experience chronic fatigue, sleep disturbances, and functional impairment.
- Pain and tenderness vary depending on stress, activity, and weather conditions.

RISK FACTORS
- Females age 30 to 50 years
- History of rheumatologic conditions, chronic fatigue syndrome, or Lyme disease
- Deep sleep deprivation

EXPECTED FINDINGS
- Mild to severe fatigue
- Sleep disturbances
- Numbness/tingling of extremities
- Sensitivity to noxious smells, loud noises, and bright lights
- Headaches
- Jaw pain
- Depression
- Concentration and memory difficulties
- GI manifestations (abdominal pain, heartburn, constipation, diarrhea)
- Genitourinary manifestations (frequency, urgency, dysuria, pelvic pain)
- Vision changes

MEDICATIONS
- Serotonin-norepinephrine reuptake inhibitors (SNRIs) and anticonvulsants
  - Pregabalin (anticonvulsant) and duloxetine (SNRI) are used to increase the release of serotonin and norepinephrine, resulting in decreased nerve pain.
  - Can cause drowsiness/sleepiness.
  - Client Education: Do not drink alcohol while on this medication.
- NSAIDs
  - Used to decrease pain and inflammation
  - Contraindicated for clients who have impaired kidney function
  - Client Education: Do not take on an empty stomach.
- Tricyclic antidepressants
  - Amitriptyline, nortriptyline, and trazodone are used to help induce sleep and decrease pain.
  - Amitriptyline and nortriptyline can cause confusion and orthostatic hypotension in older adult clients. Trazodone is often the medication of choice for the older adult client due to decreased adverse effects.

(N) *NCLEX® Connection: Physiological Adaptation, Basic Pathophysiology*

UNIT 13 NURSING CARE OF CLIENTS WHO HAVE IMMUNE SYSTEM AND CONNECTIVE TISSUE DISORDERS
SECTION: CONNECTIVE TISSUE DISORDERS

CHAPTER 78 *Rheumatoid Arthritis*

Rheumatoid arthritis (RA) is a chronic, progressive inflammatory disease that can affect tissues and organs but principally attacks the joints, producing inflammatory synovitis. It involves joints bilaterally and symmetrically, and typically affects several joints at one time. RA typically affects upper joints first.

RA is an autoimmune disease that is precipitated by WBCs attacking synovial tissue. The WBCs cause the synovial tissue to become inflamed and thickened. The inflammation can extend to the cartilage, bone, tendons, and ligaments that surround the joint. Joint deformity and bone erosion can result from these changes, decreasing the joint's range of motion and function.

RA is also a systemic disease that can affect any connective tissue in the body. Common structures affected are the blood vessels, pleura, and pericardium. Iritis and scleritis can also develop in the eyes.

The natural course of the disease is one of exacerbations and remissions.

78.1 Rheumatoid arthritis changes

HEALTH PROMOTION AND DISEASE PREVENTION

- Use adaptive devices that prevent development of deformity of inflamed joints during ADLs.
- Continue using affected joints and ambulating to maintain function and range of motion.

DATA COLLECTION

RISK FACTORS

- Female clients (3:1 compared to male clients)
- Age 20 to 50 years
- Genetic predisposition
- Epstein–Barr virus
- Stress
- Environmental factors
- Older age
  - Early manifestations of RA (fatigue, joint discomfort) are vague and can be attributed to other disorders in older adult clients. Ⓖ
  - Joint pain and dysfunction can have a greater effect on older adult clients than on younger adult clients due to the presence of other chronic conditions.
  - Older adult clients can be less able to overcome or cope with joint pain/deformity.

EXPECTED FINDINGS

Findings depend on the area affected by the disease process.
- Pain at rest and with movement
- Morning stiffness
- Pleuritic pain (pain upon inspiration)
- Xerostomia (dry mouth)
- Anorexia/weight loss
- Fatigue
- Paresthesias
- Recent illness/stressor
- Joint pain
- Lack of function
- Joint swelling and deformity
  - Joint deformities are late manifestations of RA. **(78.1)**
  - Joint swelling, warmth, and erythema are common.
  - Finger, hand, wrist, knee, and foot joints are generally affected.
  - Finger joints affected are the proximal interphalangeal and metacarpophalangeal joints.
  - Joints can become deformed merely by completing ADLs.
- Ulnar deviation, swan neck, and boutonnière deformities are common in the fingers.
- Subcutaneous nodules
- Fever (generally low-grade)
- Muscle weakness/atrophy
- Reddened sclera and/or abnormal shape of pupils
- Lymph node enlargement

LABORATORY TESTS

Anti-CCP antibodies

This test detects antibodies to cyclic citrullinated peptide (anti-CCP). The result is positive in most people who have rheumatoid arthritis, even years before manifestations develop. The test is more sensitive for RA than rheumatoid factor (RF) antibodies.

Rheumatoid factor antibody

Diagnostic level for rheumatoid arthritis is 1:40 to 1:60 (expected reference range 1:20 or less).
- High titers correlate with severe disease.
- Other autoimmune diseases also can increase RF antibody.

Erythrocyte sedimentation rate (ESR)

Elevated ESR is associated with the inflammation or infection in the body.
- 20 to 40 mm/hr is mild inflammation.
- 40 to 70 mm/hr is moderate inflammation.
- 70 to 150 mm/hr is severe inflammation.
- Other autoimmune diseases also can increase ESR antibody.

C-reactive protein: Positive

- This test may be done in place of ESR.
- This test is useful for diagnosing disease or monitoring disease activity, and for monitoring the response to anti-inflammatory therapy.

Antinuclear antibody (ANA) titer

Antibody produced against one's own DNA
- The expected finding for ANA titer is negative at 1:20 dilution.
- Rheumatoid arthritis and other autoimmune diseases produce a positive ANA titer result.

Complete blood count

- WBC count can be elevated during an exacerbation secondary to the inflammatory response.
- Decreased RBCs due to anemia.

DIAGNOSTIC PROCEDURES

Arthrocentesis

- Arthrocentesis is synovial fluid aspiration by needle.
- With RA, increased WBCs and RF are present in fluid.

NURSING ACTIONS: Monitor for bleeding or a synovial fluid leak from the needle biopsy site.

CLIENT EDUCATION: Take acetaminophen for pain.

X-ray

X-rays are used to determine the degree of joint destruction and monitor its progression. They can provide adequate visualization and reveal bony erosions and narrowed joint spaces. This negates the need for more expensive radiologic tests, such a CT scan or magnetic resonance imaging (MRI).

NURSING ACTIONS: Assist the client into position.

CLIENT EDUCATION: Minimize movement during the procedure.

PATIENT-CENTERED CARE

NURSING CARE

- Apply heat or cold to the affected areas based on client response. Q**EBP**
  - Morning stiffness (hot shower)
  - Pain in hands/fingers (heated paraffin)
  - Edema (cold therapy)
- Assist with and encourage physical activity to maintain joint mobility (within the capabilities of the client).
- Monitor for indications of fatigue.
- Reinforce teaching with the client about measures to do the following.
  - Maximize functional activity.
  - Minimize pain.
  - Monitor skin closely.
  - Conserve energy (space out activities, take rest periods, ask for additional assistance when needed).
  - Promote coping strategies.
  - Encourage routine health screenings.
- Provide a safe environment. Q**s**
  - Recommend referrals for physical therapy and occupational therapy.
  - Provide information for support organizations.
  - Facilitate the use of assistive devices.
  - Remove unnecessary equipment and supplies.
- Use progressive muscle relaxation.
- Administer medications and proper positioning.
- Monitor for medication effectiveness (reduced pain, increased mobility).
- Instruct the client regarding manifestations that need to be reported immediately (fever, infection, pain upon inspiration, substernal pain).

Nutritional teaching

- Consume foods high in vitamins, protein, and iron.
- Eat small, frequent meals.

MEDICATIONS

Nonsteroidal anti-inflammatory drugs (NSAIDs)

- Treatment begins with NSAIDs.
- NSAIDs provide analgesic, antipyretic, and anti-inflammatory effects.
- NSAIDs can cause considerable gastrointestinal (GI) distress.

NURSING ACTIONS

- Request a concurrent prescription for a GI acid-lowering agent (histamine$_2$-receptor antagonist, proton pump inhibitor) if GI distress is reported.
- Monitor for fluid retention, hypertension, and kidney dysfunction.

CLIENT EDUCATION

- Take the medication with food or with a full glass of water or milk. If taking NSAIDs routinely, an H$_2$-receptor antagonist can also be prescribed.
- Observe for GI bleeding (coffee-ground emesis; dark, tarry stools).
- Avoid alcohol, which can increase the risk of GI complications.

COX-2 enzyme blockers

Cause less GI distress but carry a risk of cardiac disease

Corticosteroids

Corticosteroids (prednisone) are strong anti-inflammatory medications that can be given for acute exacerbations or advanced forms of the disease.

They are not given for long-term therapy due to significant adverse effects (osteoporosis, hyperglycemia, immunosuppression, cataracts).

NURSING ACTIONS

- Observe for Cushingoid changes.
- Monitor weight and blood pressure.

CLIENT EDUCATION

- Observe for changes in vision, blood glucose, and impaired healing.
- Avoid crowds.
- Follow the prescription (alternate-day dosing, tapering, discontinuing medication).

Disease modifying anti-rheumatic drugs (DMARDs)

DMARDs work in a variety of ways to slow the progression of RA and suppress the immune system's reaction to RA that causes pain and inflammation. Relief of manifestations might not occur for several weeks.

Other medications

- **Antimalarial agent:** Hydroxychloroquine
- **Antibiotic:** Minocycline
- **Sulfonamide:** Sulfasalazine
- **Biologic response modifiers:** Etanercept, infliximab, adalimumab, chelator penicillamine
- **Cytotoxic medications:** Methotrexate, leflunomide, cyclophosphamide, and azathioprine can cause severe adverse effects.

THERAPEUTIC PROCEDURES

Plasmapheresis

- Removes circulating antibodies from plasma, decreasing attacks on the client's tissues
- May be done for a severe, life-threatening exacerbation

Total joint arthroplasty

Surgical repair and replacement of a joint may be done for a severely deformed joint that has not responded to medication therapy.

INTERPROFESSIONAL CARE

- Inform the client about support groups as appropriate.
- Recommend referral to occupational therapy for adaptive devices that can facilitate carrying out ADLs and prevent deformities.
- A home health aide can be necessary for assistance with ADLs. Q^{TC}

COMPLICATIONS

Sjögren's syndrome

- Triad of manifestations: dry eyes, mouth, and vagina
- Caused by obstruction of secretory ducts and glands

NURSING ACTIONS

- Provide eye drops and artificial saliva, and recommend vaginal lubricants as needed.
- Provide fluids with meals.

Secondary osteoporosis

Immobilization caused by arthritis can contribute to the development of osteoporosis.

CLIENT EDUCATION: Perform weight-bearing exercises as tolerated.

Vasculitis (organ ischemia)

Inflammation of arteries can disrupt blood flow, causing ischemia. Smaller arteries in the skin, eyes, and brain are most commonly affected in RA.

NURSING ACTIONS: Monitor for skin lesions, decrease in vision, and manifestations of cognitive dysfunction.

Application Exercises

1. A nurse in an outpatient clinic is collecting data from a client who has rheumatoid arthritis (RA). The client reports increased joint tenderness and swelling. Which of the following findings should the nurse expect? (Select all that apply.)

   A. Recent influenza

   B. Decreased range of motion

   C. Hypersalivation

   D. Increased blood pressure

   E. Pain at rest

2. A nurse is reinforcing teaching with a client who has a new diagnosis of rheumatoid arthritis. Which of the following instructions should the nurse give?

   A. "You can experience morning stiffness when you get out bed."

   B. "You can experience abdominal pain."

   C. "You can experience weight gain."

   D. "You can experience low blood sugar."

3. A nurse is reviewing the medical record of a client who has rheumatoid arthritis. The nurse should review which of the following laboratory results when monitoring this disease? (Select all that apply.)

   A. Urinalysis

   B. Erythrocyte sedimentation rate (ESR)

   C. BUN

   D. Antinuclear antibody (ANA) titer

   E. WBC count

Application Exercises Key

1. A. **CORRECT:** Some conditions, such as a recent illness like influenza, can exacerbate RA.

   B. **CORRECT:** Clients who have RA often experience a decrease in range of motion.

   C. Clients who have RA can experience xerostomia, not hypersalivation.

   D. Increased blood pressure is not indicative of RA.

   E. **CORRECT:** Clients who have RA often report pain.

   Ⓝ *NCLEX® Connection: Reduction of Risk Potential, Potential for Alterations in Body Systems*

2. A. **CORRECT:** The nurse should reinforce in the teaching that the client who has RA can experience stiffness in joints upon rising.

   B. The client who has RA can experience pleuritic pain upon inspiration, not abdominal pain.

   C. The client who has RA can experience weight loss, not weight gain.

   D. The client who has RA does not experience a low blood sugar.

   Ⓝ *NCLEX® Connection: Physiological Adaptation, Alterations in Body Systems*

3. A. A urinalysis is not a laboratory test used to diagnose RA. This test can detect kidney failure.

   B. **CORRECT:** ESR is a laboratory test used to diagnose RA. This laboratory test will show an elevated result in clients who have RA.

   C. A BUN is not a laboratory test used to diagnose RA. This test can be used for detecting kidney failure.

   D. **CORRECT:** ANA titer is a laboratory test used to diagnose RA. This laboratory test will show a positive result in clients who have RA.

   E. **CORRECT:** WBC count is a laboratory test used to diagnose RA. This laboratory test will show a decreased result in clients who have RA.

   Ⓝ *NCLEX® Connection: Reduction of Risk Potential, Laboratory Values*

PRACTICE Active Learning Scenario

A nurse is reviewing information about the adverse effects of prednisone with a client who has rheumatoid arthritis. Use the ATI Active Learning Template: Medication and the ATI Pharmacology Review Module to complete this item.

COMPLICATIONS: Identify three adverse effects of this medication, as well as related client education.

PRACTICE Answer

Using the ATI Active Learning Template: Medication

COMPLICATIONS

- Risk of infection (fever, sore throat): Notify the provider immediately if manifestations occur.
- Osteoporosis: Take calcium supplements, vitamin D, and/or bisphosphonate.
- Fluid retention: Monitor for manifestations of fluid excess (crackles, weight gain, edema).
- Adrenal suppression
  - Observe for indications of adrenal suppression and notify the provider if they occur.
  - Do not discontinue the medication suddenly.
- GI discomfort
  - Report gastrointestinal distress to the provider.
  - H_2 antagonists can be used prophylactically.
  - Report manifestations of GI bleeding (coffee-ground emesis; black, tarry stools).
- Hyperglycemia: Monitor blood glucose level. Clients who have diabetes mellitus can need to adjust hypoglycemic agents.
- Hypokalemia
  - Monitor for manifestations of low potassium.
  - Eat potassium-rich foods.
  - Take prescribed potassium supplements.

Ⓝ *NCLEX® Connection: Pharmacological Therapies, Adverse Effects/Contraindications/Side Effects/Interactions*

CHAPTER 79

CHAPTER 79 *General Principles of Cancer*

Cancer is a neoplastic disease process that involves abnormal cell growth and differentiation. Normal body cells grow, divide, and die in an orderly fashion. In cancer, dying cells grow and form new abnormal cells that grow uncontrollably. The exact cause of cancer is unknown, but viruses, physical and chemical agents, hormones, genetics, and diet are thought to be factors that trigger abnormal cell growth.

Cancer cells can invade surrounding tissues and spread to other areas of the body through lymph and blood vessels (metastasis). No matter where cancer spreads, it is named based on the site of origin. For example, colon cancer that spreads to the liver is metastatic colon cancer. Metastasis is usually diagnosed when there is onset of new findings (bone pain indicative of bone metastasis; change in bowel or bladder tone indicative of nervous system involvement).

Screening and early diagnosis are the most important aspects of health education and care. The nurse should assist with prevention, identification, and treatment of complications associated with carcinoma.

Tumors (or neoplasms) are not always cancerous. A tumor is an abnormal collection of cells that grows independently of its surrounding tissue. Noncancerous tumors are benign. They have the potential of growing large and pressing on healthy organs and tissues, but they do not invade other tissues and do not metastasize. Malignant tumors do invade other tissues and metastasize to other organs. Cancer refers to malignant tumors.

BODY TISSUES

Cancers can arise from almost any tissue in the body.
- Epithelial tissue: carcinomas
- Glandular organs: adenocarcinomas
- Mesenchymal tissue: sarcomas
- Blood-forming cells: leukemias
- Lymph tissue: lymphomas
- Plasma cells: myelomas

HEALTH PROMOTION AND DISEASE PREVENTION

- Consume a healthy diet (low-fat with increased consumption of fruits, vegetables, and lean protein).
- Limit intake of sugar and salt.
- Maintain a healthy body weight.
- Avoid smoking, tobacco, and excessive alcohol consumption.
- Avoid risky behaviors (substance use, needle sharing, unprotected sexual intercourse).
- Avoid exposure to environmental hazards (radiation, chemicals). Use personal protective equipment when available.
- Breastfeed infants exclusively for the first 6 months of life.
- Engage in physical activity or exercise routinely.
- Protect skin and eyes from UVA and UVB rays.
- Remove at-risk tissue, such as moles, to prevent conversion to skin cancer.
- Chemoprevention is the use of medications or other substances to disrupt cancer development.
  - Aspirin and celecoxib to reduce the risk of colon cancer
  - Vitamin D and tamoxifen to reduce the risk of breast cancer
- Immunize to prevent human papilloma virus (HPV), which is associated with cervical cancer.

Screening for early detection of cancer

Cancer screening guidelines are from the American Cancer Society. Refer to www.cancer.org for more information about these and other screenings.

Mammogram
- Females age 40 to 44: annual screening optional
- Females age 45 to 54: annual screening recommended
- Females age 55 and older: annual screening (can switch to every 2 years)

Pap test:
- Females age 21 to 29: every 3 years (HPV testing only if needed)
- Females age 30 to 65: every 5 years (also include an HPV test)
- Females age 65 and older and females who had a total hysterectomy: routine screening not recommended

Colonoscopy: At age 50 and then every 10 years

Fecal occult blood: Annually for adults of all ages

Digital rectal exam: Males older than 50 years; older than 45 years for African American males or males who have a family history of prostate cancer

DATA COLLECTION

RISK FACTORS

Age: Highest incidence of cancer occurs in older adults. Ⓖ
- Older adult females most commonly develop colorectal, breast, lung, pancreatic, and ovarian cancers.
- Older adult males most commonly develop lung, colorectal, prostate, pancreatic, and gastric cancers.

Immune function: Cancer incidence increases among clients who have immunosuppression.

Chronic irritation and tissue trauma: Incidence of skin cancer is increased in people who have burn scars or other types of severe skin injury.

Race
- Caucasian females are more likely to develop breast cancer than are African American females. However, the mortality rate for African American females is higher than for Caucasian females.
- Caucasian males are at an increased risk for testicular cancer, whereas African American males are at an increased risk for prostate cancer.

Genetic predisposition

Exposure to chemicals, tobacco, and alcohol

Exposure to some viruses and bacteria
- Liver cancer can develop after many years of infection with hepatitis B or hepatitis C.
- Infection with human T-cell leukemia virus increases the risk of lymphoma and leukemia.
- Infection with Epstein-Barr virus has been linked to an increased risk of lymphoma.
- HPV infection is the main cause of cervical cancer.
- HIV increases the risk of lymphoma and Kaposi's sarcoma.
- *Helicobacter pylori* can increase the risk of stomach cancer and lymphoma of the stomach lining.

Diet: A diet high in fat, red meat, processed meat, refined grains, sugar-sweetened beverages, preservatives, and additives, and low in fiber

Sun, ultraviolet light, or radiation exposure: Ionizing (radon, x-ray) and UV (sun, tanning beds)

Sexual lifestyles: Multiple sexual partners or STIs

Poverty, obesity, and chronic GERD

Substance use

Chronic disease

Air pollution

EXPECTED FINDINGS

Staging of cancer

The tumor-node-metastasis (TNM) system is used to stage cancer.

TUMOR (T)
- **TX:** Unable to evaluate the primary tumor
- **T0:** No evidence of primary tumor
- **Tis:** Tumor in situ
- **T1, T2, T3, and T4:** Size and extent of tumor involvement

NODE (N)
- **NX:** Unable to evaluate regional lymph nodes
- **N0:** No evidence of regional node involvement
- **N1, N2, and N3:** Number of nodes that are involved and/or extent of spread

METASTASIS (M)
- **MX:** Unable to evaluate distant metastasis
- **M0:** No evidence of distant metastasis
- **M1, M2, M3:** Increasing presence of distant metastasis

Grading Q_{EBP}

Grading is needed because some cancer cells are more malignant than others. **Well-differentiated** means the cells look much like normal cells and tend to grow slowly. **Undifferentiated**, or poorly differentiated, means the cells do not look like normal cells and tend to grow quickly and spread.

- **GX:** Grade cannot be determined.
- **G1:** Tumor cells are well differentiated and are the least malignant.
- **G2:** Tumor cells are moderately differentiated.
- **G3:** Tumor cells are poorly differentiated but the tissue of origin can be established.
- **G4:** Tumor cells are poorly differentiated, and determination of the tissue of origin is difficult. Most aggressively malignant cells.

Prognosis

- Early diagnosis of cancer usually results in a better prognosis. Many cancers spread or metastasize before any manifestations are noted.
- Minority populations tend to have a worse prognosis than Caucasian clients for cancer related to several factors (low socioeconomic status, lack of access to health care, reluctance to seek treatment).

COMPLICATIONS

Malnutrition

Clients who have cancer are at increased risk for weight loss and anorexia.

- The presence of carcinoma in the body increases the amount of energy required for metabolic function.
- Cancer can impair the body's ability to ingest, digest, and absorb nutrients.
- Adverse effects of cancer treatment can affect the desire for food or the ability to eat. Manifestations include nausea, vomiting, changes in taste, anorexia, pain, diarrhea, early satiety, dry mouth, thickened saliva, and irritation to the gastrointestinal tract.

NURSING ACTIONS

- Inform the client about managing the expected effects of treatment.
- Administer antiemetics and antacids.
- Monitor relevant laboratory data (albumin, ferritin, transferrin).
- Monitor for malnutrition using height-weight charts, skin-fold measurements, and body mass index.
- Encourage frequent oral hygiene.
- Incorporate client preferences into meal planning when possible. Encourage client to eat whatever is appealing regardless of nutritional value.
- Instruct the client to consume adequate protein, carbohydrates, and calories.
- Collaborate with dietary services. Q_{TC}

Constipation/gastric stasis/intestinal obstruction

- Effects can be related to cancer or cancer treatment.
- Opioids can cause delayed emptying and slowed bowel motility.

NURSING ACTIONS

- Administer a stool softener or laxative.
- Encourage fluids, fiber, and activity as tolerated.
- Encourage small, frequent meals.

Paraneoplastic syndromes

- Paraneoplastic syndromes result when T cells in the body attack normal cells rather than cancerous ones. They result in changes in neurological function (movement, sensation, mental function).
- Management includes minimizing the immune system response by administration of steroids, immune factors, plasmapheresis, or irradiation.

NURSING ACTIONS

- Recognize manifestations of paraneoplastic syndrome.
- Administer medications.
- Provide a safe environment until client returns to baseline mental status.
- Use aids for vision or hearing impairments.

ONCOLOGIC EMERGENCIES

Syndrome of inappropriate antidiuretic hormone

Syndrome of inappropriate antidiuretic hormone (SIADH) occurs when excessive levels of antidiuretic hormones are produced. Because antidiuretic hormones help the kidneys and body to conserve the correct amount of water, SIADH causes the body to retain water. This results in a dilution of electrolytes (such as sodium) in the blood. It is most commonly associated with lung and brain cancers. Key findings include nausea and vomiting (early), lethargy, hostility, seizures, and coma.

NURSING ACTIONS

- Monitor for hyponatremia and low serum osmolality.
- Assist with administration of furosemide, 0.9% sodium chloride IV, and hypertonic sodium chloride solution for severe hyponatremia.
- Monitor vital signs and serum sodium because furosemide promotes sodium excretion, and hypertonic sodium chloride can cause fluid overload.

Hypercalcemia

A common complication of breast, lung, head, and neck cancers; leukemias and lymphomas; multiple myelomas; and bony metastases of any cancer

MANIFESTATIONS: Anorexia, nausea, vomiting, shortened QT interval, kidney stones, bone pain, fatigue, polyuria, constipation, changes in mental status

NURSING ACTIONS: Assist with the administration of 0.9% sodium chloride IV, furosemide, pamidronate, and phosphates. Administration of corticosteroids and calcitonin can reduce serum calcium levels.

Superior vena cava syndrome

- Results from obstruction (metastases from breast or lung cancers) of venous return and engorgement of the vessels from the head and upper body.
- Management includes high-dose radiation therapy for emergency temporary relief and the administration of chemotherapy to reduce tumor size.

MANIFESTATIONS: Periorbital and facial edema, erythema of the upper body, dyspnea, and epistaxis. Tracheal edema can lead to respiratory compromise.

NURSING ACTIONS: Position the client in high-Fowler's initially to facilitate lung expansion.

Hematologic disorders

Hematologic problems can be caused by cancer or chemotherapy.

Anemia: When cancer invades the bone marrow, it decreases the number of red blood cells, platelets (thrombocytopenia) and white blood cells (neutropenia).

Disseminated intravascular coagulation: Secondary to leukemia or adenocarcinomas. Management includes the administration of blood clotting factors that are lost through bleeding and need replacement with plasma transfusions.

NURSING ACTIONS
- Observe for bleeding, and apply pressure as needed.
- Monitor administration of blood clotting factors that have been lost through bleeding and need replacement with plasma transfusions.

Application Exercises

1. A nurse is caring for a client who has lung cancer and is exhibiting manifestations of syndrome of inappropriate antidiuretic hormone (SIADH). Which of the following findings should the nurse report to the provider? (Select all that apply.)

   A. Behavioral changes

   B. Client report of headache

   C. Urine output 40 mL/hr

   D. Client report of nausea

   E. Increased urine specific gravity

2. A nurse is reinforcing teaching about screening for cancer. Which of the following statements by the client indicates understanding?

   A. "I will need to have a mammogram every 2 years beginning at age 45."

   B. "I should have a colonoscopy every 15 years beginning at age 60."

   C. "I will need to have a Pap test every 5 years beginning at age 30."

   D. "I should have a fecal occult test done every 3 years."

3. A nurse is contributing to the plan of care for a client who has malnutrition due to cancer. Which of the following interventions should the nurse include? (Select all that apply.)

   A. Advise the client to keep a food diary.

   B. Encourage the client to brush teeth before and after meals.

   C. Check the laboratory report of ferritin.

   D. Recommend that the client avoid foods with low nutritional value.

   E. Instruct the client to limit daily intake of carbohydrates.

4. A nurse is reviewing the health record of a client who had surgery to stage ovarian cancer. The client's pathology report states a finding of T1-N3-MX. Which of the following information explains the findings of the pathology report?

   A. The ovarian tumor is present and involves lymph nodes.

   B. No lymph nodes contain cancer cells.

   C. The tumor is receptive to current medication therapy.

   D. The cancer has metastasized to other areas in the body.

PRACTICE **Active Learning Scenario**

A nurse is preparing an in-service about identifying risk factors for cancer for a group of adults at a community health fair. What information should the nurse include? Use the ATI Active Learning Template: System Disorder to complete this item.

RISK FACTORS
- Identify two types of cancer with increased incidence in older adult females.
- Identify two types of cancer with increased incidence in older adult males.
- Identify one type of cancer with increased risk in Caucasian males.
- Identify one type of cancer with increased risk in Caucasian females.
- Describe three diet-related risk factors.
- Describe at least three lifestyle-related risk factors.

PATHOPHYSIOLOGY RELATED TO CLIENT PROBLEM: Describe at least three viruses/bacteria and the type of cancer they can cause.

Application Exercises Key

1. A. **CORRECT:** Behavioral changes can indicate cerebral edema due to SIADH. The nurse should report this finding to the provider.

   B. **CORRECT:** A client report of headache can indicate cerebral edema due to SIADH. The nurse should report this finding to the provider.

   C. Urine output of 40 mL/hr is a finding consistent with SIADH. The nurse does not need to report this finding to the provider.

   D. **CORRECT:** A client report of nausea can indicate cerebral edema due to SIADH. The nurse should report this finding to the provider.

   E. An increased urine specific gravity is a finding consistent with SIADH. The nurse does not need to report this finding to the provider

   Ⓝ *NCLEX® Connection: Health Promotion and Maintenance, Data Collection Techniques*

2. A. The American Cancer Society recommends that females consider annual mammograms beginning at age 40. Annual screenings are indicated between ages 45 to 54.

   B. The client should begin colonoscopy screening at age 50 and then every 10 years thereafter.

   C. **CORRECT:** The nurse should instruct the client to have a Pap test every 3 years from the age of 21 to 29. The American Cancer Society recommends that females age 30 to 65 have a Pap test every 5 years.

   D. The client should have a fecal occult test performed every year.

   Ⓝ *NCLEX® Connection: Health Promotion and Maintenance, Community Resources*

3. A. **CORRECT:** The use of a food diary assists in monitoring changes in eating habits that occur in malnutrition due to cancer.

   B. **CORRECT:** Oral hygiene before and after meals promotes increased salivation and improves taste perception.

   C. **CORRECT:** Ferritin is an indicator of iron and protein levels. Reduced levels result in iron deficiency anemia and protein deficiency and can indicate malnutrition in a client who has cancer.

   D. The nurse should encourage the client to eat whatever is appealing and tastes good regardless of nutritional value. This strategy helps increase the client's overall caloric and nutritional intake.

   E. The nurse should encourage the client to consume adequate protein, carbohydrates, and calories.

   Ⓝ *NCLEX® Connection: Basic Care and Comfort, Nutrition and Oral Hydration*

4. A. **CORRECT:** Using the TNM staging system, a T1 designation indicates a tumor is present, and an N3 designation confirms lymph node involvement.

   B. A N3 designation indicates that three adjacent lymph nodes show evidence of spread of cancer using the TNM staging system.

   C. The TNM diagnostic notation of the staging system does not indicate the response of a tumor to a medication therapy regimen.

   D. The MX designation indicates the inability to evaluate for distant metastasis to other areas of the body using the TNM staging system.

   Ⓝ *NCLEX® Connection: Reduction of Risk Potential, Laboratory Values*

PRACTICE Answer

Using the ATI Active Learning Template: System Disorder

RISK FACTORS
- Older adult females: Colorectal, breast, lung, pancreatic, and ovarian cancers
- Older adult male: Lung, colorectal, prostate, pancreatic, and gastric cancers
- Caucasian males: Testicular cancer
- Caucasian females: Breast cancer
- Diet-related: Diet high in fat and red meat, low in fiber

- Lifestyle-related
  - Multiple sexual partners or STIs
  - Sun, ultraviolet light, and radiation exposure
  - Use of tobacco, alcohol, and other substances
- Obesity
- Poverty
- Chronic GERD
- Air pollution

PATHOPHYSIOLOGY RELATED TO CLIENT PROBLEM
- Hepatitis B or C: Liver cancer
- Human T-cell leukemia virus: Lymphoma and leukemia
- Epstein-Barr virus: Lymphoma
- Human papilloma virus: Cervical cancer
- HIV: Lymphoma and Kaposi's sarcoma
- *Helicobacter pylori*: Stomach cancer and lymphoma of the stomach lining

Ⓝ *NCLEX® Connection: Health Promotion and Maintenance, Community Resources*

CHAPTER 80 *Cancer Screening
and Diagnostic
Procedures*

Screening and diagnostic procedures provide objective and subjective client data. Screening and diagnosis for cancer can involve hands-on assessment techniques, invasive procedures, radiography and imaging studies, and laboratory testing. The type and location of the suspected cancer dictate which methods are used. Identification of tumor cells is required for definitive diagnosis and development of a targeted treatment plan.

INDICATIONS

CLIENT PRESENTATION

Cancer
- Altered body function (fatigue, weakness, anemia, infection, fluid and electrolyte imbalances)
- Change in body structure (weight loss, masses)
- Change in body symmetry or onset of recent findings (pain, nausea, vomiting, anorexia)

Metastasis
- Secondary sites of discomfort
- Swelling and/or tenderness of lymph nodes or areas of the body
- Presence of masses
- Altered function of another body system
- Bone pain
- Bleeding from spread of tumor through blood vessels

CONSIDERATIONS

- Complete a health history and physical assessment, including client report of findings and family history of cancer or genetic disorder.
- Provide privacy.
- Consider the client's cultural preference for examination (health professional's gender, presence of support person). Qᴘᴄᴄ

- Inspect for changes in color, symmetry, muscle mass, posture, movement, or body function.
- Auscultate for adventitious sounds that indicate altered body system function.
  - Heart, lung, and bowel sounds
  - Main arteries (carotid, femoral, renal, iliac)
  - Masses or areas of discomfort
- Palpate to detect masses or tissue abnormalities.
  - Peripheral pulses, capillary refill time, edema
  - Use light, medium, and deep pressure as appropriate.
  - Note any tenderness to palpation.
  - Only the provider should perform some palpation assessments (digital rectal exam for colorectal cancer).
- Percuss for changes in expected sound over organs.
  - Dullness in the lungs or bowel can indicate areas of consolidation or tumor.
  - Increased liver size (noted by measurement of borders [dullness]) can indicate inflammation or tumor.
- Explain all procedures prior to assessment.
- Provide explanation when there is need for further testing or evaluation of unexpected findings.

CLIENT EDUCATION
- Report unexpected findings to the provider.
- Continue self-examination (breast, testicular) at home.
  - Testicular cancer is rare but most common in males age 20 to 35 years.
  - With early detection, testicular cancer has a 95% cure rate.
  - Testicular self-examination is best performed during or after a bath or shower when the scrotum is relaxed.
  - Move the penis to the side, and examine one testicle at a time.
  - Hold the testicle between the thumb and fingers of both hands, and roll it gently between the fingers.
  - Look and feel for any hard lumps; smooth rounded bumps; or change in size, shape, or consistency of the testicle.
  - It is normal for one testicle to be larger or hang lower than the other.
  - Palpation of the epididymis can feel like a lump.
  - Noncancerous conditions (hydrocele, varicocele) cause testicular lumps or swelling.
  - See **FUNDAMENTALS REVIEW MODULE CHAPTER 29: THORAX, HEART, AND ABDOMEN** for instructions on breast examination.
- Watch for the seven warning signs (CAUTION).
  - C: Change in bowel or bladder habits
  - A: A sore that doesn't heal
  - U: Unusual bleeding or discharge
  - T: Thickening or lump in the breast or elsewhere
  - I: Indigestion or difficulty swallowing
  - O: Obvious change in warts or moles
  - N: Nagging cough or hoarseness

BIOPSY

Provides definitive diagnosis indicating the site of origin (specific cell type) and cell characteristics (specific receptors on cell surface) Q**EBP**

Can be obtained during other procedures (endoscopy, laparoscopy, colonoscopy, bronchoscopy, thoracotomy)

Shave biopsy (basal or squamous cell skin cancer): Sampling of outer skin layers (raised lesions) using a scalpel or razor blade

Shedded cells (Pap smear) or secretions (sputum or urine specimens) also can provide tissue samples

Needle biopsy (fine or core): Aspiration of tumor close to the skin surface for fluid and tissue sampling. Bone marrow aspiration is a form of needle biopsy used to diagnose leukemia and lymphoma.

Incisional or excisional (open) biopsy: Cutting through skin to remove part (incisional) or all (excisional) of a tumor. Punch biopsy is a form of excisional biopsy used to diagnose skin cancer. A circular instrument punches a 2 to 6 mm sample of subcutaneous fat.

Sentinel lymph node biopsy: Removal of lymph node in proximity to the cancer. Dye is used to create a map of affected nodes.
- If lymph nodes are negative, the cancer has not likely spread.
- If lymph nodes are positive, surgical excision of remaining lymph nodes in the area is performed (lymph node dissection).

NURSING ACTIONS
- Obtain a signed informed consent form from the client.
- Assemble supplies and facilitate aseptic technique.
- Prevent bleeding. Withhold anticoagulants. Monitor findings of coagulation studies.
- Monitor for postprocedure bleeding (visible staining of dressing, hypotension, tachycardia).
- Provide a safe environment until effects of sedation are minimal. (Maintain bed rest. Withhold oral intake.)
- Ensure adequate oxygenation during the recovery period. Monitor vital signs per postprocedure protocol, or as indicated.
- Position the client in a recovery position appropriate to the procedure (on right side following liver biopsy).

LABORATORY TESTS

Performed to assess for possible cancer or effects on the body (electrolyte imbalance, altered function)

Complete blood count with differential, platelet count

Specific organ function studies: Renal function tests, pancreatic enzyme levels, thyroid hormone levels

Liver function tests: Elevation can indicate primary liver cancer or metastasis of another cancer (colorectal cancer).

Tumor marker assays detect the presence of normal body proteins at higher than expected levels (carcinoembryonic antigen, prostate-specific antigen [PSA], alpha-fetoprotein).
- Samples of urine, stool, tissue, blood, or other body fluids are tested for an excess of specific proteins or DNA patterns.
- Used to detect cancer, measure the severity of cancer, or monitor for a positive response to the cancer treatment regimen (expected finding is a decrease in the tumor marker or return to expected reference range)

Other testing: Additional to biopsy to identify tumor cell type (sputum analysis, cytology of fluid sampling)

NURSING ACTIONS: Explain the purpose of testing.

CLIENT EDUCATION: Laboratory testing can continue throughout treatment (to monitor progress) and following treatment (to screen for return of cancer).

GENETIC TESTS

To identify the presence of certain genes in a sample of blood or saliva
- Genetic overexpression or the existence of extra genes can increase the risk of cancer or cause rapid tumor growth.
- Genetic mutations can be inherited. Positive results indicate the client is at high risk for development of certain types of cancer (presence of BRCA1 and BRCA2 genes associated with breast cancer). Q**EBP**
- In most states, informed consent is required for genetic testing to protect the client from discrimination by providers or insurance company.

NURSING ACTIONS: Consult a genetic counselor to clarify misconceptions regarding positive results and cancer risk.

CLIENT EDUCATION: Genetic information is confidential.

IMAGING STUDIES

Common imaging techniques are used as secondary tools to assist in treatment of cancer. Imaging is completed around the time of diagnosis to measure the severity of cancer.

CT scan, MRI, PET scan, ultrasound, x-ray

- Provide visualization of tumors and their borders.
- Detect metastasis to organs and other body structures.
- Monitor the client during remission.

Digital imaging: Usually more accurate than x-ray. Digital storage of images and results allows for information to be easily shared among members of the interprofessional treatment team. Q**ι**

X-rays: Provide visualization of body structures (chest x-ray, mammogram)

- Clients can be given dye (IV pyelogram) or contrast (barium enema) to enhance visualization.
- With angiography, the client is injected with dye and then x-rays are taken to map vascular structures, such as arterial, venous, or lymphatic mapping.
- NURSING ACTIONS
  - Obtain signed informed consent form for x-rays that require injection of contrast.
  - Monitor for allergic reaction to contrast dye (dyspnea, tachycardia, restlessness).
  - Monitor incision or puncture site for infection or bleeding. Qs
  - Instruct the client about wound care.

Computerized axial tomography (CT) scanning combines x-ray images taken from different angles and uses computer processing to create cross-sectional images. CT scans provide more accurate diagnostic information of tumor presence than x-ray studies. CT scans can be performed with or without contrast. Contrast can be administered orally or intravenously.

MRI uses magnetic field and radio waves rather than radiation to generate pictures of tissue and organs. Contrast can be added to enhance the images. Clients who have any type of metal inside the body (clips, pacemaker, metal implants) should not have an MRI.

Ultrasound: High-energy sound waves bounce off internal tissues and organs to produce an echo pattern that can be seen as an ultrasound image. It is noninvasive and requires no exposure to radiation. Procedure allows for biopsy collection.

Nuclear imaging evaluates the function of organs and structures by detecting the presence of radiation in the body after the client is given a radioactive tracer (IV or oral). The procedure allows for detection and staging of cancer. Cancerous tissues can absorb more or less tracer than expected. These tissues are distinguishable by nuclear imaging.

Positron emission tomography (PET) measures positrons released with tissue uptake of radioactive sugar (more rapid in cancer). Mammography (PEM) can be performed this way. CT can be used with PET scans.

Electrocardiogram, echocardiogram, or multigated acquisition scan are used to evaluate heart function prior to cancer treatment or to identify damage following chemotherapy or radiation to the upper body.

Other types of imaging: Bone scan, gallium scan, thyroid scan

NURSING ACTIONS: Prepare the client as indicated according to the type of procedure.

Endoscopy

Endoscopy procedures permit visualization inside the body using flexible scopes and cameras. Tumors can be visualized in the joints (arthroscopy), respiratory system (laryngoscopy, bronchoscopy), body cavity (mediastinoscopy, thoracoscopy), or gastrointestinal system (enteroscopy, sigmoidoscopy). Organs can be visualized as well (hysteroscopy, cystoscopy). Endoscopy allows for inspection of masses and permits for collection of biopsies.

NURSING ACTIONS
- Obtain signed informed consent form.
- Prepare the client for the type of procedure to be performed.
- Provide a safe environment until effects of sedation are minimal (maintain bed rest, withhold oral intake).
- Ensure adequate oxygenation during the recovery period.

INTERPRETATION OF FINDINGS

- Findings that indicate or increase suspicion of cancer must be further evaluated.
- A variety of imaging and laboratory tests can be used to detect the following.
  - Degree of tumor involvement
  - Type and size of tumor
  - Areas of metastasis
  - Complications of cancer

NURSING ACTIONS
- Maintain knowledge of screening and diagnostic procedures.
- Educate the client about routine cancer screenings as part of health promotion and disease prevention. Qpcc
- Prepare the client for testing.
  - Withhold or restrict food or fluids.
  - Withhold medications that can alter test results or harm the client.
  - Administer preprocedure medication (sedatives, IV or PO fluids, analgesics, barium).
  - Maintain appropriate monitoring (ECG, arterial line).
  - Position the client and promote comfort.
- Provide education to the client regarding the purpose and process of procedures.
- Provide a safe environment pre-, intra-, and postprocedure.
- Reinforce teaching and provide resources for client about self-care in the home environment.

Application Exercises

1. A nurse in a clinic is caring for a client who has suspected uterine cancer. Which of the following assessment techniques should the nurse anticipate the provider performing?

   A. Bimanual pelvic examination

   B. Papanicolaou (Pap) test with cultures

   C. Digital rectal examination

   D. Percussion of upper abdominal quadrants for tympany

2. A nurse is reinforcing teaching with a client who is to have nuclear imaging for suspected cancer. Which of the following statements should the nurse make?

   A. "The test will identify the presence of liver enzymes."

   B. "You will be given an injection of a radioactive substance during the testing."

   C. "Insertion of an endoscope through your mouth will occur during the test."

   D. "Aspiration of the tumor will be part of the imaging test."

3. A nurse is collecting data from a client who has suspected cancer. Which of the following findings should the nurse expect? (Select all that apply.)

   A. Temperature 102° F (38.9° C) for more than 48 hr

   B. Presence of a sore that does not heal

   C. Difficulty swallowing

   D. Unusual discharge

   E. Weight gain of 4 lb (1.8 kg) in 2 weeks

4. A nurse is reinforcing teaching with a client who is to have a shave biopsy for suspected cancer. Which of the following statements by the client indicates understanding?

   A. "This is a test to check my bone marrow."

   B. "This examination will require the removal of a lymph node."

   C. "This procedure will include a needle insertion into the mass."

   D. "This test will involve removing a small skin sample."

5. A nurse is assisting with the plan of care for a client who is to undergo genetic testing for suspected cancer. Which of the following interventions should the nurse include?

   A. Ensure the client signs an informed consent form.

   B. Withhold all medications prior to the procedure.

   C. Verify the prescription for a tumor marker assay.

   D. Place the client in a recovery position after testing.

PRACTICE Active Learning Scenario

A nurse manager is discussing collection of findings as part of screening for cancer with a group of nurses. What information should the nurse manager include in the discussion? Use the ATI Active Learning Template: Diagnostic Procedure to complete this item.

INTERPRETATION OF FINDINGS
- Describe at least three findings indicating the presence of metastasis.
- Describe four assessment techniques and possible findings.

CLIENT EDUCATION: Include two self-assessment techniques that can identify data.

Application Exercises Key

1. A. **CORRECT:** Due to the location of uterine cancer, the provider should perform a bimanual pelvic examination to assess for uterine size, shape, and contour, which can be altered by a mass.

   B. A Pap test with cultures screens for cervical cancer.

   C. A digital rectal examination screens for prostate or rectal cancer.

   D. Percussion of the upper abdominal quadrants for tympany is a screening tool for detecting an abdominal mass.

   Ⓝ *NCLEX® Connection: Physiological Adaptation, Basic Pathophysiology*

2. A. Serum liver function tests involve the identification of altered liver enzymes, which can be present in a client who has cancer. They are not nuclear imaging tests.

   B. **CORRECT:** Nuclear imaging involves the administration of an oral or IV radioactive tracer to identify cancerous tissue.

   C. Endoscopy permits visualization inside the body. It is not a form of nuclear imaging.

   D. A needle biopsy involves aspiration of fluid and tissue samples to test for cancer. It is not a form of nuclear imaging.

   Ⓝ *NCLEX® Connection: Reduction of Risk Potential, Diagnostic Tests*

3. A. Presence of a fever for an extended period is not a warning sign for cancer.

   B. **CORRECT:** A sore that does not heal is a warning sign for cancer.

   C. **CORRECT:** Difficulty swallowing is a warning sign for cancer.

   D. **CORRECT:** The presence of unusual discharge is a warning sign for cancer.

   E. Weight gain is not a warning sign for cancer. Weight loss is more likely to occur with cancer.

   Ⓝ *NCLEX® Connection: Health Promotion and Maintenance, Health Promotion/Disease Prevention*

4. A. Bone marrow aspiration is a type of needle biopsy.

   B. Sentinel node biopsy involves excision of a lymph node.

   C. Needle biopsy involves aspiration of a tumor for fluid and tissue sampling.

   D. **CORRECT:** A shave biopsy is a sampling of the outer skin layer using a scalpel or razor blade.

   Ⓝ *NCLEX® Connection: Reduction of Risk Potential, Diagnostic Tests*

5. A. **CORRECT:** The nurse should ensure the client signs an informed consent form prior to the procedure.

   B. Medication does not affect the results of genetic testing.

   C. A tumor marker assay is a laboratory test to identify the presence of specific body proteins in blood, body secretions, and tissue. It is not a component of genetic testing.

   D. Genetic testing involves collection of blood or saliva. Recovery positioning is not required following testing.

   Ⓝ *NCLEX® Connection: Coordinated Care, Information Technology*

PRACTICE Answer

Using the ATI Active Learning Template: Diagnostic Procedure

INTERPRETATION OF FINDINGS

Metastasis
- Discomfort at secondary sites
- Swelling and/or tenderness of lymph nodes or other areas of the body
- Presence of masses
- Altered function of another body system
- Bone pain

Assessment techniques
- Inspection for changes in color, symmetry, movement, or body function
- Auscultation for adventitious sounds, which can indicate altered body system function
- Palpation to detect masses or tissue abnormalities
- Percussion to detect changes in expected sound over organs, which can indicate inflammation or tumor

CLIENT EDUCATION: Testicular and breast self-examinations

Ⓝ *NCLEX® Connection: Health Promotion and Maintenance, Health Promotion/Disease Prevention*

CHAPTER 81

UNIT 13   NURSING CARE OF CLIENTS WHO HAVE IMMUNE
            SYSTEM AND CONNECTIVE TISSUE DISORDERS
            SECTION: CANCER-RELATED DISORDERS

CHAPTER 81 *Cancer Treatment Options*

Cancer treatment is based on the cell of origin of the cancer. When metastasis occurs, treatment is still based on the primary tumor origin even though the malignancy is located elsewhere in the body. Many cancers are curable when diagnosed early.

Cancer treatment options focus on removing or destroying cancer cells and preventing the continued abnormal cell growth and differentiation. Treatment can be curative or palliative. Client-specific factors guide the treatment plan (age, childbearing desire, pregnancy, current state of health, expected lifespan) and can involve several treatment methods.

Adjuvant treatment is what is given in addition to the primary treatment standard. This can include hormone, radiation, and targeted therapies; immunotherapy; and chemotherapy.

Nursing care for clients who have cancer should include collaboration with supportive therapies and services, counseling, and transfer of care to another provider at discharge. Q_{TC}

PROCEDURES

Cancer treatment includes manipulation or removal of the tumor.

Topical procedures (cryosurgery, laser therapy, ablation) and procedures that destroy the main arteries that provide blood flow to the tumor can help reduce tumor size.

Tumor excision can be open or endoscopic (curettage and electrodissection for skin cancer).
- The surgeon removes the tumor and tissue immediately surrounding it. The anticipated outcome is for the outermost tissue from the excision is free of cancer cells.
- The purpose of surgery can include excision, biopsy (diagnosis and staging), or relief (palliation) based on findings.
- Lymph node dissection or sentinel lymph node biopsy is done to determine if the cancer has spread or there is added risk of spread.
- The surgeon sometimes forms new structures, such as a urinary or bowel stoma, to maintain body function.
- More extensive surgeries (tumors involving multiple organs or structures, lymph node involvement, deep lesions) increase the risk of complications and typically require longer recovery periods. The client can require intensive care.

NURSING ACTIONS
- Obtain a signed informed consent form.
- Prepare the client for procedures (NPO status, withholding or administering medications, monitoring laboratory findings).
- Provide postoperative care as indicated by tumor location and procedure type.
- Prevent general postoperative complications (infection, fluid or electrolyte imbalance, hemorrhage, thromboembolism, inadequate oxygenation, shock).
- Prevent and treat pain using pharmacological and nonpharmacological measures.
- Reinforce care instructions for drains, wounds, and implanted devices with the client.

CLIENT EDUCATION: Monitor for complications after discharge.

Chemotherapy

Chemotherapy involves administration of systemic or local cytotoxic medications that damage cell DNA or destroy rapidly dividing cells.

- The provider selects a chemotherapeutic agent based on the medication's effect on various stages of cell division. A combination of anticancer medications promotes more thorough destruction of cancer cells.
- Most chemotherapy agents are cytotoxic. The adverse effects of these agents are related to unintentional harm to normal cells, particularly those that reproduce rapidly, such as in the mucous membranes of the gastrointestinal (GI) tract, hair follicles, and bone marrow. The medication and dosage used influences the type of adverse effect and the severity.
- Administering agents that protect healthy cells prior to or along with chemotherapy can decrease the adverse effects on normal tissues. Examples include amifostine and mesna.
- The client can receive chemotherapy in an acute health care setting, provider's office, clinic, or the home.
- Most chemotherapy medications, including oral, are absorbed through the skin and mucous membranes. Anyone preparing, giving, or disposing of these medications must wear proper personal protective equipment.

ROUTE

- Administration routes for chemotherapy include topical (for skin lesions); oral; parenteral; IV; intra-arterial; into the ventricles of the brain; and into body cavities (abdomen, bladder, pleura, spinal cavity). Direct injection into the tumor is possible in some cases. Some agents require specialized training/certification for administration.
- Oral anticancer medications are just as toxic to the client and nurse handling the medication as standard chemotherapy medications.
- Do not crush, split, break, or allow the client to chew oral medications.
- Delivering chemotherapy through the intracavitary route reduces the risk of systemic adverse effects.

CATHETERS

- Some medications can cause serious damage to the skin and muscle tissue if they leak outside a vein (vesicants). Using a central venous catheter in a large central vein rather than a short-term peripheral IV reduces the risk that the medication will irritate the vein or leak and damage tissues. Two of the most commonly used types of central venous catheters include the peripherally inserted central catheter (PICC line) and implanted port.
- Long-term therapy often requires an implanted port. The port is comprised of a small reservoir that is covered by a thick septum.

CATEGORIES OF MEDICATIONS

- The structure and function of chemotherapy medications determines their classification. The provider selects medications based on the sensitivity of cancer cells to the medications and the stage of the cancer. Understanding the function of the medication can help predict potential adverse effects.
- Categories include alkylating agents, antimetabolites, antimitotic agents, antitumor antibiotics, topoisomerase inhibitors, hormone-related medications, and other miscellaneous medications.

INDICATIONS

- Chemotherapy can be used to cure a disease, help control its progression, or as palliative treatment for individuals who have a terminal disease.
- Chemotherapy interrupts cell division to prevent further cell reproduction.
- Cancer is the most common condition that involves chemotherapy treatment. Clients who have disorders such as autoimmune diseases can benefit from chemotherapy.

CONSIDERATIONS

- Instruct the client and family on care and use of vascular access devices.
- Extravasation of agents that are vesicants requires specific, immediate attention to minimize tissue damage. Selection of a neutralizing solution is dependent on vesicant. Closely monitor the infusion site for evidence of infiltration. Qs

PREPROCEDURE

- Because administration of chemotherapeutic medications is limited to certified individuals, monitoring and management of adverse effects during and after chemotherapy administration is the primary focus of health care personnel.
- Instruct the client on findings that indicate potential complications. The client should report findings immediately.

COMPLICATIONS

Immunosuppression/neutropenia

- Due to bone marrow suppression by cytotoxic medications
- The most significant adverse effect of chemotherapy
- Clients who have neutropenia might not develop a high fever or have purulent drainage even when an infection is present.

NURSING ACTIONS
- Monitor temperature, white blood cell (WBC) count, and absolute neutrophil count (ANC).
- Report a fever greater than 37.8° C (100° F) to the provider immediately.
- Monitor skin and mucous membranes for infection (breakdown, fissures, and abscess).

- Obtain prescribed culture specimens prior to initiating antimicrobial therapy.
- Protect skin and mucous membranes from injury (use moisturizing lotion, practice frequent position changes, provide immediate attention to skin breaks).
- Implement neutropenic precautions, including placing the client in a private room. The risk of serious infection increases as the ANC falls. An ANC less than 1,000/mm³ indicates a weakened immune system.
- **Neutropenic precautions**
  - Have the client remain in the room except to leave for a diagnostic procedure or therapy. In this case, place a mask on the client during transport.
  - Protect the client from possible sources of infection (such as plants) and change water in equipment daily.
  - Have client, staff, and visitors perform frequent hand hygiene. Restrict visitors who are ill.
  - Avoid invasive procedures that could cause a break in tissue (rectal temperatures, injections, indwelling urinary catheters) unless necessary.
  - Keep dedicated equipment (blood pressure machine, thermometer, stethoscope) in the client's room.
  - Administer colony-stimulating factors (filgrastim) to stimulate WBC production.

CLIENT EDUCATION
- Avoid crowds while undergoing chemotherapy.
- Take the client's temperature daily. Report elevated temperature to the provider.
- Avoid food sources that could contain bacteria (fresh fruits and vegetables; undercooked meat, fish, and eggs; pepper; paprika).
- Avoid yard work, gardening, or changing a pet's litter box.
- Discard beverages that have been sitting at room temperature for longer than 1 hr.
- Wash all dishes in hot, soapy water or a dishwasher. Wash glasses and cups after each use.
- Wash toothbrush daily in the dishwasher or rinse in a bleach solution.
- Do not share toiletry or personal hygiene items.
- Report fever greater than 37.8° C (100° F) or other manifestations of bacterial or viral infections to the provider immediately.

Nausea, vomiting, anorexia

- Many medications used for chemotherapy are emetogenic (induce vomiting) or cause anorexia and an altered taste in the mouth.
- Serotonin blockers, such as ondansetron, are effective at treating and preventing nausea. The client might take these along with corticosteroids, phenothiazines, and antihistamines. Q EBP
- Neurokinin receptor antagonists (aprepitant); corticosteroids (dexamethasone, methylprednisolone); dopamine antagonists (promethazine, prochlorperazine); histamine blockers (ranitidine); proton pump inhibitors (omeprazole); prokinetic agents (metoclopramide), benzodiazepines (lorazepam); and cannabinoids (dronabinol) are other examples of medications used for chemotherapy-induced nausea and vomiting (CINV).

NURSING ACTIONS
- Administer antiemetics before chemotherapy and repeat based on the response and duration of CINV.
- Administer antiemetic medications for several days after each treatment, even when CINV appears to be controlled.
- Remove vomiting cues, such as odor and supplies associated with nausea.
- Implement nonpharmacological methods to reduce nausea (visual imagery, relaxation, acupuncture, distraction).
- Perform calorie counts to determine intake, and determine client food preferences.
- Provide liquid nutritional supplements as needed. Add protein powders to food or tube feedings.
- Administer megestrol to increase appetite.
- Monitor for findings of dehydration or fluid and electrolyte imbalance.
- Perform mouth care prior to serving meals to enhance appetite.
- Instruct the client about administration of antiemetics and schedule them prior to meals.

CLIENT EDUCATION
- Eat several small meals a day if better tolerated. Low-fat dry foods (crackers, toast) and avoiding drinking liquids during meals can prevent nausea.
- Select foods that are served cold and do not require cooking. Cooking food can emit odors that stimulate nausea.
- Consume high-protein, high-calorie, nutrient-dense foods. Avoid low- or empty-calorie foods. Use meal supplements as needed.
- Use plastic eating utensils, suck on hard candy, and avoid red meats to prevent or reduce the sensation of metallic taste.
- Create a food diary to identify items that can trigger nausea, and document daily intake.

Alopecia

An adverse effect of certain chemotherapeutic medications related to their interference with the life cycle of rapidly proliferating cells

NURSING ACTIONS
- Discuss the effect of alopecia on self-image.
- Discuss options (hats, turbans, wigs) to deal with hair loss. Q PCC
- Hair loss can occur throughout the body or as mild as thinning hair of the scalp.
- Recommend soliciting information from the American Cancer Society regarding products for clients experiencing alopecia.

CLIENT EDUCATION

- Hair loss occurs 7 to 10 days after treatment begins (for some agents). Select hairpiece before treatment starts.
- Alopecia is temporary, and hair should return about 1 month after chemotherapy is discontinued. The new hair can differ from the original hair in color, texture, and thickness.
- Avoid the use of damaging hair care measures (electric rollers, curling irons, hair dye, permanent waves). A soft hair brush or wide-tooth comb for grooming is preferred.
- Cut hair short before treatment to decrease weight on the hair follicle.
- If wearing a wig, collaborate with a hairdresser to assist with selection. Wear the wig before therapy begins to reduce appearance changes.
- After hair loss, protect the scalp from sun exposure and use a diaper rash ointment/cream for itching. Qs
- Head coverings can be used to reduce body heat loss and protect skin while wearing helmets, headphones, headsets, or wigs. Choose coverings that mirror personal style preferences.

Oral effects

Mucositis refers to inflammation in the mucous lining of the upper GI tract from the mouth to the stomach.

Stomatitis refers to inflammation of tissues in the oral cavity (gums, tongue, roof and floor of the mouth, inside lips and cheeks). This common adverse effect can cause malnutrition from decreased oral intake of food and fluids.

NURSING ACTIONS

- Examine the client's mouth several times a day, and inquire about the presence of oral lesions.
- Document the location and size of lesions. Obtain cultures of new lesions and report them to the provider.
- Administer a topical anesthetic or anesthetic mouthwash prior to meals.
- Offer oral hygiene before and after each meal. Use lubricating or moisturizing agents to counteract dry mouth.

CLIENT EDUCATION

- Avoid glycerin-based mouthwashes or mouth swabs. Use nonalcoholic anesthetic mouthwashes. QEBP
- Rinse the mouth with a solution of 0.9% sodium chloride, room-temperature tap water, or salt and soda water. Frequency is guided by the intensity of the mucositis.
- Floss gently and brush using a soft-bristled toothbrush or foam swabs to avoid traumatizing the oral mucosa.
- Rinse the mouth before and after meals. Avoid mouthwash that contains alcohol or other irritants
- Take medications to control infection as prescribed (nystatin suspension, acyclovir).
- Use of coating agents, topical analgesics, topical anesthetics, or oral or parenteral analgesics can be prescribed.
- Eat cold, soft, bland foods and supplements that are high in calories (mashed potatoes, scrambled eggs, cooked cereal, milkshakes, ice cream, frozen yogurt, bananas, breakfast mixes). Avoid spicy, salty, acidic food.
- Avoid drinking alcohol and the use of tobacco.

Anemia and thrombocytopenia

Secondary to bone marrow suppression (myelosuppression)

NURSING ACTIONS

- **Anemia**
  - Monitor for fatigue, pallor, dizziness, and shortness of breath.
  - Help the client manage anemia-related fatigue by scheduling activities with rest periods between and using energy-saving measures (sitting during showers and ADLs).
  - Administer erythropoietic medications (epoetin alfa) and antianemic medications (ferrous sulfate).
  - Monitor Hgb values to determine response to medications. The client can require blood product replacement therapy.
- **Thrombocytopenia**
  - Monitor for petechiae; ecchymosis; bleeding of the gums; nosebleeds; and occult or frank blood in stools, urine, or vomitus.
  - Institute bleeding precautions.
    - Avoid IVs and injections.
    - Apply pressure for approximately 10 min after blood is obtained.
    - Handle client gently and avoid trauma.
  - Administer thrombopoietic medications such as oprelvekin to stimulate platelet production. Monitor platelet count, and be prepared to administer platelets if the count falls below 10,000/mm³.

CLIENT EDUCATION

- Manage active bleeding.
- Use measures to prevent bleeding (use electric razor and soft-bristled toothbrush, avoid blowing nose vigorously, ensure that dentures fit appropriately).
- Avoid the use of NSAIDs.
- Prevent injury when ambulating (wear closed-toes shoes, remove tripping hazards in the home) and apply cold if injury occurs. Qs

Chemotherapy-induced peripheral neuropathy

Loss of sensory or motor function of peripheral nerves is caused by exposure to certain anticancer medications. Higher doses of medication lead to greater neuropathy.

NURSING ACTIONS

- Monitor for loss of sensation in hands and feet, orthostatic hypotension, loss of taste, and constipation.
- Monitor for skin breakdown or infections in extremities.
- Monitor for orthostatic hypotension.
- Monitor for early manifestations (numbness, tingling, redness).
- Inform the client regarding the risk of erectile dysfunction and treatment options.

CLIENT EDUCATION

- Use measures to prevent injury, including falls.
- Practice good foot care.
- Protect skin because loss of sensation makes the client unaware of heat, cold, or pressure.

Radiation therapy

Radiation therapy involves ionizing radiation to target tissues and destroy cells.

- Adverse effects on tissues within the radiation path include skin changes, tissue necrosis, fistulas, hair loss, ulceration of mucous membranes, and debilitating fatigue.
- Radiation therapy typically involves a series of divided small doses on a daily basis for a set period of time.
- Cytoprotectants can protect against harmful effects of radiation therapy, such as dryness of the mouth caused by radiation treatment for head and neck cancer.
- Routes for radiation therapy include internal (brachytherapy) with an implant or external (teletherapy) with a radiation beam. The type used depends on the health of the client and shape, size, and location of the tumor.
- External beam radiation therapy does not cause the client to become radioactive.
- Internal radiation contaminates body fluids with radiation, which then require specific disposal methods to prevent exposure to others.
- The provider can prescribe radiation therapy prior to surgery to decrease the size of a tumor before excision.
- Implement measures to reduce radiation exposure to staff and visitors by limiting indirect contact time, maintaining indicated distances from sources of radiation, and preventing direct contact with the source.

Internal radiation therapy

Brachytherapy describes internal radiation that is placed close to the target tissue. This can include placing radiation in a body orifice (vagina) or body cavity (abdomen), into the tumor, or delivering it IV (such as with radionuclide iodine, which the thyroid absorbs).

- Brachytherapy provides radiation to the tumor and a limited amount to surrounding normal tissues.
- Waste products are radioactive until the isotope has been completely eliminated from the body. Dispose of waste products according to agency protocol to prevent harm to others.

NURSING ACTIONS

- Place the client in a private room away from other clients when possible. Keep the door closed as much as possible.
- Place a sign on the door warning of the radiation source. Qs
- Wear a dosimeter film badge that records personal amount of radiation exposure.
- Limit visitors to 30-min visits, and have visitors maintain a distance of 6 feet from the source.
- Restrict visitors and health care personnel who are pregnant or under the age of 18 from coming into contact with the client or radiation source.

- Wear a lead apron and lead gloves while providing care, keeping the front of the apron facing the source of radiation.
- Keep a lead container in the client's room if the delivery method could allow spontaneous loss of radioactive material. Tongs are available for placing radioactive material into this container.
- Follow protocol for proper removal of dressings and bed linens from the room.

CLIENT EDUCATION

- Remain in an indicated position to prevent dislodgement of the radiation implant.
- Call the nurse for assistance with elimination.
- Practice radiation precautions in health care and home environments.

External radiation therapy

External radiation or teletherapy involves delivery of radiation in relatively small, uniform doses over the course of several weeks from an external source. Unlike internal radiation, the client is not radioactive and is not hazardous to others.

NURSING ACTIONS

- The skin over the targeted area is marked with tattoos (markings) that guide the positioning of the external radiation source.
- Provide a well-balanced diet that does not contain red meat. Radiation can cause dysgeusia (altered taste), making foods such as red meat unpalatable.
- Help the client manage fatigue by scheduling activities with rest periods in between and using energy-saving measures (sitting during showers and ADLs).
- Monitor for radiation injury to skin and mucous membranes, and implement a skin care regimen.
  - Skin: blanching, erythema, desquamation, sloughing, hemorrhage
  - Mouth: mucositis, xerostomia (dry mouth), ulcerations
  - Neck: difficulty swallowing
  - Abdomen: gastroenteritis
- Monitor CBC (possible decreased platelets and WBCs).

CLIENT EDUCATION

- Adverse effects depend on which part of the body is exposed to radiation and how much radiation is administered.
- Nutrition considerations related to mucositis
  - Avoid spicy, salty, and acidic foods.
  - Hot foods might not be tolerated.
- Gently wash the skin over the irradiated area with mild soap and water. Dry the area thoroughly using patting motions. QEBP
- Do not remove or wash off radiation tattoos used to guide therapy. Do not apply powders, ointments, lotions, deodorants, or perfumes to the irradiated skin.
- Wear soft clothing. Avoid tight or constricting clothes.
- Do not expose the irradiated skin to sun or a heat source.
- Inspect skin for evidence of damage, and report to the provider.

Hormone therapy

Hormone therapy is effective against tumors that are supported or suppressed by hormones, such as in breast or prostate cancer.

- By giving a similar hormone, uptake of the support hormone is blocked, or production reduced. Hormone antagonists compete with the support hormone for binding sites on or in the tumor cell and are effective against tumors that require a particular hormone for support.
- Types of therapy include LH-RH agonists, androgen antagonists, estrogen receptor down-regulators, and estrogen antagonists (tamoxifen).

CLIENT EDUCATION: The type of hormone administered determines the type of adverse effect the client experiences.

- Male clients can experience impaired sexual functions (decreased libido, erectile dysfunction) and feminizing effects of hormone therapy (gynecomastia, hot flashes, bone loss). Qpcc
- Female clients can experience masculinizing effects (chest and facial hair growth, amenorrhea, decreased breast tissue) or irregular uterine bleeding.
- Other adverse effects include impaired blood cell production (anemia, leukopenia, thrombocytopenia), electrolyte imbalance, and impaired liver, cardiac, and neurologic function.

Immunotherapy

Immunotherapy (biotherapy) uses biologic response modifiers, which alter a client's biological response to cancerous tumor cells. Antibodies, cytokines, and other immune substances normally produced by the immune system can increase the body's defense against cancer by targeting and destroying cancer cells.

- Interleukins and interferons are the primary cytokines (immune response modulators) used in immunotherapy.
- **Interleukins** help coordinate the inflammatory and immune responses of the body, particularly the lymphocytes.
- **Interferons** can exert an antitumor effect by activating a variety of responses.

NURSING ACTIONS

- **Interleukins:** Monitor for influenza-like manifestations and edema.
- **Interferons:** Monitor for altered mental status and lethargy.
- Monitor for peripheral neuropathy that can affect vision, hearing, balance, and gait.
- Take precautions for orthostatic hypotension.

CLIENT EDUCATION

- Immediately report influenza-like manifestations or changes consistent with peripheral neuropathy.
- Skin rashes are common. Use of a perfume-free moisturizer can be helpful.
- Avoid sun exposure and swimming if skin manifestations develop.

Photodynamic therapy

Photodynamic therapy involves injection of a photosensitizing agent that is absorbed by all cells in the body. The agent remains in only the cancer cells 1 to 3 days later, and the tumor is then exposed to a specific wavelength of light via an endoscope. Cells are subsequently destroyed, and tumors are eliminated or reduced in size.

- Used to treat non-small cell lung cancer and esophageal cancer.
- Effective with small tumors close to body surface (within 1 cm).
- Adverse effects are related to the area of the body being treated.

CLIENT EDUCATION: Avoid sun exposure for 4 to 6 weeks until the photosensitizing agent is no longer in the body.

- Limit time outdoors.
- When outdoors, wear sunglasses, gloves, hats, and shoes.

Supportive treatment

In addition to cancer treatment, the client can require assistance for altered body function or to meet emotional and spiritual needs.

- Facilitate safe activity, providing assistive devices when necessary for clients who have altered mobility or require assistance with self-care activities. Qs
- Coordinate transfer of client care to home health, hospice, or a tertiary care setting (rehabilitation center) as appropriate.
- Provide alternate means of communication for clients who have cancer affecting the mouth, throat, larynx, or vocal cords.
- Use assistive aids and devices for clients who have visual or hearing impairments.
- Consult physical therapy, and genetic or other counseling services as indicated.
- Consult pain management for persistent or uncontrolled pain. (See **CHAPTER 83: PAIN MANAGEMENT FOR CLIENTS WHO HAVE CANCER**.)

Inadequate nutrition

Clients who have cancer are at risk for inadequate nutrition related to diagnosis or treatment. (Refer to **NUTRITION FOR NURSING REVIEW MODULE: CHAPTER 16: CANCER AND IMMUNOSUPPRESSION DISORDERS**.)

NURSING ACTIONS

- Administer nutritional supplements or substitutes.
- Encourage small, frequent meals. Incorporate client preferences.
- Provide antiemetic medications.
- Monitor feeding tube or central line.
- Encourage protein- and calorie-dense foods.
- Monitor for effectiveness of nutrition modifications (laboratory values, urine and bowel elimination, absence of GI upset).
- Monitor weight.
- Consult nutrition services.

Altered elimination

NURSING ACTIONS
- Assist with alternate means of elimination.
  - Insert indwelling or intermittent urinary catheter.
  - Apply drainage devices.
- Monitor urine and bowel output.
- Instruct the client on self-management of elimination.

Body image changes

Body image changes are a factor in clients for whom surgery is disfiguring, especially cancers of the face or sexual organs (breasts, genitalia).

NURSING ACTIONS: Assist the client with prosthetic devices.

CLIENT EDUCATION
- Express feelings about body loss or changes.
- Look at or touch affected body areas during care.
- Use positive measures to promote positive body image (makeup, clothing).

Altered sexuality

Functional impairment or body image changes following cancer treatments can cause altered sexuality patterns. Pain with sexual intercourse can also be a factor.

NURSING ACTIONS
- Encourage the client and partner to communicate feelings to each other.
- Administer hormone therapy.
- Instruct the client about medications to promote erection or manage pain sensation.

Ineffective coping

The client's ability to cope with the diagnosis and prognosis can be ineffective.

NURSING ACTIONS Qpcc
- Administer medications for anxiety or depression.
- Encourage the client to participate in a support group for clients who have similar cancers (physical or online). Recommend referral to a community resource.
- Recommend referral to counseling services for the client and family as needed.
- Instruct the client on anticipatory grief and the stages of grief.
- Recommend palliative services as indicated.
- Support the client's continued involvement in personal interests, hobbies, and employment.
- Incorporate the client's beliefs and preferences regarding spirituality and illness/death.

CLIENT EDUCATION: Express feelings verbally or through journaling and blogging.

Immunocompromise

Cancer or cancer treatment can place the client in an immunocompromised state.

CLIENT EDUCATION: Avoid individuals who have colds, infections, or viruses.

Application Exercises

1. A nurse is reviewing the plan of care for a client who has a platelet count of 10,000/mm³. Which of the following interventions should the nurse expect to implement?

   A. Apply prolonged pressure to puncture site after blood sampling.

   B. Administer epoetin alfa.

   C. Place the client in a private room.

   D. Have the client use an oral topical anesthetic before meals.

2. A nurse is caring for a client who is receiving chemotherapy and has mucositis. Which of the following actions should the nurse take?

   A. Use a glycerin-soaked swab to clean the client's teeth.

   B. Encourage increased intake of citrus fruit juices.

   C. Obtain a culture of the lesions.

   D. Provide an alcohol-based mouthwash for oral hygiene.

3. A nurse is contributing to the plan of care for a client who is undergoing chemotherapy and is on neutropenic precautions. Which of the following interventions should the nurse recommend? (Select all that apply.)

   A. Encourage a high-fiber diet.

   B. Remove plants from the room.

   C. Have the client wear a mask when leaving the room.

   D. Have client-specific equipment remain in the room.

   E. Eliminate raw foods from the client's diet.

4. A nurse is caring for a client who is undergoing chemotherapy and reports severe nausea. Which of the following statements should the nurse make?

   A. "Your nausea will lessen with each course of chemotherapy."

   B. "Hot food is better tolerated due to the aroma."

   C. "Try eating several small meals throughout the day."

   D. "Increase your intake of red meat."

5. A nurse is caring for a client who is receiving brachytherapy to treat cervical cancer. Which of the following actions should the nurse take? (Select all that apply.)

   A. Permit visitors to stay with the client 30 min at a time.

   B. Place the client on bed rest.

   C. Wear a dosimeter badge when in the client's room.

   D. Don a paper gown when providing care for the client.

   E. Inform pregnant visitors to stay 4 feet away from the client.

PRACTICE Active Learning Scenario

A nurse is communicating with a client who is receiving chemotherapy and has alopecia. What should the nurse include? Use the Active Learning Template: System Disorder to complete this item.

PATHOPHYSIOLOGY RELATED TO CLIENT PROBLEM

CLIENT EDUCATION: Describe at least four teaching points.

NURSING CARE: Describe at least two nursing actions.

Application Exercises Key

1. A. **CORRECT:** The nurse should implement bleeding precautions for the client who has thrombocytopenia.

   B. The nurse should expect to administer epoetin alfa to a client who has anemia.

   C. The nurse should place a client who has neutropenia in a private room.

   D. The nurse should recommend use of a topical oral anesthetic for a client who has mucositis.

   Ⓝ *NCLEX® Connection: Reduction of Risk Potential, Potential for Complications of Diagnostic Tests/Treatments/Procedures*

2. A. The nurse should avoid glycerin-based swabs when providing oral hygiene to a client who has mucositis.

   B. The nurse should instruct the client who has mucositis to avoid acidic foods.

   C. **CORRECT:** The nurse should obtain a culture of the oral lesions to identify pathogens and determine appropriate treatment.

   D. The nurse should recommend nonalcoholic mouthwashes for a client who has mucositis.

   Ⓝ *NCLEX® Connection: Reduction of Risk Potential, Potential for Complications of Diagnostic Tests/Treatments/Procedures*

3. A. There is no benefit to a high-fiber diet for a client who has neutropenia.

   B. **CORRECT:** Neutropenic precautions include the client avoiding contact with flowers and plants due to the presence of surface infectious agents in the water and soil.

   C. **CORRECT:** Neutropenic precautions include having the client wear a mask when leaving the room to reduce the incidence of infection.

   D. **CORRECT:** Neutropenic precautions include having equipment available that is only for use in caring for the client to reduce the incidence of infection.

   E. **CORRECT:** A client who has neutropenia should avoid consuming raw foods due to the presence of surface infectious agents on peeling and rind.

   Ⓝ *NCLEX® Connection: Reduction of Risk Potential, Potential for Complications of Diagnostic Tests/Treatments/Procedures*

4. A. Nausea usually occurs to the same extent with each session of chemotherapy.

   B. Clients usually tolerate cold foods better than warm or hot foods because odors from heated foods can induce nausea.

   C. **CORRECT:** A client who has nausea should consume several small meals a day to promote nutritional intake.

   D. A client who is undergoing chemotherapy should avoid red meat because the taste of meat is frequently altered and unpalatable.

   Ⓝ *NCLEX® Connection: Basic Care and Comfort, Nutrition and Oral Hydration*

5. A. **CORRECT:** The client who has cervical cancer will have a vaginal radiation implant. Visitors should remain for no more than 30 min at a time.

   B. **CORRECT:** The client who has cervical cancer will have a vaginal radiation implant. The client should maintain bed rest to prevent displacement of the implant.

   C. **CORRECT:** Health care personnel should wear a dosimeter badge when in the client's room to measure radiation exposure.

   D. The nurse should wear a lead apron and lead gloves while providing care for a client who has a vaginal radiation implant.

   E. The nurse should restrict pregnant visitors from entering the client's room. Adults entering the client's room should remain 6 feet away from the client to minimize radiation exposure.

   Ⓝ *NCLEX® Connection: Reduction of Risk Potential, Potential for Complications of Diagnostic Tests/Treatments/Procedures*

PRACTICE Answer

Using the Active Learning Template: System Disorder

PATHOPHYSIOLOGY RELATED TO CLIENT PROBLEM: Alopecia occurs as an adverse effect of chemotherapy medications. The medications interfere with the life cycle of rapidly proliferating cells (such as those found in hair follicles), resulting in hair loss.

CLIENT EDUCATION
- Wear hats, turbans, and wigs.
- Avoid the use of damaging hair-care measures, such as electric rollers and curling irons, hair dye, and permanent waves.
- Use a soft hairbrush or wide-tooth comb for grooming.
- Avoid sun exposure. Use a diaper rash ointment or cream for itching.
- Alopecia is temporary, and hair will return following the conclusion of the chemotherapy regimen.

NURSING CARE
- Discuss the effect of alopecia on self-image. Encourage the client to express feelings.
- Recommend use of information from the American Cancer Society on managing alopecia.
- Recommend referral to a cancer support group.

Ⓝ *NCLEX® Connection: Reduction of Risk Potential, Potential for Complications from Surgical Procedures and Health Alterations*

UNIT 13 NURSING CARE OF CLIENTS WHO HAVE IMMUNE
SYSTEM AND CONNECTIVE TISSUE DISORDERS
SECTION: CANCER-RELATED DISORDERS

CHAPTER 82 *Cancer Disorders*

The various types of cancer share general cancer principles: abnormal cell growth, tumor formation, and potential for invasion to other locations. Each type of cancer has distinguishing characteristics related to risk, manifestations, screening, and diagnosis. The prognosis and treatment varies by type.

Skin cancer

- Sunlight exposure is the leading cause of skin cancer. The most effective strategy for prevention of skin cancer is avoidance or reduction of skin exposure to sunlight.
- Precancerous skin lesions, called actinic keratoses, are common in people who have chronically sun-damaged skin or fair complexion, and older adult clients. Ⓖ

TYPES OF SKIN CANCER

Squamous cell (epidermis)

CHARACTERISTICS
- Rough, scaly lesion with central ulceration and crusting
- Occurs most often on areas of skin that are continuously exposed to ultraviolet (UV) rays and weather
- Bleeding (possible)

COURSE
- Localized most often on the head, neck, and hands; can metastasize rapidly.
- Squamous cell metastasizes and has a more rapid growth rate than basal cell cancer.

Basal cell (basal epidermis or nearby dermal cells)

CHARACTERISTICS
- Small, waxy nodule with superficial blood vessels, well-defined borders
- Erythema and ulcerations

COURSE: Invades local structures (nerves, bone, cartilage, lymphatic and vascular tissue); rarely metastatic but high rate of recurrence

Malignant melanoma (cancer of melanocytes) (82.1)

CHARACTERISTICS
- Irregular shape and borders with multiple colors; can have elevated nodules and ulcerations
- New moles or change in an existing mole (can occur in intestines or any other body structure that contains pigment cells)
- Possible itching, cracks, ulcerations, or bleeding

COURSE: Rapid invasion and metastasis with high morbidity and mortality

HEALTH PROMOTION AND DISEASE PREVENTION

- Limit exposure to sunlight, especially between 1000 and 1600.
- Apply sunscreen when near reflective surfaces (sand, snow, water, concrete).
- Use sunblock that has a sun protective factor (SPF) of at least 15, with UVA and UVB protection. Apply 30 min before exposure to sun and reapply at least every 2 hr.
- Wear protective clothing, hats, sunglasses, and lip balm that has an SPF of at least 15.
- Avoid indoor tanning (tanning beds, booths, sunlamps).
- Reinforce teaching with clients about the ABCDE system to evaluate moles.
  - **A: Asymmetry:** One side of the nevus does not match the other
  - **B: Borders**: Ragged, notched, irregular, or blurred edges
  - **C: Color:** Lack of uniformity in pigmentation (shades of tan, brown, or black)
  - **D: Diameter:** Width greater than 5 mm (about the size of a pencil eraser or a pea)
  - **E: Evolving:** Change in the lesion's appearance (shape, size, color, height, texture) or condition (bleeding, itching)
- Because of the cumulative effects of sun damage over the lifespan, screening for suspicious lesions is an essential part of the routine physical data collection of older adult clients. Ⓖ

82.1 Melanomas

normal mole

melanoma (asymmetry)

melanoma (color)

melanoma (border)

melanoma (large diameter)

5 mm

DATA COLLECTION

RISK FACTORS

- Exposure to coal tar, pitch, or creosote
- Occupational history of chemical carcinogens
- History of severe skin injury
- Immunosuppression therapy
- Exposure to UV light (natural light, indoor tanning) over long periods of time
- Chronic skin inflammation, burns, or scars
- Fair complexion (blonde or red hair, fair skin, freckles, blue eyes) with a tendency to burn easily
- Presence of several large or many small moles
- Family or personal history of melanoma
- Residing in higher elevations or in close proximity to equator (thinner layer of ozone)
- Age older than 50 years. The majority of nonmelanoma skin lesions occur on clients age 30 to 60 years.

EXPECTED FINDINGS

Report of change in appearance of mole or lesion

DIAGNOSTIC PROCEDURES

Data collection (self or clinician)

EXPECTED FINDINGS
- New or suspicious lesions
- Recent changes in size, color, or sensation of any mole, birthmark, wart, or scar

CLIENT EDUCATION
- Develop a body map (diagram of scars or lesions) and monitor monthly for changes.
- Inspect skin between fingers and toes and on scalp.

Biopsy (punch, shave, or excisional)

EXPECTED FINDINGS: Cancerous cells

CLIENT EDUCATION
- Monitor for infection.
- Perform wound care, including care of sutures (punch, excisional biopsy).

Lymph node biopsy/dissection

- If melanoma is diagnosed, blood tests are prescribed (CBC, CMP, liver function, alkaline phosphatase, aspartate aminotransferase) to check for organ involvement.
- Chest x-rays determine pulmonary involvement if the client reports difficulty breathing or hemoptysis.

EXPECTED FINDINGS: Tissue examined microscopically for the spread of cancer

NURSING ACTIONS: Monitor site of lymph node biopsy or removal for bleeding or infection.

PATIENT-CENTERED CARE

THERAPEUTIC PROCEDURES

Chemotherapy

Topical chemotherapy with 5-fluorouracil cream for treatment of actinic keratoses or for widespread superficial basal cell carcinoma.
CLIENT EDUCATION
- Extended treatment will cause the lesion to weep, crust, and erode.
- The appearance of the lesion will improve after treatment.

Interferon therapy for postoperative treatment of stage III or greater melanomas.
NURSING ACTIONS
- Report and provide relief for adverse or toxic effects of chemotherapy.
- Encourage adequate nutrition and fluid intake.
- Reinforce teaching with the client on self-injection procedure.

Targeted therapy (82.2)

Tumor-specific antigen-antibodies are biologic therapy for melanoma tumors that enhances or restores the immune system in order to destroy cancer cells. Targeted therapy is a newer molecular-based medication therapy that targets specific receptors or other processes that produce cancer cells. Because this therapy has specific targets, it often causes less adverse effects than regular cancer chemotherapy, which typically kills large numbers of normal cells along with cancer cells.
- Interleukins help coordinate the inflammatory and immune responses of the body, in particular, the lymphocytes.
- Interferons, when stimulated, can exert an antitumor effect by activating a variety of responses.

Radiation

- Limited to clients who are poor surgical candidates and older adult clients who have large, deeply invasive tumors
- Used for inoperable lesions due to size or location
- Melanoma is relatively resistant to radiation therapy.

Cryosurgery

- Cryotherapy (cryoablation) uses liquid nitrogen injected directly into the tumor to destroy the tumor.
- Procedure is used for some primary basal cell cancers and for low-risk squamous cell cancers.
- Freezes and destroys isolated lesions by applying liquid nitrogen (−200° C).
- Skin becomes edematous and tender.

CLIENT EDUCATION: Cleanse with hydrogen peroxide and apply a topical antimicrobial until healed.

Curettage and electrodessication

- Removes cancerous cells with the use of a curette to scrape away cancerous tissue, followed by the application of an electric probe to destroy remaining tumor tissue.
- Procedure is performed to remove basal cell cancer that is less than 2 cm in diameter.

Excision

The incision will be closed with sutures if possible. A skin graft can be necessary for large areas.

NURSING ACTIONS: Advise the client about postoperative wound care and care of the skin graft if used.

Mohs surgery

- Used with basal and squamous cell carcinoma
- Conserves more normal tissue and is used to determine the extent of nonmelanoma skin cancer
- Tissue is sectioned horizontally in layers and each layer is examined for presence of residual cancer. The process is continued until the samples are free from cancer.

COMPLICATIONS: Skin abscess and cellulitis

Leukemias and lymphomas

LEUKEMIAS

- Leukemias are cancers of white blood cells or of cells that develop into white blood cells. In leukemia, the white blood cells are not functional. The cancer invades and destroys bone marrow, and can metastasize to the liver, spleen, lymph nodes, testes, and brain.
- Leukemias are divided into acute (acute lymphocytic leukemia, acute myelogenous leukemia) and chronic (chronic lymphocytic leukemia, chronic myelogenous leukemia) and further classified by the type of white blood cells primarily affected.
- The goal of treatment is to eliminate all leukemic cells.
- Possible causes of leukemia are exposure to benzene (unleaded gas), radiation, HTLV-1 infection, Down syndrome, and Philadelphia chromosome.
- Overgrowth of leukemic cells prevents growth of other blood components (platelets, erythrocytes, mature leukocytes). Qs
  - Lack of mature leukocytes leads to immunosuppression. Infection is the leading cause of death among clients who have leukemia.
  - Lack of erythrocytes to produce RBCs leads to severe anemia.
  - Lack of platelets increases the risk of bleeding.

82.2 Cancer therapies at a glance

Ablation procedures

Can be used to destroy cancerous cells.

Radiofrequency ablation delivers an electric current directly to the tumor via thin needles. This current is converted into heat waves that kill the cancer cells.

Cryotherapy (cryoablation) uses liquid nitrogen injected directly into the tumor to destroy the tumor.

Microwave thermotherapy uses microwaves transmitted through a probe to heat and destroy the abnormal tissue

Chemotherapy

Chemotherapy uses anti-cancer medications administered orally or IV to destroy cancer cells.

Several courses of chemotherapy are needed because a fixed percentage of cells are killed with each course. The goal is to reduce the number of malignant cells until the body's immune system can take over. In general, the maximum amount of chemotherapy the client can tolerate is given with each course.

Photodynamic therapy

Photodynamic therapy involves the injection of a photosensitizing agent that is absorbed by all the cells in the body. When the agent remains in only the cancer cells 1 to 3 days later, the tumor is exposed to a laser light via an endoscope. Cells are subsequently destroyed and tumors are eliminated or reduced in size. Used with small, noninvasive lesions.

Radiation

With extensive disease, radiation is combined with chemotherapy.

Brachytherapy is radiation delivered inside the body. A radioactive implant is placed directly into the tumor site, delivering a high dose to the tumor and a lower dose to the tissues around it.

External beam radiation therapy (EBRT) uses radiation from a source outside of the body to destroy cancer cells.

Intensity-modulated radiation uses thousands of beams and angles of varying intensity that are even more controlled to target the cancer tissues and reduce exposure of radiation to healthy tissue.

Targeted therapy

Targeted therapy is a molecular-based medication therapy that targets specific receptors or other processes that produce cancer cells. Because this therapy has specific targets, it often causes less adverse effects than regular cancer chemotherapy, which typically kills large numbers of normal cells along with cancer cells.

Examples of targeted therapy include biologic response modifiers, monoclonal antibodies, cytokines, growth factors, and gene therapy.

Immunotherapy (biotherapy) uses biologic response modifiers (BRMs), to stimulate the immune system to target and destroy cancer cells. This alters a client's biological response to cancerous tumor cells. Cytokines work to enhance the immune system. They help the immune system recognize cancer cells and use the body's natural defenses to destroy them. Interleukins and interferons are the two primary cytokines (immune response modulators) used in immunotherapy.

- Interleukins help coordinate the inflammatory and immune responses of the body (in particular, the lymphocytes).
- Interferons, when stimulated, can exert an antitumor effect by activating a variety of responses.
- Tumor necrosis factor, a biologic response modifier, has a direct antitumor effects.

Incidence and cure rates

Acute lymphocytic leukemia (ALL): Various factors influence the prognosis for children, but the 5-year survival rate is approximately 85% (age at diagnosis, sex, cell type involved); less than 50% of adults can be cured.

Acute myelogenous leukemia (AML): Most common leukemia among adults; prognosis is poor. Toxins, genetic disorders, and cancer treatments can cause AML.

Chronic lymphocytic leukemia (CLL): Most cases involve people older than 50 years of age. Onset is slow, progressive, and chronic. CLL does not occur in children.

Chronic myeloid leukemia (CML): Most cases involve young adults. The disease is uncommon in children. Prognosis is less than 2 years of survival from the time of diagnosis.

LYMPHOMAS

- Lymphomas are cancers of lymphocytes (a type of white blood cell) and lymph nodes (which produce antibodies and fight infection).
- Lymphomas can metastasize to almost any organ.

Types of lymphoma

Hodgkin's lymphoma (HL)
- Peaks in two age groups.
  - Teens and young adults
  - Adults in their 50s and 60s
- Possible causes include viral infections and exposure to chemical agents.
- Typically starts in a single node or chain of nodes of the neck or above the clavicle.
- Untreated, HL spreads predictably from one group of lymph nodes to the next.
- One of the most treatable types of cancer.

Non-Hodgkin's lymphoma (NHL)
- More common than HL; accounts for approximately 90% of newly diagnosed cases of lymphoma.
- Most common in men and older adults.
- Possible causes include gene damage, viral infections, autoimmune disease, and exposure to radiation or toxic chemicals (pesticides, insecticides, dust).
- Generally spreads through the lymphatic system in an erratic pattern.

HEALTH PROMOTION AND DISEASE PREVENTION

- Use protective equipment, such as a mask, and ensure proper ventilation while working in environments that contain carcinogens or particles in the air.
- Influenza and pneumonia immunizations are important for all clients who are immunosuppressed.

DATA COLLECTION

RISK FACTORS

- Immunosuppression
- Exposure to chemotherapy agents or medications that suppress bone marrow
- Genetic factors (hereditary)
- Ionizing radiation (radiation therapy, environmental)

OLDER ADULT CLIENTS Ⓒ
- Often have diminished immune function and decreased bone marrow function, which increase the risk of complications of leukemia and lymphoma.
- Have decreased energy reserves and can tire more easily during treatment. Safety is a concern with ambulation.

EXPECTED FINDINGS

Acute leukemia

- Bone pain
- Joint swelling
- Enlarged liver and spleen
- Weight loss
- Fever
- Impaired WBC function leading to an infection
- Poor wound healing (infected lesions)
- Manifestations of anemia (fatigue, pallor, tachycardia, dyspnea on exertion)
- Thrombocytopenia (low platelet count) evidenced by bleeding (ecchymosis, hematuria, bleeding gums)

82.3 Phases of chemotherapy to treat leukemia

	GOAL	PROCEDURE	LENGTH OF TIME
Induction therapy: intensive combination therapy	Induce remission: absence of all findings of leukemia, including less than 5% blasts in bone marrow.	Aggressive treatment (possible continuous infusion); IV infusion; CNS and CSF infusion prophylaxis (ALL) to eradicate leukemic cells within the bone marrow high doses of chemotherapy is administered.	4 to 6 weeks (hospitalization required due to increased risk for infection and hemorrhage)
Consolidation or post-remission therapy	Cure by eradicating any residual leukemic cells after remission is attained.	Same medications as induction phase at lower dosage or different combination of medications	About 6 months
Maintenance therapy	Prevent relapse.	Lower doses of oral or IV chemotherapy	Months to years
Reinduction therapy: for a client who relapses	Place the client back in remission.	Combinations of chemotherapy used to achieve remission	Probability of relapse occurring decreases over time

Hodgkin's and non-Hodgkin's lymphoma

- Most clients only experience an enlarged lymph node (usually in the neck with HL), which is a typical finding in clients who have indolent (slow-growing) lymphomas.
- Other possible manifestations include fever, night sweats, unplanned weight loss, fatigue, and infections.

DIAGNOSTIC PROCEDURES

Staging of lymphoma involves extensive testing to ensure proper treatment is prescribed. Both Hodgkin's and non-Hodgkin's lymphoma have four stages to determine the extent and severity of the disease.

CBC

EXPECTED FINDINGS
- WBC can be high, low, or normal (leukemia)
- Hemoglobin, hematocrit, and platelets decreased

NURSING ACTIONS: Explain unexpected findings to the client.

Coagulation time

EXPECTED FINDINGS: Increased with acute leukemia

NURSING ACTIONS: Monitor for bleeding.

Biopsy of bone marrow (core or fine-needle aspiration)

EXPECTED FINDINGS
- Large quantities of immature leukemic blast cells (confirms diagnosis)
- Typing of protein markers (to differentiate myeloid or lymphoid leukemia)

NURSING ACTIONS
- Administer pain medication.
- Apply pressure for 5 to 10 min, then a pressure dressing.
- Monitor for bleeding and infection for 24 hr.

CT scan (always used for HL staging)

EXPECTED FINDINGS: Guide for lymphoma staging procedures: identify presence, size, and shape of nodes, tumors.

NURSING ACTIONS: Prepare the client for the procedure.

Biopsy of lymph nodes

EXPECTED FINDINGS
- **Hodgkin's lymphoma:** presence of Reed-Sternberg cells (cancerous B-lymphocytes)
- **Non-Hodgkin's lymphoma:** any other lymph node malignancy

NURSING ACTIONS: Provide the client with information specific to the diagnosis.

Chest x-ray, CT scan, PET scan, bone scan

Confirms diagnosis or metastatic disease

NURSING ACTIONS: Provide the client with information specific to the diagnosis.

PATIENT-CENTERED CARE

NURSING CARE

- Monitor for evidence of infection. Monitor for other physiological indicators of infection (lung crackles, cough, urinary frequency or urgency, oliguria, lesions of skin or mucous membrane).
- Manifestations that stem from the immune response (increased WBC, fever, pus, redness, inflammation) are not likely due to immunosuppression.
- Prevent infection. Implement neutropenic precautions. These interventions are especially important during chemotherapy induction and for the client who has received a bone marrow transplant. Qs
  - Frequent, thorough hand hygiene is a priority intervention.
  - Place the client in a private room. If prescribed, maintain protective isolation.
  - Allow only healthy visitors; when unavoidable, visitors who are ill must wear a mask.
  - Screen visitors carefully. Restrict visitors with cold or infections.
  - Restrict foods that can be contaminated with bacteria (no fresh or raw fruits or vegetables).
  - Monitor WBC. Report decreasing WBC levels to the charge nurse or care provider.
  - Prevent transmission of bacteria and viruses (no live plants or flowers; use high-efficiency particulate air [HEPA] filtration).
  - Eliminate standing water (humidifiers, denture cups, vases) to prevent bacteria breeding.
  - Encourage good personal hygiene.
  - Avoid crowds.
- Prevent injury.
  - Monitor platelets.
  - Check frequently for obvious and occult bleeding.
  - Protect the client from trauma. (Avoid injections and venipunctures. Apply firm pressure. Increase vitamin K intake.)
  - Reinforce teaching with the client how to avoid trauma. (Use electric shaver and soft-bristled toothbrush. Avoid contact sports.)
- Conserve the client's energy.
  - Encourage rest, adequate nutrition, and fluid intake.
  - Ensure the client gets adequate sleep.
  - Observe the client's energy resources/capability.
  - Plan activities as appropriate.

THERAPEUTIC PROCEDURES

Chemotherapy

- Chemotherapy is used to treat lymphoma in combination with other therapies.
- There are two phases of chemotherapy used to treat leukemia—induction where high doses of chemotherapy are administered, followed by post-remission therapy to eradicate the remaining leukemic cells after remission.

CLIENT EDUCATION: Report manifestations of infection or illness immediately to the provider.

Colony-stimulating medications

Medications such as filgrastim stimulate the production of leukocytes. The client receives colony-stimulating medications when there is bone marrow suppression from chemotherapy or leukemic changes.

NURSING ACTIONS
- Monitor for report of bone pain.
- Monitor CBC twice weekly to check leukocytes.
- Use cautiously with clients who have bone marrow cancer.

CLIENT EDUCATION: Report bone discomfort.

Immunotherapy (82.2)

Monoclonal antibodies are synthetic proteins that attack a specific target to treat lymphoma.

Radiation

- External lymph node radiation is the primary form of treatment for early HL. Radiation therapy or radiolabeled antibodies are part of the treatment for NHL.
- With extensive disease, radiation is combined with chemotherapy.
- Radiation is not typically used for leukemia.

Bone marrow transplantation

Bone marrow is destroyed or ablated using radiation and chemotherapy and is later replaced with healthy stem cells. The body is able to resume normal production of blood cells.
- Autologous cells are a collection of the client's own cells before chemotherapy.
- Matching of donor to recipient stem cells compares certain human leukocyte antigens (HLA) to reduce risk of rejection.
  - Syngeneic cells are donated from the client's identical twin (HLA identical).
  - Allogeneic cells are obtained from an HLA-matched donor, such as a relative or from umbilical cord blood (closely matched HLA).
- Without transplantation, the client has an increased risk of death from infection or bleeding.
- Following transplantation, the client has an increased risk of death from infection and bleeding until the transfused stem cells begin producing white blood cells and platelets again.

COMPLICATIONS

Pancytopenia

Decrease in white and red blood cells and platelets
- Neutropenia secondary to disease or treatment greatly increases the client's risk for infection.
- The risk of serious infection increases as the absolute neutrophil count (ANC) falls. ANC less than 1,000/mm³ indicates a weak immune system. ANC less than 500/mm³ indicates a severe risk of infection. Implement neutropenic precautions, including placing the client in a private room.

NURSING ACTIONS
- Maintain a hygienic environment and encourage the client to do the same.
- Monitor for infection (cough; alterations in breath sounds, urine, or feces). Report temperature greater than 37.8° C (100° F).

CLIENT EDUCATION
- Take antimicrobial, antiviral, and antifungal medications as prescribed.
- Receive blood products (granulocytes) as needed.

Thrombocytopenia

- Results from decreased platelet production, increased destruction of platelets, or accumulation of platelets in the spleen.
- Secondary to disease and/or treatment
- Greatly increases the client's risk for bleeding.
- The greatest risk is at platelet counts less than 50,000/mm³. Spontaneous bleeding can occur at less than 20,000/mm³. Qs

NURSING ACTIONS
- Monitor for petechiae; ecchymosis; bleeding of the gums; nosebleeds; and occult or frank blood in stool, urine, or vomitus.
- Monitor vital signs and level of consciousness for indications of bleeding.
- Institute bleeding precautions. (Avoid IVs and injections; apply pressure for approximately 10 min after blood is obtained; and handle client gently and avoid trauma.)
- Minimize the risk of trauma (safe environment).
- When possible, avoid invasive procedures and parenteral injections.
- Assist with administering blood products (platelets).

Hypoxemia

Anemia secondary to disease or treatment significantly increases the risk for hypoxemia.

NURSING ACTIONS
- Contribute to the plan of care to balance rest and activity and use assistive devices.
- Monitor RBC.
- Provide a diet high in protein and carbohydrates.
- Ask the charge nurse to administer colony-stimulating factors, such as epoetin alfa.
- Ask the charge nurse to administer blood products (packed red blood cells) as needed.

BONE MARROW TRANSPLANT

Stem cells in large concentrations are aspirated from the donor's anterior and posterior iliac crest, filtered, and administered to the recipient after immunosuppression is instituted.

Failure of stem cells to engraft (grow)

Bone marrow transplants are repeated when indicated.

Graft-versus-host disease (graft rejection)

CLIENT EDUCATION: Take immunosuppressants as prescribed.

Phlebitis

Blockage/inflammation of veins in the liver can occur up to 1 month after bone marrow transplant.

NURSING ACTIONS
- Monitor for jaundice, abdominal pain, and liver enlargement.
- Monitor daily weights and abdominal girth to determine fluid retention.

Thyroid cancer

As thyroid tumors increase in size or spread, they affect the function of surrounding structures (larynx, pharynx, esophagus, trachea), causing difficulty in swallowing or breathing.

Types of thyroid cancer

Papillary carcinoma grows slowly and is the most common form.

Follicular carcinoma affects blood vessels, bone, and lung tissues. It often attaches to the trachea, muscles, vasculature, and skin.

Medullary carcinoma is often the result of an endocrine disorder, which causes multiple tumors. It is most common in clients older than 50 years.

Anaplastic carcinoma replicates quickly, invading the area surrounding the tumor. It usually metastasizes before diagnosis.

HEALTH PROMOTION AND DISEASE PREVENTION

- Avoid or stop smoking.
- Wear a thyroid guard to protect the neck during upper body x-rays.

DATA COLLECTION

RISK FACTORS

- Female sex
- Diet low in iodine (follicular carcinoma)
- Radiation exposure
- Older adult clients have higher incidence of follicular and medullary carcinoma. ©

EXPECTED FINDINGS

- Dyspnea
- Hoarse voice
- Weight changes
- Depression and fatigue
- Dysphagia
- Stridor
- Change in size, shape of thyroid
- Palpable nodules or irregularities
- Dehydration (hormone imbalance)
- Thyroid bruits (possible with enlargement)

DIAGNOSTIC PROCEDURES

Serum thyroglobulin

EXPECTED FINDINGS: Elevated

CLIENT EDUCATION: The result can indicate remaining cancer cells after treatment or return of cancer.

TSH, T_3, T_4

Indicates function of the thyroid

EXPECTED FINDINGS: T_3, T_4 levels, and TSH are usually within the expected reference range in thyroid cancer.

NURSING ACTIONS: Continue to monitor thyroid laboratory levels after a thyroidectomy. Levothyroxine is a TSH suppression therapy prescribed after surgery.

CLIENT EDUCATION: Results indicate the function of the thyroid. Additional testing can be needed.

Calcitonin

EXPECTED FINDINGS: Elevated

CLIENT EDUCATION: Elevated calcitonin can indicate medullary carcinoma of the thyroid.

24-hr urine

EXPECTED FINDINGS: Altered TSH, T_3, T_4, or iodine levels

CLIENT EDUCATION: Discard the first voided urine specimen, and then save all urine for the next 24 hr.

Other laboratory testing

EXPECTED FINDINGS: Adrenocorticotropic hormone, prostaglandins, serotonin (medullary carcinoma)

NURSING ACTIONS: Reinforce information about unexpected findings to the client.

BRAF gene mutation

EXPECTED FINDINGS: Presence indicates carcinoma, possible thyroid papillary cancer.

NURSING ACTIONS: Consult genetic counseling services.

RET/PTC gene alterations

EXPECTED FINDINGS: Presence indicates high probability of papillary carcinoma.

NURSING ACTIONS: Consult genetic counseling services.

Carcinoembryonic agent (CEA)

EXPECTED FINDINGS: Positive indicates cancer, possible medullary carcinoma

CLIENT EDUCATION: CEA can represent many types of cancer.

Biopsy (fine-needle plus open or core, if indicated)

Identifies presence of cancer cells in thyroid nodules or lymph nodes

NURSING ACTIONS
- Administer pain medication.
- Apply pressure for 5 to 10 min, then a pressure dressing.
- Monitor for bleeding and infection for 24 hr.

CLIENT EDUCATION: Lesions greater than 1 cm and suspicious lymph nodes are tested.

Laryngoscopy

EXPECTED FINDINGS: Presence of cancer on vocal cords

CLIENT EDUCATION: Do not eat or drink after midnight prior to the procedure to prevent aspiration during the procedure.

Ultrasound

EXPECTED FINDINGS
- Guides biopsy procedures
- Reveals whether nodules are fluid-filled (typically benign) or solid (typically cancerous).

NURSING ACTIONS: Provide instructions to and prepare the client for the procedure.

Radioiodine thyroid scan

Not useful with medullary carcinoma

EXPECTED FINDINGS: Presence of radioactive cells (cells that retained radioiodine)

CLIENT EDUCATION
- Dye is administered (injection or oral) to scan the thyroid and other suspicious areas. Inform the provider of allergies to iodine or seafood.
- Stop taking medication containing iodine weeks before the scan as prescribed.

Chest x-ray, MRI, PET scan, CT scan

EXPECTED FINDINGS: Presence of disease or metastatic disease

PATIENT-CENTERED CARE

NURSING CARE

- Monitor airway patency in client who has a tumor affecting or compressing the trachea.
- Monitor ability to swallow in client who has a tumor affecting or compressing the esophagus.
- Administer medications to treat hypertension, dysrhythmia, or tachycardia.

MEDICATIONS

Thyroid suppression therapy

- Involves administration of synthetic thyroxine (T_4, levothyroxine sodium).
- Suppression therapy replaces T_4 needed for body function. It also prevents or slows growth of cancerous thyroid cells.
- Therapy is typically prescribed for several months following thyroid surgery.

CLIENT EDUCATION
- Never stop taking levothyroxine sodium, unless instructed by the provider. Qs
- Take levothyroxine sodium on an empty stomach.

THERAPEUTIC PROCEDURES

Radiation

- Treats anaplastic carcinoma
- With extensive disease, radiation is combined with chemotherapy

Radioactive iodine (RAI) therapy

Destroys papillary or follicular carcinoma and treats hyperthyroidism
- RAI therapy works similarly to radioactive scanning (used to diagnose thyroid cancer).
- The client ingests RAI in liquid or tablet form, which is absorbed by thyroid cells which are then destroyed.
- Client can benefit from RAI therapy following thyroid suppression therapy.

NURSING ACTIONS: Provide information on nutrition supplements for client experiencing altered taste. Consult nutrition services.

CLIENT EDUCATION
- Take radioactive precautions to reduce risk of radiation exposure.
- Chew gum or suck on hard candy to relieve dry mouth or reduced salivation.

Surgical interventions

Papillary, follicular, and medullary carcinoma are treated surgically.

- **Thyroidectomy** (total or partial) or **thyroid lobectomy** is the treatment of choice for papillary carcinoma that is limited to the thyroid gland.
- A radical neck dissection is performed when lymph nodes in the neck are involved.
- During surgery, the parathyroid glands or laryngeal nerve can be damaged.
- A wound drain can be placed intraoperatively.

NURSING ACTIONS
- Monitor and treat cardiac abnormalities.
- Support the neck with pillows or sandbags.
- Maintain a humidifier to promote airway clearance.
- Monitor for hemorrhage (incision site, hypotension, tachycardia, increased swallowing or throat "tickling").
- Monitor for respiratory distress (caused by tetany, swelling, or laryngeal nerve damage).
- Monitor for parathyroid injury (decreased PTH, hypocalcemia, tetany).
- Check for tetany (Chvostek or Trousseau sign).
- Monitor for thyroid storm (excessive release of thyroid hormone).

CLIENT EDUCATION
- Place both hands behind the neck when moving or coughing (reduces strain on the incision).
- Suppressive therapy with thyroid hormone is typically prescribed.

CLIENT EDUCATION

CARE AFTER DISCHARGE: Use strategies for managing hypothyroidism (thyroid hormone replacement therapy).

NURSING ACTIONS
- Monitor vital signs for impaired oxygenation, hypotension, or bradycardia.
- Use ECG monitoring to detect dysrhythmias.
- Determine mental status and provide a safe environment.

COMPLICATIONS

Myxedema coma

A rare, potentially lethal form of hypothyroidism resulting in decreased respiratory function (respiratory depression, cerebral hypoxia), altered cardiovascular function (bradycardia, hypotension, decreased cardiac output), endocrine abnormalities (hypoglycemia, hyponatremia), hypothermia, and stupor.

NURSING ACTIONS
- Notify provider of suspected myxedema coma.
- Provide continuous monitoring of telemetry and vital signs.
- Administer fluids, electrolytes, and medications.

Thyroid storm

- Caused by excess thyroid hormone release following surgery. This is a life-threatening emergency.
- A rapid increase in metabolic rate occurs when there is an oversecretion of thyroid hormone.
- Key findings are fever, tachycardia, and systolic hypertension. Other manifestations include GI disturbance (nausea, vomiting, diarrhea, abdominal pain), anxiety, restlessness, confusion (progresses to psychosis), and neurological alterations (tremors).
- The client's condition can progress to confusion, delirium, coma, and seizures.

NURSING ACTIONS
- Notify the provider immediately.
- Administer antithyroid medications, sodium iodide, beta adrenergic blocking agents, and glucocorticoids.
- Monitor cardiac rhythm, respiratory status, and central venous pressure.
- Reduce fever (administer antipyretics, apply cooling blanket). Do not administer aspirin during a thyroid crisis because aspirin can increase TH levels.

Lung cancer

- Lung cancer is one of the leading causes of cancer-related deaths for both men and women.
- Prognosis of lung cancer is poor because it is often diagnosed in an advanced stage, when metastasis involves the lymph system and organs. Palliative care is often the focus at the advanced stage (III, IV).
- Most lung cancers arise from bronchogenic carcinomas (arising from the bronchial epithelium)
- Most lung cancers are non-small cell lung cancer (NSCLC), which includes squamous, adeno, and large cell carcinomas.
- Small cell lung cancer (SCLC) is fast-growing and consistently linked to a history of cigarette smoking.

HEALTH PROMOTION AND DISEASE PREVENTION

- Promote smoking cessation.
- Use protective equipment (mask) and ensure proper ventilation while working in environments that can contain carcinogens or particles in the air.
- Screening (annual CT) for early detection for those at high risk for lung cancer development

DATA COLLECTION

RISK FACTORS

- Cigarette smoking (including secondhand smoke)
- Radiation or radon exposure
- Chronic exposure to inhaled environmental irritants (air pollution, asbestos, other talc dusts)
- History of tuberculosis
- Older adult clients have decreased pulmonary reserves due to normal lung changes (decreased lung elasticity, thickening alveoli), contributing to impaired gas exchange. ©
- Structural changes in the skeletal system decrease diaphragmatic expansion, thereby restricting ventilation.

EXPECTED FINDINGS

- Orthopnea
- Chronic cough
- Chronic dyspnea
- Chest wall pain
- Fatigue, weight loss, anorexia
- Clients can experience few manifestations early in the disease. Monitor for manifestations that often appear late in the disease.
  - Fever (pneumonitis or bronchitis that occurs with obstruction)
  - Persistent cough, with or without hemoptysis (rust-colored or blood-tinged sputum)
  - Hoarseness
  - Altered breathing pattern
    - Dyspnea
    - Prolonged exhalation alternated with shallow breaths (obstruction)
    - Rapid, shallow breaths (pleuritic chest pain, elevated diaphragm)
  - Altered breath sounds (wheezing)
  - Diminished or absent breath sounds (obstruction)
  - Chest pain or tightness
  - Chest wall masses
  - Muffled heart sounds
  - Pleural friction rub
  - Clubbing of fingers
  - Increased work of breathing (retractions, use of accessory muscle, stridor, nasal flaring)
  - Decreased bone density

DIAGNOSTIC PROCEDURES

Cytologic testing; thoracentesis (if pleural effusion is present)

EXPECTED FINDINGS: Sputum specimen contains cancer cells

CLIENT EDUCATION
- Provide a sputum specimen in the morning upon awakening because there is a larger accumulation of secretions.
- Cancer cells are not always found in sputum specimens even when cancer is present.

Thoracoscopy

EXPECTED FINDINGS: Presence of cancer cells

NURSING ACTIONS: Keep client NPO after midnight.

Biopsy (bronchoscopy)

EXPECTED FINDINGS: Presence of tumor

NURSING ACTIONS:
- Keep client NPO after midnight.
- Provide throat lozenges or sprays for report of a sore throat once the gag reflex returns following the procedure.

X-ray, CT scan (82.4)

EXPECTED FINDINGS: Presence of tumor

NURSING ACTIONS: Explain and prepare client for the procedure.

Needle biopsy of lymph nodes, thoracentesis with pleural biopsy, MRI, PET scan

EXPECTED FINDINGS: Presence of cancer and metastatic disease

NURSING ACTIONS: Explain and prepare client for the procedure.

Pulmonary function tests and arterial blood gases

EXPECTED FINDINGS: Compromised respiratory status

NURSING ACTIONS: Explain and prepare client for the procedure.

PATIENT-CENTERED CARE

NURSING CARE

- Determine the pack-year history (number of packs of cigarettes smoked per day times the number of years smoked) for clients who smoke. Qᴇʙᴘ
- Obtain information about the use of other tobacco products (cigars, pipes, chewing tobacco).
- Ask about exposure to secondhand smoke.
- Monitor for a cough that changes in pattern.
- Monitor nutritional status and for weight loss and anorexia.
  - Promote adequate nutrition to provide needed calories for increased work of breathing and prevention of infection.
  - Encourage fluids to promote adequate hydration.
- Maintain a patent airway, and suction as needed.
- Monitor for effective breathing and gas exchange.
- Position the client in Fowler's position to maximize ventilation.
- Provide information about planned treatments, explaining expected and side effects of each.
- Provide information for psychosocial support. Qᴘᴄᴄ

MEDICATIONS

Bronchodilators and corticosteroids are administered to help decrease inflammation and dry secretions.

Liquefying medication is administered to thin secretions and make the secretions less tenacious.

Antibiotics are administered if needed to treat infection.

Analgesics are administered to manage pain following surgery and for a client who has advanced cancer.

THERAPEUTIC PROCEDURES

Chemotherapy

Chemotherapy is the primary choice of treatment for lung cancers. It is often used in combination with radiation and surgery. A combination of two chemotherapy medications is recommended for higher stages of lung cancer.

ADVERSE EFFECTS: Nausea, vomiting, hair loss, mucositis, neutropenia, thrombocytopenia, peripheral neuropathy

Photodynamic therapy (82.2)

Photodynamic therapy is performed through bronchoscopy to treat small, accessible tumors.

Radiation therapy (82.2)

Radiation therapy is effective for lung cancer that has not spread beyond the chest wall and is used as an adjuvant therapy along with chemotherapy.

Radiation therapy is used before surgery to shrink tumors.

Radiofrequency ablation (82.2)

- Most commonly used with NSCLC
- Used to destroy cancerous cells

Targeted therapy (82.2)

Surgical interventions

- The goal of surgery is to remove all tumor cells, including involved lymph nodes.
- Often involves removal of a lung (pneumonectomy), lobe (lobectomy), segment (segmentectomy), or peripheral lung tissue (wedge resection).

NURSING ACTIONS
- Monitor vital signs, oxygenation (SaO$_2$, ABG values), and for evidence of hemorrhage.
- Manage the chest tube and drainage system.
- Administer oxygen and manage the ventilator.
- Manage pain. Reinforce teaching with the client regarding PCA use.
- Reinforce the teaching with the client about the surgical procedure and chest tube placement.

Palliative procedures

- Thoracentesis or pleurodesis to ease breathing when pleural effusion occurs
- Laser therapy and photodynamic therapy for use in treatment and palliative therapy to open airways blocked by tumors
- Pericardiocentesis or pericardial window to improve cardiac function

INTERPROFESSIONAL CARE

- Respiratory services are consulted for inhalers, breathing treatments, and suctioning for airway management.
- Rehabilitation care is consulted if the client has prolonged weakness and needs assistance with increasing the level of activity.

CLIENT EDUCATION

- Take rest periods as needed.
- Eat high-calorie foods to promote energy.
- Refrain from smoking.

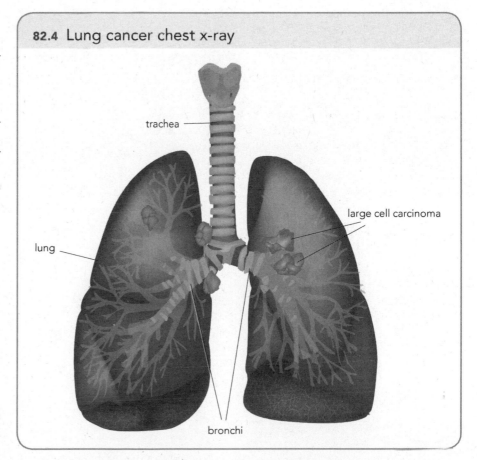

82.4 Lung cancer chest x-ray

trachea

large cell carcinoma

lung

bronchi

COMPLICATIONS

Superior vena cava syndrome

- Results from pressure placed on the vena cava by a tumor causing partial or complete obstruction of the superior vena cava. It is a medical emergency.
- Radiation and stent placement provide temporary relief. Prepare the client for radiation and stent placement.

NURSING ACTIONS
- Monitor for manifestations of superior vena cava syndrome and report to the provider immediately.
  - Early findings include facial edema, edema in neck, nosebleeds, headache, dizziness, vision changes, peripheral edema, and dyspnea.
  - Late findings include mental status changes, cyanosis, hemorrhage, and hypotension.
- Monitor vital signs and oxygenation during and after the procedure.

Oropharyngeal cancer

- Oral and pharyngeal carcinoma is more lethal than many types of cancer (cervical, testicular, thyroid, Hodgkin's lymphoma).
- Mouth lesions that do not heal within 2 weeks can be cancerous. The client should report the finding to the provider.
- Oropharyngeal cancer has a high rate of recurrence.

Main types of oropharyngeal cancer

Squamous cell carcinoma is the most common oral cancer and can be present on the lips, tongue, buccal mucosa, and oropharynx. It is a much more aggressive cancer than basal cell carcinoma.

Basal cell carcinoma affects the lips and skin around the mouth.

Kaposi's sarcoma is often found on the hard palate, gums, tongue, or tonsils and is associated with HIV infection. Raised, purple nodules or plaque lesions erupt in the lining of small blood vessels of the mucous membranes and are initially painless. As the disease progresses, the lesions can become very painful.

HEALTH PROMOTION AND DISEASE PREVENTION

- Schedule dental visits twice yearly for cleaning and inspection of mouth tissues.
- Limit exposure to UV rays (midday sun exposure, indoor tanning).
- Eliminate tobacco use (including smokeless).
- Obtain immunization for HPV.

DATA COLLECTION

RISK FACTORS

- Male sex
- Tobacco use
- Alcohol consumption (alcohol use combined with tobacco use significantly increases risk)
- Radiation exposure, including x-rays of head and neck
- Inadequate oral hygiene
- Lack of fruits and vegetables in the diet
- Occupation in textile, coal, metal, and plumbing industries
- Age older than 40 years
- Human papilloma virus (HPV16) infection
- HIV infection
- Periodontal disease with mandibular bone loss
- TP53 gene mutation
- Weakened immune system

EXPECTED FINDINGS

- Mucosal erythroplasia (red patches): earliest finding
- Oral bleeding
- Difficulty chewing or swallowing
- Speech changes
- Thick or absent saliva
- Palpable masses
- Facial paresthesia

DIAGNOSTIC PROCEDURES

Biopsy (fine-needle, incisional, excisional)

EXPECTED FINDINGS: Presence of cancer

NURSING ACTIONS: Provide diagnosis-specific information.

Cell brushing

EXPECTED FINDINGS: Presence of cancer

CLIENT EDUCATION: A brush will be used to collect cells from suspicious areas in the mouth.

MRI

EXPECTED FINDINGS
- Presence of cancer
- Thickness of lesion
- Presence of nerve involvement

NURSING ACTIONS: Reinforce teaching with and prepare the client for procedure.

PATIENT-CENTERED CARE

Protecting the airway and providing adequate nutrition are priority interventions in managing oropharyngeal cancer. Qs

NURSING CARE

- Monitor for adequate clearance of secretions. (Have the client turn, cough, deep breathe. Suction as needed.)
- Auscultate for adventitious lung sounds: wheezes (due to aspiration) or stridor (due to obstruction).
- Consult respiratory therapy to provide chest physiotherapy.
- Position the client in semi- or high-Fowler's position to promote chest expansion.
- Use a cool mist face tent to promote clearance of secretions and reduce inflammation.
- Check for difficulty swallowing.
- Administer steroids to reduce inflammation; administer antibiotic if infection is present.
- Perform oral hygiene every 2 hr. (Use an ultra-soft or foam brush for a client who has a platelet count less than 40,000/mm³.)

MEDICATIONS

- Chemotherapy when metastasis occurs
- Antibiotics for infection

INTERPROFESSIONAL CARE

- Provide alternate means of communication for clients who have impaired communication (pen and paper, picture boards). Consult speech therapy.
- Consult nutrition services to assess swallowing and provide nutrition recommendations.

THERAPEUTIC PROCEDURES

Radiation and chemotherapy are used to treat oral lesions.

Targeted therapy (82.2)

Ablation (cryotherapy, photodynamic therapy) (82.2)

Used to remove lesions

Radiation (external, implanted, or both)

Commonly used prior to surgery to reduce tumor size.
- **External radiation** is used cautiously to minimize radiation dose to the brain and spinal cord.
- **Implanted radiation** is used to cure early lesion on the floor of the mouth or anterior tongue.
- Hospitalization is typically required until radiation dosing is complete.
- Place client on radiation transmission precautions. See **CHAPTER 81: CANCER TREATMENT OPTIONS**.
- Provide tracheostomy care if needed. Tracheostomy can be required due to edema and increased oral secretions.

Tumor excision

Tumor excision removes lesions through the inside of the mouth or through external entry into the head and neck.
- The larger the tumor, the greater the risk to the client for disfigurement and loss of function.
- Composite resections are the most extensive form of oral carcinoma surgery. They can include partial or total glossectomy and partial mandibulectomy.
- Combined neck dissection, mandibulectomy, and oropharyngeal resection (commando procedure) can be used.
- Radical neck dissection can include removal of the sternocleidomastoid muscle, internal jugular vein, cranial nerve XI (accessory nerve), and all cervical lymph nodes on the affected side.
- Surgery to remove large lesions can also include placement of a tracheostomy or wound drain.

NURSING ACTIONS

- Provide clear liquid diet for 24 hr (for clients having small lesions removed locally).
- Place cold packs and elevate the head of bed to decrease edema of the neck that can cause airway obstruction.
- Maintain NPO status until intraoral suture lines heal (clients who have large tumors).
- Provide routine tracheostomy care and suctioning.
- Monitor wounds, incision sites, and donor grafting sites for evidence of infection or bleeding.
- Consult a speech language pathologist for clients who have slurred speech or difficulty speaking.
- Provide comfort to clients who have permanent loss of voice or disfigurement. Make a referral to counseling services.
- Reinforce teaching with the client about the need and options for alternate communication following surgery.

CLIENT EDUCATION

- Avoid mouthwashes containing alcohol or lemon-glycerin swabs (acidic) to prevent pain and worsening of condition. QEBP
- Rinse the mouth frequently with warm sodium bicarbonate or 0.9% sodium chloride solution.
- Keep the head of the bed elevated to reduce edema.
- Report leakage of fluid from the suture line, swallowing difficulty, or coughing once oral intake is resumed.
- Perform swallowing exercises regularly as prescribed.
- Thicken liquids prior to consumption.
- Continue thorough, frequent oral hygiene at home, cleansing the toothbrush after each use.
- Temporary or permanent loss or changes in taste (dislike of meats, metallic taste) are possible.
- Some people who are cured will later develop cancer of the lung, mouth, or throat and will need follow-up exams for the rest of their life

COMPLICATIONS

Osteonecrosis (bone death) and issues related to motor impairment of jaw structure

Colorectal cancer

- Colorectal cancer is cancer of the rectum or colon. Most colorectal cancers are adenocarcinoma, a tumor that arises from a gland in the epithelial layer of the colon.
- Colorectal cancer occurs in stages from 0 to IV according to the tissue depth of the lesion and whether it has spread to local or distant sites.
- Adenocarcinoma begins as a polyp and is benign in the early stages. If left untreated, the polyp will grow and the risk of malignancy increases.
- Colorectal cancers can spread and involve the entire bowel wall. It can metastasize through blood or lymph to the liver (most common site), lungs, brain, or bones. Metastasis can occur as a result of peritoneal seeding through the bowel wall or during surgical resection of tumor.
- The most common location of colorectal cancers is the rectosigmoidal region.

HEALTH PROMOTION/ DISEASE PREVENTION

- Consume a diet rich in calcium. (Calcium binds to free fatty acids and bile salts in the lower gastrointestinal tract.)
- Consume a diet low in fat and simple carbohydrates but high in fiber.
- Obtain age-specific regular colorectal cancer screening.
- Obtain genetic testing for familial adenomatous polyposis and hereditary nonpolyposis colorectal cancer if family members had hereditary colorectal cancer.
- Engage in healthy lifestyle (regular exercise; no smoking or excessive alcohol use).

DATA COLLECTION

RISK FACTORS

- CRC is more common in females.
- Rectal cancer is more common in males.
- Adenomatous colon polyps
- African American descent
- Inflammatory bowel disease (ulcerative colitis, Crohn's disease)
- High-fat, low-fiber diet
- Age older than 50 years; incidence in younger clients related to HPV infections
- Long-term smoking
- Physical inactivity
- Heavy alcohol consumption
- Infection exposure to *Helicobacter pylori*, *Streptococcus bovis*, John Cunningham virus, and human papilloma virus
- History of breast, ovarian, or endometrial cancer

EXPECTED FINDINGS

- Manifestations related to the location, size, and type of tumor
- Changes in stool consistency or shape (with or without noticeable blood)
- Change in bowel habits (constipation or frequent small stools)
- Blood in stool (often the only finding)
  - Left-sided tumors are more likely to produce frank bleeding and change in bowel pattern, consistency.
  - Right-sided tumors cause stools to be darker due to ulceration of the colon and intermittent bleeding.
  - Anemia occurs from occult bleeding.
- Cramps and gas
- Palpable mass (elicited by provider only through abdominal palpation or digital rectal exam)
- Weight loss and fatigue
- Vomiting
- Abdominal fullness, distention, or pain
- Abnormal bowel sounds indicative of obstruction (high-pitched tinkling bowel sounds)
- Primary complication is bowel obstruction due to tumor size.

DIAGNOSTIC PROCEDURES

- Virtual colonoscopy is performed using CT scan or MRI. Imaging is performed after air is injected into the colon. The procedure is otherwise noninvasive. No sedation is required.
- Screening for individuals who have polyps or a family history of colorectal cancer is recommended to start at an earlier age and performed more frequently.

Fecal occult blood testing (FOBT)

EXPECTED FINDINGS: Two positive stools within 3 days

NURSING ACTIONS
- To avoid false-positive results, do not use stool from digital rectal examination.
- Negative results do not completely rule out the possibility of colorectal cancer.
- Recommend annual FOBT for clients ages 50 to 75.

CLIENT EDUCATION: Avoid red meat, anti-inflammatory medications, and vitamin C for 48 hr prior to testing (to prevent false positives).

Biopsy (endoscopic)

EXPECTED FINDINGS: Definitive diagnosis

NURSING ACTIONS: Provide the client with diagnosis-specific information.

Traditional or CT-guided colonoscopy

EXPECTED FINDINGS: Visualization of lesions (CT-guided is more accurate than traditional scan)

NURSING ACTIONS
- Prepare the client for procedure.
- Reinforce instructions with the client about the diet regimen (clear liquids then NPO after midnight) and bowel preparation for colonoscopy.

Endoscopy (colonoscopy, sigmoidoscopy)

EXPECTED FINDINGS: Visualization of polyps or lesions

CLIENT EDUCATION: Receive screening between ages 50 and 75 (colonoscopy every 10 years, sigmoidoscopy every 5 years).

Double contrast (air and barium) barium enema

EXPECTED FINDINGS: Visualization and location of tumor

NURSING ACTIONS: Administer stimulant laxative following procedure (facilitates evacuation of barium, which can harden in the intestine).

CBC

EXPECTED FINDINGS: Decreased hemoglobin, hematocrit

NURSING ACTIONS: Explain unexpected findings.

Carcinoembryonic antigen (CEA)

EXPECTED FINDINGS
- Positive (denotes malignancy; not specific to colorectal cancer)
- CEA is a protein found in colorectal cancers that can determine the client's prognosis and can detect recurring tumors after surgery.

CLIENT EDUCATION: Postive CEA indicates the presence of cancer. further testing is required to determine the type.

CT, MRI

EXPECTED FINDINGS: Visualization and location of tumor and metastasis to other organs

PATIENT-CENTERED CARE

THERAPEUTIC PROCEDURES

Colon resection (colectomy): Involves the removal of a portion of the colon to excise the tumor, using open surgical or laparoscopic methods.

Colectomy: The procedure can include reconnecting the remaining colon by anastomosis (end-to-end) or by creating a colostomy (temporary or permanent) or ileostomy. To promote healing of the anastomosis, a temporary colostomy is created.

Regional lymph node removal

Abdominal-perineal (AP) resection: The sigmoid colon, rectum, and anus are removed. A permanent colostomy is created for elimination of feces.

NURSING ACTIONS
- Check the stoma (should be reddish pink, moist, small amount of blood postoperatively). Report ischemia, necrosis, or frank bleeding. (82.5)
- Manage pain. Reinforce teaching regarding PCA.
- Maintain nasogastric suction (decompression).
- Progress the diet slowly after suctioning is discontinued. Monitor the client's response (bowel sounds present; no nausea or vomiting).
- Encourage the client to turn and take deep breaths.

PREOPERATIVE CLIENT EDUCATION
- Maintain prescribed preoperative diet (clear liquids several days prior to surgery).
- Complete bowel prep with cathartics.
- Administration of antibiotics (neomycin, metronidazole) is needed to eradicate intestinal flora.

POSTOPERATIVE CLIENT EDUCATION
- Avoid heavy lifting and maintain activity limits.
- Use stool softeners to avoid straining.

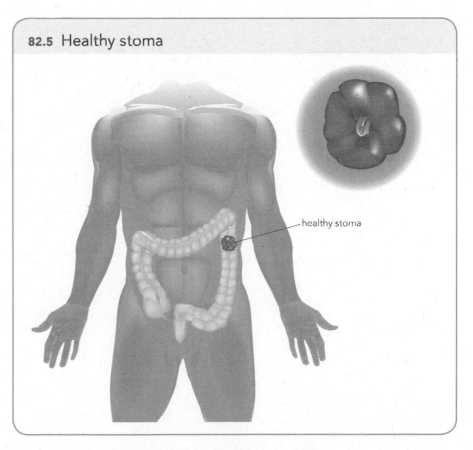

82.5 Healthy stoma

healthy stoma

- Follow instructions for incisional and ostomy care, and appliance management. Management of a colostomy can be more difficult for older adult clients due to impaired vision and a decline in fine motor skills. ⓖ
- Report manifestations of complications (incontinence, sexual dysfunction, ischemia) to the provider.

Chemotherapy

Given for stage IV cancer as an adjunctive therapy for colorectal cancer

Radiation therapy

- Radiation therapy is given in conjunction with chemotherapy to improve prognosis (usually used for rectal cancer to prevent lymph node involvement and recurrence). Radiation can also be used as a palliative measure to control pain, hemorrhage, bowel obstruction, or metastatic disease.
- With extensive disease, radiation is combined with chemotherapy.

INTERPROFESSIONAL CARE

- Ostomy nurse referral for instruction on care of colostomy
- Referral to ostomy support group
- Referral to cancer support group as needed
- Case manager or social worker for ongoing patient and family support

COMPLICATIONS

- Secondary primary colorectal tumors
- Complete intestinal obstruction
- Perforation of the bowel

Pancreatic cancer

- Pancreatic carcinoma has vague manifestations and is usually diagnosed in late stages after liver or gall bladder involvement.
- Tumors are usually adenocarcinoma, originate in the pancreatic head, and grow rapidly in glandular patterns.
- Pancreatic cancer has a high mortality rate; 5-year survival rates are low.

DATA COLLECTION

RISK FACTORS

- Possible inherited risk
- Age older than 45 years
- Male sex
- African American descent
- Tobacco use
- Chronic pancreatitis
- Cirrhosis
- High intake of red meat (especially processed)
- Long-term exposure to gasoline and pesticides

- Diabetes mellitus
- Family history of pancreatic cancer
- Metastasis from other cancer (breast, lung, kidney, skin)

EXPECTED FINDINGS

- Pain that radiates to the back and is unrelieved by change in position, and is more severe at night
- Fatigue
- Anorexia
- Pruritus

PHYSICAL FINDINGS

- Weight loss
- Flatulence
- Dull epigastric pain
- Palpable abdominal mass
- Enlarged gallbladder and liver
- Hepatomegaly
- Jaundice (late finding)
- Clay colored stools
- Dark, frothy urine
- Ascites
- Pruritus (buildup of bile salt)
- Early satiety or anorexia

DIAGNOSTIC PROCEDURES

Biopsy (percutaneous or laparoscopic)

EXPECTED FINDINGS: Presence of cancer cells; holds some risk of seeding (not always performed if imaging shows tumor can be surgically removed)

NURSING ACTIONS: Provide diagnosis-specific information to the client.

Endoscopic retrograde cholangiopancreatography (ERCP)

EXPECTED FINDINGS: Definitive diagnosis of tumor

CLIENT EDUCATION: A biliary drain or stent can be placed during the procedure.

Abdominal paracentesis

EXPECTED FINDINGS: Malignant cells in abdominal fluid

NURSING ACTIONS: Instruct the client on care of the dressing at the puncture site and activity restrictions.

Tumor markers

EXPECTED FINDINGS: Positive (denotes non-specific malignancy)

CLIENT EDUCATION: CA 19-9, carcinoembryonic antigen (CEA) can indicate many types of cancer.

Other laboratory testing

EXPECTED FINDINGS: Elevated amylase, lipase, alkaline phosphatase, and bilirubin

NURSING ACTIONS: Elevated liver enzymes, albumin, and bilirubin can indicate primary or metastatic cancer.

Imaging

Ultrasound or computerized tomography-visualization (CT scan) of the tumor with or without biopsy

NURSING ACTIONS: Prepare the client and explain unexpected findings.

Endoscopic ultrasound

EXPECTED FINDINGS: Visualization of tumor for the client who has a strong family history or genetic syndrome that increases the client's risk.

NURSING ACTIONS: Prepare the client and explain unexpected findings.

PATIENT-CENTERED CARE

NURSING CARE

- Care of a client who has pancreatic cancer usually focuses on palliation and not curative measures. Pain management is the priority intervention. Advise clients to ask for analgesics before the pain becomes severe.
- Monitor blood glucose and administer insulin.
- A jejunostomy is often placed to provide enteral feedings (prevents reflux, promotes absorption). Provide nutritional support (enteral supplements, TPN).
- Treat and prevent malnutrition.
- Increase supplemental feedings as tolerated, and monitor for frequency of diarrhea. Possibly initiate total parenteral feedings.

THERAPEUTIC PROCEDURES

Chemotherapy (82.2)

- Chemotherapy can be used to shrink tumor size. Several medications are given to improve the results.
- **Targeted therapy** can be included.
- **Radiation**
  ○ Used to shrink tumor size
  ○ Radioactive iodine seeds implanted in combination of chemotherapy
- **Ablation procedures**
  ○ Procedures are used to destroy cancerous cells.
  ○ Embolization therapy severs the blood supply to the tumor.
  ○ Cyberknife treatment targets the tumor through image-guided radio-surgery with little disruption of healthy tissue.

Surgical interventions

- Surgical procedure is open or laparoscopic. Q**EBP**
- Surgical interventions can be considered potentially curative or palliative.

Partial pancreatectomy: Used to remove tumors less than 3 cm in diameter

Total pancreatectomy: Removes the entire pancreas

Whipple procedure (pancreaticoduodenectomy): Removal of the head of the pancreas, duodenum, parts of the jejunum and stomach, gallbladder, and possibly the spleen. The pancreatic duct is connected to the common bile duct, and the stomach is connected to the jejunum.

NURSING ACTIONS
- Monitor NG tube and surgical drains for color and amount.
- Monitor for bloody or bile-tinged drainage, which could indicate anastomotic disruption.
- Place the client in semi-Fowler's position to facilitate lung expansion and prevent stress on the suture line.
- Monitor blood glucose and administer insulin as needed.
- Instruct the client about support measures for pain, anorexia, weight loss, and community resources.

Palliative to relieve or prevent manifestations

Stent placement: A stent is placed to keep the bile duct open and resist compression from the surrounding cancer.

Bypass surgery: Reroutes the flow of bile from the common bile duct, bypassing the pancreas and into the small intestines.

COMPLICATIONS

Fistulas

Breakdown of a site of anastomosis

NURSING ACTIONS: Report drainage that is not serosanguineous from the drain or drainage from the wound to the provider immediately.

Peritonitis

- Results from internal leakage of corrosive pancreatic fluid that causes inflammation of the peritoneum.
- Paralytic ileus can also develop.

NURSING ACTIONS
- Monitor for manifestations of peritonitis (fever, WBC, abdominal pain, boardlike abdominal rigidity, abdominal tenderness/rebound tenderness, alteration in bowel sounds, shoulder pain).
- Ask the charge nurse to administer IV antibiotics.

Thromboembolism

Due to hypercoagulable state caused by release of necrotic products from the tumor, or immobility postoperatively

NURSING ACTIONS
- Report findings of thromboembolism to the provider.
- Administer anticoagulants.
- Maintain bed rest as indicated.

Liver cancer

Cancers can be primary tumors originating in the liver or bile duct, or metastatic cancers that spread from other organ to the liver.

Hepatocellular carcinoma (HCC) is the most frequently occurring type of primary liver cancer. Primary liver cancer can also originate in the bile duct or liver vasculature.

Hepatoma arises from the hepatocytes and can develop in the client who has cirrhosis.

Intrahepatic cholangiocarcinomas starts in the cells that line the small bile ducts.

Hepatocellular carcinoma increases due to hepatitis C.

HEALTH PROMOTION AND DISEASE PREVENTION

- Avoid excessive alcohol intake.
- Eat a low-fat diet and maintain a BMI less than 30.
- Receive a hepatitis B vaccine.
- Take precautions against hepatitis B and C. (Recognize that multiple sexual partners, IV drug use, and the sharing of needles increase risk.)

DATA COLLECTION

RISK FACTORS

- Older age Ⓖ
- Cirrhosis
  - Chronic hepatitis B or C infection
  - Alcohol-related liver disease
  - Hemochromatosis (inability to breakdown iron)
- Male sex
- Tobacco use
- Asian descent (particularly Vietnamese)
- African American descent

EXPECTED FINDINGS

- Right upper abdominal pain
- Epigastric fullness
- Loss of appetite
- Weakness and fatigue
- Fever

PHYSICAL FINDINGS

- Weight loss
- Enlarged liver upon palpation
- Jaundice
- Ascites
- Pruritus
- Encephalopathy
- Bleeding or bruising

DIAGNOSTIC PROCEDURES

Biopsy

Percutaneous or through the jugular to the hepatic veins (via fluoroscopy). Biopsy results can establish a diagnosis.

EXPECTED FINDINGS: Presence of cancerous cells

NURSING ACTIONS
- Position the client to the right side for 1 to 2 hr to ensure hemostasis.
- Monitor for hemorrhage (coagulation studies, frank bleeding).

CLIENT EDUCATION: Biopsy through venous route reduces the risk of hemorrhage.

Alpha-fetoprotein (AFP)

EXPECTED FINDINGS
- Elevated AFP is a serum marker.
- High probability of primary hepatocellular cancer (false positive: cirrhosis, hepatitis).
- Elevated CEA along with elevated AFP can discriminate metastatic from primary cancer.

CLIENT EDUCATION: False positives are possible.

Other laboratory testing

EXPECTED FINDINGS: Elevated alkaline phosphatase (ALP), serum aspartate aminotransferase (AST), albumin, and bilirubin

NURSING ACTIONS: Educate the client about other reasons liver function tests might be elevated.

Imaging (contrast-enhanced ultrasound , MRI, CT scan)

EXPECTED FINDINGS: Visualization of tumor

NURSING ACTIONS: Reinforce instructions for the procedure and prepare the client for procedure.

PATIENT-CENTERED CARE

NURSING CARE

- Observe for potential bleeding complications (frank bleeding, decreased hemoglobin and hematocrit, altered coagulation findings). Ⓠpcc
- Administer blood products (packed red blood cells, fresh frozen plasma) to replace blood volume and clotting factors.
- Replace vitamins due to the inability of the liver to store them (vitamin pills or vitamin-enriched supplements).
- Restrict fluids and sodium for clients who have ascites.
- Measure abdominal girth daily (indicates increased ascites).
- Monitor I&O and daily weight (impaired fluid balance).
- Check for adequate nutrition (fluid, electrolytes, weight loss, anorexia).

- Monitor for worsening hepatic function (liver function tests, jaundice).
- Monitor and treat pain and abdominal discomfort.
- Provide medications. Medications are administered sparingly (especially opioids, sedatives, and barbiturates) due to impaired liver function (reduced ability to metabolize medications).

CLIENT EDUCATION
- Consume small, frequent meals that are high-calorie, moderate-fat, and high-protein (unless the client has hepatic encephalopathy).
- Benefits of avoiding alcohol include preventing further damage, allowing for healing and regeneration of the liver, and decreasing the risk of bleeding and other life-threatening complications.

MEDICATIONS

Targeted therapy (sorafenib)

- Targeted therapy is a newer molecular-based medication therapy that targets specific receptors or other processes that produce cancer cells. Because this therapy has specific targets, it often causes fewer adverse effects than regular cancer chemotherapy, which typically kills large numbers of normal cells along with cancer cells.
- Examples of targeted therapy include biologic response modifiers, monoclonal antibodies, cytokines, growth factors, and gene therapy.
- Sorafenib is a multi-tyrosine kinase inhibitor taken orally and used to treat advanced liver cancer.

CLIENT EDUCATION: Report bleeding, heart palpitations, and chest pain.

Hepatic arterial infusion

- Systemically delivered chemotherapy is largely ineffective in treating tumors of the liver or prolonging life. Therefore, more direct delivery methods are used.
- The direct infusion of chemotherapy via a catheter into the tumor. The client can go home with a catheter in place if continuous infusion is desired. Systemic adverse effects of chemotherapy are avoided through this delivery method. Q EBP

CLIENT EDUCATION: Watch for evidence of infection at the catheter site, hepatic toxicity (jaundice, liver function tests), and immunosuppression (fatigue, decreased WBC).

THERAPEUTIC PROCEDURES

Hepatic artery embolization

Using a catheter threaded through the femoral artery and up to the liver, particles are injected into the arteries that supply blood to the tumor to block blood flow. If a chemotherapeutic medication is included, this procedure is called **chemoembolization**. If radiation is included, this procedure is called **radioembolization**.

NURSING ACTIONS: Monitor for bleeding.

Ablation procedures (82.2)

- Assists in destroying cancerous cells.
- Percutaneous alcohol (ethanol) injections directly into the tumor mass cause cell death.

NURSING ACTIONS
- Monitor for hypothermia, bile leak, and hemorrhage.
- Monitor urine for myoglobinuria.

Tunneled abdominal drain

Often placed and then used at home to remove excess ascetic fluid

NURSING ACTIONS: Reinforce with the client and family how to empty the drain and maintain the system.

CLIENT EDUCATION: Do not remove more than 2,000 mL at one time to prevent hypovolemia shock.

External radiation

Although liver cancer cells are sensitive to radiation, the treatment cannot be used at very high doses because normal liver tissue is also easily damaged.

Surgical interventions

Surgical resection or liver transplantation is required for long-term survival. Q EBP

Surgical resection: If liver cancer involves only one lobe of the liver and has not spread beyond the liver, surgical removal is often indicated. A liver-lobe resection can result in a survival rate of up to 5 years. Most liver tumors are not resectable.

Liver transplantation is an option for clients who have small primary tumors.
- Immunosuppressants administered after the transplant can increase the risk for recurrence of cancer and for development of secondary infection.
- For interprofessional care, see **CHAPTER 81: CANCER TREATMENT OPTIONS**.

NURSING ACTIONS
- Monitor for altered blood glucose due to stress on the liver caused by surgery.
- Monitor for bleeding. Replace fluids and blood as necessary.

CLIENT EDUCATION: Diagnostic tests to determine if the liver cancer has metastasized include chest x-ray, PET scan, MRI, and laparoscopy.

COMPLICATIONS

- Acute graft rejection following liver transplantation
- Liver failure or kidney failure (due to impaired blood flow to the kidneys)

Kidney and renal pelvis cancer

- Adenocarcinoma of the kidney, or renal cell cancer, is the most common form of kidney cancer.
- Paraneoplastic syndromes (syndromes resulting from cancer in the body) can occur with renal cell cancer. The tumor can produce hormones or prevent hormone production, causing imbalance in the body. Effects include the following.
  - Anemia (reduced erythropoietin)
  - Erythrocytosis (excess erythropoietin)
  - Hypercalcemia (tumor production of parathyroid hormone)
  - Liver dysfunction
  - Increased sedimentation rate
  - Hypertension (increased renin)
- Renal cell cancer is discovered when imaging studies or exploratory surgery are performed for other reasons.
- Renal cell cancer that spreads to the inferior vena cava has a poor prognosis.

HEALTH PROMOTION AND DISEASE PREVENTION

Minimize exposure to chemicals (environmental).

DATA COLLECTION

RISK FACTORS

- Von Hippel-Lindau syndrome
- Exposure to lead, cadmium, or phosphate
- Age (55 to 60 years: highest incidence)
- Family history of kidney, bladder, ureter, prostate gland, uterus, ovary, or appendix cancer.
- Genetic and hereditary risk factors
- African American and American Indian descent

EXPECTED FINDINGS

- Smoky or cola-colored urine Q̲EBP
- Hematuria (late finding)
- Inability to urinate or weak urine stream (urinary tract obstruction)
- Abdominal or flank pain (often dull, aching)
- Palpable mass
- Renal bruit (possible)
- Weight loss
- Fever
- Hypertension
- Hypercalcemia
- Hyperglycemia
- Fatigue
- Anemia or polycythemia

DIAGNOSTIC PROCEDURES

Biopsy (percutaneous through the flank)

EXPECTED FINDINGS: Positive for cancer

NURSING ACTIONS
- Provide the client with diagnosis-specific information.
- Place a pressure dressing over the puncture site.
- Maintain client activity restrictions (bed rest laying supine for at least 6 hr).
- Monitor for bleeding by checking vital signs, biopsy site, hemoglobin and hematocrit, flank pain, and color of urine for the first 24 hr.

Urinalysis

Urine cytology checks for cancer cells.

EXPECTED FINDINGS: Hematuria (possible)

NURSING ACTIONS
- Inform the client of other reasons for hematuria.
- Reinforce information with the client about the role of the kidneys in red blood cell production.

CLIENT EDUCATION: Elevated ESR is related to chronic kidney disease.

Nuclear imaging (IV urogram with nephrograms)

EXPECTED FINDINGS: Presence of tumor

NURSING ACTIONS
- Prepare the client for the procedure. (Keep NPO. Check for contrast dye allergy.)
- Inform the client of other reasons for increased LFTs.

Imaging (CT, MRI, PET scans)

Identifies tumor borders and presence in surrounding tissue

NURSING ACTIONS: Prepare the client for imaging.

Hematologic studies

EXPECTED FINDINGS
- **Hgb/Hct:** decreased
- **Ca:** elevated
- **ESR:** elevated with chronic kidney disease
- **ACTH:** elevated
- **hCG:** elevated
- **BUN/creatinine:** elevated
- **LFTs:** increases

NURSING ACTIONS: Inform clients regarding lab-specific findings.

PATIENT-CENTERED CARE

NURSING CARE

Monitor urine output and laboratory findings (BUN, serum creatinine, urinalysis) to check renal function of the unaffected kidney.

THERAPEUTIC PROCEDURES

Radiation

With extensive disease, radiation is combined with chemotherapy.

Targeted therapy (82.2)

Immunotherapy (biotherapy) (82.2)

Ablation therapy for kidney cancer (82.2)

- Administered to destroy cancerous cells
- Arterial embolization is performed through a catheter to deliver material to block the artery that feeds the kidney with the tumor.

Chemotherapy

Kidney cancer cells are usually resistant to chemotherapy. However, chemotherapy can be used after targeted medication or immunotherapy.

Surgical interventions

The client who undergoes surgery for renal cell cancer (RCC) is at increased risk for bleeding due to the highly vascular nature of RCC.

Nephrectomy is the standard of treatment for RCC.
- Removal of ribs during surgery allows better access to the kidney or tumor.
- Surgical entry includes one of three approaches: transthoracic, lumbar, or abdominal with placement of a wound drain.
- Adrenal glands are left intact when possible.
- The unaffected kidney should sustain adequate renal function.

NURSING ACTIONS

- Monitor vital signs and daily weight.
- Monitor lung sounds, respiratory effort, or presence of sputum production.
  - Monitor for evidence of bleeding (hypotension, decreased urine output, altered level of consciousness). Blood can pool under the client's back.
  - Monitor for adrenal insufficiency (nausea, vomiting, diarrhea, hypoglycemia, hypotension).
  - Monitor hemoglobin, hematocrit, and WBC every 6 to 12 hr for first 24 to 48 hr.
  - Monitor urine output to determine remaining kidney function (25 to 30 mL/hr).
  - Monitor incision drainage.
  - Label, secure with tape, and monitor all drainage tubes (catheters, stents, nephrostomy tubes or drains).
- Administer opioid analgesics for pain (PCA, intercostal blocks).

CLIENT EDUCATION

- Avoid lifting more than 5 lb or engaging in strenuous activity.
- Care for the incision and any remaining drainage tubes, catheters, or stents.
- Report manifestations of UTIs and other complications to the provider.
- Protect the function of the remaining kidney. (Control blood pressure. Drink adequate fluids. Limit NSAID use. Stop smoking.) **Qs**

COMPLICATIONS

Adrenal insufficiency

Manifestations of adrenal insufficiency are similar to those of hemorrhage (hypotension, decreased urine output, altered level of consciousness).

Spinal cord decompression

- RCC can expand and compress the spinal cord.
- Key manifestations include sharp, severe, band-like pain.

NURSING ACTIONS

- Report pain findings to the provider.
- Prepare the client for imaging studies to determine spinal cord decompression.

Urinary bladder cancer

- Bladder cancer begins most often in the transitional cell layer.
- There are four layers of the bladder wall: transitional epithelium (innermost layer), lamina propria, muscularis propria, and fatty connective tissue. As cancer advances, it grows through the next layer.
- Bladder cancer can be invasive (cancer cells grow outside of the transitional epithelium) or noninvasive (cancer cells remain in the transitional epithelium layer). Bladder cancer is often described based on how far it invades the bladder wall.
- Transitional cell carcinoma can be further classified as papillary or flat based on how it grows.

HEALTH PROMOTION AND DISEASE PREVENTION

- Use personal protective equipment (PPE) when handling chemicals, paints, fertilizers, gases, or items that contain specific environmental chemicals.
- When working with chemicals is unavoidable, shower and don clean clothing after task completion.

DATA COLLECTION

RISK FACTORS

- Frequent contact with rubber, paint, electric cable, leather processing, or nitrates
- Inhalation of gas, fumes, or chemical compounds
- Tobacco use
- Schistosoma haematobium (parasite) infection
- Long-term cyclophosphamide use
- Male sex
- Chronic urinary tract inflammation
- Caucasian clients
- Age older than 55

CAUSES OF CHRONIC BLADDER IRRITATION: UTI, kidney and bladder stones, chronic bladder catheters

EXPECTED FINDINGS

- Hematuria
- Dysuria, frequency, urgency (infection or obstruction)
- Weight loss
- Anorexia

DIAGNOSTIC PROCEDURES

Biopsy (cystoscopic)

EXPECTED FINDINGS: Presence of cancer or bladder lesions

NURSING ACTIONS: Prepare the client for cystoscopy.

Bladder wash

EXPECTED FINDINGS: Presence of cancerous cells in saline wash solution (definitive diagnosis)

CLIENT EDUCATION: Saline will be instilled into the bladder, then retrieved for microscopic examination.

Imaging (CT scan, MRI)

EXPECTED FINDINGS
- CT scan: extent of tumor invasion
- MRI: depth and spread of tumor

NURSING ACTIONS: Prepare the client for imaging.

Nuclear imaging

IV (excretory) urography and pyelography

EXPECTED FINDINGS: Possible changes in structure or function of the urinary tract

NURSING ACTIONS: Prepare the client for the procedure. (Keep NPO. Check for contrast allergy.)

Urinalysis

Urine cytology is used to check for cancer cells.

EXPECTED FINDINGS: Microscopic or gross hematuria

NURSING ACTIONS: Inform the client of other possible reasons for hematuria.

82.6 Urinary diversions

	URETER DIVERSION	PORTAL OF EXIT	URINARY ELIMINATION
Ileal conduit	Ileum segment separated and formed into tubular pouch to drain ureters	Abdominal stoma-tubular pouch brought to skin surface	Continuous drainage into external pouch
Continent urinary diversion	Pouch created from ileum or terminal ileum combined with the ascending colon	Abdominal stoma	Penrose drain and catheter might be present until sutures heal. Client performs intermittent urinary catheterization.
Bladder reconstruction (neobladder)	Pouch created from small intestine	Urethra	Client performs intermittent urinary catheterization.
Ureterosigmoidostomy		Anus	During bowel movement

PATIENT-CENTERED CARE

THERAPEUTIC PROCEDURES

Intravesical treatments

Intravesical chemotherapy: Chemotherapy medications are administered directly into the bladder. Many of these medications are administered systemically during chemotherapy.

Intravesical immunotherapy uses biologic response modifiers (BRMs) to stimulate the immune system to target and destroy cancer cells.
- Bacillus Calmette-Guérin (BCG)
  - BCG is a live virus compound commonly used to vaccinate high-risk individuals against tuberculosis.
  - BCG is infused into the bladder and retained for 2 hr.
- Other BRM medications frequently administered for bladder cancer are mitomycin and thiotepa directly in to the bladder and in combination with other chemotherapy medications.

NURSING ACTIONS Qpcc
- Ask the client to void, then insert an indwelling urinary catheter for therapy infusion.
- After infusion, position the client on the back, abdomen, and each side for 15 min in each position.
- Assist the client to a standing position. Ensure the client can safely stand for the second hour.
- After the 2 hr dwell time, the urinary catheter is removed and the client is instructed to sit to void. This position prevents urine splashing and reduces the risk of contamination.
- Provide or assist with perineal cleansing.

CLIENT EDUCATION
- Restrict fluids for 4 hr prior to infusion therapy.
- Use precautions to prevent exposure of others to BCG over the following 24 hr. After each voiding (sitting position), perform the following.
  - Cleanse the genitals.
  - Disinfect the urine by pouring 10% bleach solution (in an amount equal to the void) into the toilet prior to flushing.
  - Cleanse the seat and toilet surfaces.
- Wash clothing and linen that comes in contact with urine within 24 hr following infusion.
- Avoid sexual intercourse for 24 hr following the infusion.
- Possible adverse reactions to intravesical chemotherapy include bladder irritation, frequency, dysuria, and contact dermatitis.

Systemic chemotherapy

Often used alone or in combination with radiation. Chemotherapy is often administered before surgery (neoadjuvant) or after surgery (adjuvant). Several courses of chemotherapy are needed because a fixed percentage of cells are killed with each course. The goal is to reduce the number of malignant cells until the body's immune system can take over. In general, the maximum amount of chemotherapy the client can tolerate is given with each course.

External beam radiation (82.2)

- Often used to shrink tumors before surgery, or together with chemotherapy to reduce the risk of tumor recurrence.
- EBRT can cause radiation cystitis.

Surgical interventions

- Surface excision, transurethral resection of bladder tumors, and partial cystectomy (removal of part of the bladder) are used to treat small, confined tumors.
- Radical cystectomy with removal of surrounding tissue or muscle is used for large, invasive, or recurrent tumors. Intensive care can be required following extensive bladder repair. Ureters are diverted to another location. (82.6)
- Internal or external drains or catheters can be placed intraoperatively.
- Clients who have neobladder surgery are at risk for extreme weight loss.
- Radical cystectomy with lymph node dissection includes the removal of other pelvic structures.
  - In males, the removal of the seminal vesicles and prostate with possible urethrectomy, resulting in impotence
  - In females, the removal of the ovaries, fallopian tubes, uterus, cervix, anterior vaginal wall, and urethra, resulting in sterility

NURSING ACTIONS
- Consult enterostomal therapy to assist with management and client/family education related to urinary diversion. Qpcc
- Provide adequate nutrition, snacks, and supplements to clients who have bladder reconstruction. Consult nutrition services as needed.
- Monitor output from drains or catheters for expected color and amount.
- Notify the provider if urine is decreased or absent in a client who has an external pouch.
- Secure the external drainage catheter. Notify the provider if it becomes dislodged or removed.

CLIENT EDUCATION
- Plan to self-catheterize at timed intervals, because of lack of bladder sensation when the bladder is full (neobladder, continent pouch).
- Monitor peristomal skin for redness, excoriation, or infection (ileal conduit, continent pouch).

COMPLICATIONS

Hydronephrosis

- Inability to eliminate urine causes dilation of the renal pelvis.
- A tumor that blocks the urinary tract can prevent urinary elimination.

NURSING ACTIONS: Notify the provider if urine output is decreased or absent.

Breast cancer

- Breast cancer is the second-leading cause of cancer deaths in females in the U.S.
- Breast cancer in males is rare.
- Breast cancer can be invasive (most common) or noninvasive.
- Common sites of metastasis are bone, lung, brain, and liver. Q**EBP**

Noninvasive breast cancers

Ductal carcinoma in situ (DCIS)
- Cancer cells are located in the duct and have not invaded surrounding tissue.
- DCIS cells lack the biologic capacity to metastasize.

Lobular carcinoma in situ (LCIS)
- Abnormal cell growth occurs in the milk-producing glands.
- Can increase risk of developing a separate invasive breast cancer at a later time.
- Managed with observation.
- When other risk factors exist, prophylactic treatment (tamoxifen, raloxifene, mastectomy) can be considered. Cancer originates in the mammary ducts and grows in the epithelial cells lining the ducts.

Invasive breast cancers

Infiltrating ductal carcinoma
- Can present as a lump, skin dimpling, or edematous thickening and pitting of breast skin (orange peel).
- Staging of the disease determines the prognosis and treatment plan.
- Invasive breast cancers can metastasize to other areas of breast tissue, lymph, and blood vessels.

Inflammatory breast cancer (IBC)
- Can present as swelling, skin redness, warmth, and breast pain
- Seldom presents as a lump and might not be present on a mammogram

HEALTH PROMOTION AND DISEASE PREVENTION

- Consume at least five servings of fruits and vegetables daily.
- Perform breast self-exam (BSE) and clinical breast exam (CBE).
- Obtain screening mammography.
- Maintain healthy weight.
- Engage in regular physical exercise.
- Minimize alcohol intake.
- Breastfeeding for 1 year or more decreases breast cancer risk.
- Avoid hormone replacement therapy.
- Avoid environmental estrogens.

DATA COLLECTION

RISK FACTORS

- High genetic risk
  - Inherited mutations of BRCA1 and BRCA2
  - History of previous breast cancer
  - Dense breast tissue Q**EBP**
  - Biopsy confirmed atypical hyperplasia
  - Early age at diagnosis
  - Female sex
- Age older than 50 years
- First-degree relative who has breast cancer
- Early menarche
- Late menopause
- Nulliparity or first pregnancy after age 30
- Early or prolonged use of oral contraceptives
- Low-fiber diet
- Excessive alcohol intake (possibly related to folic acid depletion)
- Cigarette smoking
- Exposure to low-level radiation
- Hormone replacement therapy
- Recent oral birth control use
- Obesity
- Breast cancer rates are expected to increase over the next 50 years due to the increase of the older adult population. **ⓖ**
- Older adult clients are at greater risk of complications following surgery for cancer.

EXPECTED FINDINGS

- Breast change (appearance, texture, presence of lumps)
- Breast pain or soreness
- Persistent skin rash near the nipple area.

PHYSICAL FINDINGS
- Skin changes (*peau d'orange*) **(82.7)**
- Dimpling
- Breast tumors (usually small, irregularly shaped, firm, nontender, and nonmobile)
- Increased vascularity
- Nipple discharge
- Nipple retraction or ulceration
- Enlarged lymph nodes above the collarbone or in the armpit

DIAGNOSTIC PROCEDURES

MALES: Breast cancer is often diagnosed later, with a poorer prognosis. Clients at increased risk should discuss a screening plan with the provider.

FEMALES: Early, frequent screening and an MRI are necessary for clients who have breast changes or who are at high risk.

Breast self-exam, clinical breast exam

EXPECTED FINDINGS: Palpable tumors or lesions

CLIENT EDUCATION
- Perform BSE monthly.
- Premenopausal clients should perform BSE after their menstrual period.
- Have regular CBE (every 3 years from age 20 to 39; yearly over 40 years of age).

Mammography

EXPECTED FINDINGS: Visualization of the lesion

NURSING ACTIONS: Reinforce information for the client regarding additional diagnostic testing if needed.

Biopsy (open or fine-needle)

EXPECTED FINDINGS: Definitive diagnosis of cancer cell type

NURSING ACTIONS: Provide diagnosis-specific information.

Genetic testing

EXPECTED FINDINGS
- **BRCA1 and BRCA2:** Gene mutation increases breast cancer risk.
- **HER2:** Excess HER2 (normal gene that causes cell replication) indicates the need for targeted therapy.

CLIENT EDUCATION: Genetic testing is recommended for BRCA1 and BRCA2 for clients at risk (two first-degree relatives diagnosed with breast cancer prior to age 50 or family history of breast and ovarian cancer).

MRI

EXPECTED FINDINGS: Better visualization of lesions in the client who has dense breasts.

NURSING ACTIONS: Prepare client for imaging.

Nuclear imaging: breast-specific gamma imaging

EXPECTED FINDINGS: Visualization of the lesion

CLIENT EDUCATION: Scanning will display the uptake of the radioactive substance injected prior to the procedure.

Positron emission mammography (PEM)

Type of PET scan

EXPECTED FINDINGS: Visualization of the lesion

CLIENT EDUCATION: PEM provides consistent images despite hormone fluctuations.

Ultrasound (US)

Ultrasound determines if a lesion is a solid or cystic mass.

EXPECTED FINDINGS: Visualization of the lesion

CLIENT EDUCATION: An ultrasound provides better visualization of lesions in clients who have dense breasts.

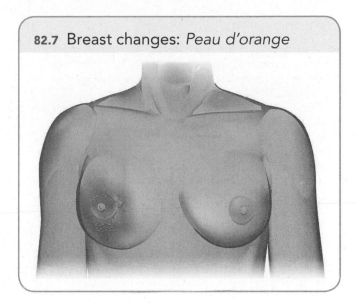

82.7 Breast changes: *Peau d'orange*

X-ray

EXPECTED FINDINGS: Visualization of the lesion (digital mammography is more accurate)

CLIENT EDUCATION: If older than 40 years, schedule an annual mammogram.

Other tests

Chest x-ray, CT scan, MRI, liver enzymes, serum calcium and alkaline phosphatase

EXPECTED FINDINGS: Metastatic disease

NURSING ACTIONS: Provide diagnosis-specific information.

PATIENT-CENTERED CARE

THERAPEUTIC PROCEDURES

Adjuvant therapy follows surgery to decrease the risk of reoccurrence.

Hormone therapy

Most effective in cancer cells with estrogen or progesterone receptors. This type of cancer has a better prognosis.

Ovarian ablation to stop the production of estrogen
- Inhibits estrogen synthesis.
- Used in premenopausal women to stop or prevent the growth of breast tumors.

Selective estrogen receptor modulators (SERMs): Toremifene (tamoxifen and raloxifene)
- Used in clients who are have a high risk for developing breast cancer or who have advanced breast cancer. Q EBP
- Suppress the growth of remaining cancer cells postoperatively following mastectomy or lumpectomy by blocking estrogen.
- Tamoxifen has been found to increase the risk of endometrial cancer, deep-vein thrombosis, and pulmonary embolism. Raloxifene does not share these adverse effects.

Chemotherapy/radiation therapy

- Chemotherapy and radiation can augment or replace a mastectomy, depending on several factors (client's age, hormone status related to menopause, genetic predisposition, staging of disease).
- Clients who undergo chemotherapy are usually given a combination of several medications.
- Radiation therapy is usually reserved for clients who had a lumpectomy or breast-conserving procedure to decrease or destroy cells that have metastasized.
    - Whole or partial breast radiation can be prescribed. Skin care is a priority concern due to radiation damage and generalized fatigue.
    - Brachytherapy with radioactive seeds can also be an option.
    - Intraoperative radiation therapy allows an intense dose of radiation to be delivered directly to the surgical site.

Surgical interventions

Surgical procedures include lumpectomy (breast-conserving), wide excision or partial mastectomy, total mastectomy, modified radical mastectomy (lymph nodes removed), radical mastectomy (lymph nodes and muscle removed), and reconstructive surgery. (82.8)

NURSING ACTIONS

- Ask the client to sit with the head of the bed elevated 30° when awake and support the arm on the affected side on a pillow. Lying on the unaffected side can relieve pain.
- Tell the client to wear a sling while ambulating (to support the arm).
- Avoid administering injections, taking blood pressure, or obtaining blood from the affected arm. Place a sign above the bed regarding these precautions. Qs
- Emphasize the importance of a well-fitted breast prosthesis for a client who had a mastectomy.
- Provide emotional support to the client and family.

- Encourage the client to express feelings related to perception of sexuality and body image.
- Reinforce teaching with the client on how to care for the incision and drainage tubes. (Drains are usually left in for 1 to 3 weeks.)
- Reinforce teaching regarding BSE.

CLIENT EDUCATION

- Avoid placing the arm on the affected side in a dependent position. This position will interfere with wound healing.
- Engage in early arm and hand exercises (squeezing a rubber ball, elbow flexion and extension, hand-wall climbing) to prevent lymphedema and to regain full range of motion.
- Do not wear constrictive clothing, and avoid cuts and injuries to the arm on the affected side.
- Avoid lifting heavy objects with arm on the affected side.
- Report excessive bleeding to the provider.
- Report numbness, pain, heaviness, or impaired motor function of the affected arm to the surgeon.
- Discuss breast reconstruction alternatives with the surgeon.
    - Reconstruction can begin during the original breast removal procedure or after some healing occurs.
    - A tissue expander (saline-filled implant that has a port through which additional saline can be injected, gradually expanding the tissue prior to permanent implant) is often placed during the original procedure.
    - Saline or silicone implants are used for permanent placement.
    - Autologous flaps can also be used for reconstruction.
    - Nipple reconstruction is performed using tissue from the labia, abdomen, or inner thigh or by using tissue from the opposite nipple.
- Genetic counseling for the client who tests positive for the BRCA1/BRCA2 genetic mutation includes recommendation of bilateral mastectomy and oophorectomy to prevent cancer occurrence. The client who does not choose this option should have early, frequent, thorough screening for breast and ovarian cancer. QTC

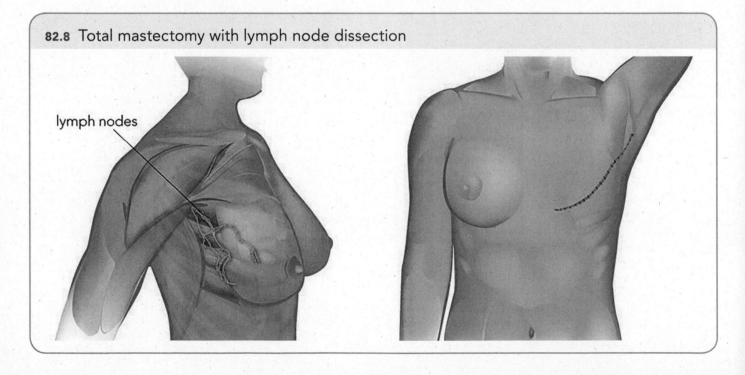

82.8 Total mastectomy with lymph node dissection

lymph nodes

Other procedures

The client who is at high risk for recurrence or who has advanced disease can have stem cell (autologous or allogeneic) implantation.

COMPLICATIONS

A common complication is disfigurement of part of the chest wall and mastitis.

Ovarian cancer

- Ovarian cancers are epithelial tumors that grow on the surface of the ovaries.
- The tumors grow quickly and are often bilateral.
- Metastases frequently occur before the primary ovarian malignancy is diagnosed.
- Ovarian cancer is the leading cause of death from female reproductive cancers.
- The exact etiology of ovarian cancer is unknown. However, the more times a clients ovulates in a lifetime, the greater the risk. Ovarian cancer is more prevalent in clients who have early menarche, late-onset menopause, or nulliparity, and those who use infertility agents.

HEALTH PROMOTION AND DISEASE PREVENTION

- Birth control pills and pregnancy can offer protection against ovarian cancer (reduced estrogen exposure).
- Risk-reducing or prophylactic bilateral salpingo-oophorectomy helps protect clients who have BRCA1 or BRCA2 mutations against ovarian cancer.
- Although regular exams are recommended, it is difficult to palpate ovarian tumors during a pelvic exam.

DATA COLLECTION

RISK FACTORS

- Age greater than 40 years
- Nulliparity or first pregnancy after 30 years of age
- Family history of ovarian, breast, or genetic mutation for hereditary nonpolyposis colon cancer (HNPCC)
- BRCA1 or BRCA2 gene mutations
- Diabetes mellitus
- Early menarche/late menopause
- History of dysmenorrhea or heavy bleeding
- Endometriosis
- High-fat diet
- Hormone replacement therapy
- History of infertility
- European American females
- Use of infertility medications
- Older adult clients following surgery for cancer Ⓖ

EXPECTED FINDINGS

- Abdominal pain or swelling
- Abdominal discomfort (dyspepsia, indigestion, gas, distention) Ⓠᴇʙᴾ
- Abdominal mass
- Constipation
- Urinary frequency
- Unexpected weight loss
- Vaginal bleeding
- Urinary frequency or incontinence
- Enlarged ovary

DIAGNOSTIC PROCEDURES

- There is no specific test for ovarian cancer.
- Staging of ovarian cancer is determined at the time of the hysterectomy or exploratory laparotomy when the tumor is removed and examined by the pathologist.

Biopsy through laparoscopy

EXPECTED FINDINGS: Presence of cancer cells

CLIENT EDUCATION: Biopsy is usually performed during surgery to remove the tumor.

Genetic testing

EXPECTED FINDINGS: **BRCA1** and **BRCA2** gene mutation increases ovarian cancer risk.

CLIENT EDUCATION: Genetic testing is often used to determine risk of developing ovarian cancer, but it is not used to diagnose or monitor treatment.

Tumor markers

EXPECTED FINDINGS: Elevated CA125 measurement can indicate ovarian cancer but can indicate cancer from another source.

Transvaginal ultrasound, chest x-ray, CT or PET scan

EXPECTED FINDINGS: Metastatic disease

NURSING ACTIONS: Reinforce teaching with the client regarding implications of metastatic disease, and offer emotional support.

PATIENT-CENTERED CARE

THERAPEUTIC PROCEDURES

Chemotherapy (traditional or intraperitoneal)

Chemotherapy is always given for ovarian cancer, even if surgery is performed. Cisplatin and carboplatin are the most common chemotherapeutic medications used for ovarian cancer.

NURSING ACTIONS: Monitor temperature, white blood cell (WBC) count, and absolute neutrophil count.

CLIENT EDUCATION
- Side effects of chemotherapy include nausea, vomiting, loss of appetite, mouth and vaginal sores, and hair loss.
- Report findings of infection, including peritonitis.

Surgical interventions

Exploratory laparotomy can be performed to diagnose, treat, and stage ovarian tumors. Debulking (cytoreduction) of very large tumors can be done laparoscopically.

A total abdominal hysterectomy (TAH) with bilateral salpingectomy and oophorectomy (BSO) is the usual treatment for ovarian cancer. TAH with BSO also helps determine the extent of the disease as well as local and distant metastases. Staging of the cancer is done at this time with inspection of other organs for metastasis.

NURSING ACTIONS
- Observe for urinary retention and difficulty voiding.
- Check for bowel sounds. Paralytic ileus can occur due to manipulation of the bowel during surgery.
- Discuss sexuality, surgically induced menopause, and other self-image issues with the client.

CLIENT EDUCATION
- Avoid straining, driving, lifting more than 5 lb, douching, and participating in sexual intercourse until the provider gives release.
- Immediately report evidence of infection, as well as vaginal discharge that is excessive or has a foul odor.

COMPLICATIONS

Abdominal ascites and intestinal obstruction

Uterine (endometrial) cancer

- Endometrial cancer is the most common gynecological cancer.
- Endometrial cancer is more common in older adult clients (related to prolonged exposure to estrogen). Ⓖ
- Estrogen therapy in postmenopausal clients who have a uterus should include progesterone to decrease the risk of endometrial cancer.
- Endometrial cancer is curable. The client who is diagnosed and treated early can have a 5-year survival rate greater than 90%.

HEALTH PROMOTION AND DISEASE PREVENTION

Avoid the use of unopposed estrogen when considering postmenopausal hormone replacement therapy.

DATA COLLECTION

RISK FACTORS

- Family history of endometrial or colorectal cancer
- Personal history of breast or ovarian cancer
- Diabetes mellitus
- Genetic mutation for HNPCC
- Age greater than 50 years
- Obesity (due to fat cell production of estrogen)
- Unopposed estrogen hormone replacement therapy
- Nulliparity
- Use of tamoxifen to prevent or treat breast cancer
- Late menopause (longer-term exposure to significant estrogen levels)

EXPECTED FINDINGS

- Irregular and postmenopausal bleeding
- Vaginal discharge
- On pelvic examination, uterus enlargement
- Low-back, abdominal, or low pelvic pain

DIAGNOSTIC PROCEDURES

Biopsy

EXPECTED FINDINGS: Endometrial biopsy: presence of carcinoma

CLIENT EDUCATION: Biopsy is usually performed through transvaginal ultrasound.

Pathology testing for staging

EXPECTED FINDINGS: Extent, size of tumor, metastasis

CLIENT EDUCATION: Staging occurs after exploratory laparotomy or hysterectomy following tumor removal.

Tumor markers

EXPECTED FINDINGS: **Cancer antigen-125 (CA-125):** positive

CLIENT EDUCATION: Results indicate some type of carcinoma.

Transvaginal ultrasound and endometrial biopsy

Endometrial thickness and presence of carcinoma

Other tests to determine metastatic cancer

Chest x-ray, intravenous pyelography, abdominal ultrasound, CT of the pelvis, MRI of abdomen/pelvis, and liver and bone scans

PATIENT-CENTERED CARE

THERAPEUTIC PROCEDURES

Radiation therapy (82.2)

- Given as adjuvant therapy, usually after a hysterectomy.
- Brachytherapy and external radiation therapy can be options for cancer that is no longer limited to the uterus.

Brachytherapy: Low dose rate involves the use radioactive implants that are left in place for about 1 to 4 days.

External beam radiation therapy (EBRT)
- Can be used in combination with surgery, brachytherapy, and/or chemotherapy
- Often given 5 days/week for 4 to 6 weeks on an outpatient basis
- Treatment area is marked with permanent ink or injected dye.
- A mold of the pelvis and lower back is used to maintain the exact position for treatment.
- NURSING ACTIONS: Reinforce teaching regarding radiation cystitis and proctitis. Q̇EBP
- CLIENT EDUCATION
  - Side effects include fatigue, nausea, vomiting, loose stool, and vaginal dryness.
  - Monitor for signs of skin breakdown in the perineal area.
  - Avoid sunbathing.
  - Avoid washing treatment areas marked with ink.

Chemotherapy (82.2)

- Often given in cycles (a period of treatment, followed by a rest period).
- Combination treatment is better than one medication alone.
- Common chemotherapy agents for endometrial cancer include doxorubicin, cisplatin, paclitaxel, and carboplatin.

CLIENT EDUCATION: Side effects of chemotherapy include nausea, vomiting, loss of appetite, mouth and vaginal sores, and hair loss.

NURSING ACTIONS: Monitor temperature, WBC count, and ANC.

Surgical interventions

Total hysterectomy with bilateral salpingectomy/oophorectomy is the standard treatment. The vagina is spared.
- An open, laparoscopic, or vaginal approach can be used.
- Peritoneal fluid sampling during this procedure allows for testing of metastasis to the peritoneal cavity.

NURSING ACTIONS
- Observe for urinary retention and difficulty voiding due to proximity to the urethra (more common after vaginal hysterectomy).
- Monitor bowel sounds for paralytic ileus (more common due to manipulation of the bowel during surgery).
- Discuss sexuality, surgically induced menopause, and other self-image issues with the client.
- Discuss hormone replacement therapy options with the client if premenopausal.

CLIENT EDUCATION
- Avoid straining, driving, lifting more than 5 lb, douching, and sexual intercourse until the provider gives release.
- Immediately report evidence of infection, excess vaginal discharge, or foul-smelling drainage.

COMPLICATIONS

Anemia and uterine perforation

Cervical cancer

Cervical cancer is slow-growing. With proper screening, it is detected early and treated with good results.

Early cervical cancer is often undetected. Manifestations do not occur until the cancer has become invasive.

Human papillomavirus (HPV) is the leading cause of cervical cancer. Most cervical cancers are related to infection of the cervix with HPV.

HEALTH PROMOTION AND DISEASE PREVENTION

- Receive vaccine series with HPV vaccine between 9 and 26 years of age, before first sexual contact. Ⓖ
- Obtain Pap and pelvic exams for cervical cancer screening.
- Obtain HPV screening (co-testing) every 5 years for women aged 30 to 65 years.
- Limit the number of sexual partners.
- Use condoms during sexual intercourse.

DATA COLLECTION

RISK FACTORS

- Infection with high-risk HPV types (strains 16 and 18), which is associated in 90% of cases Q**EBP**
- Chronic cervical inflammation/infections
- Infection with HIV or other immunosuppressive disorder
- History of sexually transmitted infections
- Sexual activity before 18 years of age
- Client or male partner who had multiple sexual partners
- Male partner who had a partner with cervical cancer
- Family history of cervical cancer
- African American descent
- Cigarette smoking

EXPECTED FINDINGS

- Painless vaginal bleeding between menses
- Dysuria, hematuria
- Watery, blood-tinged, or white vaginal discharge
- Unexplained weight loss
- Pelvic pain
- Pain during and after vaginal sexual intercourse
- Rectal bleeding or bloody stools
- Hematuria
- Chest pain, coughing

DIAGNOSTIC PROCEDURES

Simultaneous PAP test and HPV testing improves the accuracy of the reading.

Papanicolaou (Pap) test

EXPECTED FINDINGS: Abnormal cells

CLIENT EDUCATION
- Begin Pap screening by 21 years of age (or 3 years following first sexual intercourse). Frequency of screening depends on many factors (age, results, presence of a cervix).
- The Pap is a screening tool and not diagnostic. An abnormal Pap requires additional testing.

Biopsy

EXPECTED FINDINGS: Abnormal cells (follow-up to Pap test)

NURSING ACTIONS: Provide diagnosis-specific information to the client.

HPV typing: DNA test

EXPECTED FINDINGS: Presence of HPV on cervical cells

CLIENT EDUCATION: HPV increases the risk of cervical cancer.

Chest x-ray, MRI, CT, PET

EXPECTED FINDINGS: Metastatic/advanced disease

NURSING ACTIONS: Reinforce preprocedure instructions.

PATIENT-CENTERED CARE

NURSING CARE

Administer antibiotics for pelvic, vaginal, or urinary tract infections.

THERAPEUTIC PROCEDURES

Removal of the lesion

- By conization, cryotherapy, laser ablation, hysterectomy, or a loop electrosurgical excision procedure.
- Conization (removal of a cone-shaped wedge of cervical tissue) is used as either a diagnostic procedure or treatment in early cancer.

CLIENT EDUCATION
- Report heavy vaginal bleeding, foul-smelling drainage, or fever to the provider. Q**PCC**
- Vaginal discharge is normal.
- Take showers rather than tub baths.
- Avoid heavy lifting, vaginal penetration, douches, and tampons for the prescribed time (typically 3 weeks).

Radiation

Brachytherapy and external radiation therapy is an option for cancer that is not limited to local invasion.

NURSING ACTIONS
- Monitor for skin damage, especially in the perineal area.
- Chemotherapy can be used along with radiation.

Surgical interventions

Hysterectomy: The client who has early stage cervical cancer can require a **simple hysterectomy** (removes the uterus and cervix) or a **radical hysterectomy** (removes the uterus, upper third of the vagina, uterosacral uterovesical ligaments, and pelvic nodes). The choice to have a hysterectomy can be guided by the client's condition and desire for future childbearing.

Exenteration: Clients who have more extensive cancer can require this more extensive pelvic surgery.
- **Anterior exenteration** involves removal of the uterus, cervix, fallopian tubes, vagina, ovaries, bladder, urethra, and pelvic lymph nodes. An ileal conduit is established for urinary diversion.
- **Posterior exenteration** involves removal of the uterus, cervix, fallopian tubes, vagina, ovaries, anal canal, rectum, and descending colon. A colostomy is established for bowel diversion.
- **Total exenteration** involves removal of all of the above organs and establishment of both urinary and bowel diversions.

NURSING ACTIONS

- Manage drains as well as urinary and bowel diversions.
- Check for body image disturbance and encourage the client to speak openly about it.
- Reinforce teaching with the client about findings of wound infection and how to care for drains that can remain after discharge.
- Reinforce teaching with the client about how to care for urinary and bowel diversion.
- Reinforce teaching with the client about how to care for perineal wounds and expectations regarding discharge.

COMPLICATIONS

- Fistula development can occur after pelvic exenteration or radiation.
- Kidney infections are also common secondary to the urinary diversion.

Prostate cancer

- This is the second most common type of cancer in males.
- Prostate cancer is slow-growing. Conservative treatment is the treatment of choice, based on how fast the cancer is growing, if it has spread, and the client's age and life expectancy. Treatment can be delayed up to 10 years following diagnosis.
- The posterior lobe or outer gland epithelium are sites of origin for most prostate cancer. It is usually slow-growing in response to androgen (testosterone and dihydrotestosterone).
- Manifestations are often similar to those of benign prostatic hyperplasia.

HEALTH PROMOTION AND DISEASE PREVENTION

- Consume a diet low in animal fat. Include omega-3 fatty acids (fish), fruits, and vegetables.
- Engage in regular exercise.
- Discuss prostate-specific antigen (PSA) screening with a provider.

DATA COLLECTION

RISK FACTORS

- History of vasectomy
- Age greater than 65 years (risk increases with age) ©
- Family history
- African American descent
- High-fat, complex-carbohydrate, low-fiber diet
- Prostate cancer antigen gene (PCA3) is associated with an increased risk
- Rapid growth of the prostate (benign high-grade prostatic intraepithelial neoplasia)
- Exposure to environmental toxins, such as arsenic and some chemicals

EXPECTED FINDINGS

- Usually no manifestations in early stages
- Urinary manifestations: hesitancy, weak stream, urgency, frequency, nocturia
- Recurrent bladder infections
- Urinary retention
- Blood in urine and semen (late manifestation)
- Painful ejaculation
- Erectile dysfunction
- Pain, particularly bone or joint (pelvis, spine, hips, ribs)
- Unexplained weight loss
- Loss of sexual desire or function
- Penile discharge or scrotal pain/swelling
- Significant residual urine after voiding a small amount of urine
- Swollen lymph nodes, especially in the groin

DIAGNOSTIC PROCEDURES

- Regular screening can begin as early as age 40 for individuals who have high risk.
- PSA levels increase when the client has prostate cancer and should reduce within a few days postoperatively.
- Early prostate cancer antigen (EPCA-1 tissue test and EPVA-2 blood test) is highly sensitive; if positive, biopsy then is excluded.

Digital rectal examination (DRE)

EXPECTED FINDINGS: Hard enlarged prostate with palpable irregularities

NURSING ACTIONS: Ask the client to discuss prostate screening after age 50.

Needle or transrectal ultrasound-guided biopsy

EXPECTED FINDINGS
- Presence of cancer
- Staging is based on biopsy result.

NURSING ACTIONS: Provide diagnosis-specific information to the client.

CLIENT EDUCATION: PSA, age, race, and family history are used to determine if biopsy is needed.

Genetic testing

EXPECTED FINDINGS: PCA3

CLIENT EDUCATION: The presence of the PCA3 gene increases cancer risk.

Prostate specific antigen (PSA)

EXPECTED FINDINGS: Greater than 4 ng/mL indicates possible prostate disease (not specific to carcinoma).

NURSING ACTIONS
- Ask the client to discuss prostate screening after age 50.
- Ensure that the client's PSA is checked prior to DRE to promote accuracy of results.

EPCA-1 and EPCA-2

EXPECTED FINDINGS: Positive (tissue and serum maker for prostate cancer)

CLIENT EDUCATION: Positive results are highly indicative for prostate cancer.

Renal function testing

EXPECTED FINDINGS: BUN and serum creatinine elevated (renal damage)

NURSING ACTIONS: Support the client when unexpected findings are reported.

Transrectal ultrasonography (TRUS)

EXPECTED FINDINGS: Visualization of lesions and biopsy if needed

NURSING ACTIONS: Reinforce instructions with the client regarding possible complications and postprocedure care (extra fluids, no strenuous exercise, manifestations to report).

CLIENT EDUCATION: An enema will be administered prior to procedure.

Urinalysis

EXPECTED FINDINGS: Hematuria, bacteriuria

NURSING ACTIONS: Reinforce teaching with the client about causes of hematuria and bacteriuria.

Bone scan, MRI, or CT scans are performed to identify possible tumor metastasis.

PATIENT-CENTERED CARE

MEDICATIONS

Hormone therapy

Leuprolide acetate, goserelin, triptorelin: luteinizing hormone-releasing hormone (LH-RH) agonists
- Used in advanced prostate cancer to produce chemical castration.
- CLIENT EDUCATION
  - Hot flashes, gynecomastia, impotence, and decreased libido are adverse effects.
  - Have testing performed for osteoporosis, which can occur due to testosterone suppression.

Flutamide, bicalutamide, nilutamide: androgen receptor blocker
- Used alone or in conjunction with a LH-RH agonist.
- CLIENT EDUCATION
  - Gynecomastia is an adverse effect.
  - Liver function tests are periodically monitored.

Chemotherapy

Can be used on clients whose cancer has spread or who have had minimal improvement with other therapies

CLIENT EDUCATION: Routine blood tests are performed to monitor for neutropenia, leukopenia, thrombocytopenia, and anemia.

THERAPEUTIC PROCEDURES

Radiation (82.2)

Internal (brachytherapy) or external beam (EBRT): Not likely to be beneficial if the cancer has spread to the lymph nodes, bones, or other organs

Surgical interventions

Radical prostatectomy is the treatment of choice to remove the cancer. It is not likely to be beneficial if the cancer has spread to the lymph nodes, bones, or other organs.
- It involves the removal of the prostate gland, along with the seminal vesicles, the cuff at the bladder neck, and the regional lymph nodes.
- Open or laparoscopic surgery can be done using a suprapubic, perineal, or retropubic approach.
- Laparoscopic is used if PSA is less than 10 ng/mL and the client has had no previous hormone or abdominal surgery.
- Perineal nerves are seldom disrupted, so the client should not experience sexual dysfunction. However, dry climax can occur. Removal of tissue at the bladder neck allows seminal fluid to travel upward rather than down the urethral tract, resulting in retrograde ejaculation.

NURSING ACTIONS
- PREOPERATIVE: Ensure the client understands the procedure and what to expect postoperatively. Qᴘᴄᴄ
- POSTOPERATIVE
  - Provide care consistent with other types of abdominal surgery.
  - Manage pain with analgesics and cold therapy.
  - Observe for evidence of infection.
  - If the client has a suprapubic surgical approach, a suprapubic catheter is inserted (in addition to the urethral catheter).
    - Provide catheter care and administer bladder antispasmodics.
    - Monitor suprapubic catheter output (usually removed when residual urine measurements are less than 75 mL).
    - Reinforce teaching catheter care if the client is home with a catheter in place.
  - Provide information regarding availability of a sex therapist or intimacy counselor if needed.
  - Reinforce teaching with the client on how to use the pump and how to determine if the device is functioning properly. The mechanism is located in the scrotum.

CLIENT EDUCATION
- Report manifestations of infection.
- Avoid heavy lifting (up to 6 weeks), strenuous activity (up to 12 weeks), or straining during bowel movements.
- Avoid tub baths for at least 2 to 3 weeks (open radical surgery).
- Engage in Kegel exercises to reduce urinary incontinence.
- For urinary incontinence, the client can require insertion of an artificial urinary sphincter.

COMPLICATIONS

Urinary incontinence

Erectile dysfunction

Radiation cystitis or proctitis
- Some clients can have a transurethral resection of the prostate if obstruction occurs in the early stages of cancer before treatment is initiated.
- Bilateral orchiectomy palliative measures can slow the rate of tumor growth (decreases testosterone levels).
- Active surveillance is an option for older clients who are asymptomatic. Treatment is given only when manifestations become bothersome.

PRACTICE Active Learning Scenario

A nurse is reinforcing teaching with a client who has a new diagnosis of prostate cancer. What information should the nurse include in the teaching? Use the Active Learning Template: System Disorder to complete this Item.

MEDICATIONS: Describe at least four medications and their uses.

THERAPEUTIC PROCEDURES: Describe a prostatectomy.

NURSING INTERVENTIONS: Describe at least three nursing actions.

Application Exercises

1. A nurse is caring for a client who has leukemia and has developed thrombocytopenia. Which of the following actions should the nurse take first?
   - A. Plan for the client to take rest periods throughout the day.
   - B. Encourage the client to cough, turn, and deep breathe every 2 hr.
   - C. Measure temperature every 4 hr.
   - D. Monitor platelet counts.

2. A nurse is reviewing the health record of a client who has suspected ovarian cancer. Which of the following findings supports this diagnosis? (Select all that apply.)
   - A. Previous treatment for endometriosis
   - B. Family history of colon cancer
   - C. First pregnancy at age 24
   - D. Report of scant menses
   - E. Use of oral contraceptives for 10 years

3. A nurse is caring for a client 24 hr following a liver lobectomy for hepatocellular carcinoma. Which of the following laboratory reports should the nurse monitor?
   - A. Urine specific gravity
   - B. Blood glucose
   - C. Serum amylase
   - D. D-dimer

4. A nurse is assisting with teaching about colon cancer to a group of female clients. Which of the following statements should the nurse include in the teaching?
   - A. "Colonoscopies for individuals with no family history of cancer should begin at age 40."
   - B. "A sigmoidoscopy is recommended every 5 years beginning at age 60."
   - C. "Fecal occult blood tests should be done annually beginning at age 50."
   - D. "An endoscopy provides a definitive diagnosis of colon cancer."

5. A nurse is caring for a client who has multiple types of skin lesions. Which of the following skin lesions are indicative of a malignant melanoma? (Select all that apply.)
   - A. Diffuse vesicles
   - B. Uniformly colored papule
   - C. Area with asymmetric borders
   - D. Rough, scaly patch
   - E. Irregular colored mole

Application Exercises Key

1. A. The nurse should offer the client rest periods throughout the day to prevent fatigue. However, another action is the priority.

   B. The nurse should encourage the client to cough, turn, and deep breathe every 2 hr to prevent atelectasis. However, another action is the priority.

   C. The nurse should measure the client's temperature every 4 hr to determine if the client has a fever. However, another action is the priority.

   D. **CORRECT:** The greatest risk to the client who has thrombocytopenia is injury due to bleeding. The priority action for the nurse to take is to initiate bleeding precautions, such monitoring platelet count.

   Ⓝ *NCLEX® Connection: Physiological Adaptation, Basic Pathophysiology*

2. A. **CORRECT:** Endometriosis is a risk factor for ovarian cancer.

   B. **CORRECT:** A family history of breast, ovarian, or colon cancer is a risk factor for ovarian cancer.

   C. A first pregnancy after 30 years of age or nulliparity is a risk factor for ovarian cancer.

   D. Dysmenorrhea or heavy bleeding is a risk factor for ovarian cancer.

   E. Birth control pills offer protection against ovarian cancer. However, hormone replacement therapy is a risk factor for ovarian cancer.

   Ⓝ *NCLEX® Connection: Coordinated Care, Performance Improvement (Quality Improvement)*

3. A. Alterations in urine specific gravity following a liver lobectomy are not expected.

   B. **CORRECT:** Blood glucose should be monitored during the first 24 to 48 hr following a liver lobectomy due to decreased gluconeogenesis and stress to the liver from surgery.

   C. Alterations in serum amylase following a liver lobectomy are not expected.

   D. Alterations in the D-dimer following a liver lobectomy are not expected.

   Ⓝ *NCLEX® Connection: Reduction of Risk Potential, Laboratory Values*

4. A. A colonoscopy is recommended every 10 years beginning at age 50 for a client who has no family history of cancer.

   B. A sigmoidoscopy is recommended every 5 years beginning at age 50.

   C. **CORRECT:** Fecal occult blood tests should be done annually by clients ages 50 to 75.

   D. A biopsy performed during an endoscopic procedure confirms this diagnosis.

   Ⓝ *NCLEX® Connection: Health Promotion and Maintenance, Community Resources*

5. A. Diffuse vesicles are consistent with an allergic reaction.

   B. A uniformly colored papule is consistent with a birthmark or skin injury.

   C. **CORRECT:** A lesion with asymmetric borders is considered suspicious for a melanoma.

   D. A rough, scaly patch is consistent with squamous cell skin cancer.

   E. **CORRECT:** A lack of uniformity of pigmentation of a mole is considered suspicious for a melanoma.

   Ⓝ *NCLEX® Connection: Physiological Adaptation, Basic Pathophysiology*

PRACTICE Answer

Using the Active Learning Template: System Disorder

MEDICATIONS
- Hormone therapy: luteinizing hormone-releasing hormone agonists (leuprolide acetate)
- Androgen receptor blocker: flutamide
- Chemotherapy: docetaxel
- Antifungal: ketoconazole
- Estrogen: diethylstilbestrol

THERAPEUTIC PROCEDURES: Prostatectomy is the surgical removal of the prostate gland, seminal vesicles, bladder cuff, and regional lymph nodes. It can be done by an open surgery or laparoscopic approach in the suprapubic, perineal, or retropubic area. Perineal nerves are usually not disrupted, so the client should not experience sexual dysfunction.

NURSING INTERVENTIONS
- Reinforce preoperative teaching.
- Implement care consistent with abdominal surgery.
- Monitor pain. Administer analgesics and cold therapy.
- Monitor for evidence of infections.
- Provide catheter care (suprapubic or urethral). Administer bladder antispasmodics.

Ⓝ *NCLEX® Connection: Physiological Adaptation, Alterations in Body Systems*

CHAPTER 83 *Pain Management for Clients Who Have Cancer*

Management of cancer pain can be necessary to optimize quality of life for a client who has cancer. Not all clients who have cancer have pain.

Either the tumor or the treatment can cause cancer pain. Tumor pressure or cell invasion can cause direct tissue, bone, and nerve pain. Surgery, radiation, chemotherapy, and inactivity can also contribute to cancer pain.

PAIN

- Pain is subjective and can indicate existing or impending tissue injury.
- Pain can have physical and emotional components.
- The reaction to pain varies from person to person. Age, gender, and culture can influence the reaction to pain.
- Pain can be acute or chronic.
  - **Acute pain** occurs suddenly, is localized, and is short-term. Acute cancer pain can be the result of surgery.
  - **Chronic pain** results from nerve changes after the condition causing the pain has resolved, and lasts longer than 3 months. Tumor growth and the effects on surrounding tissue (destruction or pressure) can cause chronic cancer pain.

TYPES OF PAIN

Neuropathic
- Due to nerve damage
- Numb, tingling, shooting, burning, or radiating

Visceral/Deep
- Occurs in internal organs
- Can be difficult to identify or localize
- Deep, sharp, or dull pain
- Can radiate or be referred to a different location of the body

Somatic
- Occurs in bone or connective tissues
- Throbbing or dull and diffuse

DATA COLLECTION

- The most reliable indicator of pain is the client's verbal expression of pain.
- Use standard pain measures (location, quality, intensity, timing, setting, associated manifestations, aggravating or relieving factors) to assess pain.
- Pain assessment involves observing and documenting nonverbal indicators and physiological changes.
- Use a standard pain assessment tool.

NONVERBAL INDICATORS OF ACUTE PAIN
- Agitation, grimacing, muscle tension
- Elevated heart rate
- Rapid, shallow breathing
- Increased blood pressure
- Diaphoresis, pallor, pupil dilation
- Guarding of an area

NONVERBAL INDICATORS OF CHRONIC PAIN
- Depression
- Lethargy
- Anger, frustration
- Decreased sleep
- Decreased appetite
- Weakness

BARRIERS TO EFFECTIVE PAIN MANAGEMENT
- Inadequate pain assessment
- Inadequate knowledge of the client about analgesic use
- Inadequate knowledge of the health care professional regarding pharmacological pain management
- Reluctance by the client to report pain
- Fear of addiction to analgesics leading to nonadherence
- Inadequate dosing

MANAGEMENT

Palliative care is based on cancer pain and manifestation management; its purpose is to provide comfort and reduce pain rather than to cure the cancer.

The goal of palliative pain management is to reduce pain to improve quality of life while maintaining dignity and mental clarity.

METHODS OF PAIN MANAGEMENT: Surgery, chemotherapy, and radiation therapy can reduce pain by removing the tumor or reducing its size, which can alter pressure on adjacent tissues or organs.

NURSING ACTIONS Qpcc
- Actions are specific to each surgery or procedure.
- Reinforce information regarding the specific procedure or treatment.
- Include the family in care and management.
- Provide information about support groups and professional organizations, such as the American Cancer Society.
- **Radiation:** Instruct the client about specific skin care and to avoid sun exposure.
- **Chemotherapy:** Reinforce information about avoiding infection and managing adverse effects.

MEDICATIONS

Pharmacological management of pain includes NSAIDs, opioids, antidepressants, anticonvulsants, corticosteroids, and local anesthetics. Some clients who have cancer pain require regular use of analgesics for pain control.

Nonopioid medications and NSAIDs

- Acetaminophen
- Ketorolac
- Aspirin (acetylsalicylic acid)
- Ibuprofen
- Celecoxib
- Naproxen

THERAPEUTIC INTENT: For mild to moderate pain

NURSING ACTIONS
- Monitor for gastrointestinal (GI) bleeding, such as bloody stools or coffee-ground emesis.
- Monitor for bruising and bleeding.
- Do not administer acetaminophen to clients who have liver disease. Clients who have a healthy liver should take no more than 4 g/day. For long-term treatment, adults should take no more than 3 g/day.
- Monitor for tinnitus and hearing loss with NSAIDs.

CLIENT EDUCATION
- Take with food to prevent GI upset.
- These medications have an "analgesic ceiling." Taking more than the prescribed or recommended dosage does not increase the pain relief effect.
- Monitor for GI bleeding and bruising.
- Do not crush or chew enteric-coated products.

Opioids

- Morphine
- Codeine
- Meperidine
- Hydromorphone
- Oxycodone
- Fentanyl (available for transdermal use as well as a lozenge/sucker, buccal film and tablets, and nasal and sublingual spray)
- Combinations, such hydrocodone with acetaminophen, for breakthrough pain

THERAPEUTIC INTENT
- Moderate to severe pain
- Breakthrough pain

NURSING ACTIONS
- Use with caution for older adult clients.
- Manage acute severe pain with short-term (24 to 48 hr) around-the-clock administration of opioids rather than following a PRN schedule.
- The parenteral route is best for immediate, short-term relief of acute pain. The oral route is better for chronic, nonfluctuating pain.

- Monitor and intervene for adverse effects of opioid use (constipation, orthostatic hypotension, urinary retention, nausea, vomiting, sedation).
- Monitor for respiratory depression.
- Have naloxone available to reverse effects.
- Administer stimulant laxatives to prevent opioid-induced constipation.

CLIENT EDUCATION
- Avoid driving and using hazardous equipment until the effects of the opioid are known.
- Do not drink alcohol while taking opioids.
- Use strategies to prevent constipation, such as stool softeners and dietary changes (increased fiber and fluids).
- Nausea can subside after a few days.
- Reduce the risk of orthostatic hypotension by rising slowly from a lying or sitting position.

Antidepressants

Tricyclic antidepressants (TCAs)
- Amitriptyline
- Desipramine
- Imipramine

Selective norepinephrine reuptake inhibitors (SNRIs)
- Venlafaxine
- Duloxetine

Selective serotonin reuptake inhibitors (SSRIs)
- Fluoxetine
- Paroxetine
- Sertraline

THERAPEUTIC INTENT
- Reduce depression
- Promote normal sleep patterns in clients who have chronic pain
- Increase serotonin levels to improve feelings of well-being
- Decrease neuropathic pain

ADVERSE EFFECTS
- **TCAs:** Dry mouth, dizziness, mental clouding, weight gain, constipation
- **SNRIs:** Nausea, headache, sedation, insomnia, weight gain, impaired memory, sweating, tremors
- **SSRIs:** Nausea, vomiting, nervousness, agitation, decreased libido, insomnia

NURSING ACTIONS
- Use with caution for older adult clients.
- Use with caution for young adult clients and those who are at risk for suicide, because antidepressants can increase suicide risk. Qs
- **TCAs:** Do not administer to clients who have seizure disorders or a history of cardiac problems.

CLIENT EDUCATION
- Notify the provider if depression increases or if thoughts of suicide occur.
- Therapeutic effects can take 2 to 3 weeks.

Anticonvulsants

- Gabapentin
- Valproic acid
- Pregabalin
- Carbamazepine

THERAPEUTIC INTENT: Neuralgia and neuropathic pain

NURSING ACTIONS
- Monitor electrolytes, liver function, blood cell counts, and medication levels.
- Monitor for rash (life-threatening) and tremors.

CLIENT EDUCATION
- Medication can cause sleepiness and dizziness.
- Avoid alcohol.
- Do not drive at the start of therapy.
- Notify the provider if rash or tremors occur.

Corticosteroids

- Prednisolone (syrup)
- Dexamethasone

THERAPEUTIC INTENT: Reduce pain by reducing swelling

NURSING ACTIONS
- Reduce dosage gradually.
- Monitor for muscle weakness, joint pain, or fever.
- Monitor glucose levels.
- Monitor for changes in behavior or confusion.
- Monitor for indications of infection.

CLIENT EDUCATION
- Do not discontinue the medication suddenly.
- Take the medication with food.
- The medication weakens the immune system.
- Report any indications of infection.

Adjunctive agents: Sympatholytic agents

Clonidine

THERAPEUTIC INTENT
- Neuropathic pain
- Administered with bupivacaine in epidural or other local infusions.

NURSING ACTIONS: Monitor for hypotension.

CLIENT EDUCATION: Change positions slowly because these medications can cause orthostatic hypotension.

Adjunctive agents: Skeletal muscle relaxants

Baclofen

THERAPEUTIC INTENT: With other pain medications for muscle spasms accompanying cancer pain

NURSING ACTIONS: Monitor for seizure activity.

CLIENT EDUCATION
- Take the medication with food.
- Use caution when driving or operating machinery.
- These medications can cause drowsiness and dizziness.

Systemic local anesthetics

- Lidocaine
- Bupivacaine
- Ropivacaine

THERAPEUTIC INTENT: Administered via an infusion pump directly into the area of pain (intrathecal, intra-articular, intrapleural) to provide pain relief.

NURSING ACTIONS
- Monitor for hypotension.
- Monitor for infection at the catheter insertion site.
- Evaluate pain status.
- Monitor for motor impairment and level of sedation.
- Administered with an opioid or another medication, such as clonidine.

CLIENT EDUCATION
- Observe the infusion site for indications of infection, such as redness and swelling.
- Watch for fever.
- Notify the provider of increased pain or decreased movement that can indicate a motor block.

Topical local anesthetics

Lidocaine (patch)

THERAPEUTIC INTENT: Provides medication through a patch at a continuous level. Blocks generation and conduction of nerve impulses that transmit pain

NURSING ACTIONS: Monitor for pain relief and local skin reactions.

CLIENT EDUCATION: Use the medication only on intact skin.

ADMINISTRATION METHODS

Oral

- First choice for administration
- Short- and long-acting formulations

Transdermal

Fentanyl
- Easy to administer
- Slow onset, consistent dosing
- Long duration (48 to 72 hr)

Rectal

- Effective for clients who have impaired swallowing ability, nausea, vomiting, or who are unable to swallow oral medication due to confusion
- Low WBC and platelet counts are contraindications.

NURSING ACTIONS: Insert above the level of the rectal sphincter.

Intravenous

- Requires collaboration with the RN
- Can be administered by continuous IV infusion, IV bolus, or patient-controlled analgesia (PCA)
- Risk of infiltration
- Rapid onset

Epidural or intrathecal

- Risk of infection, pruritus, sedation, respiratory depression, and urinary retention
- Invasive and requires an RN to monitor and provide care, especially with increases in dosage
- More effective than IV analgesia during the immediate postoperative period and with severe cancer pain

Sublingual/buccal

Forms include tablets, films, and sprays.

NURSING ACTIONS
- Place sublingual forms under the tongue for absorption.
- Place buccal forms between the gum and cheek.

CLIENT EDUCATION: Refrain from drinking, eating, or smoking when taking the medication.

Topical/local

- Produces minimal systemic absorption and adverse effects
- Lidocaine patch on for 12 hr, off for 12 hr

NURSING ACTIONS
- Place patches directly over or adjacent to the painful area.
- Monitor for local skin reactions.
- Monitor for breakthrough pain.

ANESTHETIC INTERVENTIONS

Regional nerve blocks

Involves injecting an anesthetic agent, such as bupivacaine, and a corticosteroid directly into or near a nerve root to provide pain relief.
- For identifying or treating an isolated area of pain. For example, an intercostal nerve block treats chest or abdominal wall pain.
- The procedure can take from 15 min to 1 hr, depending on the area receiving the block.

NURSING ACTIONS
- Measure baseline vital signs. Monitor blood pressure and vital signs during the procedure and for at least 1 hr following the procedure (follow established guidelines).
- Assist with establishing IV access before the procedure.
- Monitor for manifestations of systemic infusion (metallic taste, ringing in ears, perioral numbness, seizures).
- Check the insertion site for redness and swelling.
- Protect the area of numbness from injury.
- Monitor for effectiveness of pain relief.

CLIENT EDUCATION
- Observe the injection site for swelling, redness, or drainage.
- Protect the area of numbness from injury, and notify the provider of increased pain or manifestations of systemic infusion.

Epidural or intrathecal catheters

- Involves injecting a local anesthetic or analgesic into the epidural space (the area outside the dura mater of the spinal cord) or intrathecal space (the subarachnoid area within the spinal cord sheath that contains cerebrospinal fluid)
- Involves surgically placing an external catheter under the skin with an external port for long-term use
  - For chronic pain management
  - Allows administration of a continuous infusion or injection PRN
  - For upper abdominal pain, thoracic pain, and pain below the umbilicus

NURSING ACTIONS
- Monitor during and for at least 1 hr following insertion or injection for hypotension, anaphylaxis, muscle weakness, seizures, and dura puncture. Qs
- Monitor oxygenation status.
- Monitor for respiratory depression and sedation.
- Monitor the insertion site for hematoma and infection.
- Evaluate leg strength prior to ambulating.

CLIENT EDUCATION
- Notify the provider of manifestations of infection (fever, swelling, redness, increase in pain, severe headache).
- Notify the provider of sudden weakness of the lower extremities or decreases in bowel or bladder control.
- Notify the provider of manifestations of systemic infusion.
- Long-term reactions can include sexual dysfunction and amenorrhea.

OTHER INVASIVE TECHNIQUES

Neurolytic ablation

Involves interrupting the nerve pathway or destroying the nerve roots that are causing pain
- For example, celiac plexus nerve ablation can be effective for pancreatic, stomach, abdominal, small bowel, and proximal colon pain.
- The procedure is irreversible.
- Nerve ablation can provide relief for several months until nerve fibers regenerate.
- Nerve ablation can cause loss of sensory, motor, and autonomic function.
- Use only when noninvasive methods are ineffective.

Radiofrequency ablation

Electrical current creates heat on a probe that the provider guides to the tumor or nerves to destroy cancer cells or ablate nerve endings (for lung and bone tumors).

Cryoanalgesia

Uses a needlelike probe to deliver extreme cold to interfere with pain conduction via nerve pathways

NURSING ACTIONS
- Monitor vital signs, especially blood pressure, for at least 1 hr following the procedure.
- Monitor for manifestations of bleeding (tachycardia, hypotension).
- Monitor for skin irritation.
- Monitor for other adverse effects (diarrhea, loss of bladder or bowel control, extremity weakness).
- Assess pain relief.

CLIENT EDUCATION
- Apply cold for pain at the insertion site.
- Continue to use pain medications PRN.
- Notify the provider of an increase in pain or weakness of extremities.

ALTERNATIVE APPROACHES

Use alternative approaches to pain management in addition to pain medications or other techniques. Many of these provide some pain reduction with minimal adverse effects. Qpcc

Transcutaneous electrical nerve stimulation (TENS)

Skin electrodes near or over the area of pain transmit low-voltage electrical impulses. The client regulates the voltage to achieve the perception of pins and needles or a vibrating sensation (sensory perception) rather than pain. Often used for chronic and acute postoperative pain.

NURSING ACTIONS
- Use with conductive gel.
- Monitor electrode sites for burns and rash.
- Offer other pain medications.
- Do not use for clients who have pacemakers, infusion pumps, or cardiac dysrhythmias.

CLIENT EDUCATION
- Place the electrodes on clean, intact skin.
- Inspect the skin under the electrodes for burns or irritation.
- Do not use if pregnant.
- Do not use near the head or over the heart.

Relaxation techniques and imagery QEBP

Useful during a procedure or a period of increased pain
- Relaxation techniques include deep breathing, diaphragmatic breathing, progressive muscle relaxation, and meditation.
- Positive (guided) imagery involves visualizing a peaceful image or scene with or without audio recordings.
- Relaxation and imagery can reduce anxiety, stress, and pain, and they can assist the client to feel more in control of the pain.

Distraction

Music, television, exercise, and family and friends can be effective distractions from pain and stress. A change of scenery can offer a distraction from pain.

Heat, cold

- Heat increases blood flow, relaxes muscles, and reduces joint stiffness.
- Cold decreases inflammation and causes local analgesia.
- Do not use heat or cold directly on skin that has radiation damage. Qs

Massage, vibration

Massage and vibration can promote pain relief through relaxation, distraction, and increased surface circulation.

Acupuncture

Acupuncture uses vibration or electrical stimulation to specific points on the body by inserting small needles into the skin and subcutaneous tissues at different depths to stimulate and alter nerve pathways and enhance the flow of energy. It can also increase the client's pain threshold.

Hypnosis

Hypnosis involves using an altered state of awareness to redirect the perception of pain. It can help induce positive imagery, reduce anxiety, and improve coping ability.

Peer group support

A support group helps provide emotional support for the client and family. Other benefits include the presence of a social network, availability of information, and help in strengthening coping skills.

Application Exercises

1. A nurse is caring for a client who has chronic cancer pain and a permanent epidural catheter for administration of a fentanyl/bupivacaine solution. The nurse should monitor for which of the following adverse effects of epidural analgesics? (Select all that apply.)

    A. Respiratory depression

    B. Hypotension

    C. Sedation

    D. Muscle spasticity

    E. Incontinence

2. A nurse is caring for a client who is scheduled to undergo a neurolytic ablation. The client asks the nurse the reason for this procedure. Which of the following responses should the nurse make?

    A. "It attempts to provide long-term pain relief."

    B. "It treats adverse effects of pain medication."

    C. "It treats decreases in immunity."

    D. "It treats decreases in cells that stop bleeding."

3. A nurse is caring for a client who has cancer and a prescription for transcutaneous electrical nerve stimulation (TENS) for pain management. Which of the following actions should the nurse take?

    A. Apply a conductive gel before applying the electrodes from the TENS unit on the skin.

    B. Apply alcohol to the skin before attaching the electrodes from the TENS unit.

    C. Attach the electrodes from the TENS unit over painful incisions or skin damage.

    D. Avoid other pain medications when using the TENS unit.

4. A nurse is contributing to the plan of care for a client who has cancer and is scheduled to undergo cryoanalgesia. Which of the following interventions should the nurse recommend? (Select all that apply.)

    A. Monitor blood pressure following the procedure.

    B. Instruct the client to apply heat to the insertion site.

    C. Check for skin irritation following the procedure.

    D. Evaluate bladder control after the procedure.

    E. Instruct the client to continue to use pain medications PRN.

5. A nurse is discussing analgesics and routes of administration with a nurse who is orienting to the oncology unit. Which of the following information should the nurse include? (Select all that apply.)

    A. Oral analgesics are the first choice for administration.

    B. Transdermal fentanyl has a duration of 8 to 12 hr.

    C. Rectal administration is preferred if the client has thrombocytopenia.

    D. Buccal analgesics are placed between the client's gum and cheek.

    E. Topical patches are placed at least 15.2 cm (6 in) from the painful area.

PRACTICE Active Learning Scenario

A nurse is assisting with a discussion for a group of nurses on the oncology unit about alternative approaches to pain management. What information should the nurse include? Use the ATI Active Learning Template: Basic Concept to complete this item.

RELATED CONTENT: Describe four approaches. Include two nursing interventions and one teaching point for each approach.

Application Exercises Key

1. A. **CORRECT:** Respiratory depression is an adverse effect of epidural analgesics.

   B. **CORRECT:** Hypotension is an adverse effect of epidural analgesics that can be corrected by administration of fluids.

   C. **CORRECT:** Sedation is an adverse effect of epidural analgesics. Other adverse effects include anaphylaxis and severe headache.

   D. Muscle weakness, not spasticity, is an adverse effect of epidural analgesics.

   E. **CORRECT:** Decreases in bowel and bladder control are adverse effects of epidural analgesics.

   Ⓝ *NCLEX® Connection: Pharmacological Therapies, Pharmacological Pain Management*

2. A. **CORRECT:** Neurolytic ablation causes destruction of the nerves that transmit pain from a specific area and is a last resort after other methods have been unsuccessful. Nerve ablation can provide relief for several months until nerve fibers regenerate.

   B. Neurolytic ablation should reduce the need for analgesics and thus the adverse effects that result from them. However, it is not a treatment for the adverse effects themselves.

   C. Neurolytic ablation does not treat myelosuppression, an adverse effect of cancer treatment.

   D. Neurolytic ablation does not treat thrombocytopenia, an adverse effect of cancer treatment.

   Ⓝ *NCLEX® Connection: Reduction of Risk Potential, Therapeutic Procedures*

3. A. **CORRECT:** The nurse should apply a conductive gel before applying the electrodes from the TENS unit to the skin.

   B. The nurse should ensure that the skin is clean and intact before applying the electrodes, but it is not necessary to cleanse it with alcohol.

   C. The nurse should apply the electrodes over intact skin that is over or near the site of pain, but not over incisions or areas of damage.

   D. The nurse should administer pain medication while the client is using the TENS unit.

   Ⓝ *NCLEX® Connection: Reduction of Risk Potential, Therapeutic Procedures*

4. A. **CORRECT:** The nurse should monitor blood pressure for at least 1 hr following cryoanalgesia. Hypotension is a manifestation of bleeding following the procedure.

   B. The nurse should instruct the client to apply cold to the insertion site for pain after cryoanalgesia.

   C. **CORRECT:** The nurse should monitor the skin for irritation following cryoanalgesia.

   D. **CORRECT:** The nurse should monitor for loss of bladder or bowel control, which are adverse effects of cryoanalgesia.

   E. **CORRECT:** The nurse should instruct the client to continue to use pain medications PRN following cryoanalgesia to promote effective pain relief.

   Ⓝ *NCLEX® Connection: Reduction of Risk Potential, Potential for Complications from Surgical Procedures and Health Alterations*

5. A. **CORRECT:** Oral analgesics are the first choice for routes of administration of analgesics for the treatment of cancer pain.

   B. Transdermal fentanyl has a duration of 48 to 72 hr.

   C. The rectal route of administration is contraindicated if the client has a low platelet count (thrombocytopenia) or a low WBC count.

   D. **CORRECT:** Buccal analgesics are placed between the gum and cheek.

   E. Topical patches should be placed directly over or adjacent to the painful area.

   Ⓝ *NCLEX® Connection: Pharmacological Therapies, Expected Actions/Outcomes*

PRACTICE Answer

Using the ATI Active Learning Template: Basic Concept

RELATED CONTENT

Transcutaneous electrical nerve stimulation (TENS)
- Use with conductive gel.
- Monitor electrode sites for burns or rash.
- Offer pain medications.
- Do not use on clients who have pacemakers, infusion pumps, or dysrhythmias.
- Place electrodes on clean, intact skin. Inspect skin under the electrodes for burns or irritation.
- Do not use if the client is pregnant.
- Do not use near the head or over the heart.

Relaxation and positive (guided) imagery
- Use during a procedure or during a period of increased pain. Encourage deep breathing, diaphragmatic breathing, progressive muscle relaxation, meditation, or a focus on a peaceful image or scene.
- Use with or without audio recordings.
- These approaches reduce stress, anxiety, and pain, and promote a feeling of control of the pain.

Application of heat, cold
- Apply heat to increase blood flow, relax muscles, and reduce joint stiffness.
- Apply cold to decrease inflammation and produce local analgesia.
- Do not apply heat or cold directly to skin that has radiation damage.

Massage or vibration
- Massage can cause relaxation, distraction, and increased surface circulation.
- Avoid further skin irritation from excessive massage or vibration.

Distraction
- Offer music.
- Encourage watching television, exercising, and activities with family and friends.
- Use repetitive actions or movements, focused breathing, a visual focal point, and a change of scenery.

Acupuncture
- Make referrals to community resources.
- Involves inserting small needles into the skin at different depths to stimulate and alter nerve pathways and enhance the flow of energy. This affects the pain threshold.

Hypnosis
- Helps redirect the client's perception of pain.
- Make referrals to community resources.
- Use to induce positive imagery, reduce anxiety, and improve coping ability.

Peer group
- Make referrals to community resources.
- Encourage family participation.
- Groups provide emotional support for family members and clients.
- Groups offer the presence of a social network, availability of information, and strengthening of coping skills.

Ⓝ *NCLEX® Connection: Pharmacological Therapies, Medication Administration*

NCLEX® Connections

When reviewing the following chapters, keep in mind the relevant topics and tasks of the NCLEX outline, in particular:

Coordinated Care

INFORMED CONSENT: Recognize that informed consent was obtained (completed consent form, client understanding of procedure).

Reduction of Risk Potential

POTENTIAL FOR COMPLICATIONS FROM SURGICAL PROCEDURES AND HEALTH ALTERATIONS
Identify the client's response to surgery or health alterations.

Provide care for the client before surgical procedures and reinforce education.

Provide intra-operative care (positioning client for surgery, maintaining sterile field, providing operative observation).

Reinforce client teaching to prevent complications due to surgery or health alterations (cough and deep breathing, elastic stockings).

THERAPEUTIC PROCEDURES: Assist with the performance of a diagnostic or invasive procedure.

Physiological Adaptation

ALTERATIONS IN BODY SYSTEMS
Perform care for the client after surgical procedures.

Remove wound sutures or staples.

Remove the client's wound-drainage device.

CHAPTER 84

CHAPTER 84 *Preoperative Nursing Care*

Surgery can take on many forms, including curative, palliative, cosmetic, and functional.

There are three categories of inpatient surgical procedures based on acuity: emergent, urgent, and elective.

Outpatient or ambulatory surgery generally is an elective surgery (cataract removal, hernia repair) that is not considered acute.

Preoperative care takes place from the time a client is scheduled for surgery until care is transferred to the operating suite. Collecting data about risk factors is one of the major aspects of preoperative care. Preoperative care also includes thorough data collection regarding physical, emotional, and psychosocial status.

RISK FACTORS

OF SURGERY
- Infection (risk of sepsis)
- Anemia (malnutrition, oxygenation, effect on healing)
- Hypovolemia from dehydration or blood loss (circulatory compromise)
- Electrolyte imbalance through inadequate diet or disease process (dysrhythmias)

FOR SURGICAL COMPLICATIONS
- **Pregnancy:** Fetal risk with anesthesia
- **Respiratory disease:** COPD, pneumonia, asthma
- **Cardiovascular disease:** Heart failure, myocardial infarction, hypertension, dysrhythmias
- **Diabetes mellitus:** Decreased intestinal motility, altered blood glucose levels, delayed healing
- **Liver disease:** Altered medication metabolism, increased risk for bleeding
- **Kidney disease:** Altered elimination and medication excretion
- **Endocrine disorders:** Hypothyroidism, hyperthyroidism, Addison's disease, Cushing's syndrome
- **Immune system disorders:** Immunocompromised
- **Coagulation defect:** Increased risk of bleeding
- **Malnutrition:** Delayed healing
- **Obesity:** Pulmonary complications due to hypoventilation, effect on anesthesia, elimination, and wound healing

- **Medications:** Antihypertensives, anticoagulants, NSAIDs, tricyclic antidepressants, herbal medications, over-the-counter medications
- **Substance use:** Tobacco, alcohol
- **Family history:** Malignant hyperthermia
- **Allergies:** Latex, anesthetic agents
- **Inability to cope,** lack of support system
- **Disease processes** involving multiple body systems
- **Comorbidities:** Chronic disease processes, use of multiple medications
- **Sensory limitations** (poor eyesight, hearing loss): Maintain a safe environment for these clients.
- **Oral alterations** (dentures, bridges, loose teeth) can pose problems during intubation.
- **Older adult clients** Ⓖ
  - Age-related changes to hepatic and renal function alter clearance of anesthetic agents and opioids.
  - Older adult clients have a greater risk of adverse reactions to preoperative medications.
  - Older adult clients have less physiologic reserve than younger clients, which can cause decreased immune system response and decreased wound healing
  - Reduction of muscle mass and the amount of body water places older adult clients at risk for dehydration.
  - Older adult clients perspire less, which leads to dry, itchy skin that becomes fragile and easily abraded. Take precautions when moving and positioning these clients.
  - Older adult clients have decreased subcutaneous fat, which makes them more susceptible to temperature changes.

PREOPERATIVE DATA COLLECTION

Detailed history: Medical history, surgical history, tolerance of anesthesia, medication use, complementary or alternative practices (herbals), substance use, psychosocial history, and cultural considerations

Allergies: Medications, latex, contrast agents, food products
- Allergies to banana or kiwi can indicate the client is at risk for a reaction to latex.
- Allergy to eggs or soybean oil is a contraindication to the use of propofol for anesthesia.
- Allergies to shellfish can result in a reaction to povidone-iodine.

Anxiety level: Regarding the procedure, support systems, and coping mechanisms

> Older adult clients can be more fearful due to financial concerns and lack of social support. Ⓖ

Baseline data: Head-to-toe data collection, vital signs, oxygen saturations

Venous thromboembolism risk: Evaluation is based on surgical procedure, client history, and anticipated time the client will be immobilized following surgery

DIAGNOSTIC PROCEDURES

INDICATIONS

- Urinalysis: Renal function, rule out infection
- Blood type and cross match: Transfusion readiness
- CBC: Fluid status, anemia, infection/immune status
- Pregnancy test: Fetal risk of anesthesia
- Clotting studies: PT, INR, aPTT, platelet count
- Electrolyte levels: Electrolyte imbalances
- Serum creatinine and BUN: Renal status
- Chest x-ray: Heart and lung status
- 12-lead ECG: Baseline heart rhythm, dysrhythmias, history of cardiac disease, all clients receiving general anesthesia, age older than 40 years

PATIENT-CENTERED CARE

NURSING CARE

- Verify that the informed consent is accurately completed, signed, and witnessed.
- Administer enemas or laxatives the night before or the morning of bowel surgery.
- Regularly check scheduled medication prescriptions. Some medications (antihypertensives, anticoagulants, antidepressants) can be held until after the procedure.
- Ensure that the client remains NPO for at least 6 hr for solid foods and 2 hr for clear liquids before surgery with general anesthesia (3 to 4 hr with local anesthesia) to avoid aspiration. Note on the chart the last time the client ate or drank. Q_{EBP}
- Perform skin preparation, which can include cleansing with antimicrobial soap. If necessary, use electric clippers or chemical depilatories to remove hair in areas that will be involved in the surgery.
- Ensure that jewelry, dentures, prosthetics, makeup, nail polish, and glasses are removed. These items can be given to the family or stored safely.
- Cover the client with a lightweight cotton blanket heated in a warmer to prevent hypothermia. Hypothermia increases the chance for surgical wound infections, alters metabolism of medication, and causes coagulation problems and cardiac dysrhythmias.
- Maintain IV access using a large-bore (18-gauge) catheter for easier infusing of IV fluids or blood products.
- Administer preoperative medications (prophylactic antimicrobials, antiemetics, sedatives).
  - Prophylactic antibiotics are administered within 1 hr of surgical incision.
  - If the client previously took a beta blocker, administer a beta blocker prior to surgery to prevent a cardiac event and mortality.
  - Have the client void prior to administration.
  - Monitor response to medications.
  - Raise side rails following administration to prevent injury.

- Ensure that the preoperative checklist is complete. **(84.1)**
- Confirm and verify the correct surgical site with the client and all health care team members before clearly marking the surgical site.
- Instruct the client regarding the purpose and effects of preoperative medications that will be administered.
- Explain care and restrictions relative to the surgical procedure performed.

Informed consent

- Once surgery has been discussed as treatment with the client and partner, family member, or friend, it is the responsibility of the provider to obtain consent after discussing the risks and benefits of the procedure. The nurse shall not obtain the consent for the provider in any circumstance.
- The nurse can clarify any information that remains unclear after the provider's explanation of the procedure. The nurse may not provide any information not previously given by the provider.
- The nurse's role is to witness the client's signing of the consent form after the client acknowledges understanding of the procedure.
- The nurse should determine if the client is
  - 18 years of age or emancipated.
  - Mentally capable of understanding the risks, reason, and options for surgery and anesthesia.
  - Under the influence of medication that affects decision-making or judgment (opioids, benzodiazepines, sedatives).

> ! Do not have the client sign the informed consent if these types of medications have been administered.

- A legal guardian can sign the surgical consent form if the client is not capable of providing consent or if there is no family.
- Informed consent is required for surgical procedures, invasive procedures (biopsy, paracentesis, scopes), and any procedure requiring sedation or anesthesia, involving radiation, or that places the client at increased risk for complications.

PROVIDER RESPONSIBILITIES
- Obtain informed consent.
- To obtain informed consent, the provider must give the client the following.
  - Complete description of the treatment/procedure
  - Description of the professionals who will be performing and participating in the treatment
  - Information on the risks of anesthesia
  - Description of the anticipated benefits of the treatment/procedure
  - Description of the potential harm, pain, and discomfort that can occur
  - Options for other treatments
  - The right to refuse treatment

Preoperative Checklist	Yes	No	N/A	Initials
Allergies (list below)				
Operative permit correct/signed, dated, timed				
Authorization for treatment signed				
Anesthesia consent/signed, dated, timed				
Blood consent/signed, dated, timed				
ID bracelet correct and on client				
Blood bracelet correct and on client				
Height and weight recorded (height _____ /weight _____)				
Preoperative laboratory reports on chart				
ECG report on chart				
Chest x-ray report on chart				
Correct operative site marked with an X				
MAR/home medications				
History and physical report on chart				
Old records with chart				
Undergarments removed				
Hospital gown on client				
Operative area preparation				
Colored nail polish removed				
Foley catheter placed				
Body piercing removed, if applicable				
Emboli stockings/elastic bandages applied				
Contact lens/glasses removed-deposition				
Dentures/partial plates removed-deposition				
Valuable jewelry removed-deposition				
Preoperative antibiotic given				
Preoperative teaching completed by _____				
Oxygen _____ liters per nasal cannula, _____% per face mask				

Allergies		
Preoperative medication given		
NPO since	Date	Time
Preoperative vital signs		
Comments		
Transported to OR per _____	Date	Time
Signed		

CLIENT RESPONSIBILITIES

- Give informed consent.
- To give informed consent, the client must do the following.
  - Give it voluntarily (no coercion involved).
  - Receive enough information to make a decision based on an understanding of what is expected.
  - Be competent and of legal age or be an emancipated minor. When the client is unable to provide consent, another authorized person must give consent.

NURSE RESPONSIBILITIES: Witness informed consent.

- Ensure that the provider gave the client the necessary information.
- Ensure that the client understood the information and is competent to give informed consent.
- Notify the provider if the client has more questions or seems to not understand any of the information provided. (The provider is then responsible for clarifying.)
- Have the client sign the informed consent document.
- Document questions the client has and notify the provider. Also document any additional reinforcement of teaching.
- Provide a trained medical interpreter (not a family member or friend) and record the use of an interpreter in the medical record.

CLIENT EDUCATION

- Use postoperative pain control techniques (medications, immobilization, patient-controlled analgesia pumps).
- Use splinting, coughing, and deep breathing.
- Use range-of-motion exercises and early ambulation for prevention of thrombi and respiratory complications.
- The purpose of antiembolism stockings and pneumatic compression devices is to prevent deep-vein thrombosis.
- Bowel and skin preparations will be completed (cleansing enema, preoperative shower with medicated soap).
- Invasive devices can be used during the procedure (drains, catheters, IV lines).
- Follow postoperative diet.
- Follow instructions for use of the incentive spirometer.
- Preoperative instructions include avoiding cigarette smoking, medications to hold, bowel preparation.
  - Clients who are taking acetylsalicylic acid should stop taking it for 1 week before an elective surgery to decrease the risk of bleeding.
  - Clients who take herbal medications (ginkgo biloba, ginseng, feverfew) should stop taking them 2 weeks before surgery to prevent
- Hemorrhage is a possible adverse effect to the anesthetic.
- Medications for cardiovascular disease, pulmonary disease, seizures, and diabetes mellitus, some antihypertensive medications, and eye drops for glaucoma may be taken prior to surgery or a procedure.
- Use a pain scale to rate pain level postoperative.

COMPLICATIONS

Complications during the postoperative period usually are related to the medications given preoperatively.

- Note the following medications and their potential complications.
  - **Sedatives (benzodiazepines, barbiturates):** Respiratory depression, drowsiness, dizziness
    - NURSING ACTIONS
      - Monitor respiratory rate and oxygen saturation.
      - Administer oxygen.
      - Ensure the administration of a reversal agent, flumazenil.
  - **Opioids:** Respiratory depression, drowsiness, dizziness, constipation, urinary retention
    - NURSING ACTIONS
      - Monitor respiratory rate and oxygen saturation.
      - Administer oxygen.
      - Ensure the administration of a reversal agent, naloxone.
      - Perform intermittent catheterization.
  - **IV infusions (0.9% NaCl, lactated Ringer's):** Fluid overload, hypernatremia
    - NURSING ACTIONS
      - Obtain preoperative cardiac and pulmonary history.
      - Monitor I&O closely.
      - Monitor the IV fluid rate of infusion.
      - Ensure the administration of a diuretic.
  - **Gastrointestinal medications (antiemetics, antacids, H2 receptor blockers):** Alkalosis, cardiac abnormalities (some H2 receptor blockers), drowsiness
    - NURSING ACTIONS
      - Obtain preoperative cardiac history.
      - Monitor for electrolyte abnormalities.
- For clients encountering severe anxiety and panic, reassurance is necessary and sedation medications may be given. Nonpharmacological interventions (distraction, imagery, music therapy) can be initiated.
- Ensure that measures are taken to prevent postoperative deep-vein thromboembolism by continuing anticoagulation therapy and/or antiembolism stockings, pneumatic compression devices, and range-of-motion exercises.
- Be alert for any allergic reactions the client has to medications.

Application Exercises

1. A nurse is reviewing a client's laboratory values before surgery. Which of the following results should the nurse report to the provider? (Select all that apply.)

   A. Potassium 3.9 mEq/L

   B. Sodium 145 mEq/L

   C. Creatinine 2.8 mg/dL

   D. Blood glucose 235 mg/dL

   E. WBC 17,850/mm³

2. A nurse is reinforcing preoperative teaching with a client who is to have abdominal surgery. Which of the following statements should the nurse make? (Select all that apply.)

   A. "Take your heart medication with a sip of water before surgery."

   B. "Splint the abdominal incision with a pillow when coughing and deep breathing."

   C. "Bed rest is recommended for the first 48 hr."

   D. "Antiembolism stockings are applied before surgery."

   E. "You may eat solid foods up to 4 hr before surgery."

3. A nurse is verifying informed consent for a client who is having a paracentesis. Which of the following actions should the nurse take? (Select all that apply.)

   A. Explain the purpose of the procedure.

   B. Inform the client of risks of the procedure.

   C. Ensure the client understands information about the procedure.

   D. Witness the client signing the informed consent form.

   E. Determine if the client is capable of understanding the reason for the procedure.

4. A nurse is caring for a client who is scheduled for an exploratory laparotomy. The client's temperature is 39° C (102.2° F) orally. Which of the following actions should the nurse take?

   A. Inform the surgeon of the elevated temperature.

   B. Transfer the client to the preoperative unit.

   C. Apply ice packs to the groin.

   D. Encourage the client to increase intake of clear liquids.

5. A nurse is caring for a client who is having a colon resection. Which of the following actions should the nurse take?

   A. Encourage the client to void after preoperative medication administration.

   B. Administer antibiotics 2 hr prior to surgical incision.

   C. Remove hair using a manual razor.

   D. Remove nail polish on fingers and toes.

PRACTICE Active Learning Scenario

A nurse is assisting with the plan of care for a client who is having a surgical procedure. What potential complications should the nurse include? Use the ATI Active Learning Template: Basic Concept to complete this item.

RELATED CONTENT: List three potential complications. Explain the related cause and include one intervention for each complication.

Application Exercises Key

1. A. The potassium level is within the expected reference range.

    B. The sodium level is within the expected reference range.

    C. **CORRECT:** The nurse should report an elevated creatinine level, which can indicate impaired renal function.

    D. **CORRECT:** The nurse should report an elevated blood glucose, which needs treatment prior to surgery.

    E. **CORRECT:** The nurse should report an elevated WBC count, which indicates a need for antibiotic therapy before surgery.

    (N) *NCLEX® Connection: Reduction of Risk Potential, Laboratory Values*

2. A. **CORRECT:** The nurse should reinforce teaching with the client to take some cardiac and other medications as prescribed with a sip of water before surgery.

    B. **CORRECT:** The nurse should reinforce teaching with the client about how to splint with a pillow to support the incision when coughing and deep breathing postoperatively.

    C. The nurse should reinforce teaching with the client about the importance of early ambulation following abdominal surgery to prevent complications.

    D. **CORRECT:** The nurse should inform the client of the application of antiembolism stockings to prevent deep-vein thrombosis.

    E. The nurse should inform the client to stop eating solid food for 6 hr or more before surgery.

    (N) *NCLEX® Connection: Reduction of Risk Potential, Potential for Complications from Surgical Procedures and Health Alterations*

3. A. The provider should explain the purpose of the procedure.

    B. The provider should inform the client of risks of the procedure.

    C. **CORRECT:** The nurse should ensure the client understands the information about the procedure.

    D. **CORRECT:** The nurse should witness the client sign the informed consent.

    E. **CORRECT:** The nurse should determine if the client is capable of understanding the reason for the procedure.

    (N) *NCLEX® Connection: Coordinated Care, Client Rights*

4. A. **CORRECT:** The nurse should immediately notify the surgeon of the elevated temperature to determine if canceling the surgery is necessary due to an underlying infection.

    B. Transferring the client to the preoperative unit is not an appropriate nursing action when there is a possible underlying infection.

    C. Applying ice packs to the client's groin is not an appropriate action for a temperature of 39° C (102.2° F).

    D. Increasing intake of clear liquids is not an appropriate action because the client should be NPO for at least 2 hr before surgery.

    (N) *NCLEX® Connection: Reduction of Risk Potential, Potential for Complications of Diagnostic Tests/Treatments/Procedures*

5. A. The client should void before administration of medication for relaxation or sedation to prevent the risk for falls.

    B. The nurse should administer antibiotics within 1 hr prior to the surgical incision as a prophylactic measure to prevent infection.

    C. The nurse should remove hair at the surgical site with electric clippers or use a chemical depilatory to prevent traumatizing the skin and increasing the risk for infection.

    D. **CORRECT:** The nurse should ensure the nail beds are visible for color and circulation by removing nail polish before surgery.

    (N) *NCLEX® Connection: Reduction of Risk Potential, Potential for Complications from Surgical Procedures and Health Alterations*

PRACTICE Answer

Using the ATI Active Learning Template: Basic Concept

RELATED CONTENT

Respiratory depression
- Caused by overmedication with benzodiazepines, barbiturates, or opioids.
- Ensure the administration of a reversal agent, and monitor closely.

Fluid overload
- Caused by too much IV fluids and inability to readily excrete the fluids.
- Obtain a preoperative cardiac and pulmonary history, monitor I&O closely, monitor the rate of IV fluids, and ensure the administration of a diuretic.

Deep-vein thrombosis
- Caused by blood stasis in lower extremities due to absent muscle contractility.
- Apply antiembolism stockings or pneumatic compression devices, administer anticoagulants, and reinforce teaching about range-of-motion exercises.

Infection
- Caused by micro-organisms contaminating the surgical wound.
- Administer a prophylactic antibiotic within 1 hr before the surgical incision is made.

(N) *NCLEX® Connection: Reduction of Risk Potential, Potential for Complications from Surgical Procedures and Health Alterations*

Transferring a client who is postoperative from the operating suite to the postanesthesia care unit (PACU) is the responsibility of the anesthesia provider, who is an anesthesiologist or certified registered nurse anesthetist. The circulating nurse will give the verbal hand-off report to the PACU nurse.

Postoperative care is usually provided initially in the PACU, where skilled nurses who are certified in advanced cardiac life support can monitor recovery from anesthesia. In some instances, a client is transferred from the operating suite directly to the intensive care unit.

Initial postoperative care involves data collection, administering medications, managing pain, preventing complications, and determining when a client is ready to be discharged from the PACU. During the immediate postoperative stage, maintaining airway patency and ventilation and monitoring circulatory status are the priorities for care. Postoperative clients who receive general anesthesia require frequent data collection of their respiratory status. Postoperative clients who receive epidural or spinal anesthesia require ongoing data collection of motor and sensory function.

A client who is stable and able to breathe spontaneously is discharged to a postsurgical unit or home if an outpatient surgical procedure was performed. A client discharged home must demonstrate ability to swallow and safely ambulate to the bathroom and wheelchair with assistance. A client who had an outpatient surgery should be accompanied by someone who can receive discharge instructions and transport the client home.

RISK FACTORS FOR COMPLICATIONS

Immobility: Respiratory compromise, thrombophlebitis, pressure ulcer

Anemia: Blood loss, inadequate/decreased oxygenation, impaired healing factors

Hypovolemia: Tissue perfusion

Hypothermia: Risk of surgical wound infection, altered absorption of medication, coagulopathy, cardiac dysrhythmia

Cardiovascular diseases: Fluid overload, deep-vein thrombosis, arrhythmia

Respiratory disease: Respiratory compromise

Immune disorder: Risk for infection, delayed healing

Diabetes mellitus: Gastroparesis, delayed wound healing

Coagulation defect: Increased risk of bleeding

Malnutrition: Delayed healing

Obesity: Respiratory compromise, postoperative nausea and vomiting, wound healing, dehiscence, evisceration

Age-related: Respiratory, cardiovascular, and renal changes necessitate specific attention to the postoperative recovery of older adults. ©

Older adult clients are more susceptible to cold temperatures, so additional warm blankets in the PACU can be required.
- Responses to medications and anesthetics can delay return of orientation postoperatively.
- Age-related physiologic changes (decreased liver and kidney function) can affect response to and elimination of postoperative medications. Monitor for appropriate response and possible adverse effects.
  ○ Older adults perspire less, which leads to dry, itchy skin that becomes fragile and easily abraded. The use of paper tape for wound dressings can be appropriate, as well as lifting precautions.
  ○ Older adults can be at risk for delayed wound healing because of possible compromised nutrition.

DIAGNOSTIC PROCEDURES

CBC: WBC (infection/immune status), Hgb, Hct (fluid status, anemia)

Metabolic profile: Serum electrolytes (electrolyte imbalances), BUN, creatinine (renal function)

ABGs: Oxygenation status

Additional laboratory tests: Serum glucose, prothrombin time, INR (based on procedure and associated health problems)

UNIT DATA COLLECTION

Upon receiving the client from the PACU, the nurse should immediately perform full-body data collection with priority given to airway, breathing, and circulation. This serves as a baseline to identify changes in postoperative status.

MONITORING AND MANAGEMENT

Airway

Contraindications to coughing include cosmetic, eye, and intracranial surgeries.

NURSING ACTIONS
- Monitor oxygen saturation using a pulse oximeter.
- Assist with coughing and deep breathing at least every 1 hr while awake, and provide a pillow or folded blanket so the client can splint as necessary for abdominal incision.
- Assist with the use of an incentive spirometer at least every 2 hr while awake to encourage expansion of the lungs and prevent atelectasis.
- Reposition every 2 hr, and ambulate early and regularly.

Positioning

Do not put pillows under knees or elevate the knee gatch on the bed (decreases venous return).

NURSING ACTIONS: Encourage early ambulation with adequate rest periods to prevent cardiovascular disorders, deep-vein thrombosis, and pulmonary complications.

Fluid status and oral comfort

A client who returns to the medical-surgical unit receives a prescription IV solution based on needs (hydration, electrolytes).

NURSING ACTIONS
- Check skin turgor, and monitor for diaphoresis.
- Encourage ice chips and fluids.
- Provide frequent oral hygiene.

Pain

A preventative approach using around-the-clock scheduling is more effective than PRN medication delivery during the first 24 to 48 hr postoperatively.

NURSING ACTIONS
- Provide continuous pain relief through the use of a patient-controlled analgesia pump. Epidural and intrathecal infusions are also used postoperatively.
- Monitor pain level frequently, using a standardized pain scale.
- Encourage the client to ask for pain medication before pain gets severe.
- Monitor for manifestations of pain (increased heart rate, respirations, or blood pressure; restlessness; wincing or moaning during movement).
- Monitor for adverse effects of opioids (respiratory depression, nausea, urinary retention, constipation). Encourage the client to change positions slowly
- Provide analgesia 30 min before ambulation or painful procedures.
- Monitor for effectiveness of pain medication after administration.

Kidney function

- Output should equal intake.
- A bladder scan is used to check for retention of urine.

NURSING ACTIONS
- Monitor and report urinary output less than 30 mL/hr.
- Palpate bladder following voiding to collect data regarding distention.

85.1 Closed suction drain with bulb

tubing

emptying cap

emptying port

collection reservoir

Bowel function

NURSING ACTIONS

- Maintain the client NPO until return of gag reflex (risk of aspiration) and peristalsis (risk of paralytic ileus). Qs
- Irrigate NG suction tubes with saline as needed to maintain patency. Do not move NG tubes in clients who are postoperative following gastric surgery (risk to incision).
- Monitor bowel sounds in all four quadrants as well as ability to pass flatus.
- Advance diet (clear liquids to regular).

Thromboembolism prevention

NURSING ACTIONS

- Apply pneumatic compression devices and/or antiembolism stockings.
- Reposition the client every 2 hr.
- Ambulate the client early and regularly.
- Administer anticoagulants or antiplatelet medications.
- Monitor extremities for calf pain, warmth, erythema, and edema.

Incisions and drain sites

In most instances, the surgeon performs the first dressing change. The nurse can perform subsequent dressing changes using surgical aseptic technique.

NURSING ACTIONS

- Monitor drainage (should progress from sanguineous to serosanguineous to serous).
- Monitor the incision site. Expected findings include pink wound edges, slight swelling under sutures/staples, and slight crusting of drainage. Report any evidence of infection (redness, excessive tenderness, purulent drainage).

- Monitor wound drains each time vital signs are measured. Empty closed-suction drainage collection devices as needed to maintain compression. Report increases in drainage (possible hemorrhage).
  (85.1, 85.2, 85.3)
- Use an abdominal binder for clients who are obese or debilitated.
- Encourage splinting with position changes, coughing, and deep breathing.
- Administer prophylactic antibiotics.
- Remove sutures or staples in 5 to 10 days.

Wound healing

NURSING ACTIONS

- Encourage the client to consume a diet high in calories, protein, and vitamin C.
- If the client has diabetes mellitus, maintain appropriate glycemic control.

Discharge teaching

CLIENT EDUCATION

- The purpose, administration guidelines, and adverse effects of medications
- Activity restrictions (driving, stairs, weight limits on lifting, sexual activity)
- Dietary guidelines, if applicable
- Treatment instructions (wound care, catheter care, use of assistive devices)
- Emergency contact information and findings to report

85.2 Penrose drain

85.3 Closed-drain system with spring evacuator

COMPLICATIONS

Airway obstruction

Swelling or spasm of the larynx or trachea, mucus in the airway, or relaxation of the tongue into the nasopharynx can cause airway obstruction, often manifesting as stridor or snoring.

NURSING ACTIONS
- Monitor for choking; noisy, irregular respirations; decreased oxygen saturation values; and cyanosis. Intervene accordingly.
- Implement a head-tilt/chin-lift maneuver to pull the tongue forward and open the airway.
- Keep emergency equipment (resuscitation bag, suction equipment, airways) at the bedside in the PACU.
- Notify the anesthesiologist, elevate head of bed if not contraindicated, provide humidified oxygen, and assist with the plan for reintubation with endotracheal tube.

Hypoxia

Hypoxia is evidenced by a decrease in oxygen saturation.

NURSING ACTIONS
- Monitor oxygenation status, and administer oxygen.
- Position the client with the head of bed elevated, and turn every 2 hr to facilitate chest expansion.

CLIENT EDUCATION: Coughing and deep breathe to prevent atelectasis.

Hypovolemic shock

Postoperative shock can result from a massive loss of circulating blood volume.

NURSING ACTIONS
- Monitor for decreased blood pressure and urinary output, increased heart and respiratory rates, narrowing of pulse pressure, and slow capillary refill.
- Monitor postoperative laboratory values (hemoglobin, hematocrit, creatinine, BUN).
- Administer oxygen.
- Place the client in a supine position with legs elevated.
- Assist with the administration of IV fluids and vasopressors.

Paralytic ileus

Can occur due to the absence of GI peristaltic activity caused by abdominal surgery or other physical trauma

NURSING ACTIONS
- Monitor bowel sounds.
- Encourage ambulation.
- Advance the diet as tolerated when bowel sounds or flatus are present.
- Administer prokinetic agents, such as metoclopramide.

CLIENT EDUCATION: An NG tube can be inserted to empty stomach contents.

Wound dehiscence or evisceration

- Caused by spontaneous opening of the incisional wound (dehiscence)
- Can progress to the protrusion of the internal organs through the incision (evisceration)

NURSING ACTIONS
- Monitor risk factors (obesity, coughing, moving without splinting, poor nutritional status, diabetes mellitus, infection, hematoma, steroid use).
- If wound dehiscence or evisceration occurs, call for help, stay with the client, cover the wound with a sterile towel or dressing that is moistened with sterile saline, place in a low-Fowler's position with hips and knees bent, monitor for shock, and notify the provider immediately. Do not attempt to reinsert organs.

Deep-vein thrombosis

- Caused by dehydration; stress response that leads to hypercoagulability of the blood, immobility, obesity, trauma, malignancy, history of thrombosis, hormones, and use of indwelling venous catheter
- Prophylactic measures include administration of low-molecular-weight heparin, low-dose heparin, or low-dose warfarin; antiembolism stockings; pneumatic compression devices; range-of-motion exercises; and early ambulation.

NURSING ACTIONS
- Avoid any form of pressure behind the knee with a pillow or blanket, which can cause constriction of blood vessels and decreased venous return.
- Avoid dangling the client's legs for long periods of time.
- Provide adequate hydration by monitoring the administration of IV fluids or encouraging increased oral fluid intake.

Application Exercises

1. A nurse is reviewing health records of several clients scheduled for a surgical procedure to identify risk factors that can lead to postoperative complications. Which of the following clients are at risk for complications? (Select all that apply.)

   A. A client who has a WBC of 22,500/uL

   B. A client who uses an insulin pump

   C. A client who takes warfarin daily

   D. A client who has heart failure

   E. A client who has a BMI of 26

2. A nurse is caring for a client who is postoperative and manifests indications of hypovolemia while in the PACU. Which of the following findings requires action by the nurse? (Select all that apply.)

   A. Urine output less than 25 mL/hr

   B. Hematocrit 48%

   C. BUN 24 mg/dL

   D. Tenting of skin over the sternum

   E. Heart rate 62/min

3. A nurse is assisting with the plan of care for a client to prevent postoperative atelectasis. Which of the following interventions should the nurse include? (Select all that apply.)

   A. Encourage use of the incentive spirometer every 2 hr.

   B. Instruct the client to splint the incision when coughing and deep breathing.

   C. Reposition the client every 2 hr.

   D. Administer antibiotic therapy.

   E. Assist with early ambulation.

4. A nurse is caring for a client who reports nausea and vomiting 2 days postoperative following hysterectomy. Which of the following actions should the nurse perform first?

   A. Check for bowel sounds.

   B. Administer antiemetic medication.

   C. Ensure IV fluids are initiated.

   D. Insert a nasogastric tube.

5. A nurse is caring for a client who is postoperative following a gastric resection. Which of the following actions should the nurse take? (Select all that apply.)

   A. Reposition the client every 4 hr.

   B. Apply pneumatic compressing stockings bilaterally.

   C. Place pillows under the client's knees when in the supine position.

   D. Administer pain medication 30 min prior to ambulation

   E. Encourage the client to perform leg exercises every 1 hr.

PRACTICE Active Learning Scenario

A nurse is reviewing the health records of several clients to identify postoperative complications. What information should the nurse expect to find? Use the ATI Active Learning Template: Basic Concept to complete this item.

RELATED CONTENT: List three possible complications. Describe one cause and one intervention for each complication.

Application Exercises Key

1. A. **CORRECT:** An increased WBC indicates an underlying infection and places the client at risk for postoperative complications.

B. **CORRECT:** An insulin pump indicates the client has type 1 diabetes mellitus and places the client at risk of postoperative complications, such as delayed wound healing.

C. **CORRECT:** A client who takes warfarin daily is at risk for bleeding and postoperative complications, such as hemorrhage.

D. **CORRECT:** A client who has a history of heart failure is at risk for complications (fluid overload, dysrhythmias).

E. A BMI of 26 is within the expected reference range and does not place the client at risk for postoperative complications.

Ⓝ *NCLEX® Connection: Reduction of Risk Potential, Potential for Complications of Diagnostic Tests/Treatments/Procedures*

2. A. **CORRECT:** Urine output less than 25 mL/hr is a manifestation of hypovolemia and requires intervention by IV fluid therapy.

B. **CORRECT:** Hematocrit 48% indicates concentrated blood volume and is a manifestation of hypovolemia, requiring intervention by IV fluid therapy.

C. **CORRECT:** BUN 24 mg/dL indicates decreased kidney function and can be a manifestation of hypovolemia, requiring intervention with IV fluid therapy.

D. **CORRECT:** Tenting of skin indicates decreased or absent skin turgor due to dehydration, requiring intervention with IV fluid therapy.

E. A heart rate of 62/min is not a manifestation of hypovolemia.

Ⓝ *NCLEX® Connection: Physiological Adaptation, Fluid and Electrolyte Imbalances*

3. A. **CORRECT:** Use of the incentive spirometer every 2 hr expands the lungs and prevents atelectasis.

B. **CORRECT:** Incisional splinting with a pillow or blanket supports the incision during coughing and deep breathing, which prevents atelectasis.

C. **CORRECT:** Repositioning the client every 2 hr will mobilize secretions and allow the client to deep breathe and expand the lungs to prevent atelectasis.

D. Antibiotic therapy is used to prevent or treat infection and does not prevent atelectasis.

E. **CORRECT:** Early ambulation expands the lungs through deep breathing and prevents atelectasis.

Ⓝ *NCLEX® Connection: Reduction of Risk Potential, Potential for Complications of Diagnostic Tests/Treatments/Procedures*

4. A. **CORRECT:** Using the nursing process, the first step is to collect data from the client. Checking for bowel sounds is the priority action by the nurse.

B. Administering an antiemetic medication can alleviate nausea and vomiting, but it is not the first nursing action.

C. Ensuring IV fluids are initiated will prevent dehydration, but it is not the first nursing action.

D. Inserting a nasogastric tube can alleviate nausea and vomiting, but it is not the first nursing action.

Ⓝ *NCLEX® Connection: Reduction of Risk Potential, Potential for Complications of Diagnostic Tests/Treatments/Procedures*

5. A. The client should be repositioned at least every 2 hr.

B. **CORRECT:** Pneumatic compression stockings promote venous return and prevent venous thromboembolism.

C. Placing pillows under the client's knees will impede venous return.

D. **CORRECT:** Administering pain medication can help promote mobility by decreasing the client's pain level with activity.

E. **CORRECT:** Leg exercises will promote venous return and prevent venous thromboembolism.

Ⓝ *NCLEX® Connection: Physiological Adaptation, Basic Pathophysiology*

PRACTICE Answer

Using the ATI Active Learning Template: Basic Concept

RELATED CONTENT

Paralytic ileus
- Caused by abdominal surgery or other physical trauma and absent gastrointestinal peristaltic activity
- Monitor bowel sounds.
- Encourage ambulation.
- Insert nasogastric tube to empty stomach contents.

Wound evisceration
- Protrusion of the abdominal contents through the incisional wound of the abdominal cavity, caused by failure to splint when moving or coughing, delayed healing due to obesity or diabetes mellitus
- Call for help.
- Cover the wound with sterile saline soaked dressings or towel.
- Position the client in semi-Fowler's position with hips and knees bent.

Airway obstruction
- Swelling or spasm of the larynx or trachea, mucus in the airway, or relaxation of the tongue into the nasopharynx can cause airway obstruction, often manifesting as stridor or snoring.
- Notify the anesthesiologist.
- Provide humidified oxygen.
- Elevate the head of the bed if not contraindicate.
- Perform a head-tilt/chin-lift maneuver to open the airway.
- Assist with the plan for reintubation of the endotracheal tube.

Hypovolemic shock
- Caused by blood loss
- Monitor for decreased blood pressure and urinary output, increased heart and respiratory rates, narrowing of the pulse pressure, and slow capillary refill.
- Monitor postoperative laboratory values (hemoglobin, hematocrit, creatinine, BUN).
- Administer oxygen.
- Place the client in a supine position with the legs elevated.
- Assist with the administration of IV fluids and vasopressors as indicated.

Ⓝ *NCLEX® Connection: Physiological Adaptation, Basic Pathophysiology*

References

American Heart Association. (n.d.). *Healthy living.* Retrieved from https://healthyforgood.heart.org/

Berman, A., Snyder, S., & Frandsen, G. (2016). *Kozier & Erb's fundamentals of nursing: Concepts, process, and practice* (10th ed.). Upper Saddle River, NJ: Prentice-Hall.

Burchum, J. R., & Rosenthal, L. D. (2016). *Lehne's pharmacology for nursing care* (9th ed.). St. Louis, MO: Elsevier.

Burke, K., Mohn-Brown, L., Eby, L. (2016). *Medical-surgical nursing care* (4th ed.). Upper Saddle River, NJ: Prentice-Hall.

Centers for Disease Control and Prevention (2017). *Diseases and conditions.* Retrieved from https://www.cdc.gov/diseasesconditions/index.html

Centers for Disease Control and Prevention. (2017). *Vaccines and immunizations.* Retrieved from https://www.cdc.gov/vaccines/index.html

deWit, S. C., Stromberg, H. K., & Dallred, C. V. (2017). *Medical-surgical nursing: Concepts and practice* (3nd ed.). St. Louis, MO: Saunders

Dudek, S. G. (2014). *Nutrition essentials for nursing practice* (7th ed.). Philadelphia: Lippincott Williams & Wilkins.

Eliopoulos, C. (2014). *Gerontological nursing* (8th ed.). Philadelphia: Lippincott Williams & Wilkins.

Grodner, M., Escott-Stump, S., & Dorner, S. (2016). *Nutritional foundations and clinical applications of nutrition: A nursing approach* (6th ed.). St. Louis, MO: Mosby.

Halter, M. J. (2014). *Varcarolis' foundations of psychiatric mental health nursing: A clinical approach* (7th ed.). St. Louis, MO: Saunders.

Hinkle, J. L., & Cheever, K. H. (2014). *Brunner and Suddarth's textbook of medical-surgical nursing* (13th ed.). Philadelphia: Lippincott Williams & Wilkins.

Ignatavicius, D. D., & Workman, M. L. (2016). *Medical-surgical nursing* (8th ed.). St. Louis, MO: Elsevier.

Immunization Action Coalition. (2017). *Advisory Committee on Immunization Practice.* Retrieved from http://www.immunize.org/acip/

Lilley, L. L., Rainforth-Collins, S., & Snyder, J. S. (2017). *Pharmacology and the nursing process* (8th Ed.). St. Louis, MO: Elsevier.

Pagana, K. D., & Pagana, T. J. (2014). *Mosby's manual of diagnostic and laboratory tests* (5th ed.). St. Louis, MO: Elsevier.

Potter, P. A., Perry, A. G., Stockert, P., & Hall, A. (2017). *Fundamentals of nursing* (9th ed.). St. Louis, MO: Elsevier

Touhy, T. A., & Jett, K. F. (2016) *Ebersole & Hess' toward healthy aging: Human needs and nursing response* (9th ed.). St. Louis, MO: Elsevier.

Vallerand, A. H., & Sanoski, C. A. (2017). *Davis's drug guide for nurses* (15th Ed.). Philadelphia, PA: Elsevier.

STUDENT NAME _____

CONCEPT_____ REVIEW MODULE CHAPTER_____

Related Content

(E.G., DELEGATION,
LEVELS OF PREVENTION,
ADVANCE DIRECTIVES)

Underlying Principles

Nursing Interventions

WHO? WHEN? WHY? HOW?

STUDENT NAME _____

PROCEDURE NAME _____ REVIEW MODULE CHAPTER_____

Description of Procedure

Indications

CONSIDERATIONS

Nursing Interventions (pre, intra, post)

Interpretation of Findings

Client Education

Potential Complications

Nursing Interventions

Growth and Development

STUDENT NAME _____

DEVELOPMENTAL STAGE _____ REVIEW MODULE CHAPTER_____

EXPECTED GROWTH AND DEVELOPMENT

Physical Development	Cognitive Development	Psychosocial Development	Age-Appropriate Activities

Health Promotion

Immunizations	Health Screening	Nutrition	Injury Prevention

ACTIVE LEARNING TEMPLATE: *Medication*

STUDENT NAME _____

MEDICATION _____ REVIEW MODULE CHAPTER_____

CATEGORY CLASS_____

PURPOSE OF MEDICATION

Expected Pharmacological Action

Therapeutic Use

Complications

Medication Administration

Contraindications/Precautions

Interactions

Nursing Interventions

Client Education

Evaluation of Medication Effectiveness

STUDENT NAME _____

SKILL NAME_____ REVIEW MODULE CHAPTER_____

Description of Skill

Indications

CONSIDERATIONS

Nursing Interventions (pre, intra, post)

Outcomes/Evaluation

Client Education

Potential Complications

Nursing Interventions

STUDENT NAME _____

DISORDER/DISEASE PROCESS _____ REVIEW MODULE CHAPTER_____

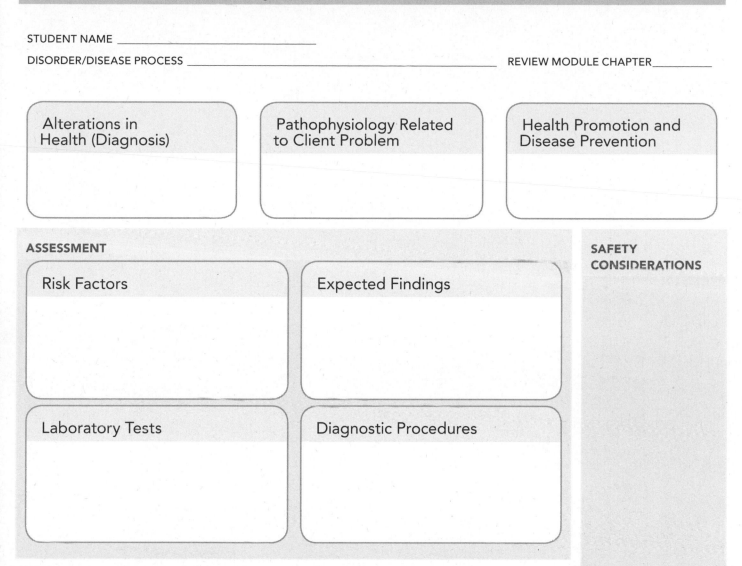

| Alterations in Health (Diagnosis) | Pathophysiology Related to Client Problem | Health Promotion and Disease Prevention |

ASSESSMENT

Risk Factors

Expected Findings

Laboratory Tests

Diagnostic Procedures

SAFETY CONSIDERATIONS

PATIENT-CENTERED CARE

Nursing Care

Medications

Client Education

Therapeutic Procedures

Interprofessional Care

Complications

STUDENT NAME _____

PROCEDURE NAME _____ REVIEW MODULE CHAPTER_____

Description of Procedure

Indications

CONSIDERATIONS

Nursing Interventions (pre, intra, post)

Outcomes/Evaluation

Client Education

Potential Complications

Nursing Interventions